PROGRESS IN BRAIN RESEARCH

VOLUME 69

PHOSPHOPROTEINS IN NEURONAL FUNCTION

Recent volumes in PROGRESS IN BRAIN RESEARCH

PROGRESS IN BRAIN RESEARCH

VOLUME 69

PHOSPHOPROTEINS IN NEURONAL FUNCTION

Proceedings of the
Second International Workshop at the State University of Utrecht,
September 1985

EDITED BY

WILLEM HENDRIK GISPEN

*Professor of Molecular Neurobiology, Rudolf Magnus Institute for
Pharmacology and Institute of Molecular Biology, Padualaan 8,
3584 CH Utrecht (The Netherlands)*

and

ARYEH ROUTTENBERG

*Professor of Psychology and Neurobiology, Cresap Neuroscience
Laboratory, 2021 Sheridan Road, Evanston, IL 60201 (U.S.A.)*

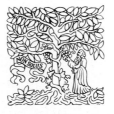

ELSEVIER
AMSTERDAM – NEW YORK – OXFORD
1986

LC

ISBN 0 444 80781 0 (volume)
ISBN 0 444 80104 9 (series)

Published by:
Elsevier Science Publishers B.V. (Biomedical Division)
P.O. Box 211
1000 AE Amsterdam
The Netherlands

Sole distributors for the USA and Canada:
Elsevier Science Publishing Company, Inc.
52 Vanderbilt Avenue
New York, NY 10017
USA

Library of Congress Cataloging-in-Publication Data

Phosphoproteins in neuronal function.

   (Progress in brain research; v. 69)
   Second International Workshop on "Phosphoproteins in
Neuronal Function" was held under the auspices of the
Air Force Office of Scientific Research, and others.
   Includes bibliographies and index.
   1. Neural transmission—Congresses.
2. Phosphoproteins—Physiological effect—Congresses.
3. Ion channels—Congresses.   4. Neural receptors—
Congresses.   5. Neuroplasticity—Congresses.
I. Gispen, Willem Hendrik.   II. Routtenberg, Aryeh.
III. International Workshop on "Phosphoproteins in
Neuronal Function" (2nd: 1985: State University of Utrecht)   IV. United States. Air Force. Office of
Scientific Research.   V. Series. [DNLM: 1. Neurons—
physiology—congresses.   2. Phosphoproteins—metabolism
—congresses.   W1 PR667J v.69 / WL 104 P5755 1985]
QP376.P7   vol. 69   612'.82 s   86–16501
[QP364.5]   [599'.01'88]
ISBN 0-444-80781-0 (U.S.)

Printed in the Netherlands

8-28-87

Preface

This volume contains the contributions of participants in the Second International Workshop on "Phosphoproteins in Neuronal Function", which took place at the State University of Utrecht, September 2–5, 1985.

The impetus for the second meeting was based on our belief that the field had matured considerably since our first meeting in September 1981. Moreover, discoveries made in the interim such as the effect of phorbol diesters on protein kinase C, the calcium-releasing effect of inositol trisphosphate and direct evidence for the participation of protein kinases in regulating ion channels, made it auspicious for us to review progress made in the past four years as well as to integrate these new discoveries within the existing database. It seemed rather clear to the editors that the field has shifted from the early emphasis on characterization of substrates and kinases to issues of function. While some thinking along these lines was apparent in the 1981 meeting, the present one was rich with specific empirical detail and a few detailed models of phosphoprotein function.

We wish to thank the participants for their enthusiastic participation at the workshop and their cooperation in the final steps of preparing this volume. The entire meeting was one of spirited discussion, frank and at times critical, but with a good collegiality of spirit. This was in no small way contributed to by the members of the Molecular Biology Institute in Utrecht. One of us, Aryeh Routtenberg, wishes to acknowledge the truly outstanding leadership of Willem Hendrik Gispen for making the participants feel welcome and allowing for a spirit of shared comradeship throughout the meeting. He was ably assisted by the members of the local committee Pierre De Graan, Loes Schrama and Lia Claessens and by Jan Brakkee (technical assistance) and Ed Kluis (artwork and photography).

The meeting would not have been possible without support from agencies in both The Netherlands and the United States. Under the auspices of the Air Force Office of Scientific Research (Dr. William Berry, Program Director), the US Office of Naval Research, London Branch (Dr. C. Neurath-Zomzeli), the 'Pharmacologisch Studiefonds' (Utrecht), the Dr. Saal van Zwanenberg Foundation, the State University of Utrecht (Board of Trustees and Medical Faculty) and the Royal Dutch Academy of Sciences (KNAW), we were able to invite the current leaders in the field to contribute to the volume.

We note with sadness the passing of Henry Mahler, an important contributor to the phosphoprotein field, and a cherished colleague who provided both the wit and wisdom that lent depth and perspective to our studies of brain phosphoproteins.

The past four years has seen the realization of a hope expressed in our earlier volume that brain protein phosphorylation represents a critical step in relating neuronal function to brain chemistry. Such functions were at that time vaguely defined as signaling capacity related to synaptic transmission. The present volume illustrates the specificity achieved in defining particular physiological processes in brain that are closely related to the phosphorylation state of brain proteins. Through this specificity one imagines that the next four years will bring fresh insights into the central role of brain phosphoproteins in understanding the physiological chemistry of nerve cells.

February 1986

Utrecht, Willem Hendrik Gispen
Evanston, Aryeh Routtenberg

Participants

A.A. Abdel-Latif, School of Medicine, Dept. of Cell and Molecular Biology, Medical College of Georgia, Augusta, GA 30912 (USA).

B.W. Agranoff, University of Michigan, Neuroscience, Laboratory Building, 1103 East Huron, Ann Arbor, MI 48104-1687 (USA).

K. Albert, Laboratoy of Molecular and Cellular Neuroscience, Rockefeller University, 1230 York Avenue, New York, NY 10021-6388 (USA).

F. Benfenati, Dept. of Human Physiology. University of Modena, Via Campi, 287, 41100 Modena (Italy).

P.J. Blackshear, Dept. of Medicine, Duke University, Medical Center, P.O. Box 3897, Durham, NC 27710 (USA).

M. Cimino, University of Milano, Inst. for Pharmacology, Via A. Del Sarto, 21, Milan (Italy).

B. Defize, International Embryological Institute, Royal Dutch Academy of Sciences, Uppsalalaan 8, 3584 CT Utrecht (NL).

P.N.E. De Graan, Div. of Molecular Neurobiology, Inst. of Molecular Biology and Rudolf Magnus Inst. for Pharmacology, State University of Utrecht, Padualaan 8, 3584 CH Utrecht (NL).

R. De Kloet, Rudolf Magnus Inst. for Pharmacology, State University of Utrecht, Vondellaan 6, 3521 GD Utrecht (NL).

S.W. De Laat, International Embryological Institute, Royal Dutch Academy of Sciences, Uppsalalaan 8, 3585 CT Utrecht (NL).

I. Diamond, School of Medicine, Dept. of Neurology, University of California, Bldg 1, Room 101, San Francisco, CA 94110 (USA).

L.A. Dokas, Dept. of Biochemistry, Medical College of Ohio, 3000 Arlington Avenue, Toledo, OH 43699 (USA).

R. Drawbaugh, Chief Life Sciences, EOARD, 223/231 Old Marleybone Road, London NW1 5TH (UK).

P.R. Dunkley, Faculty of Medicine, Univ. of Newcastle, New South Wales, 2308, Australia.

P.M. Edwards, Div. of Molecular Neurobiology, Inst. of Molecular Biology, State University of Utrecht, Padualaan 8, 3584 CH Utrecht (NL).

Y.H. Ehrlich, Dept. of Psychiatry, Medical Alumni Bldg, Burlington, VT 05405 (USA).

J. Eichberg, Dept. of Biochemical and Biophysical Sciences, Univ. of Houston, Houston, TX 77004 (USA).

J. Elands, Rudolf Magnus Inst. for Pharmacology, State University of Utrecht, Vondellaan 6, 3521 GD Utrecht (NL).

P. Friedrich, Inst. of Enzymology, Biological Research Center, Hungarian Academy of Sciences, Budapest, P.O. Box 7, F-1502 (Hungary).

W.E.J.M. Ghijsen, University of Amsterdam, Animal Physiology, Kruislaan 318, 1098 SA Amsterdam (NL).

W.H. Gispen, Div. of Molecular Neurobiology, Inst. of Molecular Biology and Rudolf Magnus Inst. of Pharmacology, State University of Utrecht, Padualaan 8, 3584 CH Utrecht (NL).

J.R. Goldenring, Dept. of Neurology, Yale University of Medicine, 333 Cedar Street, New Haven, CT 06510 (USA).

A.S. Gordon, School of Medicine, Dept. of Neurobiology, Univ. of California, Bldg 1, Room 101, San Francisco, CA 94110 (USA).

P. Greengard, Lab. of Molecular and Cellular Neuroscience, Rockefeller University, 1230 York Avenue, New York, NY 10021-6399 (USA).

I. Hanbauer, Section Biochemical Pharmacology, NHLBI, NIH, Bldg 10, Room 7N244, Bethesda, MD 20205 (USA).

H. Horstmann, Dept. of Neurobiology, TROPONWERKE, Neurather Ring 1, 5000 Cologne 80 (FRG).

L.K. Kaczmarek, Dept. of Pharmacology, Yale University, School of Medicine, Sterling Hall of Medicine 333 Cedar Street, New Haven, CT 06510-8066 (USA).

G.I. Kristjansson, Max-Planck-Institut für Biophysikalischer Chemie, Karl-Friedrich-Bon-höffer Institut, Abt. Neurochemie, D-3400 Göttingen, Postfach 2841 (FRG).

I.B. Levitan, Graduate Dept. of Biochemistry, Brandeis University, Waltham, MA 02254 (USA).

L. Lovinger, Northwestern University, Cresap Neuroscience Lab., 2021 Sheridan Road, Evanston, IL 60201 (USA).

K. Murakami, Northwestern University, Cresap Neuroscience Lab., 2021 Sheridan Road, Evanston, IL 60201 (USA).

A. Nairn, Lab. of Molecular and Cellular Neuroscience, Rockefeller University, 1230 York Avenue, New York, NY 10021-6399 (USA).

J.T. Neary, Dept. of Health and Human Services, NIH, Lab. of Biophysics, IRP, NINCDS, Marine Biology Lab., Woods Hole, MA 02543 (USA).

E.J. Nestler, Dept. of Psychiatry, Connecticut Mental Health Center, 34 Park Street, New Haven, CT 06508 (USA).

Y. Nishizuka, Dept. of Biochemistry, Kobe University, School of Medicine, Kobe 650 (Japan).

A.B. Oestreicher, Div. of Molecular Neurobiology, Inst of Molecular Biology and Rudolf Magnus Inst. for Pharmacology, State University of Utrecht, Padualaan 8, 3584 CH Utrecht (NL).

A. Pauloin, Lab. des Protéines Unité CNRS No 102 à l'INSERM, Univ. de Paris V, 45, rue des Saints-Pères, F-75270 Paris Cedex 06 (France).

K.H. Pfenninger, College of Physicians and Surgeons, Columbia University, Dept. of Anatomy and Cell Biology, 630 West 168th Street, New York, NY 10032 (USA).

R. Rodnight, Inst. of Psychiatry, De Crespigny Park, Denmark Hill, London SE5 8AF (UK).

J.A.P. Rostas, Faculty of Medicine, Discipline of Medical Biochemistry, University of Newcastle, New South Wales, 2308 (Australia).

A. Routtenberg, Northwestern University, Cresap Neuroscience Lab., 2021 Sheridan Road, Evanston, IL 60201 (USA).

P. Schotman, Div. of Molecular Neurobiology, Inst. of Molecular Biology and Lab. for Physiological Chemistry, State University of Utrecht, Padualaan 8, 3584 CH Utrecht (NL).

L.H. Schrama, Div. of Molecular Biology, Inst. of Molecular Biology, State University of Utrecht, Padualaan 8, 3584 CH Utrecht (NL).

M.J. Shuster, Dept. of Pharmacology and Center for Neurobiology and Behavior, College of Physicians and Surgeons, Columbia University, 630 West 168th Street, New York, NY 10032 (USA).

A.P.N. Themmen, Medical Faculty, Erasmus University, Dept. of Biochemistry II, P.O. Box 1738, 3000 TR Rotterdam (NL).

A.B. Vaandrager, Medical Faculty, Erasmus University, Dept. of Biochemistry II, P.O. Box 1738, 3000 TR Rotterdam (NL).

C.O.M. Van Hooff, Div. of Molecular Neurobiology, Inst. of Molecular Biology, State University of Utrecht, Padualaan 8, 3584 CH Utrecht (NL).

L.A.A. Van Rooijen, Dept. of Neurobiology, TROPONWERKE, Neurather Ring 1, 5000 Cologne 80 (FRG).

J. Verhaagen, Div. of Molecular Neurobiology, Inst. of Molecular Biology, State University of Utrecht, Padualaan 8, 3584 CH Utrecht (NL).

V.M. Wiegant Rudolf Magnus Inst. for Pharmacology, State University of Utrecht, Vondellaan 6, 3521 GD Utrecht (NL).

J.E. Wilson, School of Medicine, Dept. of Biochemistry and Nutrition, University of North Carolina at Chapel Hill, Faculty Lab. Office, Bldg 231H, Chapel Hill, NC 27514-7231 (USA).

K.W.A. Wirtz, Dept. of Biochemistry, State University of Utrecht, Padualaan 8, 3584 CH Utrecht (NL).

Contents

Section III– Receptors

Section IV– Plasticity

Protein Phosphorylation and Polyphosphoinositide Metabolism

W.H. Gispen and A. Routtenberg (Eds.)
Progress in Brain Research, Vol. 69
© 1986 Elsevier Science Publishers B.V. (Biomedical Division)

CHAPTER 1

Ligand-stimulated turnover of inositol lipids in the nervous system

Bernard W. Agranoff and Stephen K. Fisher

Neuroscience Laboratory and Departments of Biological Chemistry, and Pharmacology, University of Michigan, Ann Arbor, MI 48104-1687, U.S.A.

Introduction

The stimulated turnover of inositol-related lipids (STI) following ligand interaction with plasma membrane receptor sites is common to numerous hormones, neurotransmitters and modulators in a variety of tissues (Michell, 1975; Hawthorne and Pickard, 1979; Abdel-Latif, 1983; Berridge and Irvine, 1984; Fisher and Agranoff, 1985). The initial metabolic consequence of receptor–ligand interaction is increased breakdown of phosphatidylinositol 4,5-bisphosphate (PIP_2)* via a Ca^{2+}-dependent phosphodiesterase (Fig. 1), yielding diacylglycerol (DG) and inositol trisphosphate (IP_3), each of which may affect protein phosphorylation: the DG moiety by direct activation of protein kinase C (Nishizuka, 1983, 1984), and the IP_3 moiety indirectly through liberation of intracellular Ca^{2+} stores (Berridge and Irvine, 1984). That the inositide phosphodiesterase requires the presence of Ca^{2+} to prime a reaction that leads in turn to additional Ca^{2+} release has been a source of some confusion (Hawthorne, 1982; Michell, 1982). It is likely that sufficient Ca^{2+} for initiation of phosphodiesterase action is bound to the inner membrane surface, perhaps as the salt of PIP_2, a lipid known to bind

divalent cations (Kerr et al., 1964; Eichberg and Dawson, 1965; Hendrickson and Reinertsen, 1971). In some instances the rise in intracellular Ca^{2+} that follows the receptor–ligand interaction results from the opening of plasma membrane Ca^{2+} channels, rather than from the mobilization

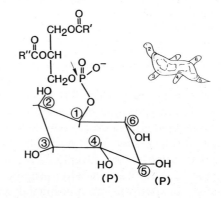

Fig. 1. The inositides. Phosphatidylinositol (PI) and its phosphorylated derivates phosphatidylinositol 4-phosphate (PIP) and phosphatidylinositol 4,5-bisphosphate (PIP_2). All three inositides are cleaved by a Ca^{2+}-activated phosphodiesterase at a site designated by the arrow. PIP_2 is believed to be selectively cleaved following receptor–ligand activation, with the liberation of diacylglycerol (DG) and inositol trisphosphate (IP_3). R′ and R″ are predominantly 18:0 (stearate) and 20:4ω6 (arachidonate) esters, respectively. The turtle (inset) is a convenient representation of inositol to emphasize that its favored chair conformation consists of one axial (the head) and 5 equatorial (the legs and tail) hydroxyls. In all three inositides, the phosphatidate moiety (PA) is attached to inositol via the right front leg (D-1). In PIP there is an additional phosphate on the left hind leg and in PIP_2, at the tail as well.

---

*The abbreviations used for inositol lipids and inositol phosphates are those recommended at the Chilton Conference on Inositol and Phosphoinositides, Dallas, TX, January, 1984 (see Agranoff et al., 1985).

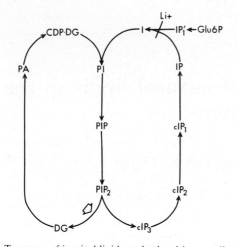

Fig. 2. Turnover of inositol lipids and related intermediates. As currently viewed, the activated breakdown of PIP$_2$ (arrow) leads to formation of DG, which is converted, via PA and CDP-DG intermediates, to PI. Sequential phosphorylations to PIP and PIP$_2$ complete the cycle. The phosphodiesteratic cleavage of PIP$_2$ also produces IP$_3$, here postulated to be the cyclic intermediate, which is then sequentially degraded by phosphatases to inositol and inorganic phosphate. This view must be considered highly speculative at present, since there is as yet little documentation for the presence of cIP$_3$ in tissue. The last step in this sequence, the hydrolysis of inositol D-1 phosphate, can be blocked by Li$^+$. The Li$^+$-blocked step also prevents breakdown of inositol D-3 phosphate formed from the cyclization of glucose.

of intracellular stores (Rasmussen and Barrett, 1984).

Under conditions in which STI has been observed via ^{32}P$_i$ incorporation into lipids, no increase in de novo lipid synthesis is seen (Schacht and Agranoff, 1974; Fisher and Agranoff, 1981), a finding that supports the concept of a regenerative cycle (Fig. 2). It was initially proposed that stimulated breakdown of phosphatidylinositol (PI) rather than of PIP$_2$ occurred (Hokin and Hokin, 1964; Durell et al., 1969), and it remains possible that stimulated breakdown of PI and phosphatidylinositol 4-phosphate (PIP) also occurs, since the same phosphodiesterase cleaves all three of the inositides (Wilson et al., 1984, 1985). Since PI is present in membranes in higher amounts than is PIP or PIP$_2$, it constitutes a potentially rich source of intracellular DG. It should be noted that cleavage of PI or of PIP leads to release of DG but not of IP$_3$, thus offering

the possibility of a cycle in which only one of the two STI-associated second messengers is liberated. Experimental designs to establish at which inositide level DG is released are based on establishing whether IP$_3$, inositol bisphosphate (IP$_2$) or inositol 1-phosphate (IP) is formed simultaneously with DG. Unfortunately, breakdown of IP$_3$ to IP$_2$ and then to IP also proceeds rapidly. In most systems which have been carefully examined with appropriate techniques, the evidence favors carbon flow through PIP$_2$ prior to phosphodiesteratic cleavage, with release of DG and an equal amount of IP$_3$, which in turn may be rapidly dephosphorylated (Berridge, 1983; Downes and Wusteman, 1983; Aub and Putney, 1984).

While cytidine diphosphodiacylglycerol (CDP-DG) formation is an obligatory step in the regenerative phase of the cycle, it is seldom seen in ^{32}P labeling studies, because its formation is rate-limiting. Cellular inositol levels are generally high, permitting rapid conversion of the liponucleotide as it is formed. In pineal cell preparations, the addition of α-adrenergic agonists to the medium in the absence of added inositol results in the accumulation of CDP-DG (Hauser and Eichberg, 1975). This can be considered an exceptional situation, since in other cell preparations examined thus far, intracellular inositol cannot be readily washed out. While the enzymatic formation of CDP-DG from CTP and phosphatidate (PA) is irreversible. CDP-DG pyrophosphatase activity that cleaves CDP-DG to CMP and PA has been detected in bacterial preparations as well as in brain (Raetz et al., 1972; Rittenhouse et al., 1981). The enzyme is competitively inhibited by 5' AMP, a finding of possible regulatory significance.

While *myo*-inositol is one of nine possible isomers of hexahydroxy-cyclohexane, it is by far the most prevalent form in nature and the favored substrate of PI synthase, which transfers PA from CDP-DG to the D-1 hydroxyl group of inositol (Benjamins and Agranoff, 1969; Agranoff, 1978). There is no evidence that the synthase will react with phosphorylated derivatives of inositol. Sequential phosphorylation of PI on the D-4' and 5' positions in inositol (see Fig. 1) to PIP and thence to PIP_2 also appear to be stereospecific.

A cycle complementary to that proposed for the DG backbone of the inositides has been envisioned for inositol and its phosphates, in which IP_3 released from PIP_2 is sequentially degraded to free inositol (Fig. 2). While inositol has often been considered to be a growth factor or vitamin, it is now known that inositol D-3 phosphate (L-1) can be formed from glucose 6-phosphate via a cyclization reaction in a number of tissues, including brain (Hawthorne and White, 1975; Eisenberg and Maeda, 1985). Phosphatase activity then releases free inositol. Biosynthesis is likely the major source of brain inositol, since it does not readily cross the blood–brain barrier (Spector and Lorenzo, 1975). While the availability of intracellular inositol is thought not to have regulatory significance in STI, this may be the case when Li^+ is present, as is discussed below.

Significance of STI in the nervous system

Historically, polyphosphoinositides have been linked with neurochemistry, and were in fact first identified and characterized in brain (Folch, 1949; Brockerhoff and Ballou, 1961, 1962; Eichberg and Dawson, 1965). The enzymes of phosphoinositide turnover are also enriched in brain (Fisher and Agranoff, 1985), as is the machinery for the relevant second messenger systems, e.g. protein kinase C and other Ca^{2+}-mediated phosphorylation systems (Nishizuka, 1983, 1984; Berridge, 1984a; Berridge and Irvine, 1984). The brain has also played a key role in the elucidation of the inositol lipid turnover cycle, primarily from studies with cholinergic ligands. In early studies, it was demonstrated (Hokin and Hokin, 1955) that the addition of carbamoylcholine to tissue slices from pancreas and brain could elicit STI. However, whereas the effect required the maintenance of cell integrity in the pancreas, a robust muscarinic STI later shown to be mediated by the nerve ending fraction of total homogenate (Schacht and Agranoff, 1972; Yagihara and Hawthorne, 1972), could be observed in cell-free preparations from brain. Since nerve endings, or synaptosomes, are pinched-off and resealed nerve terminals that maintain vectorial inside/outside

relationships, they can be considered to be anucleate neurons and thus do not contradict the generalization that intact cells are required for demonstration of ligand-stimulated labeling. The availability of this 'simpler' neuronal preparation facilitated our understanding of the underlying biochemical mechanism of STI.

In view of the known information processing and transfer functions of the brain and its rich anatomical heterogeneity, it is not surprising that it has proven to be a veritable treasure trove of ligands and their receptors. To add to this complexity, it is becoming increasingly clear that the same neurotransmitter can have different receptor interactions in different brain regions, a circumstance that has given rise to a thriving industry in receptor subtype and sub-subtype identification.

Interest in STI in brain has also been employed as a functional probe. As our sophistication in evaluating chemoreception in the brain grows, we find that we can rely less and less solely on binding of radiolabeled agents to membranes as measures of receptor physiology. To demonstrate that a ligand-binding protein is truly a receptor requires measurement of a physiological consequence of the binding. Hence, STI, as well as subsequent events, including elevation of intracellular Ca^{2+} and protein phosphorylation that may ultimately lead to either secretion, depolarization, or possibly to contraction, bring us one step closer to the understanding of higher brain function.

Experimental approaches

The STI is seen in whole brain (in vivo), brain slices, subcellular fractions and also in two CNS-related tissues, the pineal and anterior pituitary (Table I). In the peripheral nervous system, both the superior cervical ganglion and adrenal medulla support a readily demonstrable STI. Recently there has been much interest in ligands that support STI in transformed cell lines of neural origin, e.g. neuroblastoma and astrocytoma.

For many years, the enhanced turnover of PA and inositol lipids has been detected through the increased incorporation of added $^{32}P_i$ into PA

TABLE I

Neuroeffector-linked inositide turnover

Preparation	^{32}P		^{3}H
	PA/PI↑	PIP/PIP$_2$↓	IP↑
Whole brain (in vivo)	+		
Brain slices or minces	+		+
Subcellular fractions			
Nerve ending preparations	+	+	
Synaptic plasma membranes		+	
Dissociated cells or slices			
Adrenal medulla	+	+	+
Pineal	+		+
Pituitary	+		
Superior cervical ganglion	+		+
	+		+
Transformed cells			
Neuroblastoma	+		+
Astrocytoma			+
GH$_3$ pituitary cells		+	+
PC-12 cells	+		+

For details, see Fisher and Agranoff (1985) and references therein.

and PI, following ligand addition. Using this approach, 2 to 5-fold increases in the labeling of PA and PI have been observed in the absence of appreciable increases in the labeling of the quantitatively major phospholipids, phosphatidylcholine and phosphatidylethanolamine, or of phosphatidylserine (Fisher and Agranoff, 1985). Alternatively, tissue preparations can be prelabeled with ^{32}P$_i$ or [^{3}H]inositol and stimulated loss of label from individual lipids monitored following ligand addition. Using this approach, a role for polyphosphoinositide breakdown in STI was indicated in nerve ending preparations (Fisher and Agranoff, 1981), in GH$_3$ pituitary cells (Martin, 1983) and in the adrenal medulla (Table I). Both the initial labeling and prelabeling approaches are open to criticism: by measurement of increased [^{32}P]PA and [^{32}P]PI labeling, the restorative phase of the STI cycle is being monitored, several enzymatic steps away from the initial site of the receptor–ligand inter-

action; in the case of prelabeling studies, the loss of radioactivity from prelabeled polyphosphoinositides indicates the likelihood of their primary involvement, but the observed effect is often of small magnitude, can be obfuscated by an accompanying stimulated resynthesis in response to the agonist and does not unequivocally differentiate between inhibition of lipid synthesis and increased lipid breakdown (Fisher et al., 1984b). The problems of interpretation encountered with either the labeling or prelabeling approach are largely circumvented by measurement of the release of labeled water-soluble inositol phosphates. Under normal circumstances, inositol phosphates are rapidly hydrolyzed by phosphatases, thus rendering their detection difficult or impossible. However, the observation that Li$^+$ inhibits the myo-inositol l-phosphatase (Allison et al., 1976; Hallcher and Sherman, 1980) has made possible the development of a specific and rapid method for assessing the ligand-induced breakdown of inositol lipids (Berridge et al., 1982). When brain slices are incubated in the presence of [^{3}H]inositol and Li$^+$, the further addition of selective agonists results in a several-fold accumulation of IP derived primarily from IP$_3$ degradation (Berridge et al., 1983; Brown et al., 1984; Fisher and Bartus, 1985; Jacobson et al., 1985). The fact that in some tissue preparations (e.g. astrocytoma) increased IP$_3$ and IP$_2$ release can also consistently be detected, may reflect a lower activity of the phosphatases that sequentially remove the 5′ and 4′ phosphates from the inositol phosphates in this tissue relative to other phosphatases (Masters et al., 1984).

Pharmacological characteristics and transduction

The CNS and other neural preparations are particularly enriched in receptors linked to inositide turnover (Table II). To date, coupling to fourteen pharmacologically distinct receptors has been demonstrated, including muscarinic, α_1-adrenergic, H$_1$-histaminergic, 5-hydroxytryptamine(5HT)$_2$-serotonergic and receptors specific for a variety of neuropeptides. Most detailed information has been obtained for the muscarinic cholinergic receptor (mAChR). The involvement of the

TABLE II

Neuro-receptors linked to inositide turnover

Receptor	In vivo	Brain slices	Nerve ending preparations	Transformed cells[a]	Dissociated cells or slices (PNS)[b]
Muscarinic cholinergic	+	+	+	+	+
α_1-Adrenergic	+	+	+	+	+
H_1-Histaminergic	+	+		+	
$5HT_2$-Serotonergic		+			
$ACTH_{1-24}$			+		
β-Endorphin			+		
Substance P		+			+
V_1-Vasopressin		+			+
Thyrotropin-releasing hormone				+	
CCK		+			
Neurotensin		+		+	+
Bradykinin				+	
Nerve growth factor					+
Ibotenate		+			

For details, see Fisher and Agranoff (1985) and references therein.
[a]Neuroblastoma, GH_3 pituitary cells, astrocytoma or PC-12 cells.
[b]Superior cervical ganglion, adrenal medulla or pineal cells.

mAChR in STI, first indicated by Hokin and Hokin (1955), has been confirmed by several groups using either an in vivo approach in the CNS, or in vitro techniques with brain slices, nerve ending preparations, dissociated cells from the PNS or transformed cells (for review, see Fisher and Agranoff, 1985). In all systems studied thus far, low concentrations of classical antagonists such as atropine or scopolamine potently inhibit the response with K_i values similar to the dissociation constants for the mAChR-antagonist complex. In contrast, the addition of nicotinic antagonists even at high concentrations is without effect on STI. Within the category of muscarinic agonists, there are considerable differences in efficacy. Thus the CNS Group 'A' agonists — acetylcholine, muscarine, metacholine or carbamoylcholine (Fisher et al., 1983, 1984a; see also Brown et al., 1984; Gonzales and Crews, 1984; Jacobson et al., 1985) — are considerably more effective as enhancers of inositide turnover than are the Group 'B' agonists — oxotremorine, bethanechol, pilocarpine or arecoline. Not only are the Group B agonists less effective when added alone, but when present in incubations containing the Group A agonists,

block the stimulatory effect of the latter, i.e. they act as 'partial' agonists. An explanation for these differences in efficacy is to be found in the complexity with which an agonist interacts with the mAChR. Group A agonists bind to both 'high' and 'low' affinity forms of the mAChR, whereas Group B agonists bind predominantly to a single high affinity form (Fisher et al., 1983, 1984a). Thus, Group A agonists appear to induce a conformational change in the receptor which then results in the appearance of its low affinity form. From examination of dose–response curves, it is evident that the agonist concentrations required for STI are those required to occupy the low affinity sites. Thus, the magnitude of STI reflects both the ability of an agonist to induce the appearance of the low affinity form of the receptor and the concentration requirements for its occupancy. Regional differences in mAChR coupling characteristics also exist. In the guinea pig CNS, the muscarinic STI in the neostriatum is atypical in that selective partial agonists are more efficacious, full agonists are more potent and the antagonist pirenzepine inhibits the response only weakly (Fisher and Bartus, 1985). The differences in the sensitivity of the muscarinic STI to pirenzepine observed in neural tissues such as guinea pig brain, rat brain and astrocytoma cells (Gonzalez and Crews, 1984; Brown et al., 1985; Fisher and Bartus, 1985; Gil and Wolfe, 1985; Lazareno et al., 1985) as well as in non-neural tissues (Brown et al., 1985; Gil and Wolfe, 1985; Snider et al., 1986) militate against a simple M_1 (pirenzepine-sensitive) or M_2 (pirenzepine-insensitive) classification (Watson et al., 1982, 1983) for STI. The relatively high concentrations of muscarinic agonists required for a maximal STI might be considered to argue against a physiological role for inositide turnover. However, it is now recognized that these high agonist concentrations are precisely those required to occupy all of the available receptors, a result consistent with the original suggestion that STI represents a biochemical mechanism for signal amplification of muscarinic receptors (Michell et al., 1976).

The adrenergic STI response is limited to the α rather than the β receptor, and in particular to the α_1 subtype. This conclusion is derived from studies in both the pineal gland and CNS in which the addition of norepinephrine elicits a large increase in STI, which can be blocked by inclusion of prazosin or phentolamine, two α_1 antagonists, but not by propranolol, a β-antagonist (Friedel et al., 1973; Hauser et al., 1974; Nijjar et al., 1980; Berridge et al., 1982; Schoepp et al., 1984). In addition, agonists which preferentially act on α_2-adrenergic receptors (e.g. clonidine) have little or no effect (Smith et al., 1979; Schoepp et al., 1984). The histaminergic response in CNS is mediated through the H_1 receptor, since it can be blocked by inclusion of pyrilamine (H_1-antagonist), but not by cimetidine (H_2-antagonist; Friedel and Schanberg, 1975; Subramanian et al., 1980, 1981; Daum et al., 1984). The magnitude of the histamine response correlates well with the appearance of brain H_1 receptors and of histaminergic neurotransmission (Subramanian et al., 1980, 1981). Only recently has the detailed pharmacology of the serotonin-induced STI come under close scrutiny. The addition of 5HT to brain slices results in an accumulation of [^{3}H]inositol phosphates, with a pharmacological profile characteristic of the $5HT_2$ subtype, but with some differences. Thus, while addition of 8-hydroxy-2-(di-N-propylamino)tetralin, a $5HT_1$ agonist, is without effect, and ketanserin, a potent $5HT_2$ antagonist, blocks the response in the cerebral cortex, the latter has little effect and is less potent in other brain areas such as the hippocampus and limbic forebrain regions (Conn and Sanders-Bush, 1984, 1985; Janowsky et al., 1984; Kendall and Nahorski, 1985). Moreover, there is no correlation between regional differences in the density of $5HT_2$ binding sites as determined by radioligand binding studies, and the magnitude of the STI. The possibility remains that STI is coupled to distinct 5HT receptor subtypes in different brain regions, or alternatively, that the effect is a reflection of the activation of a novel serotonergic receptor. Neuropeptide receptors linked to STI have also been demonstrated in the CNS, initially through the studies of Gispen and colleagues with adrenocorticotropic hormone (ACTH) and analogs (Jolles et al., 1980, 1981a,b) and more recently from the studies of Downes and colleagues (Downes, 1983; Watson and Downes, 1983; Mantyh et al., 1984). While the effects are relatively modest in comparison to those elicited by muscarinic and adrenergic stimuli, STI-mediated responses of substance P, neurotensin, vasopressin and cholecystokinin (CCK) receptors in STI have now been established. In addition, bradykinin has been shown to elicit a robust STI in the neuroblastoma X glioma hybrid (NG 108-15 cells; Yano et al., 1984). A recent and unexpected finding is that addition of ibotenate, a structural analog of glutamate, results in a large STI – apparently due to the stimulation of a receptor shared by L-glutamate (Nicoletti et al., 1985). This result was not anticipated, since it had widely been assumed that glutamate receptors couple directly to plasma membrane ionophores, without involvement of second-messenger molecules.

A major unresolved question for all of these receptors is that of the transduction process that intervenes between the changes in receptor conformation and activation of PIP_2 phosphodiesterase. There is presently little information on this topic, but one candidate is a guanine nucleotide binding protein, in a manner analogous to that seen for a group of receptors that operate through activation (G_s) or inhibition (G_i) of adenylate cyclase. A possibility that merits further attention is the involvement of G_o protein(s) in STI, since it is distinct from G_s or G_i and is highly enriched in the CNS (Sternweis and Robishaw, 1984).

Synaptic localization of STI

Since stimulation of a number of muscarinically innervated exocrine glands leads to STI and secretion, one might predict by analogy that the site of the muscarinic STI in brain is postsynaptic. However, since synaptosomal preparations support a muscarinic STI measured by increased incorporation of $^{32}P_i$, we are faced with a problem: synaptosomes are generally considered to be pinched-off presynaptic terminals, and the lipids are presumably labeled by $[^{32}P]ATP$ formed intrasynaptosomally. Even if there were attached fragments of postsynaptic membrane, they would be unavailable for lipid phosphorylation from $[^{32}P]ATP$ because of their separation by the synaptic cleft. To resolve this matter, we examined muscarinic STI from guinea pig hippocampus preparations a week after one of two lesioning procedures. In the first instance, the fimbria–fornix was cut, thus removing the cholinergic input to the hippocampus from the septal nuclei. As anticipated, choline acetyl-transferase activity (CAT) in the hippocampus was greatly diminished, while binding of the muscarinic antagonist quinuclidinyl benzilate (QNB) was not. This result indicated that pre-synaptic inputs had been removed without affecting postsynaptic sites. The muscarinic STI in this preparation was not impaired, a result consistent with a postsynaptic locus of the effect (Fisher et al., 1980). In the second instance, the excitatory neurotoxin ibotenate was injected into the hippocampus one week prior to synaptosome preparation. In this case, CAT remained unchanged while QNB binding was greatly diminished, as was the muscarinic STI, confirming a postsynaptic locus of the STI (Fisher et al., 1981).

How then does one resolve the clear indication from these experiments of a postsynaptic locus of the muscarinic STI with our preconceived notion of the synaptosome as a pinched-off presynaptic terminal? We proposed that the stimulated labeling could be mediated by pinched-off post-synaptic terminals, i.e. 'dendrosomes', or alternatively that the synaptosomes that support stimulated labeling are actually 'intersomes,' i.e. terminals having both pre- and postsynaptic membranes as integral plasma membrane components (Fig. 3; Fisher and Agranoff, 1985). The second possibility but not the first is supported by the immunohistochemical report that protein kinase C is presynaptic (Girard et al., 1985). Interpretation of the muscarinic STI relative to protein kinase C assumes that protein kinase C action is intimately, if not exclusively, linked with STI. While there is evidence to support this concept (Nishizuka, 1984), it should also be noted that in platelets, DG released from PIP_2 as well as from PIP and even from the more abundant PI may not constitute a sufficiently large reservoir of DG to account for the large amount released upon cell activation. Other

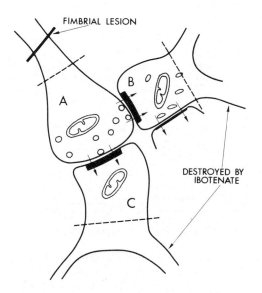

Fig. 3. Synaptic interrelationships in the hippocampus may explain the results of lesions on stimulated labeling in nerve-ending fractions. A:A cholinergic nerve terminal whose cell body is outside of the hippocampus. It forms a synapse with intrinsic neurons of the hippocampus axoaxonally (B) or axoden-dritically (C). On homogenization these fragments break off and are resealed, as indicated by the dashed lines. (From *Phospholipids in the Nervous Tissues*, J. Eichberg, Ed., John Wiley and Sons, New York, 1985.)

possible sources for DG unrelated to STI are: PA phosphatase action on newly biosynthesized PA; biosynthesis of sphingomyelin from ceramide and phosphatidylcholine; and degradation of triacylglycerol. A firmer causal link between protein kinase C activation by the DG released from STI would be the demonstration that 1-stearoyl, 2-arachidonoyl DG was uniquely effective. There is no indication that this will be the case (Mori et al., 1982). The inferred postsynaptic locus of STI (and therefore of IP_3-mediated Ca^{2+} release) is, on the other hand, consistent with the reported site of another protein kinase – calcium/calmodulin-dependent protein kinase II (Ouimet et al., 1985).

Functional significance of STI

Much progress has been made, primarily in non-neural systems, to indicate that receptor-mediated STI leads to increased Ca^{2+}-mediated phosphorylation reactions, which in turn leads to a physiological response (Berridge, 1984a). The use of phorbol esters as agonists of the DG-binding site for protein kinase C has been particularly convenient, since one can examine in whole cells how DG regulates other second messenger systems or the STI itself (see Fig. 4). Of special interest in the nervous system is the recent convergence of results from a number of laboratories regarding a protein variously known as GAP 43 (Skene and Willard, 1981; Heacock

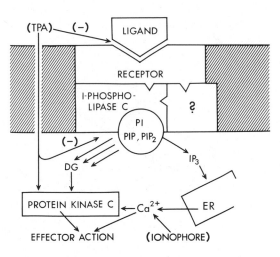

Fig. 4. Proposed relationship of a receptor and the stimulated turnover of inositides. Receptor–ligand interaction at the cell surface results in activation of PIP_2 phosphodiesterase on the inner surface of the plasma membrane, possibly via the mediation of an additional membrane protein (?), resulting in the release into the cytosol of inositol phosphates. IP_3 (or cIP_3) then stimulates release of Ca^{2+} from the endoplasmic reticulum (ER). Intracellular Ca^{2+} can also be increased by addition of ionophore. Phorbol esters such as TPA can inhibit the receptor–ligand interaction, the inositide phosphodiesterase, or can bind, like DG, to protein kinase C.

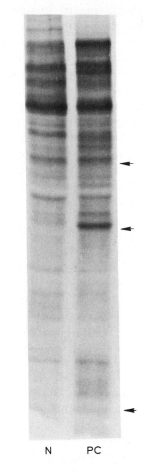

N   PC

Fig. 5. Fluorography of labeled axonally transported proteins in normal (N) and regenerating (postcrush: PC) optic nerve 6 h following intraocular injection of [³H]proline. The PC band just below the middle arrow (a 45 000 M_r standard) is the GAP-43 protein, known to be phosphorylated in a number of neural systems. See text. (From Heacock, A.M. and Agranoff, B.W. (1982) Protein synthesis and transport in the regenerating goldfish visual system, *Neurochem. Res.* 7:771–778).

and Agranoff, 1982; Benowitz and Lewis, 1983), B-50 (Gispen et al., 1985), PP46 (Katz et al., 1985), or F1 (Nelson and Routtenberg, 1985). It is axonally transported and is seen in developing or regenerating tissues, but is normally undetectable (Fig. 5). That it is present in growth cones, is regulated by hormones, appears to be involved in neuroplasticity, and last but not least, is phosphorylated by protein kinase C, assures that it will be a popular topic for some time. A pharmacological probe for demonstration of IP_3 effects in whole cells, analogous to phorbol ester for investigating DG is not available. It must be tested by addition of IP_3 to permeabilized cells or by intracellular injection, procedures which are both heroic and artifactual. The addition of ionophores to elevate intracellular Ca^{2+} provides an alternative, indirect way of examining the effects of IP_3. The mechanism by which IP_3 releases Ca^{2+} from intracellular stores (presumably the endoplasmic reticulum) is not known. The report of a potentially relevant calcium-independent IP_3-dependent protein phosphorylation (Whitman et al., 1984) is at present controversial. Of current interest is the possibility that 1,2 cyclic, 4,5-IP_3 (cIP_3) is the initial product of PIP_2 cleavage, leading to the hypothesis that the cyclic derivative is the true intracellular messenger, rather than 1,4,5-IP_3. Since a specific and highly active 5′-phosphohydrolase inactivates IP_3 (Storey et al., 1984; Connolly et al., 1985) one can speculate that the enzyme also acts on cIP_3 to yield cIP_2, and is more rapid than a postulated phosphodiesterase that opens the cyclic bond. If so, cIP_3 would be converted to cIP_2 without the intermediate formation of the 1,4,5-trisphosphate.

Neuropharmacological aspects of STI

There are a number of sites at which STI could be disrupted experimentally. From the standpoint of drug development, one must look to the receptor site, since it is extracellular and therefore more accessible to drugs than intracellular sites, and also because interference with subsequent steps may not retain specificity, inasmuch as second messenger systems are shared by multiple receptor types. Nevertheless, identification and development of agents that block one or another of these subsequent steps would be particularly useful in dissecting out regulatory aspects of this complex dual second messenger system. At present, there is not a good blocker of the inositide phosphodiesterase. Elsewhere in the lipid regenerative cycle, the liponucleotide step would appear to be very amenable for disruption because of its rate-limiting nature. At the level of PI synthase, inositol analogs might prove effective. PI and PIP kinases appear to be regulated steps, both in regard to negative feedback (protein kinase C) and positive feedback (oncogenes; see review by Berridge, 1984b).

Pharmacological manipulation of STI via inositol phosphate turnover may be the basis of the therapeutic action of Li^+. As IP_3 is degraded to IP_2 and then to IP_1 (the D-1 phosphate), it must then be cleaved to free inositol prior to reincorporation into PI. It is this step that is blocked by Li^+. Since the blood–brain barrier is relatively impermeable to inositol and since Li^+ is also an effective blocker of breakdown of inositol D-3-phosphate, the precursor of biosynthetic brain inositol, STI could become limited by inositol availability. Since accumulation of the inositol monophosphates and thus depletion of free inositol are a function of the rate of STI, it has been postulated that Li^+ will have little effect on cells that are undergoing normal rates of receptor–ligand interaction, but will selectively block STI in cells that are being highly stimulated. In this way Li^+ is proposed to have a normalizing action in hyperactive cells in manic psychosis (Berridge et al., 1982; Honchar et al., 1983). While this is a rather simplistic model, it deserves careful consideration, particularly in view of the observation that the levels of Li^+ required to inhibit the phosphohydrolase are in the therapeutic range, and that in animals treated chronically with Li^+, brain free inositol is lowered and inositol monophosphate is increased several-fold (Allison et al., 1976). At the very least, Li^+ has provided us with an enormously valuable tool for the study of intracellular regulation of the events following receptor-stimulated inositide turnover.

References

Abdel-Latif, A.A. (1983) Metabolism of phosphoinositides. In A. Lajtha (Ed.), *Handbook of Neurochemistry, Vol. 3*, Plenum, New York, pp. 91–131.

Agranoff, B.W. (1978) Cyclitol confusion. *Trends Biochem. Sci.*, 3:N283–N285.

Agranoff, B.W., Eisenberg, F., Jr., Hauser, G., Hawthorne, J.N. and Michell, R.H. (1985) Comment on abbreviations. In J. Bleasdale, J. Eichberg and G. Hauser (Eds.), *Inositol and Phosphoinositides, Metabolism and Regulation*, Humana Press, Clifton, NJ, pp. xxi–xxii.

Allison, J.H., Blisner, M.E., Holland, W.H., Hipps, P.P. and Sherman, W.R. (1976) Increased brain myo-inositol 1-phosphate in lithium-treated rats. *Biochem. Biophys. Res. Commun.*, 71:664–670.

Aub, D.L. and Putney, J.W., Jr. (1984) Metabolism of inositol phosphates in parotid cells: Implications for the pathway of the phosphoinositide effect and for the possible messenger role of inositol trisphosphate. *Life Sci.*, 34:1347–1355.

Benjamins, J.A. and Agranoff, B.W. (1969) Distribution and properties of CDP-diglyceride: Inositol transferase from brain. *J. Neurochem.*, 16:513–527.

Benowitz, L.I. and Lewis, E.R. (1983) Increased transport of 44,000- to 49,000-dalton acidic proteins during regeneration of the goldfish optic nerve: A two-dimensional gel analysis. *J. Neurosci.*, 3:2153–2163.

Berridge, M.J. (1983) Rapid accumulation of inositol trisphosphate reveals that agonists hydrolyze polyphosphoinositides instead of phosphatidylinositol. *Biochem. J.*, 212:849–858.

Berridge, M.J. (1984a) Inositol triphosphate and diacylglycerol as second messengers. *Biochem. J.*, 220:345–360.

Berridge, M.J. (1984b) Oncogenes, inositol lipids and cellular proliferation. *Biotechnology*, 2:541–546.

Berridge, M.J. and Irvine, R.F. (1984) Inositol trisphosphate, a novel second messenger in cellular signal transduction. *Nature*, 312:315–321.

Berridge, M.J., Downes, C.P. and Hanley, M.R. (1982) Lithium amplifies agonist-dependent phosphatidylinositol responses in brain and salivary glands. *Biochem. J.*, 206:587–595.

Berridge, M.J., Dawson, R.M.C., Downes, C.P., Heslop, J.P. and Irvine, R.F. (1983) Changes in the levels of inositol phosphates after agonist-dependent hydrolysis of membrane phosphoinositides. *Biochem. J.*, 212:473–482.

Brockerhoff, H. and Ballou, C.E. (1961) The structure of the phosphoinositide complex of beef brain. *J. Biol. Chem.*, 236:1907–1911.

Brockerhoff, H. and Ballou, C.E. (1962) Phosphate incorporation in brain phosphoinositides. *J. Biol. Chem.*, 237:49–52.

Brown, E., Kendall, D.A. and Nahorski, S.R. (1984) Inositol phospholipid hydrolysis in rat cerebral cortical slices. I. Receptor characterisation. *J. Neurochem.*, 42:1379–1387.

Brown, J.H., Goldstein, D. and Masters, S.B. (1985) The putative M1 muscarinic receptor does not regulate phosphoinositide hydrolysis: Studies with pirenzepine and McN-A-343 in chick heart and astrocytoma cells. *Mol. Pharmacol.*, 27:525–531.

Conn, P.J. and Sanders-Bush, E. ((1984) Selective 5HT-2 antagonists inhibit serotonin stimulated phosphatidylinositol metabolism in cerebral cortex. *Neuropharmacology*, 23:993–996.

Conn, P.J. and Sanders-Bush, E. (1985) Serotonin-stimulated phosphoinositide turnover: Mediation by the S_2 binding site in rat cerebral cortex but not in subcortical regions. *J. Pharmacol. Exp. Ther.*, 234:195–203..

Connolly,, T.M., Bross, T.E. and Majerus, P.W. (1985) Isolation of a phosphomonoesterase from human platelets that specifically hydrolyzes the 5-phosphate of inositol 1,4,5-trisphosphate. *J. Biol. Chem.*, 260:7868–7874.

Daum, P.R., Downes, C.P. and Young, J.M. (1984) Histamine stimulation of inositol 1-phosphate accumulation in lithium-treated slices from regions of guinea pig brain. *J. Neurochem.*, 43:25–32.

Downes, C.P. (1983) Inositol phospholipids and neurotransmitter-receptor signalling mechanisms. *Trends Neurosci.*, 6:313–316.

Downes, C.P. and Wusteman, M.M. (1983) Breakdown of polyphosphoinositides and not phosphatidylinositol accounts for muscarinic agonist stimulated inositol phospholipid metabolism in rat parotid glands. *Biochem. J.*, 216:633–640.

Durell, J., Garland, J.T. and Friedel, R.O. (1969) Acetylcholine action: Biochemical aspects. *Science*, 165:862:866.

Eichberg, J. and Dawson, R.M.C. (1965) Polyphosphoinositides in myelin. *Biochem. J.*, 96:644–650.

Eisenberg, F., Jr. and Maeda, T. (1985) The mechanism of enzymatic isomerization of glucose 6-phosphate to L-myo-inositol 1-phosphate. In J.E. Bleasdale, J. Eichberg, and G. Hauser (Eds.), *Inositol and Phosphoinositides, Metabolism and Regulation*, Humana Press, Clifton, NJ, pp. 3–11.

Fisher, S.K. and Agranoff, B.W. (1981) Enhancement of the muscarinic synaptosomal phospholipid labeling effect by the ionophore A23187. *J. Neurochem.*, 37:968–977.

Fisher, S.K. and Agranoff, B.W. (1985) The biochemical basis and functional significance of enhanced phosphatidate and phosphoinositide turnover. In J. Eichberg (Ed.), *Phospholipids in Nervous Tissues*, John Wiley, New York, pp. 241–295.

Fisher, S.K. and Bartus, R.T. (1985) Regional differences in the coupling of muscarinic receptors to inositol phospholipid hydrolysis in guinea pig brain. *J. Neurochem.*, 45:1085–1095.

Fisher, S.K., Boast, C.A. and Agranoff, B.W. (1980) The muscarinic stimulation of phospholipid labeling is indepedent of its cholinergic input. *Brain Res.*, 189:284–288.

Fisher, S.K., Frey, K.A. and Agranoff, B.W. (1981) Loss of muscarinic receptors and of stimulated phospholipid labeling in ibotenate-treated hippocampus. *J. Neurosci.*, 1:1407–1413.

Fisher, S.K., Klinger, P.D. and Agranoff, B.W. (1983) Muscarinic agonist binding and phospholipid turnover in brain. *J. Biol. Chem.*, 258:7358–7363.

Fisher, S.K., Figueiredo, J.C. and Bartus, R.T. (1984a) Differential stimulation of inositol phospholipid turnover in brain by analogs of oxotremorine. *J. Neurochem.*, 43:1171–1179.

Fisher, S.K., Van Rooijen, L.A.A. and Agranoff, B.W. (1984b) Renewed interest in the polyphosphoinositides. *Trends in Biochem. Sci.*, 9:53–56.

Folch, J. (1949) Brain diphosphoinositide, a new phosphatide having inositol metadiphosphate as a constituent. *J. Biol. Chem.*, 177:505–519.

Friedel, R.O. and Schanberg, S.M. (1975) Effects of histamine on phospholipid metabolism of rat brain in vivo. *J. Neurochem.*, 24:819–820.

Friedel, R.O., Johnson, J.R. and Schanberg, S.M. (1973) Effects of sympathomimetic drugs on incorporation in vivo of intracisternally injected $^{32}P_i$ into phospholipids of rat brain. *J. Pharmacol. Exp. Ther.*, 184:583–589.

Gil, D.W. and Wolfe, B.B. (1985) Pirenzepine distinguishes between muscarinic receptor-mediated phosphoinositide breakdown and inhibition of adenylate cyclase. *J. Pharmacol. Exp. Ther.*, 232:608–616.

Girard, P.R., Mazzei, G.J., Wood, J.G. and Kuo, J.F. (1985) Polyclonal antibodies to phospholipid/Ca^{2+}-dependent protein kinase and immunocytochemical localization of the enzyme in rat brain. *Proc. Natl. Acad. Sci U.S.A.*, 82:3030–3034.

Gispen, W.H., Leunissen, J.L.M., Oestreicher, A.B., Verkleij, A.J. and Zwiers, H. (1985) Presynaptic localization of B-50 phosphoprotein: The (ACTH)-sensitive protein kinase substrate involved in rat brain polyphosphoinositide metabolism. *Brain Res.*, 328:381–385.

Gonzales, R.A. and Crews, F.T. (1984) Characterization of the cholinergic stimulation of phosphoinositide hydrolysis in rat brain slices. *J. Neurosci.*, 4:3120–3127.

Hallcher, L.M. and Sherman, W.R. (1980) The effects of lithium ion and other agents on the activity of *myo*-inositol-1-phosphatase from bovine brain. *J. Biol. Chem.*, 255:10896–10901.

Hauser, G. and Eichberg, J. (1975) Identification of cytidine diphosphate-diglyceride in the pineal gland of the rat and its accumulation in the presence of DL-propranolol. *J. Biol. Chem.*, 250:105–112.

Hauser, G., Shein, H.M. and Eichberg, J. (1974) Relationship of α-adrenergic receptors in rat pineal gland to drug-induced stimulation of phospholipid metabolism. *Nature*, 252:482–483.

Hawthorne, J.N. (1982) Is phosphatidylinositol now out of the calcium gate? *Nature*, 295:281–282.

Hawthorne, J.N. and Pickard, M.R. (1979) Phospholipids in synaptic function. *J. Neurochem.*, 32:5–14.

Hawthorne, J.N. and White, D.A. (1975) Myo-inositol lipids. *Vitamins Hormon.*, 33:529–573.

Heacock, A.M. and Agranoff, B.W. (1982) Protein synthesis and transport in the regenerating goldfish visual system. *Neurochem. Res.*, 7:771–788.

Hendrickson, H.S. and Reinertsen, J.L. (1971) Phosphoinositide interconversion: A model for control of Na^+ and K^+ permeability in the nerve axon membrane. *Biochim. Biophys. Res. Commun.*, 44:1258–1264.

Hokin, L.E. and Hokin, M.R. (1955) Effects of acetylcholine on the turnover of phosphoryl units in individual phospholipids of pancreas slices and brain cortex slices. *Biochim. Biophys. Acta*, 18:102–110.

Hokin, M.R. and Hokin, L.E. (1964) Interconversions of phosphatidylinositol and phosphatidic acid involved in the response to acetylcholine in the salt gland. In R.M.C. Dawson and D.N. Rhodes (Eds.), *Metabolism and Physiological Significance of Lipids*, John Wiley and Sons, New York, pp. 423–434.

Honchar, M.P., Olney, J.W. and Sherman, W.R. (1983) Systemic cholinergic agents induce seizures and brain damage in lithium-treated rats. *Science*, 220:323–325.

Jacobson, M.D., Wusteman, M. and Downes, C.P. (1985) Muscarinic receptors and hydrolysis of inositol phospholipids in rat cerebral cortex and parotid gland. *J. Neurochem.*, 44:465–472.

Janowsky, A., Labarca, R. and Paul, S.M. (1984) Characterization of neurotransmitter receptor-mediated phosphatidylinositol hydrolysis in the rat hippocampus. *Life Sci.*, 35:1953–1961.

Jolles, J., Zwiers, H., Van Dongen, C., Schofman, P., Wirtz, K.W.A. and Gispen, W.H. (1980) Modulation of brain polyphosphoinositide metabolism by ACTH-sensitive protein phosphorylation. *Nature*, 286:623–625.

Jolles, J., Bar, P.R. and Gispen, W.H. (1981a) Modulation of brain polyphosphoinositide metabolism by ACTH and β-endorphin: Structure-activity studies. *Brain Res.*, 224:315–326.

Jolles, J., Zwiers, H., Dekker, A., Wirtz, K.W.A. and Gispen, W.H. (1981b) Corticotropin-(1-24)-tetracosapeptide affects protein phosphorylation and polyphosphoinositide metabolism in rat brain. *Biochem. J.*, 194:283–291.

Katz, F., Ellis, L. and Pfenninger, K.H. (1985) Nerve growth cones isolated from fetal rat brain. III. Calcium-dependent protein phosphorylation. *J. Neurosci.*, 5:1402–1414.

Kendall, D.A. and Nahorski, S.R. (1985) 5-Hydroxytryptamine-stimulated inositol phospholipid hydrolysis in rat cerebral cortex slices: Pharmacological characterization and effects of antidepressants. *J. Pharmacol. Exp. Ther.*, 233:473–479.

Kerr, S.E., Kfoury, G.A. and Djibelian, L.G. (1964) Preparation of brain polyphosphoinositides. *J. Lipid Res.*, 5:481–483.

Lazareno, S., Kendall, D.A. and Nahorski, S.R. (1985) Pirenzepine indicates heterogeneity of muscarinic receptors linked to cerebral inositol phospholipid metabolism. *Neuropharmacology*, 24:593–595.

Mantyh, P.W., Pinnock, R.D., Downes, C.P., Goedert, M. and Hunt, S.P. (1984) Correlation between inositol phospholipid hydrolysis and substance P receptors in rat CNS. *Nature*, 309:795–797.

Martin, T.F.J. (1983) Thyrotropin releasing hormone rapidly activates the phosphodiester hydrolysis of polyphosphoinositides in GH_3 pituitary cells. *J. Biol. Chem.*, 258:14816–14822.

Masters, S.B., Quinn, M.T. and Brown, J.H. (1985) Agonist-induced desensitization of muscarinic receptor-mediated calcium efflux without concomitant desensitization of phosphoinositide hydrolysis. *Mol. Pharmacol.*, 27:325–332.

Michell, R.H. (1975) Inositol phospholipids and cell surface receptor function. *Biochim. Biophys. Acta*, 415:81–147.

Michell, R.H. (1982) Is phosphatidylinositol really out of the calcium gate? *Nature*, 296:492–493.

Michell, R.H., Jafferji, S.S. and Jones, L.M. (1976) Receptor occupancy dose-response curve suggests that phosphatidylinositol breakdown may be intrinsic to the mechanism of the muscarinic cholinergic receptor. *FEBS Lett.*, 69:1–5.

Mori, T., Takai, Y., Yu, B., Takahashi, J., Nishizuka, Y. and Fujikara, T. (1982) Specificity of the fatty acyl moieties of diacylglycerol for the activation of calcium-activated, phospholipid-dependent protein kinase. *J. Biochem.*, 91:427–431.

Nelson, R.B. and Routtenberg, A. (1985) Characterization of protein F1 (47 kDa, 4.5 p*I*): A kinase C substrate directly related to neural plasticity. *Exp. Neurol.*, 89:213–224.

Nicoletti, F., Meek, J.L., Chuang, D.M., Iodarola, M., Roth, B.L. and Costa, E. (1985) Ibotenic acid stimulates inositol phospholipid turnover in rat hippocampal slices: An effect mediated by 'APB-sensitive' receptors, *Fed. Proc.*, 44:Abstr. 480.

Nijjar, M.S., Smith, T.L. and Hauser, G. (1980) Evidence against dopaminergic and further support for α-adrenergic receptor involvement in the pineal phosphatidylinositol effect. *J. Neurochem.*, 34:813–821.

Nishizuka, Y. (1983) Phospholipid degradation and signal translation for protein phosphorylation. *Trends Biochem. Sci.*, 8:13–16.

Nishizuka, Y. (1984) Turnover of inositol phospholipids and signal transduction. *Science*, 225:1365–1370.

Ouimet, C.C., McGuinness, T.L. and Greengard, P. (1984) Immunocytochemical localization of calcium/calmodulin-dependent protein kinase II in rat brain. *Proc. Natl. Acad. Sci. U.S.A.*, 81:5604–5608.

Raetz, C.R.H., Hirschberg, C.B., Dowhan, W., Wickner, W.T. and Kennedy, E.P. (1972) A membrane-bound pyrophosphatase in *Escherichia coli* catalyzing the hydrolysis of cytidine diphosphate-diglyceride. *J. Biol. Chem.*, 247:2245–2247.

Rasmussen, H. and Barrett, P.Q. (1984) Calcium messenger system: An integrated view. *Physiol. Rev.*, 64:938–984.

Rittenhouse, H.G., Seguin, E.B., Fisher, S.K. and Agranoff, B.W. (1981) Properties of a CDP-diglyceride hydrolase from guinea pig brain. *J. Neurochem.*, 36:991–999.

Schacht, J. and Agranoff, B.W. (1972) Effects of acetylcholine on labeling of phosphatidate and phosphoinositides by [^{32}P]orthophosphate in nerve-ending fractions of guinea pig cortex. *J. Biol. Chem.*, 247:771–777.

Schacht, J. and Agranoff, B.W. (1974) Stimulation of hydrolysis of phosphatidic acid by cholinergic agents in guinea pig synaptosomes. *J. Biol. Chem.*, 249:1551–1557.

Schoepp, D.D., Knepper, S.M., and Rutledge, C.O. (1984) Norepinephrine stimulation of phosphoinositide hydrolysis in rat cerebral cortex is associated with the alpha$_1$-adrenoceptor. *J. Neurochem.*, 43:1758–1761.

Skene, J.H.P. and Willard, M. (1981) Changes in axonally transported proteins during axon regeneration in toad re-

tinal ganglion cells. *J. Cell Biol.*, 89:86–95.

Smith, T.L., Eichberg, J. and Hauser, G. (1979) Postsynaptic localization of the alpha receptor-mediated stimulation of phosphatidylinositol turnover in pineal gland. *Life Sci.*, 24:2179–2184.

Snider, R.M., Roland, R.M., Lowy, R.J., Agranoff, B.W. and Ernst, S.A. (1986) Muscarinic receptor-stimulated Ca^{2+} signalling and inositol lipid metabolism in avian salt gland cells. *Biochim. Biophys. Acta*, in press.

Spector, R. and Lorenzo, A.V. (1975) Myo-inositol transport in the central nervous system. *Am. J. Physiol.*, 228:1510–1518.

Sternweis, P.C. and Robishaw, J.D. (1984) Isolation of two proteins with high affinity for guanine nucleotides from membranes of bovine brain. *J. Biol. Chem.*, 259:13806–13813.

Storey, D.J., Shears, S.B., Kirk, C.J. and Michell, R.H. (1984) Stepwise enzymatic dephosphorylation of inositol 1,4,5-trisphosphate to inositol in liver. *Nature*, 312:374–376.

Subramanian, N., Whitmore, W.L., Seidler, F.J. and Slotkin, T.A. (1980) Histamine stimulates brain phospholipid turnover through a direct H-1 receptor-mediated mechanism. *Life Sci.*, 27:1315–1319.

Subramanian, N., Whitmore, W.L., Seidler, F.J. and Slotkin, T.A. (1981) Ontogeny of histaminergic neurotransmission in the rat brain: Concomitant development of neuronal histamine, H-1 receptors, and H-1 receptor- mediated stimulation of phospholipid turnover. *J. Neurochem.*, 36:1137–1141.

Watson, S.P. and Downes, C.P. (1983) Substance P induced hydrolysis of inositol phospholipids in guinea-pig ileum and rat hypothalamus. *Eur. J. Pharmacol.*, 93:245–253.

Watson, M., Roeske, W.R. and Yamamura, H.I. (1982) [^{3}H]Pirenzepine selectively identifies a high affinity population of muscarinic cholinergic receptors in the rat cerebral cortex. *Life Sci.*, 31:2019–2023.

Watson, M., Yamamura, H.I. and Roeske, W.R. (1983) A unique regulatory profile and regional distribution of [^{3}H]pirenzepine binding in the rat provides evidence for distinct M1 and M2 muscarinic receptor subtypes. *Life Sci.*, 32:3001–3011.

Whitman, M.R., Epstein, J. and Cantley, L. (1985) Inositol 1,4,5-trisphosphate stimulates phosphorylation of a 62,000-dalton protein in monkey fibroblast and bovine brain cell lysates. *J. Biol. Chem.*, 259:13652–13655.

Wilson, D.B., Bross, T.E., Hoffman, S.L. and Majerus, P.W. (1984) Hydrolysis of polyphosphoinositides by purified sheep seminal vesicle phospholipase C enzymes. *J. Biol. Chem.*, 259:11718–11724.

Wilson, D.B., Neufeld, E.J. and Majerus, P.W. (1985) Phosphoinositide interconversion in thrombin-stimulated human platelets. *J. Biol. Chem.*, 260:1046–1051.

Yagihara, Y. and Hawthorne, J.N. (1972) Effects of acetylcholine on the incorporation of [^{32}P]orthophosphate in vitro into the phospholipids of nerve-ending particles from guinea-pig brain. *J. Neurochem.*, 19:355–367.

Yano, K., Higashida, H., Inoue, R. and Nozawa, Y. (1984) Bradykinin-induced rapid breakdown of phosphatidylinositol 4,5-bisphosphate in neuroblastoma X glioma hybrid NG 108-15 cells. *J. Biol. Chem.*, 259:10201–10207.

W.H. Gispen and A. Routtenberg (Eds.)
Progress in Brain Research, Vol. 69
© 1986 Elsevier Science Publishers B.V. (Biomedical Division)

CHAPTER 2

The role of inositol phosphates in intracellular calcium mobilization

J. Eichberg and L.N. Berti-Mattera

Department of Biochemical and Biophysical Sciences, University of Houston, Houston, TX 77004, U.S.A.

Introduction

The responses of cells to changes in their environment depend upon mechanisms that detect external cues and transduce the information into decipherable internal signals able to initiate appropriate alterations in cellular performance. The cues involved, primarily neurotransmitters. hormones, growth factors or light, activate cell surface receptors as the first step in a transmembrane cascade of events leading to production of second messenger molecules which serve as intracellular currencies to modify cellular activities such as secretion, phototransduction, cell growth and transmission or modulation of electrical signals. The most extensively studied cellular transduction system to date is that using cyclic AMP and is one which invariably evokes enhanced protein phosphorylation in response to a receptor-mediated rise in the intracellular concentration of this cyclic nucleotide. This chapter will focus on the state of our knowledge of what is increasingly coming to be recognized as another important cellular transduction pathway that employs inositol phosphates derived from inositol-containing phospholipids. Particular attention will be paid to the role of this signalling mechanism in the alteration of intracellular Ca^{2+} levels.

The phosphoinositide cycle

Over 30 years ago, Hokin and Hokin (1953) observed that ^{32}P incorporation into phospho-lipids of pancreatic slices was greatly stimulated when acetylcholine was present in the incubation medium. The enhanced labeling was subsequently found to be confined to two minor membrane lipids, phosphatidylinositol (PI) and phosphatidic acid and was blocked in the presence of atropine (Hokin and Hokin, 1955). These findings were the first to implicate changes in the turnover of inositol-containing phospholipids in response to activation of a cell surface receptor and proved to be the seed from which a vast flowering of similar observations was recorded. A plethora of agonists have since been shown to activate a wide variety of receptors and thereby to stimulate PI (and often phosphatidic acid) labeling in numerous cell and tissue types, including diverse neural preparations (Berridge and Irvine, 1984; Fisher and Agranoff, 1985).

In ensuing years, the polyphosphoinositides, phosphatidylinositol 4-phosphate (PIP) and phosphatidylinositol 4,5-bisphosphate (PIP_2), which are quantitatively trace components of many cells, were characterized and enzymatic pathways for the metabolism of all three phosphoinositides were clarified. As may be seen in Fig. 1, phosphatidic acid is converted to the liponucleotide intermediate, CMP-phosphatidic acid (CDP-diacylglycerol), which reacts with *myo*-inositol to form PI. The polyphosphoinositides are formed by stepwise phosphorylation of PI with ATP as phosphate donor to produce first PIP and then PIP_2. Each phosphoinositide can undergo phospholipase C-catalyzed degradation to form 1,2 diacylglycerol (primarily the 1-stearoyl-2-arach-

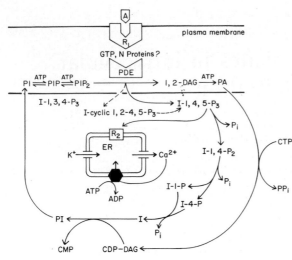

Fig. 1. The phosphoinositide cycle and intracellular Ca^{2+} release. An agonist (A) interacts with its receptor (R_1) at the cell surface and stimulates polyphosphoinositide phosphodiesterase (PDE) by a coupling mechanism possibly involving GTP-binding proteins (N proteins). The accelerated breakdown of PIP_2 yields IP_3 and 1,2-diacylglycerol, the former perhaps arising via a *myo*-inositol-1,2 cyclic-4,5-trisphosphate intermediate. *Myo*-Inositol-1,3,4-trisphosphate is also generated via an unknown mechanism (see text). IP_3 then interacts at a hypothetical specific site (R_2) on the endoplasmic reticulum (ER) to activate a distinct Ca^{2+} channel through which the cation passes into the cytosol by a process requiring K^+ uptake. Liberated Ca^{2+} can re-enter the endoplasmic reticulum by the ATP-dependent Ca^{2+} pump. IP_3 in the cytosol is degraded by a series of phosphatases to *myo*-inositol. 1,2-Diacylglycerol in the plasma membrane is phosphorylated to form phosphatidic acid which is then converted via CDP-diacylglycerol to PI. Successive phosphorylations then transform PI to PIP_2. The mono-esterified phosphate groups of PIP and PIP_2 can also be rapidly removed and replaced by a combination of phosphatases and kinases. The sum of these reactions comprises a futile cycle.

idonyl species) and the corresponding inositol phosphate. In the case of PIP_2, the D-*myo*-inositol 1,4,5-trisphosphate (IP_3) produced can be degraded by removal of phosphate groups successively to D-*myo*-inositol 1,4-bisphosphate (IP_2), D-*myo*-inositol 1-phosphate (IP) and *myo*-inositol. The liberated inositol can then be reutilized in the synthesis of PI so as to replenish the supply of polyphosphoinositides. The lipids can also be degraded to PI by phosphomonesterase activities and the dephosphorylations in conjunction with the kinase-catalyzed reactions can be considered to constitute a futile cycle. Finally, the

1,2-diacylglycerol released by phospholipase C action can be reincorporated via conversion to phosphatidic acid into the phosphoinositides. Taken together, these reactions comprise the phosphoinositide cycle in which the polar head groups of these phospholipids may be continually renewed.

Intracellular distribution of phosphoinositide-metabolizing enzymes

It is pertinent to consider briefly the localization of some of the enzymes which metabolize phosphoinositides and inositol phosphates within the cell. PI synthesis, like that of most phospholipids, occurs almost entirely in the endoplasmic reticulum (Benjamins and Agranoff, 1969). The location of PI kinase appears diverse, since this enzyme is enriched not only in plasma membrane, but at least in liver is largely concentrated in the Golgi apparatus and lysosomes as well (Downes and Michell, 1982; Jergil and Sundler, 1983; Collins and Wells, 1983; Cockcroft et al., 1985). PIP kinase was originally reported to be a largely cytosolic enzyme in brain (Kai et al., 1968), but recently it was found in liver to be nearly exclusively confined to the plasma membrane (Cockcroft et al., 1985). Thus the possibility must be considered that PIP kinase, at least in some tissues, is a loosely bound membrane enzyme that is readily displaced during cell fractionation. Evidence that the plasma membrane is an exceptionally active site of polyphosphoinositide synthesis was furnished by Seyfred and Wells (1984a) who observed that ^{32}P incorporation by a liver plasma membrane fraction into PIP and PIP_2 was 5–10 and 25–50 times faster, respectively, than for any other subcellular fraction.

The nature and distribution of the phosphodiesterase(s) which hydrolyze the phosphoinositides are far from clear. In early studies, separate Ca^{2+}-dependent enzyme activities which degraded PI and the polyphosphoinositides were identified (for review, cf. Irvine, 1982; Irvine et al., 1985a). The PI phosphodiesterase was long considered to be exclusively cytosolic, although more recent evidence suggests that a Ca^{2+}-independent PI phosphodiesterase activity is present in lysosomes

(Irvine et al., 1978). Much less attention has been paid to phosphodiesteratic cleavage of polyphosphoinositides, but recently both soluble and membrane-bound activities have been studied (Allen and Michell, 1978; Van Rooijen et al., 1983; Cockcroft et al., 1984; Irvine et al., 1984a; Seyfred and Wells, 1984b).

While the enzymatic hydrolysis of PIP_2 and PIP generally displays dependence on Ca^{2+}, manipulation of reaction conditions can dramatically reduce this requirement (Irvine et al., 1984a). Indeed, there is a distinct possibility that the same phosphodiesterase is capable of hydrolyzing all three phosphoinositides and that the avidity and specificity of the enzyme for a particular phosphoinositide may be dependent on its own environment and/or that of the substrate. Thus when PIP_2 is present in nonbilayer configuration obtained by incorporating it into phosphatidylethanolamine-rich vesicles, it is vigorously degraded by the soluble brain phosphodiesterase at approximately physiological concentrations of Ca^{2+}, Mg^{2+} and K^+ (Irvine et al., 1984a). In contrast, PIP_2 as part of a lipid mixture with a composition similar to the inner monolayer of rat liver plasma membrane is not attacked under these ionic conditions. Majerus and coworkers (Wilson et al., 1984) found that each of two purified and immunologically distinct phospholipase C enzymes from sheep seminal vesicles can hydrolyze all three phosphoinositides. When phosphoinositides were presented to the enzymes as constituents of vesicles with a lipid composition resembling the cytoplasmic leaflet of the membrane, polyphosphoinositides were preferentially hydrolyzed, especially at low Ca^{2+} levels. These studies indicate that there is still much to be learned regarding the properties and factors that influence the activities of enzymes which hydrolyze the phosphoinositides.

Enzymes which degrade IP_3 to IP_2 have been characterized in erythrocyte membranes (Downes et al., 1982), liver plasma membranes (Storey et al., 1984; Seyfred et al., 1984) and, after purification, in soluble form from platelets (Connolly et al., 1985). These activities are completely dependent on Mg^{2+} but are unaffected by Li^+ which markedly inhibits IP_2 phosphatase and IP phosphatase, both of which are soluble enzymes (Hallcher and Sherman 1980; Storey et al., 1984; Seyfred et al., 1984).

Thus it seems likely that enzymatic machinery for the synthesis and phosphodiesteratic degradation of PIP_2 is present in or adjacent to the plasma membrane and that IP_3 can be readily degraded to *myo*-inositol. Once the cyclitol is reincorporated into phospholipid in the endoplasmic reticulum the PI formed must be transported to the plasma membrane, presumably by the PI-specific exchange protein (Helmkamp et al., 1974). We have not considered here the extent of reutilization of the other product of PIP_2 hydrolysis, 1,2-diacylglycerol. Its fate is unclear; some speculative schemes envision that the compound is rephosphorylated at the plasma membrane by diacylglycerol kinase and the resulting phosphatidic acid is then transferred to the endoplasmic reticulum for use in phospholipid synthesis. Such movement of phosphatidic acid is at best poorly documented.

Regulation of cellular Ca^{2+} levels

In a resting cell the cytosolic Ca^{2+} concentration is 0.1–0.2 µM. Since high amounts of Ca^{2+} can be toxic (Rasmussen, 1985), this level is maintained in part by controlling the flux of cation into and out of the cell by means of a Ca^{2+}-dependent ATPase pump and a Na^+/Ca^{2+} exchange process, both located at the plasma membrane (Rasmussen and Barrett, 1984). In addition, both endoplasmic reticulum and mitochondria can sequester or release Ca^{2+}. The uptake mechanism for endoplasmic reticulum utilizes a Ca^{2+}-ATPase distinct from that at the plasma membrane, whereas mitochondria employ a specific carrier and a mechanism dependent on the proton-motive force. The liberation of Ca^{2+} from intracellular stores is much less well understood, but accumulating evidence, discussed further below, suggests that the endoplasmic reticulum is the major source of bound Ca^{2+} released into the cytosol under physiological conditions (Burgess et al., 1983). When receptor activation by an appropriate agonist occurs, there is a rapid (within seconds) 2–5-fold rise in cytosolic Ca^{2+} concentration above the resting level; mobilized Ca^{2+} is swiftly extruded through the plasma membrane and, since the internal stores of cation are limited, a receptor-mediated event which relied solely on elevated levels of intracellular Ca^{2+} would be of short duration. However, in the case of pancreatic acinar cells, addition of carbamylcholine to cells in a Ca^{2+}-containing medium elicits a burst of Ca^{2+} release into the cytosol followed by a much slower return to the prestimulated level (Schulz et al., 1985). This is evidently due to the onset of increased Ca^{2+} permeability of the plasma membrane by an unknown mechanism and the increase in cytosolic Ca^{2+} sustained by influx of extracellular cation prolongs the Ca^{2+}-mediated physiological response.

A discussion of the means by which Ca^{2+} exerts its action is for the most part beyond the scope of this chapter. As covered extensively elsewhere in this volume, increased phosphorylation of target proteins mediated either by Ca^{2+}-calmodulin-dependent protein kinases or by Ca^{2+}- and phospholipid-dependent protein kinase C is a mandatory component of many physiological responses in nervous tissue. Similar events are widespread in non-neural systems (cf. Berridge and Irvine, 1984; Exton, 1985).

Receptor activation and stimulated phosphoinositide breakdown

Approximately 12 years ago, evidence began to emerge that the earliest response to activation of muscarinic cholinergic and α_1 adrenergic receptors was an increased breakdown of phosphoinositides. Initially, cellular phosphatidylinositol levels were found to decline over a period of minutes following initiation of receptor stimulation (Jones and Michell, 1974). In this context, enhanced incorporation of ^{32}P or [^3H]inositol into PI, first observed by the Hokins, was interpreted as a secondary phenomenon that reflects resynthesis of a depleted PI pool. Much of this pioneering work was spearheaded by Michell, who published an influential review that summarized what was then known concerning the linkage between enhanced phosphoinositide metabolism and cellular responses and in which he pointed out

that those receptors associated with stimulated phosphoinositide turnover were also implicated in the regulation of intracellular Ca^{2+} levels (Michell, 1975). Accumulated observations in the literature led Michell to propose that accelerated PI breakdown precedes and is required for increased Ca^{2+} influx ('gating') into the cell.

There is little doubt that for most cellular systems examined, this general hypothesis has held up very well, although significant changes in its formulation have occurred. For one, the idea that the primary event in Ca^{2+} regulation following stimulated phosphoinositide breakdown is increased Ca^{2+} entry into the cell has been displaced by the concept that Ca^{2+} is mobilized from intracellular stores; in this connection, a persistent criticism of the hypothesis has been that removal of Ca^{2+} from the external medium can sometimes diminish the extent of receptor-mediated stimulation of PI labeling, which is commonly taken as a measure of increased phosphoinositide breakdown (e.g. Prpić et al., 1982; Eichberg and Harrington, 1983). Many previous studies employed EGTA to deplete Ca^{2+} and it is now generally recognized that this chelator may exhibit variable potency in removing intracellular Ca^{2+}, sometimes including that small amount presumably required for activation of membrane-associated enzymes which degrade phosphoinositides. Thus, while enhanced phosphoinositide turnover is dependent on a minimal concentration of Ca^{2+}, it is most unlikely to be regulated by changes in intracellular Ca^{2+} associated with physiological responses.

A further difficulty with the hypothesis as originally presented is that the rise in cytosolic Ca^{2+} concentration occurs more rapidly than the time required for a fall in PI or rise in IP to be detected as measured either chemically or following prelabeling with ^{32}P or [^3H]inositol (Thomas et al., 1984; Berridge et al., 1984). Efforts to demonstrate a receptor-mediated change in polyphosphoinositide metabolism in conjunction with enhanced PI labeling were for a time unsuccessful (cf. Fisher and Agranoff, 1985). Initial indications that accelerated breakdown of polyphosphoinositides occurs as a consequence of muscarinic cholinergic or α_1-adrenergic receptor activation were obtained for iris smooth muscle and nerve ending preparations (Durrell et al., 1969; Abdel-Latif et al., 1977; Fisher and Agranoff, 1981; Abdel-Latif, 1983). Using hepatocytes in which polyphosphoinositides had been labeled to equilibrium with ^{32}P, Michell et al., (1981) found that on addition of vasopression an extremely rapid hydrolysis of both PIP_2 and PIP occurred (within seconds) and that polyphosphoinositide concentrations were then swiftly restored to prestimulated levels. These findings made it clear that the involvement of polyphosphoinositides had previously been missed because of their brief and transient metabolic response following receptor activation. Numerous reports soon followed of both rapid phosphodiesteratic degradation of PIP_2 and PIP and appearance of their inositol-containing hydrolysis products, IP_2 and IP_3, in a variety of cellular systems (Berridge, 1983; Berridge et al., 1983; Agranoff et al., 1983; Aub and Putney, 1984; Thomas et al., 1984; Berridge and Irvine, 1984). The hydrolysis of PIP_2 is now widely accepted as the primary receptor-stimulated event, and it is generally assumed that resynthesis of the depleted pool of this compound takes place via phosphorylation of PI resulting in a gradual loss of this substance (cf. Fig. 1). However, there remain disagreements concerning the precise time course of phosphoinositide breakdown in response to stimulation as well as the origin of the 1,2-diacylglycerol, which is released together with inositol phosphates (see below).

Role of IP_3 in intracellular Ca^{2+} mobilization

Careful measurements established that in several systems (Berridge et al., 1984; Thomas et al., 1984; Drummond et al., 1985) the appearance of IP_3 following receptor stimulation precedes the elevation of intracellular Ca^{2+} and led to the suggestion that IP_3 itself was the trigger for liberation of the cation into the cytosol. Evidence that this could be the case has been gathered through studies of a variety of cells permeabilized by the absence of external Ca^{2+}, ATP, digitonin or saponin treatment and was presented first for pancreatic acinar cells (Streb et al., 1983) and later for a number of other cell types (e.g. Burgess et al.,

1984a; Joseph et al., 1984; Biden et al., 1984; Brown and Rubin, 1984; Volpe et al., 1985; cf. Berridge and Irvine, 1984). In these investigations, cells were incubated at a low Ca^{2+} concentration and allowed to sequester Ca^{2+} until an equilibrium between the internal uptake and release of the ion was achieved. Upon addition of micromolar amounts of IP_3, a rapid release of Ca^{2+} was observed and was followed by a slower re-uptake of cation. Subsequent repeated additions of IP_3 elicited similar several-fold elevations of Ca^{2+} consistent with the existence of an IP_3-sensitive Ca^{2+} pool which is emptied and then rapidly refilled, perhaps as IP_3 is removed by enzymatic degradation. In further support of this concept, not only did blockage of IP_3 production in permeabilized pancreatic cells by neomycin-induced inhibition of polyphosphoinositide (PPI) phosphodiesterase abolish Ca^{2+} release, but when IP_3 breakdown was hindered by addition of 2,3-diphosphoglycerate or reduction of Mg^{2+} levels, increased Ca^{2+} liberation resulted (Streb et al., 1985).

The rate of IP_3 generation in intact cells appears to be such that it could reach concentrations of 20–30 µM within 1 minute (Aub and Putney 1984; Burgess et al., 1984a). Since half-maximal response of Ca^{2+} release in permeabilized cell systems is expressed from 0.1–1.0 µM IP_3, it seems likely that the levels of IP_3 could rise sufficiently rapidly so that it could act as a signal for Ca^{2+} liberation.

The site at which IP_3 acts has been shown to be a vesicular ATP-dependent nonmitochondrial pool of Ca^{2+}. This has been established by showing that Ca^{2+} can be released by IP_3 after loading permeabilized cells with Ca^{2+} in the presence of ATP and at low concentrations of the cation, conditions in which uptake was unaffected by mitochondrial poisons (Burgess et al., 1984a). In contrast, if the ambient Ca^{2+} concentration was raised so that Ca^{2+} sequestration was greatly increased and accounted for almost entirely by mitochondrial uptake, IP_3 elicited no significant Ca^{2+} release. Experiments utilizing subcellular fractions indicate that the most likely source of mobilized Ca^{2+} is the endoplasmic reticulum. The cation is released from isolated liver microsomes substantially free of mitochondria in the presence of IP_3 (Dawson and Irvine, 1984). Moreover, fractionation of pancreatic microsomes reveals that IP_3-induced liberation of Ca^{2+} is most evident in those subfractions enriched in enzyme markers for endoplasmic reticulum and not for plasma membrane (Prentki et al., 1984a; Streb et al., 1985). Some heterogeneity in the response of microsomal vesicle populations has been detected, but the significance if any of these observations for the localization of IP_3-triggered Ca^{2+} release in the cell is unclear.

Studies of structural features of those inositol phosphates able to release Ca^{2+} has established that adjacent phosphates at the 4 and 5 positions of the inositol are essential for activity. Thus glycerophosphoinositol 4,5-bisphosphate and inositol-2,4,5-trisphosphate are nearly as potent as IP_3. Inositol 4,5-bisphosphate is much less effective, suggesting the phosphate at position 1 of the cyclitol also plays a role perhaps in enhancing binding of the molecule to a specific site. Inactive compounds include *myo*-inositol, IP_2, IP and inositol 1,2-cyclic phosphate (Berridge and Irvine, 1984).

While the ability of IP_3 to liberate sequestered intracellular Ca^{2+} in permeabilized cells seems well established, only in the case of leaky pancreatic acinar cells has evidence been presented that an agonist, carbachol, acts on the same pool of Ca^{2+} that is susceptible to the direct effects of IP_3 (Streb et al., 1983). Alternative and less damaging methods for introducing IP_3 into cells may be necessary so that the physiological relevance of Ca^{2+} release by immediate application of this substance to increases in cytosolic Ca^{2+} elicited by a variety of external stimuli via receptor-mediated processes can be more clearly demonstrated for additional cell types.

Recent developments and unsolved problems

Although much support now exists for the concept that IP_3 is essential for intracellular Ca^{2+} mobilization, a considerable number of unanswered or incompletely resolved questions remain concerning the metabolism of phosphoinositides, the mechanism of Ca^{2+} release and regulation of the entire process. Among the most important of these are the following.

What is the molecular linkage between receptor–agonist interaction and PIP_2 hydrolysis?

The binding of ligand to receptor has been proposed to evoke a transmembrane conformational change that increases the degree of accessibility between membrane domains containing PIP_2 and polyphosphoinositide phosphodiesterase so that stimulated phosphoinositide breakdown can be initiated (Agranoff and Bleasdale, 1978; Irvine et al., 1984a). Whether or not this is true, there are now several indications that a GTP-binding protein may provide an essential link in the coupling of the receptors to PIP_2 phosphodiesterase. Permeabilized blood platelets loaded with either GTP or its nonhydrolyzable analogs, GTP-γ-S or $G\rho\rho NH_P$, display increased Ca^{2+} mobilization and 1,2-diacylglycerol accumulation (Haslam and Davidson, 1984). Permeabilized mast cells exposed to GTP-γ-S secrete histamine when Ca^{2+} is present in the medium (Gomperts, 1983) and this Ca^{2+}-dependent secretion is abolished when neomycin is allowed to enter the cells (Cockcroft and Gomperts, 1985). The indication from these results that PPI phosphodiesterase is regulated by a GTP-binding protein was strengthened by the demonstration that the enzyme in neutrophil plasma membranes could be activated by GTP analogs (but not ATP or its analogs) at physiological levels of Ca^{2+} (Cockcroft and Gomperts, 1985). Somewhat similar results were obtained by Fain and coworkers using a cell-free system from blowfly salivary gland capable of degrading phosphoinositides to inositol phosphates in the presence of serotonin or 5-methyl tryptamine (Litosch et al., 1985). When added to membranes from the gland, GTP analogs markedly increased both the basal and hormone-stimulated production of inositol phosphates. This group has also reported that GTP-γ-S stimulates phospholipase C-catalyzed degradation of phosphoinositides in hepatocyte plasma membranes (Wallace and Fain, 1985).

Thus, analogous to the activation of adenylate cyclase, a putative GTP-binding protein may play a role in the activation of PPI phosphodiesterase or alternatively modulate the accessibility within the membrane of the enzyme for its substrate. It is not yet clear whether the same or related but distinct families of GTP-binding proteins are coupled to receptors that activate PPI phosphodiesterase and adenylate cyclase. Pertussis toxin, which blocks the agonist-mediated inhibition of adenylate cyclase by ADP-ribosylation of the $41\,000\,M_r$ component of the GTP-binding protein termed N_i (Gilman, 1984), did not abolish either the muscarinic receptor-mediated stimulation of phosphoinositide hydrolysis or Ca^{2+} mobilization (Masters et al., 1985). However, other reports indicate that the toxin does inhibit Ca^{2+} mobilization as well as enhanced PIP_2 breakdown and PI synthesis associated with certain other agonists (Moreno et al., 1983; Nakamura and Ui, 1985; Smith et al., 1985; Brandt et al., 1985).

What reactions of the phosphoinositide cycle participate in stimulated production of 1,2-diacylglycerol and inositol phosphates?

In many systems, it has been clearly demonstrated that IP_3 is the first inositol phosphate formed following receptor activation (Berridge, 1983; Downes and Wusteman, 1983). However, in others the rate of appearance of IP_2 and decline of PIP is as fast or faster than corresponding changes in IP_3 and PIP_2 (Aub and Putney, 1984; Berridge et al., 1984). Since IP_2 can be generated either by phosphodiesteratic cleavage of PIP or through action of IP_3 phosphatase, the significance of kinetic data for this compound is difficult to evaluate. In any case, rapid production of IP_2 which is ineffective in mobilizing Ca^{2+} would itself constitute a modulatory mechanism if it competed for intracellular sites to which IP_3 binds.

It is now generally accepted that a decline in PI following stimulation occurs only after a considerable delay, although some data suggest that the absolute rates of breakdown of all three phosphoinositides are similar (Thomas et al., 1983; Litosch et al., 1983). Most commonly, the decline in PI, which is present in much larger amounts than the polyphosphoinositides, has been inter-

preted as caused entirely by its utilization to replenish depleted stores of PIP_2 and PIP in the plasma membrane (Downes and Wusteman, 1983; Berridge, 1984). The relatively slow accumulation of IP as compared to IP_3 and IP_2 which has been observed in a number of systems has also been taken to mean that this compound arises wholly or mainly by successive dephosphorylations of IP_3 (Aub and Putney, 1984).

In order to validate the idea that changes in PI levels are indeed accounted for by its phosphorylation to form polyphosphoinositides, the rate of conversion of this molecule to PIP and PIP_2 must be comparable to the rate of appearance of IP_3. At least in thrombin-stimulated platelets, calculation of the flux of PI to polyphosphoinositides by measurement of changes in the specific activities of the monoesterified phosphate groups under nonequilibrium conditions indicates that this is not the case. Less than 15% of the decline in PI mass seen during the first 30 seconds can be accounted for by transformation of the molecule to PIP (Wilson et al., 1985b). It was therefore suggested that for this system phospholipase C-catalyzed hydrolysis is the major route of PI utilization, an explanation which would rationalize the origin of the much greater quantity of 1,2-diacylglycerol liberated as compared to IP_3 (Wilson et al., 1985b; Majerus et al., 1985). Thus the initial hydrolysis of PIP_2 is envisioned as leading to the mobilization of sufficient intracellular Ca^{2+} to activate a phospholipase C (possibly the same enzyme) which then degrades a much greater amount of PI. Whether this model is generally applicable or is restricted to the platelet in which an unusually high proportion of cellular PI disappears upon stimulation awaits further study.

What is the significance of other inositol trisphosphates?

Recently, evidence has been put forward that inositol trisphosphates other than IP_3 may be formed in response to agonists. A compound identified by chemical degradation studies as D or L *myo*-inositol 1,3,4-trisphosphate (cf. Fig. 2) is generated following carbamylcholine stimulation of parotid gland fragments (Irvine et al., 1984b).

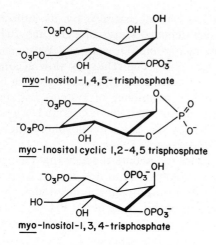

myo-Inositol-1,4,5-trisphosphate

myo-Inositol cyclic 1,2-4,5 trisphosphate

myo-Inositol-1,3,4-trisphosphate

Fig. 2. Structures of inositol trisphosphates with demonstrated or possible biological activity. *Myo*-Inositol-1,4,5-trisphosphate (IP$_3$) is formed by phosphodiesteratic hydrolysis of PIP$_2$ and can mobilize intracellular Ca^{2+}. *Myo*-Inositol-1,2-cyclic-4,5-triphosphate has been shown to be formed enzymatically from PIP$_2$ in a cell-free preparation and could be a short-lived intracellular second messenger. *Myo*-Inositol-1,3,4-trisphosphate accumulates to a greater extent than IP$_3$ following stimulation of several cell types. The precursor of the compound is unknown and it has no known physiological action. See text for further details.

The appearance of this compound lags behind that of IP$_3$, but with increasing time a progressively greater proportion of total inositol trisphosphate is inositol 1,3,4-trisphosphate, which is much less readily degraded than IP$_3$ (Irvine et al., 1985b). Thus it seems quite likely that much if not most of the inositol trisphosphate which accumulates in a variety of systems following receptor stimulation is, except for very early times, the more slowly metabolized isomer. Given this fact, much previously published kinetic data on IP$_3$ production may need to be reevaluated. Efforts to date have failed to reveal the metabolic origins of inositol 1,3,4-trisphosphate; for example, no phosphatidylinositol 3,4-bisphosphate, a possible precursor, could be detected (Irvine et al., 1985b). The significance of inositol 1,3,4-trisphosphate remains entirely speculative, although its relatively slow appearance makes it unlikely that it is associated with rapid Ca^{2+} mobilization.

Very recently, Majerus and coworkers have found evidence that, in addition to IP$_3$, a cyclic inositol trisphosphate, which they propose is inositol 1,2-cyclic-4,5-trisphosphate (Fig. 2), is formed in vitro by action of a purified seminal vesicle phospholipase C on PIP$_2$ (Wilson et al., 1985a). Indications for production of a cyclic inositol trisphosphate depicted in Fig. 2 was obtained by performing the enzyme hydrolysis of PIP$_2$ in the presence of ^{18}O. This result is analogous to the formation of substantial amounts of both IP and inositol 1,2-cyclic phosphate on phosphodiesteratic degradation of PI (Dawson et al., 1971), although the cyclic inositol trisphosphate comprises only 6–15% of the water-soluble products. The cyclic inositol trisphosphate could constitute an extremely labile second messenger involved in generating transient Ca^{2+} signals and would be rapidly hydrolyzed, presumably to IP$_3$ by analogy with the enzymatic conversion of inositol 1,2-cyclic phosphate to IP (Dawson and Clarke, 1972). Proper evaluation of this hypothesis requires proof that cyclic inositol trisphosphate can actually be formed in response to receptor stimulation in intact cells.

How does IP$_3$ release sequestered Ca^{2+}?

Although there is persuasive evidence that newly liberated cytosolic Ca^{2+} arises from a pool predominantly associated with endoplasmic reticulum, the precise mechanism by which IP$_3$ brings this about is obscure. A conclusion that the process involves mobilization of sequestered Ca^{2+} rather than inhibition of Ca^{2+} uptake seems warranted because when the latter was prevented in permeabilized cells either by the ATPase inhibitor, vanadate, or by removal of ATP, Ca^{2+} release not only occurred upon addition of IP$_3$ but its magnitude was markedly increased (Prentki et al., 1984b). The results of structure–activity studies on the ability of inositol phosphates to release Ca^{2+} is consistent with the idea of a 'receptor' for IP$_3$ (Burgess et al., 1984b), but direct evidence for such a specific binding site associated with endoplasmic reticulum is lacking. Recently, Muallem et al. (1985) have reported that IP$_3$ added to a liver rough endoplasmic reticulum vesicle preparation activates a Ca^{2+} channel that is distinct from the electrogenic ATP-dependent Ca^{2+} pump and allows Ca^{2+} efflux into the cytosol in exchange for K^+ uptake as shown in Fig. 1.

How are IP$_3$ levels regulated?

While the enzymatic machinery by which IP$_3$ is generated and removed has been identified and is being characterized, much less is known concerning the regulatory mechanisms that govern the moment-to-moment levels of IP$_3$ in the cell. Presumably such modulation is important to avoid excessively prolonged elevation of intracellular Ca^{2+} as well as to control other possible actions of this second messenger molecule. Once formed, the IP$_3$ concentration in parotid gland fragments either continuously exposed to carbamylcholine or treated with atropine after carbamylcholine stimulation decreases to control levels within 1–3 minutes (Irvine et al., 1985b). The rate of IP$_3$ decline is consonant with the time during which physiological effects thought to be mediated by Ca^{2+} are manifested in this tissue (Poggioli and Putney, 1982) and the disappearance of IP$_3$ parallels the re-uptake of liberated Ca^{2+} in saponin-permeabilized hepatocytes (Joseph et al., 1984).

The rate of IP$_3$ production could be affected both by the activity of PPI phosphodiesterase and the maintenance of the precursor PIP$_2$ pool in the plasma membrane. The former may well be determined by a variety of as yet poorly understood factors which determine the efficiency of coupling between activated receptor and the enzyme through putative GTP-binding proteins analogous to the regulation of adenylate cyclase.

The regulation of phosphoinositide metabolism has been considered by several investigators to involve protein kinase C which is activated by 1,2-diacylglycerol released upon PIP$_2$ hydrolysis (Nishizuka, 1984; Chapter 3). In synaptic plasma membranes, decreased phosphorylation of a 48-kDa protein, termed B-50, a substrate of protein kinase C, accompanied by increased PIP kinase activity (Gispen et al., 1985). This has prompted the hypothesis that release of 1,2-diacylglycerol upon receptor activation results in protein kinase

C-mediated increased phosphorylation of B-50. Such an effect would decrease PIP kinase activity and hence diminish PIP$_2$ formation by a negative feedback mechanism (Gispen et al., 1986; Chapter 4). In possible support of this concept are several reports that certain phorbol esters, which are well-known protein kinase C activators, reduce the formation of inositol phosphates under stimulatory conditions in both neural and nonneural systems (Labarca et al., 1984; Vicentini et al., 1985; Rittenhouse and Sasson, 1985; Watson and Lapetina, 1985; Orellana et al., 1985). However, phorbol esters can also increase the synthesis of polyphosphoinositides (de Chaffoy de Courcelles et al., 1984; Halenda and Feinstein, 1984; Watson and Lapetina, 1985; Boon et al., 1985). It is conceivable that phorbol esters exert their effects via protein kinase C at more than one locus so as to alter the activity of synthetic enzymes and also to inactivate some component involved in coupling the receptor–agonist complex to phospholipase C. A recent report has suggested that PIP$_2$ may also diminish PIP kinase activity by product inhibition (Van Rooijen et al., 1985). Hopefully this confusing picture and its implications for regulation of polyphosphoinositide metabolism will be clarified in the near future.

In an investigation of possible feedback regulation of intracellular Ca^{2+} levels partially mediated by IP$_3$, Drummond (1985) found that low concentrations of thyrotropin-releasing hormone (TRH) elicited a relatively prolonged elevation of IP$_3$ and cytosolic Ca^{2+} in GH$_3$ pituitary tumor cells, whereas higher concentrations produced a larger but more short-lived rise in Ca^{2+} levels. This decreased duration of the Ca^{2+} response was interpreted as due to the operation of an inhibitory component. The inhibition was seen after addition of either the stimulatory peptide in the presence of high K^+ (which opens voltage-sensitive Ca^{2+} channels) or phorbol esters, conditions which would be expected to activate protein kinase C. A similar reduction in intracellular Ca^{2+} was produced by addition of exogenous phospholipase C in the presence of high K^+, a treatment which rapidly released 1,2-diacylglycerol with little or no appearance of IP$_3$. It is considered likely that protein kinase C regulates

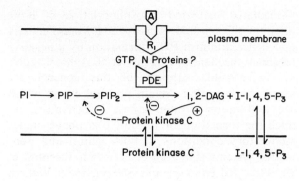

Fig. 3. Hypothetical mechanisms for negative feedback control of PIP$_2$ levels and IP$_3$ formation. Following agonist (A)–receptor (R$_1$) interaction and stimulation of polyphosphoinositide phosphodiesterase (PDE), the increased production of 1,2-diacylglycerol activates protein kinase C in part by promoting its translocation from the cytosol to a plasma membrane site. Stimulated protein kinase C diminishes the rate of hydrolysis of PIP$_2$ by an unknown mechanism and may diminish PIP$_2$ formation possibly via enhanced phosphorylation of an intermediate protein such as the synaptic membrane protein B-50 (Gispen et al., 1986). IP$_3$ initially released in the plasma membrane is shown exchanging with a cytosolic pool of the substance.

the expression of IP$_3$ effects and, whatever the mechanism, IP$_3$ is not directly involved in the process underlying the rapid decrease of elevated Ca^{2+} concentrations seen at high levels of TRH. Thus an inhibition of IP$_3$ formation may constitute a means of limiting information transmitted by means of phosphoinositide turnover in conditions of chronic rather than acute cell stimulation.

A provocative recent finding is that upon stimulation of GH$_3$ cells by TRH there is a very rapid and transient redistribution of substantial protein kinase C from the cytosol to membranous structures (Durst and Martin, 1985) so that particulate enzyme activity following stimulation rose up to 9 fold after brief exposure to the hormone. Other agents, including 1-oleyl-2-arachidonylglycerol and a phorbol ester, compounds that stimulate the enzyme directly or stimulate phospholipase C so as to elevate 1,2-diacylglycerol levels, had similar effects. Prior depletion of Ca^{2+} in the cells by EGTA did not abolish the phenomenon, suggesting that IP$_3$ is not essential for transloca-

tion. These observations provide a rationale for how protein kinase C, ordinarily a cytosolic enzyme, could quickly modify the activity of one or more membrane-bound enzymes of phosphoinositide metabolism to effect negative feed-back as illustrated schematically in Fig. 3.

Concluding remarks

This chapter has concentrated on reviewing what must now be considered compelling evidence that hydrolysis of plasma membrane polyphosphoinositides in response to receptor–agonist interaction produces a second messenger molecule, IP$_3$, which triggers the release of a burst of intracellular sequestered Ca^{2+} into the cytosol. It is probable that many of the gaps in our understanding of the steps in this process will be bridged in the next few years and, in particular, aspects of the synergistic actions between liberated inositol phosphates and 1,2-diacylglycerol (via protein kinase C) on cellular calcium modulation will be much better elucidated.

An additional potentially exciting area for research is the identification of other as yet unknown cellular functions for inositol phosphates. For example, IP$_3$ has been claimed to stimulate protein phosphorylation (Whitman et al., 1984; Lapetina et al., 1984), although this could not be confirmed (Gispen et al., 1985b). The possible role of the relatively stable inositol 1,3,4-trisphosphate in longer-term cellular proliferative responses might be a fruitful field for exploration. It seems certain that the advances of the past few years in our knowledge of the role in cellular signal transduction played by phosphoinositide metabolism merely presage many more future discoveries concerning the functions of this unique and flexible signalling system

Addendum (May 1986)

In recent months, the pace of new discoveries concerning the metabolism and function of IP$_3$ has continued unabated. Particularly significant progress has been made toward answers for two of the questions posed in this review. Further evidence has rapidly accumulated which firmly implicates a GTP-binding protein in the coupling mechanism between receptor activation and stimulated IP$_3$ production in membrane preparations from liver, brain, salivary gland and GH$_3$ pituitary cells (Gonzales and Crews, 1985; Litosch and Fain, 1985; Uhing et al., 1986; Straub and Gershengorn, 1986). The demonstration of these effects in several cell-free preparations should greatly expedite the characterization of the GTP-binding protein that is likely involved. A major advance has been achieved in our knowledge of inositol phosphate metabolism with the finding that inositol-1,3,4,5-tetraphosphate (IP$_4$) is formed in stimulated animal tissues (Batty et al., 1985; Heslop et al., 1985) and can be synthesized by action of an IP$_3$ kinase (Irvine et al., 1986). Since IP$_4$ can be degraded by a 5-phosphatase, presumably the same enzyme that converts IP$_3$ to IP$_2$, this pathway accounts for the generation of inositol-1,3,4-trisphosphate and provides for rapid removal of IP$_3$. Whether IP$_4$ possesses Ca^{2+}-mobilizing or other physiological activity remains to be tested.

Acknowledgement

This chapter was prepared with support from NIH grant AM30577.

References

Abdel-Latif, A.A. (1983) Metabolism of phosphoinositides. In Handbook of Neurochemistry, Vol. 3, 2nd Edn., Abel Lajtha (Ed.), Plenum, New York, pp. 91–131.

Abdel-Latif, A.A., Akhtar, R.A. and Hawthorne, J.N. (1977) Acetylcholine increases the breakdown of triphosphoinositide of rabbit iris muscle prelabeled with [^{32}P]-phosphate. Biochem. J., 162:61–73.

Agranoff, B.W. and Bleasdale, J.E. (1978) The acetylcholine-phospholipid effect. What has it told us; what is it trying to tell us? In Wells, W.W. and Eisenberg, F. Jr. (Eds.), Cyclitols and Phosphoinositides, Academic Press, New York. pp. 105–120.

Agranoff, B.W., Murthy, P. and Seguin, E.B. (1983) Thrombin-induced phosphodiesteratic cleavage of phosphatidylinositol-bisphosphate in human platelets. J. Biol. Chem., 258:2076–2078.

Allen, D. and Michell, R.H. (1978) A calcium-activated polyphosphoinositide phosphodiesterase in the plasma membrane of human and rabbit erythrocytes. Biochim. Biophys. Acta, 508:277–286.

Aub, D.L. and Putney, J.W. (1984) Metabolism of inositol phosphates in parotid cells: Implications for the pathway of the phosphoinositide effect and for the possible messenger role of inositol trisphosphate. Life Sci., 34:1347–1355.

Batty, I.R., Nahorski, S.R. and Irvine, R.F. (1985) Rapid formation of inositol 1,3,4,5-tetrakisphosphate following muscarinic receptor stimulation of rat cerebral cortical slices. Biochem. J., 232:211–215.

Benjamins, J.A. and Agranoff, B.W. (1969) Distribution and properties of CDP-diglyceride inositol transferase from brain. J. Neurochem. 16:513–527.

Berridge, M.J. (1983) Rapid accumulation of inositol trisphosphate reveals that agonists hydrolyze polyphosphoinositides instead of phosphatidylinositol. Biochem. J., 212:849–858.

Berridge, M.J. (1984) Inositol trisphosphate and diacylglycerol as second messengers. Biochem. J., 220:345–360.

Berridge, M.J. and Irvine, R.F. (1984) Inositol trisphosphate, a novel second messenger in cellular signal transduction. Nature, 312:315–321.

Berridge, M.J., Buchan, P.B. and Heslop, J.P. (1984) Relationship of polyphosphoinositide metabolism to the hormonal activation of the insect salivary gland by 5-hydroxytryptamine. Mol. Cell. Endocrinol., 36:37–42.

Berridge, M.J., Dawson, R.M.C., Downes, C.P., Heslop, J.P. and Irvine, R.F. (1983) Changes in the levels of inositol phosphates after agonist-dependent hydrolysis of membrane phosphoinositides. Biochem. J., 212:473–482.

Biden, T.J., Prentice, M., Irvine, R.F., Berridge, M.J. and Wollheim, C.B. (1984) Inositol 1,4,5-trisphosphate mobilizes intracellular Ca^{2+} from permeabilized insulin-secreting cells. Biochem. J., 223:467–473.

Boon, A.M., Beresford, B.J. and Mellors, A. (1985) A tumor promoter enhances the phosphorylation of polyphosphoinositides while decreasing phosphatidylinositol labeling in lymphocytes. Biochem. Biophys. Res. Commun., 129:431–438.

Brandt, S.J., Dougherty, R.W., Lapetina, E.G. and Niedel, J.E. (1985) Pertussis toxin inhibits chemotactic peptide-stimulated generation of inositol phosphates and lysosomal enzyme secretion in human (HL-60) cells. Proc. Natl. Acad. Sci. U.S.A., 82:3277–3280.

Brown, J.E. and Rubin, L.J. (1984) A direct demonstration that inositol trisphosphate induces an increase in intracellular calcium in Limulus photoreceptors. Biochem. Biophys. Res. Commun., 125:1137–1142.

Burgess, G.M., Godfrey, P., McKinney, J.S., Berridge, M.J., Irvine, R.F. and Putney, J.W. Jr (1984a) The second messenger linking receptor activation to internal Ca release in liver. Nature, 309:63–66.

Burgess, G.M., Irvine, R.F., Berridge, M.J., McKinney, J.S. and Putney, J.W. Jr (1984b) Actions of inositol phosphates on Ca^{2+} pools in guinea-pig hepatocytes. Biochem. J., 224:741–746.

Burgess, G.M., McKinney, J.S., Fabiato, A., Leslie, B.A. and Putney, J.W. Jr. (1983) Calcium pools in saponin-permeabilized guinea pig hepatocytes. J. Biol. Chem., 258:15336–15345.

Cockcroft, S. and Gomperts, B.D. (1985) Role of guanine nucleotide binding protein in the activation of polyphosphoinositide phosphodiesterase. Nature, 314:534–536.

Cockcroft, S., Baldwin, J.M. and Allan, D. (1984) The Ca^{2+}-activated polyphosphoinositide phosphodiesterase of human and rabbit neutrophil membranes. *Biochem. J.*, 221:477–482.

Cockcroft, S., Taylor, J.A. and Judah, J.D. (1985) Subcellular localisation of inositol lipid kinases in rat liver. *Biochim. Biophys. Acta*, 845:163–170.

Collins, C.A. and Wells, W.W. (1983) Identification of phosphatidylinositol kinase in rat liver lysosomal membranes. *J. Biol. Chem.*, 258:2130–2134.

Connolly, T.M., Bross, T.E. and Majerus, P.W. (1985) Isolation of a phosphomonoesterase from human platelets that specifically hydrolyzes the 5-phosphate of inositol-1,4,5-trisphosphate. *J. Biol. Chem.*, 260:7868–7874.

Dawson, A.P. and Irvine, R.F. (1984) Inositol(1,4,5)trisphosphate-promoted Ca^{2+} release from microsomal fractions of rat liver. *Biochem. Biophys. Res. Commun.*, 120:858–864.

Dawson, R.M.C. and Clarke, N.G. (1972) D-*myo*-Inositol 1:2-cyclic phosphate 2-phosphohydrolase. *Biochem. J.*, 127:113–118.

Dawson, R.M.C., Freinkel, N., Jungalwala, F. and Clarke, N. (1971) The enzymic formation of *myo*-inositol 1:2-cyclic phosphate from phosphatidylinositol. *Biochem. J.*, 122:605–607.

De Chaffoy de Courcelles, D., Roevens, P. and Van Belle, H. (1984) 12-*O*-Tetradecanoylphorbol 13-acetate stimulates inositol lipid phosphorylation in intact human platelets. *FEBS Letters*, 123:389–393.

Downes, C.P. and Michell, R.H. (1982) Phosphatidylinositol-4-phosphate and phosphatidylinositol-4,5-bisphosphate: lipids in search of a function. *Cell Calcium*, 3:467–502.

Downes, C.P. and Wuseman, M. (1983) Breakdown of polyphosphoinositides and not phosphatidylinositol accounts for muscarinic agonist-stimulated inositol phospholipid metabolism in rat parotid glands. *Biochem. J.*, 216:633–640.

Downes, C.P., Mussat, M.C. and Michell, R.H. (1982) The inositol trisphosphate phosphomonoesterase of the human erythrocyte membrane. *Biochem. J.*, 203:169–177.

Drummond, A., Knox, R.J. and Macphee, C.H. (1985) The role of inositol lipids in hormonal mobilization of cell-associated Ca^{2+}. *Biochem. Soc. Trans.*, 13:58–60.

Drummond, A. (1985) Bidirectional control of cytosolic free calcium by thyrotropin-releasing hormone in pituitary cells. *Nature*, 315:752–757.

Drust, D.S. and Martin, T.F.J. (1985) Protein kinase C translocates from cytosol to membrane upon hormone activation: effects of thyrotropin-releasing hormone in GH_3 cells. *Biochem. Biophys. Res. Commun.*, 128:531–537.

Durrell, J., Sodd, M.A. and Friedel, R.O. (1968) Acetylcholine stimulation of the phosphodiesteratic cleavage of guinea pig brain phosphoinositides. *Life Sci.*, 7:363–368.

Eichberg, J. and Harrington, C.A. (1985) Receptor-mediated changes in hepatocyte phosphoinositide metabolism: mechanism and significance. In R.P. Rubin, G.B. Weiss and J.W. Putney Jr. (Eds.), *Calcium in Biological Systems*, Plenum Press, New York, pp. 53–60.

Exton, J.H. (1985) Role of calcium and phosphoinositides in the actions of certain hormones and neurotransmitters. *J. Clin. Invest.*, 75:1753–1757.

Fisher, S.K. and Agranoff, B.W. (1981) Enhancement of the muscarinic synaptosomal phospholipid labeling effect by the ionophore A23187. *J. Neurochem.*, 37:968–977.

Fisher, S.K. and Agranoff, B.W. (1985) The biochemical basis and functional significance of enhanced phosphatidate and phosphoinositide turnover. In J. Eichberg (Ed.), *Phospholipids in Nervous Tissues*, John Wiley and Sons, New York, pp. 241–295.

Gilman, A.G. (1984) G proteins and dual control of adenylate cyclase. *Cell* 36:577–579.

Gispen, W.H., Van Dongen, C.J., de Graan, P.N.E. Oestreicher, A.B. and Zwiers, H. (1985) The role of phosphoprotein B-50 in phosphoinositide metabolism in brain synaptic plasma membranes. In J.E. Bleasdale, J. Eichberg, and G. Hauser (Eds.), *Inositol and Phosphoinositides: Metabolism and Regulation*, Humana Press, Clifton NJ, pp. 399–414.

Gispen, W.H., de Graan, P.N.E., Schrama, L.H. and Eichberg, J. (1986) Phosphoprotein B-50 and polyphosphoinositide-dependent signal transduction in brain. In L.A. Horrocks, L. Freys and G. Toffano, *Phospholipids in the Nervous System III. Biochemical and Molecular Pharmacology*, Livania Press, Padova, Italy (in press).

Gomperts, B.D. (1983) Involvement of guanine nucleotide-binding protein in the gating of Ca^{2+} by receptors. *Nature*, 306:64–66.

Gonzales, R.A. and Crews, F.T. (1985) Guanine nucleotides stimulate production of inositol trisphosphate in rat cortical membranes. *Biochem. J.*, 232:799–804.

Hallcher, L.M. and Sherman, W.R. (1980) The effects of lithium and other agents on the activity of *myo*-inositol-1-phosphatase from bovine brain. *J. Biol. Chem.*, 255:10896–10901.

Haslam, R.J. and Davidson, M.M.L. (1984) Guanine nucleotides decrease the free $[Ca^{2+}]$ required for secretion of serotonin from permeabilized blood platelets: Evidence of a role for a GTP-binding protein in platelet activation. *FEBS Letters*, 174:90–95.

Helmkamp, G.M., Harvey, M.S., Wirtz, K.W.A. and Van Deenen, L.L.M. (1974) Phospholipid exchange between membranes: purification of bovine brain proteins that preferentially catalyze the transfer of phosphatidylinositol. *J. Biol. Chem.*, 249:6382–6389.

Heslop, J.P., Irvine, R.F., Tashjian, A.H. Jr. and Berridge, M.J. (1985) Inositol tetrakis- and pentakisphosphates in GH_4 cells. *J. Exp. Biol.*, 119:395–401.

Hokin, L.E. and Hokin, M.R. (1955) Effects of acetylcholine on the turnover of phosphoryl units in individual phospholipids of pancreas slices and brain cortex slices. *Biochim. Biophys. Acta*, 18:102–110.

Hokin, M.R. and Hokin, L.E. (1953) Enzyme secretion and the incorporation of ^{32}P into phospholipids of pancreas slices. *J. Biol. Chem.*, 203:967–977.

Irvine, R.F. (1982) The enzymology of stimulated inositol lipid turnover. *Cell Calcium*, 3:295–309.

Irvine, R.F., Letcher, A.J. and Dawson, R.M.C. (1984a) Phosphatidylinositol-4,5-bisphosphate phosphodiesterase and phosphomonoesterase activities of rat brain. *Biochem. J.*, 218:177–185.

Irvine, R.F., Letcher, A.J., Lander, D.J. and Downes, C.P. (1984b) Inositol triphosphates in carbachol-stimulated rat parotid glands. *Biochem. J.*, 223:237–243.

Irvine, R.F., Letcher, A.J., Lander, D.J. and Dawson, R.M.C. (1985a) The enzymology of phosphoinositide catabolism with particular reference to phosphatidyl-4,5-bisphosphate phosphodiesterase. In J. Bleasdale, J. Eichberg, and G. Hauser (Eds.), *Inositol and Phosphoinositides: Metabolism and Regulation.* Humana Press, Clifton NJ, pp. 123–135.

Irvine, R.F., Änggard, E.A., Letcher, A.J. and Downes, C.P. (1985b) Metabolism of inositol (1,4,5) trisphosphate and inositol(1,3,4)trisphosphate in rat parotid glands. *Biochem. J.*, 229:505–511.

Irvine, R.F., Letcher, A.J., Heslop, J.P. and Berridge, M.J. (1986) The inositol tris/tetrakisphosphate pathway-demonstration of Ins(1,4,5)P$_3$ 3-kinase activity in animal tissues. *Nature*, 320:631–634.

Irvine, R.F., Hemington, N. and Dawson, R.M.C. (1978) The hydrolysis of phosphatidylinositol by lysosomal enzymes of rat liver and brain. *Biochem. J.*, 176:475–484.

Jergil, B. and Sundler, R. (1983) Phosphorylation of phosphatidylinositol in rat liver Golgi. *J. Biol. Chem.*, 258:7968–7973.

Jones, L.M. and Michell, R.H. (1974) Breakdown of phosphatidylinositol provoked by muscarinic cholinergic stimulation of rat parotid gland fragments. *Biochem. J.*, 142:583–590.

Joseph, S.K., Thomas, A.P., Williams, R.J., Irvine, R.F. and Williamson, J.R. (1984) *myo*-Inositol 1,4,5-trisphosphate. *J. Biol. Chem.*, 259:3077–3081.

Kai, M., Salway, J.G. and Hawthorne, J.N. (1968) The diphosphoinositide kinase of rat brain. *Biochem. J.*, 106:791–801.

Labarca, R., Janowsky, A., Patel, J. and Paul, S.M. (1984) Phorbol esters inhibit agonist-induced [^{3}H]inositol-1-phosphate accumulation in rat hippocampal slices. *Biochem. Biophys. Res. Commun.*, 123:703–709.

Lapetina, E., Watson, S.P. and Cuatrecasas, P. (1984) *myo*-Inositol-1,4,5-trisphosphate stimulates protein phosphorylation in saponin-permeabilized human platelets. *Proc. Natl. Acad. Sci. U.S.A.*, 81:7431–7435.

Litosch, I. and Fain, J.N. (1985) 5-Methyltryptamine stimulates phospholipase C-mediated breakdown of exogenous phosphoinositides by blowfly salivary gland membranes. *J. Biol. Chem.*, 260:16052–16055.

Litosch, I., Lin, S-H. and Fain, J.N. (1983) Rapid changes in hepatocyte phosphoinositides induced by vasopressin. *J. Biol. Chem.*, 258:13727–13732.

Litosch, I., Wallis, C. and Fain, J.N. (1985) 5-Hydroxytryptamine stimulates inositol phosphate production in a cell-free system from blowfly salivary glands. *J. Biol. Chem.*, 260:5464–5471.

Majerus, P.W., Wilson, D.B., Connolly, T.M., Bross, T.E. and Neufeld E.J. (1985) Phosphoinositide turnover provides a link in stimulus–response coupling. *Trends in Biochem. Sci.* 10:168–171.

Masters, S.B., Martin, M.W., Harden, K.T. and Brown, J.H. (1985) Pertussis toxin does not inhibit muscarinic receptor-mediated phosphoinositide hydrolysis or calcium mobilization. *Biochem. J.*, 227:933–937.

Michell, R.H. (1975) Inositol phospholipids and cell surface receptor function. *Biochim. Biophys. Acta*, 415:81–147.

Michell, R.H., Kirk, C.J., Jones, L.M., Downes, C.P. and Creba, J.A. (1981) The stimulation of inositol lipid metabolism that accompanies calcium mobilization in stimulated cells: defined characteristics and unanswered questions. *Phil. Trans. R. Soc. London Ser. B.* 296:123–137.

Moreno, F.J., Mills, I., Garcia-Sainz, J.A. and Fain, J.N. (1983) Effects of pertussis toxin treatment on the metabolism of rat adipocytes. *J. Biol. Chem.*, 258:10938–10943.

Muallem, S., Schoeffield, M., Pandol, S. and Sachs, G. (1985) Inositol trisphosphate modification of ion transport in rough endoplasmic reticulum. *Proc. Nat. Acad. Sci. U.S.A.*, 82:4433–4437.

Nakamura, T. and Ui, M. (1985) Simultaneous inhibitions of inositol phospholipid breakdown, arachidonic acid release, and histamine secretion in mast cells by islet-activating protein, pertussis toxin. *J. Biol. Chem.*, 260:3584–3593.

Nishizuka, Y. (1984) The role of protein kinase C in cell surface signal transduction and tumor promotion. *Nature*, 308:693–698.

Orellana, S.A., Solski, P.A. and Brown, J.H. (1985) Phorbol ester inhibits phosphoinositide hydrolysis and calcium mobilization in cultured astrocytoma cells. *J. Biol. Chem.*, 260:5236–5239.

Poggioli, J. and Putney, J.W. Jr. (1982) Net calcium fluxes in rat parotid acinar cells. Evidence for a hormone-sensitive pool in or near the plasma membrane. *Pflug. Arch.*, 392:239–243.

Prentki, M., Biden, T.J., Janjic, D., Irvine, R.F., Berridge, M.J. and Wollheim, C.B. (1984a) Rapid mobilization of Ca^{2+} from rat insulinoma microsomes by inositol-1,4,5-trisphosphate. *Nature* 309:562–564.

Prentki, M., Wollheim, C.B. and Lewis, D.P. (1984b) Ca^{2+} homeostasis in permeabilized human neutrophils. *J. Biol. Chem.*, 259:13777–13782.

Prpić, V., Blackmore, P.F. and Exton, J.H. (1982) Phosphatidylinositol breakdown induced by vasopressin and epinephrine in hepatocytes is calcium-dependent. *J. Biol. Chem.*, 257:11323–11331.

Rasmussen, H. and Barrett, P.Q. (1984) Calcium messenger systems: an integrated view. *Physiol. Rev.*, 64:938–984.

Rasmussen, H. (1985) Calcium ion: a synarchic and mercurial but minatory messenger. In R.P. Rubin, G.B. Weiss and J.W. Putney Jr. (Eds.), *Calcium in Biological Systems*, Plenum Press, New York, pp. 13–22.

Rittenhouse, S.E. and Sasson, J.P. (1985) Mass changes in *myo*-inositol trisphosphate in human platelets stimulated by thrombin: inhibitory effects of phorbol esters. *J. Biol. Chem.*, 260:8657–8660.

Rooijen, L.A.A. Van, Rossowska, M. and Bazan, N.G. (1985) Inhibition of phosphatidylinositol-4-phosphate kinase by its product phosphatidylinositol-4,5-bisphosphate. *Biochem. Biophys. Res. Commun.*, 126:150–155.

Rooijen, L.A.A. Van, Seguin, E.B. and Agranoff, B.W. (1983) Phosphodiesteratic breakdown of endogenous polyphosphoinositides in nerve ending membranes. *Biochem. Biophys. Res. Commun.*, 112:919–926.

Schulz, I., Streb, H., Bayerdörffer, E. and Imamura, K. (1985) Hormonal and neurotransmitter regulation of Ca^{2+} movements in pancreatic acinar cells. In J.E. Dumont, B. Hamprecht, and J. Numez, (Eds.), *Hormones and Cell Regulation, Vol. 9*, Elsevier, Amsterdam, pp. 325–342.

Seyfred, M.A. and Wells, W.W. (1984a) Subcellular incorporation of ^{32}P into phosphoinositides and other phospholipids in isolated hepatocytes. *J. Biol. Chem.*, 259:7659–7665.

Seyfred, M.A. and Wells, W.W. (1984b) Subcellular site and mechanism of vasopressin-stimulated hyrolysis of phosphoinositides in rat hepatocytes. *J. Biol. Chem.*, 259:7666–7672.

Seyfred, M.A., Farrell, L.E. and Wells, W.W. (1984) Characterization of D-*myo*-inositol 1,4,5-trisphosphate phosphatase in rat liver plasma membranes. *J. Biol. Chem.*, 259:13204–13208.

Smith, C.D., Lane, B.C., Kusaka, I., Verghese, M.W. and Snyderman, R. (1985) Chemoattractant receptor-induced hydrolysis of phosphatidylinositol-4,5-bisphosphate in human polymorphonuclear leukocyte membranes: requirement for a guanine nucleotide regulatory protein. *J. Biol. Chem.?* 260:5875–5878.

Storey, D.J., Shears, S.B., Kirk, C.J. and Michell, R.H. (1984) Stepwise enzymatic dephosphorylation of inositol 1,4,5-trisphosphate to inositol in liver. *Nature*, 312:374–376.

Straub, R.E. and Gershengorn, M.C. (1986) Thyrotropin-releasing hormone and GTP activate inositol trisphosphate formation in membranes isolated from rat pituitary cells. *J. Biol. Chem.*, 261:2712–2717.

Streb, H., Heslop, J.P., Irvine, R.F., Schulz, I. and Berridge, M.J. (1985) Relationship between secretagogue-induced Ca^{2+} release and inositol polyphosphate production in permeabilized pancreatic acinar cells. *J. Biol. Chem.*, 260:7309–7315.

Streb, H., Irvine, R.F., Berridge, M.J. and Schulz, I. (1983) Release of Ca^{2+} from a nonmitochondrial intracellular store in pancreatic acinar cells by inositol-1,4,5-trisphosphate. *Nature*, 306:67–69.

Thomas, A.P., Alexander, J. and Williamson, J.R. (1984) Relationship between inositol polyphosphate production and the increase of cytosolic free Ca^{2+} induced by vasopressin in isolated hepatocytes. *J. Biol. Chem.*, 259:5574–5584.

Thomas, A., Marks, J.S., Coll, K.E. and Williamson, J.R. (1983) Quantitation and early kinetics of inositol lipid changes induced by vasopressin in isolated and cultured hepatocytes. *J. Biol. Chem.*, 258:5716–5725.

Uhing, R.J., Prpić, V., Jiang, H. and Exton, J.H. (1986) Hormone-stimulated polyphosphoinositide breakdown in rat liver plasma membranes: Roles of guanine nucleotides and calcium. *J. Biol. Chem.*, 261:2140–2146.

Vicentini, L.M., Di Virgilio, F., Ambrosini, A., Pozzan, T. and Meldolesi, J. (1985) Tumor promotor phorbol 12-myristate, 13-acetate inhibits phosphoinositide hydrolysis and cytosolic Ca^{2+} rise induced by the activation of muscarinic receptors in PC12 cells. *Biochem. Biophys. Res. Commun.*, 127:310–317.

Volpe, P., Salvati, G., Di Virgilio, F. and Pozzan, T. (1985) Inositol-1,4,5-trisphosphate induces calcium release from sarcoplasmic reticulum of skeletal muscle. *Nature* 316:347–349.

Wallace, M.A. and Fain, J.N. (1985) Guanosine-5'-*O*-thiotriphosphate stimulates phospholipase C activity in plasma membranes of rat hepatocytes. *J. Biol. Chem.*, 260:9527–9530.

Watson, S.P. and Lapetina, E.G. (1985) 1,2-Diacylglycerol and phorbol ester inhibit agonist-induced formation of inositol phosphates in human platelets: possible implications for negative feedback regulation of inositol phospholipid hydrolysis. *Proc. Natl. Acad. Sci. U.S.A.*, 82:2623–2626.

Whitman, M.R., Epstein, J. and Cantley, L. (1984) Inositol-1,4,5-trisphosphate stimulates phosphorylation of a 62 000-dalton protein in monkey fibroblast and bovine brain cell lysates. *J. Biol. Chem.*, 259:13652–13655.

Wilson, D.B., Bross, T.E., Hofmann, S. and Majerus, P.W. (1984) Hydrolysis of polyphosphoinositides by purified sheep seminal vesicle phospholipase C enzymes. *J. Biol. Chem.*, 259:11718–11724.

Wilson, D.B., Bross, T.E., Sherman, W.R., Berger, R.A. and Majerus, P.W. (1985a) Inositol cyclic phosphates are produced by cleavage of phosphatidylphosphoinositols (polyphosphoinositides) with purified sheep seminal vesicle phospholipase C enzymes. *Proc. Natl. Acad. Sci. U.S.A.*, 82:4013–4017.

Wilson, D.B., Neufeld, E.J. and Majerus, P.W. (1985b) Phosphoinositide interconversion in thrombin-stimulated human platelets. *J. Biol. Chem.*, 260:1046–1051.

W.H. Gispen and A. Routtenberg (Eds.)
Progress in Brain Research, Vol. 69
© 1986 Elsevier Science Publishers B.V. (Biomedical Division)

CHAPTER 3

Possible roles of protein kinase C in signal transduction in nervous tissues

U. Kikkawa, T. Kitano, N. Saito, H. Fujiwara, H. Nakanishi, A. Kishimoto, K. Taniyama, C. Tanaka and Y. Nishizuka

Departments of Biochemistry and Pharmacology, Kobe University School of Medicine, Kobe 650, Japan

Introduction

The mechanism of transduction of various informational signals such as those from a group of hormones and some neurotransmitters across the cell membrane has attracted great attention. It is proposed that inositol 1,4,5-trisphosphate that is produced from the receptor-mediated hydrolysis of phosphatidylinositol 4,5-bisphosphate mobilizes Ca^{2+} from its internal stores (Berridge and Irvine, 1984). There has been growing evidence that, at an early phase of cellular responses, 1,2-diacylglycerol, which is transiently produced from inositol phospholipids in membranes, activates protein kinase C, and that the activation of this enzyme and Ca^{2+} mobilization are both essential for evoking many physiological responses such as exocytosis and release reactions, including neurotransmitter release from nerve endings. It is also suggestive that the signal transduction via this protein kinase C pathway appears to modulate several neuronal functions such as membrane conductance, and potentiation or inhibition of other signalling systems. The present article will briefly review the evidence on the possible roles of this unique protein kinase in nervous tissues. Some aspects of protein kinase C have been outlined elsewhere (Nishizuka, 1984a,b).

Release reactions and exocytosis

Under physiological conditions diacylglycerol is almost absent from membranes but is produced

only transiently in a signal-dependent manner. Tumor-promoting phorbol esters such as 12-*O*-tetradecanoylphorbol-13-acetate (TPA) are intercalated into the membrane and substitute for diacylglycerol, thereby activating protein kinase C without mobilization of Ca^{2+} (Castagna et al., 1982). It is also shown that some synthetic diacylglycerols such as 1-oleoyl-2-acetylglycerol are permeable to the membrane and directly activate this enzyme in intact cells (Kaibuchi et al., 1983). Thus, it is possible to open the two signal pathways, protein kinase C activation and Ca^{2+} mobilization (by which information flows from the cell surface into the cell interior), by the selective application of such a permeable synthetic diacylglycerol or tumor promoter for the former and a Ca^{2+} ionophore such as A23187 for the latter as schematically shown in Fig. 1. By using these procedures the two pathways are shown to act synergistically for serotonin release from platelets (Nishizuka, 1983), and later for release reactions

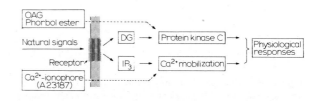

Fig. 1. Bifurcation signal pathways for the activation of cellular functions. OAG, 1-oleoyl-2-acetyl-glycerol; DG, 1,2-diacylglycerol; and IP$_3$, inositol-1,4,5-trisphosphate.

and exocytosis of a variety of tissues and cell types (for reviews, see Nishizuka, 1984b; Kikkawa and Nishizuka, 1985).

In peripheral nerves, the release of acetylcholine from the cholinergic nerve endings of guinea pig ileum is fully induced by the simultaneous application of TPA and A23187 (Tanaka et al., 1985). The experiments summarized in Fig. 2 were designed to show that the synergistic role of protein kinase C and Ca^{2+} mobilization may be extended to the release reaction of neurotransmitters in central nervous tissues. The tissue slices of guinea pig caudate nucleus were preincubated with radioactive choline, and then stimulated under the electrical fields as indicated. The release reaction of acetylcholine was found to be markedly potentiated by the addition of TPA to the incubation media (Fig. 2A), and the half maximum potentiation was observed at less than 50 nM TPA (Fig. 2B). TPA alone did not induce the release reaction, and 4α-phorbol-12,13-didecanoate, an inactive phorbol ester analog, was inert in this capacity. Similar potentiation by TPA was also noted for the release reactions induced by high potassium as well as by A23187 instead of electrical stimulation, and the effect of TPA was counteracted by the co-existense of polymyxin B, a protein kinase C inhibitor. These results imply that the two signal pathways, protein kinase C activa-

tion and Ca^{2+} mobilization, are essential for the release of neurotransmitters such as acetylcholine in the central nervous tissues. However, a possibility may not be excluded that diacylglycerol and TPA act as membrane fusigens, particularly at higher concentrations (Nishizuka, 1984a), and the biochemical basis of this release reaction remains to be substantiated.

Modulation of membrane conductance

In nervous tissues, protein kinase C phosphorylates several endogenous proteins, particularly those associated with membranes. It has been proposed that protein kinase C may play a role in extrusion of Ca^{2+} immediately after it mobilizes into the cytosol, and Ca^{2+}-transport ATPase is a possible target of protein kinase C (Limas, 1980; Movsesian et al., 1984). Kinetic studies with some cell types such as vascular smooth muscle (Morgan and Morgan, 1982) and platelets (Johnson et al., 1985; Nishizuka et al., 1985) have shown that, once the receptors are stimulated, the rise of Ca^{2+} is only transient, and the Ca^{2+} thus increased is immediately extruded as measured by aequorin. In the experiment given in Fig. 3, the amount of aequorin loaded is not limited since this Ca^{2+} spike may be repeatedly shown by subsequent stimulations by thrombin. It is possible that protein kinase C may be involved in this extrusion process. This assumption is based primarily on the observations in intact cell systems where the cytosolic Ca^{2+} concentration is frequently decreased by the addition of TPA (Tsien et al., 1982; Moolenaar et al., 1984; Lagast et al., 1984; Sagi-Eisenberg et al., 1985; Drummond, 1985). In addition, it is attractive to imagine that the role of protein kinase C may be extended to the enhancement of Ca^{2+} channel, since it has been reported that the microinjection of TPA or protein kinase C itself into bag cell neurons of *Aplysia* enhances the voltage-sensitive Ca^{2+} current (DeRiemer et al., 1985). Analogously, a possible role of protein kinase C in activating Na^+-transport ATPase in nervous tissues has been proposed (Greene and Lattimer, 1985). Several lines of evidence so far described are compatible with the supposition that protein

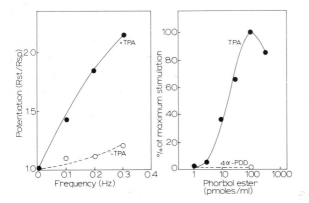

Fig. 2. Potentiation by tumor-promoting phorbol ester of acetylcholine release from guinea pig caudate nucleus induced by electrical stimulation. The detailed experimental conditions are described by Tanaka et al. (1986). 4αPDD, 4α-phorbol-12, 13-didecanoate.

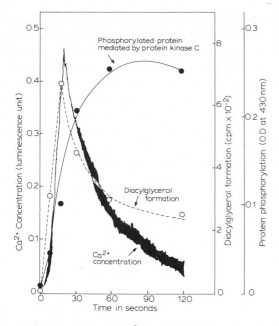

Fig. 3. Transient rise of Ca^{2+} and diacylglycerol and persistance of phosphate covalently linked to 47K protein, a specific substrate of protein kinase C in human platelets stimulated by thrombin. Human platelets were isolated, labeled with either [^{3}H]arachidonate or ^{32}Pi, and stimulated by thrombin at 37°C. The radioactive diacylglycerol and 47K protein were determined as described by Kaibuchi et al. (1983). In a separate set of experiments human platelets were loaded by aequorin under the conditions described by Johnson et al. (1985), and stimulated by thrombin. The detailed experimental procedures will be described elsewhere. (Adapted from Nishizuka et al., 1985).

kinase C may modulate membrane conductance by phosphorylating such proteins as those related to channels and pumps therein involved. In fact, it was recently found that a protein kinase C-positive immunoreactive material is abundant in nerve endings as well as many regions of the neuronal cell, including axons and dendrites. Fig. 4 illustrates a unique feature of rat Purkinje cells which are stained by monoclonal antibodies against protein kinase C. It is clear that a protein kinase C-like material is present throughout the cytoplasm and that the cell nucleus apparently lacks protein kinase C. A definitive biochemical basis for such an attractive role of protein kinase C in modulating membrane conductance may be obtained by further investigations.

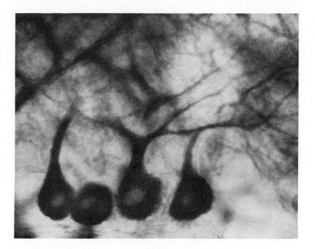

Fig. 4. Rat Purkinje cells stained by monoclonal antibodies against protein kinase C. The black tone represents the immunoreactive material. The detailed properties of the antibodies used and the conditions of staining will be described elsewhere by U. Kikkawa et al.

It is worth noting that, as also shown in Fig. 3, the phosphate attached to the substrate proteins of protein kinase C appears to be often resistant to phosphatases and, therefore, the consequence of this phosphorylation reaction may be a longer persistence in time. This may provide a basis for dual functions of this enzyme; on the one hand negative feedback control as discussed above, and on the other hand positive forward and sustained control of cellular functions as schematically given in Fig. 5. Presumably, Ca^{2+} may initiate the cel-

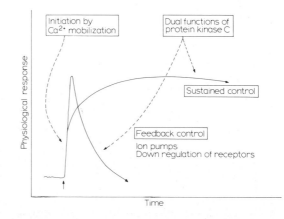

Fig. 5. Schematical representation of dual functions of protein kinase C.

lular responses by its transient increase, and protein kinase C may support the persistence of these responses. Crucial information of the target proteins related to such persistence is still limited, but it is proposed that B-50 protein (F1 protein) is one of the proteins, whose phosphorylation may be related to plasticity (Gispen et al., 1985; Routtenberg, 1985).

Interaction with other signalling systems

With some exceptions in bovine adrenal medullary cells (Swilem and Hawthorne, 1983) and certain presynaptic muscarinic receptors (Starke, 1980), it is generally the case that, when stimulation of receptors leads to inositol phospholipid breakdown, Ca^{2+} is mobilized simultaneously. The mode of cellular responses may be tentatively divided into several groups shown schematically in Fig. 6. In some tissues, such as platelets, the signal that induces the turnover of inositol phospholipids promotes the activation of cellular functions, whereas the signal that produces cyclic AMP usually antagonizes such activation. In an

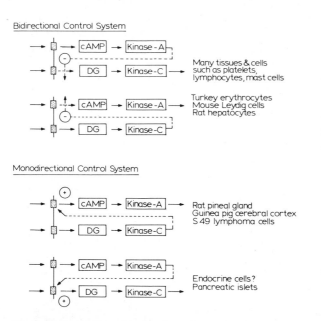

Fig. 6. Various types of interaction of two signal-tranducing systems. cAMP, cyclic AMP; DG, diacylglycerol; Kinase-A, protein kinase A; Kinase-C, protein kinase C.

earlier report from our laboratories (Kaibuchi et al., 1982) it has been shown that in such tissues the signal-induced breakdown of inositol phospholipids and subsequent events leading to physiological responses are all blocked profoundly by cyclic AMP. Inversely, in another group of tissues such as mouse Leydig cells (Mukhopadhyay et al., 1984), turkey erythrocytes (Kelleher et al., 1984), and rat hepatocytes (Heyworth et al., 1984), protein kinase C inhibits and desensitizes adenylate cyclase. In several tissues such as rat pineal gland (Sugden et al., 1985), guinea pig cerebral cortex (Hollingsworth et al., 1985), and S49 lymphoma cells (Bell et al., 1985), protein kinase C greatly potentiates cyclic AMP formation. On the other hand, no obvious example has been presented for tissues in which cyclic AMP potentiates signal-induced turnover of inositol phospholipids. However, these two signal transduction pathways often act in concert in some endocrine cells such as pancreatic islets (Tamagawa et al., 1985). The evidence presented thus far is still incomplete, but it is reasonable to assume that various combinations of the two receptor signalling systems may operate in controlling a wide variety of neuronal functions. It is also noted that protein kinase C has been recently proposed to exert feedback control over its own receptors and to block inositol phospholipid breakdown (Labarca et al., 1984; Vicentini et al., 1985; MacIntyre et al., 1985; Orellana et al., 1985; Watson and Lapetina, 1985; Lynch et al., 1985; Zavoico et al., 1985). Nicotinic acetylcholine receptor has also been proposed to serve as a substrate of protein kinase C (Nairn et al., 1985).

Specificity of protein kinase C and control of metabolic processes

Protein kinase C and cyclic AMP-dependent protein kinase (protein kinase A) appear to transduce distinctly different pieces of information into the cell interior, but these two receptor signaling systems sometimes cause apparently similar cellular responses. To assess one of the basic problems, the substrate specificity of protein kinase C, bovine myelin basic protein is employed for a model substrate, since this protein is phosphory-

Protein kinase C specific sites	-Phe -Phe -Gly -Ser⁴⁶- Asp -[Arg]-Gly - -Gly -Thr -Leu-Ser-[Lys]¹⁵¹- Ile -Phe-
Protein kinase A specific sites	-His -[Arg]-Asp-Thr-Gly³⁴ - Ile -Leu- -Ser -[Arg]-Phe-Ser-Try¹¹⁵ -Gly -Ala -
Common sites	-[Lys -Arg]-Pro-Ser⁸-Gln -[Arg]-Ser- -Ser -Gln -[Arg]-Ser¹¹-[Lys] -Tyr -Leu- -[Lys -Arg]-Gly -Ser⁵⁵-Gly -[Lys]-Asp- -[Arg]- Gly -Leu-Ser¹¹⁰- Leu - Ser -[Arg]- - Gly -[Arg]-Ala-Ser¹³²-Asp -Tyr -[Lys]- - Gly -[Arg]-Asp-Ser¹⁶¹-[Arg] -Ser -Gly-

Fig. 7. Major phosphorylation sites of bovine myelin basic protein for protein kinases C and A. The detailed experimental conditions are described elsewhere (Kishimoto et al., 1985).

lated at multiple sites by both protein kinases C and A. The results summarized in Fig. 7 indicate that, contrary to protein kinase A, protein kinase C reacts with seryl residues that are located at the amino-terminal side close to lysine or arginine. The seryl residues that are commonly phosphorylated by these two enzymes have basic amino acids at both amino- and carboxyl-terminal sides. The result provides some clues to understand the rationale that these two protein kinases may show normally different but sometimes similar functions depending upon the structure of the target phosphate acceptor protein (Kishimoto et al., 1985).

In nervous tissues many undefined endogenous proteins are shown to serve as substrates for protein kinase C, but little is known about the molecular events occurring as a consequence of such protein phosphorylation reactions (Nishizuka, 1980; Wrenn et al., 1980; Wu et al., 1982). In addition to B-50 (F1) protein (Gispen et al., 1985; Routtenberg, 1985) noted above, GABA-modulin (Wise et al., 1983), tyrosine hydroxylase (Albert et al., 1984; Vuilliet et al., 1985) and guanylate cyclase (Zwiller et al., 1985) have been proposed as targets of this enzyme. It is possible that protein kinase C may have a role in the control of other neuronal functions and metabolic processes such as neurotransmitter biosynthesis.

Coda

Although evidence is accumulating to suggest the

potential importance of protein kinase C in nervous tissues, still little is known about a molecular basis of its physiological functions. Presumably, the protein phosphorylation reactions catalyzed by protein kinase C may exert 'modulation' rather than 'prerequisite' of neuronal processes such as neurotransmitter release, membrane conductance, interaction of receptors, and metabolic processes as reviewed briefly in this article. The problem of crucial importance in the next few years is to establish the biochemical basis of many observations outlined above, particularly to clarify the target proteins of protein kinase C.

Acknowledgements

The authors are indebted to Dr. Y. Ichimori and Dr. Y. Sugino, (Biotechnology Laboratories, Central Research Division, Takeda Chemical Industries Ltd.) for their great efforts in preparing monoclonal antibodies against protein kinase C. This investigation has been supported in part by research grants from the Scientific Research Fund of the Ministry of Education, Science and Culture (1985), the Science and Technology Agency (1985), the Yamanouchi Foundation for Research on Metabolic Disorders (1985), the Foundation for the Promotion of Research on Medical Resources (1985), the Muscular Dystrophy Association (1985–1986), Merck, Sharp and Dohme Research Laboratories (1985), and Biotechnology Laboratories of Takeda Chemical Industries (1985).

References

Albert, K.A., Helmer-Matyjek, E., Nairn, A.C., Muller, T.H., Haycock, J.W., Greene, L.A., Goldstein, M. and Greengard, P. (1984) Calcium/phospholipid-dependent protein kinase (protein kinase C) phosphorylates and activates tyrosine hydroxylose. Proc. Natl. Acad. Sci. U.S.A., 84:7713–7717.

Bell, J.D., Buxton, I.L.O. and Brunton, L.L. (1985) Enhancement of adenylate cyclase activity in S49 lymphoma cells by phorbol esters. J. Biol. Chem., 260:2625–2628.

Berridge, M.J. and Irvine, R.F. (1984) Inositol trisphosphate, a novel second messenger in cellular signal transduction. Nature, 312:315–321.

Castagna, M., Takai, Y., Kaibuchi, K., Sano, K., Kikkawa, U. and Nishizuka, Y. (1982) Direct activation of calcium-activated, phospholipid-dependent protein kinase by tumor-promoting phorbol esters. J. Biol. Chem., 257:7847–7851.

34

DeRiemer, S.A., Strong, J.A., Albert, K.A., Greengard, P. and Kaczmarek, L.K. (1985) Enhancement of calcium current in *Aprisia* neurones by phorbol ester and protein kinase C. *Nature*, 313:313–316.

Drummond, A.H. (1985) Bidirectional control of cytosolic free calcium by thyrotropin-releasing hormone in pituitary cells. *Nature*, 315:752–755.

Gispen, W.H., de Graan, P.N.E., Schrama, L.H. and Eichberg, J. (1985) Synaptic plasticity, phosphoprotein B-50 and poly-phosphoinositide-dependent signal transduction. In L.A. Horrocks, G. Toffano and L. Freysz (Eds.), *Phospholipids in the Nervous System*, Liviana Press, Padova, in press.

Greene, D.A. and Lattimer, S.A. (1986) Protein kinase C agonists actually normalize decreased ouabain-inhibitable respiration in diabetic rabbit nerve: implications for (Na, K)-ATPase regulation and diabetic complications. *Diabetes*, 35: 242–245.

Heyworth, C.M., Whetton, A.D., Kinsella, A.R. and Houslay, M.D. (1984) The phorbol ester, TPA inhibits glucagon-stimulated adenylate cyclase activity. *FEBS Lett.* 170:38–42.

Hollingsworth, E.B., Sears, E.B. and Daly, J.W. (1985) An activator of protein kinase C (phorbol-12-myristate-13-acetate) augments 2-chloroadenosine-elicited accumulation of cyclic AMP in guinea pig cerebral cortical particulate preparations. *FEBS Lett.* 184:339–342.

Johnson, P.C., Ware, J.A., Cliveden, P.B., Smith, M., Dvorak, A.M. and Salzman, E.W. (1985) Measurement of ionized calcium in blood platelets with photoprotein aequorin. *J. Biol. Chem.*, 260:2069–2076.

Kaibuchi, K., Takai, Y., Ogawa, Y., Kimura, S. and Nishizuka, Y. (1982) Inhibitory action of adenosine 3′,5′-monophosphate on phosphatidylinositol turnover: difference in tissue responses. *Biochem. Biophys. Res. Commun.*, 104:105–112.

Kaibuchi, K., Takai, Y., Sawamura, M., Hoshijima, M., Fujikura, T. and Nishizuka, Y. (1983) Synergistic functions of protein phosphorylation and calcium mobilization in platelet activation. *J. Biol. Chem.*, 258:6701–6704.

Kelleher, D.J., Pessin, J.E., Ruoho, A.E. and Johnson, G.L. (1984) Phorbol ester induces desensitization of adenylate cyclase and phosphorylation of the β-adrenergic receptor in turkey erythrocytes. *Proc. Natl. Acad. Sci. U.S.A.*, 81:4316–4320.

Kikkawa, U. and Nishizuka, Y. (1986) Protein kinase C. In E.G. Krebs and P.D. Boyer (Eds.), *The Enzymes, Vol. 17*. Academic Press, Orlando, FL, in press.

Kishimoto, A., Nishiyama, K., Nakanishi, H., Uratsuji, Y., Nomura, H., Takeyama, Y. and Nishizuka, Y. (1985) Studies on the phosphorylation of myelin basic protein by protein kinase C and adenosine-3′,5′-monophosphate-dependent protein kinase. *J. Biol. Chem.*, 260:12492–12499.

Labarca, R., Janowsky, A., Patel, J. and Paul, S.M. (1984) Phorbol ester inhibit agonist-induced [^{3}H]inositol-1-phosphate accumulation in rat hippocampal slices. *Biochem. Biophys. Res. Commun.*, 123:703–709.

Lagast, H., Pozzan, T., Waldvogel, F.A. and Lew, P.D. (1984) Phorbol myristate acetate stimulates ATP-dependent calcium transport by the plasma membrane of neutrophils. *J. Clin. Invest.*, 73:878–883.

Limas, C.J. (1980) Phosphorylation of cardiac sarcoplasmic reticulum by a calcium-activated, phospholipid-dependent protein kinase. *Biochem. Biophys. Res. Commun.*, 96:1378–1383.

Lynch, C. J., Charest, R., Bocckino, S.B., Exton, J.H. and Blackmore, P.F. (1985) Inhibition of hepatic α_1-adrenergic effects and binding by phorbol myristate acetate. *J. Biol. Chem.*, 260:2844–2851.

MacIntyre, D.E., McNicol, A. and Drummond, A.H. (1985) Tumor-promoting phorbol esters inhibit agonist-induced phosphatidate formation and Ca^{2+} flux in human platelets. *FEBS Lett.*, 180:160–164.

Moolenaar, W.H., Tertoolen, L.G.J. and de Laat, S.W. (1984) Phorbol ester and diacylglycerol mimic growth factors in raising cytoplasmic pH. *Nature*, 313:371–373.

Morgan, J.P. and Morgan, K.G. (1982) Vascular smooth muscle: the first recorded Ca^{2+} transients. *Pfluegers Arch.*, 395:75–77.

Movsesian, M.A., Nishikawa, M. and Adelstein, R.S. (1984) Phosphorylation of phospholamban by calcium-activated, phospholipid-dependent protein kinase. *J. Biol. Chem.*, 259:8029–8032.

Mukhopadhyay, A.K., Bohnet, H.G. and Leidenberger, F.A. (1984) Phorbol ester inhibit LH stimulated steroidogenesis by Leydig cells in vitro. *Biochem. Biophys. Res. Commun.*, 119:1062–1067.

Nairn, A.C., Hemmings, H.C. Jr. and Greengard, P. (1985) Protein kinases in the brain. *Annu. Rev. Biochem.*, 54:931–976.

Nishizuka, Y. (1980) Three multifunctional protein kinases in transmembrane control. *Mol. Biol. Biochem. Biophy.*, 32:113–135.

Nishizuka, Y. (1983) Calcium, phospholipid turnover and protein phosphorylation. *Phil. Trans. R. Soc. Lond. Ser. B* 302:101–112.

Nishizuka, Y. (1984a) The role of protein kinase C in cell surface signal transduction and tumor promotion. *Nature*, 308:693–698.

Nishizuka, Y. (1984b) Turnover of inositol phospholipids and signal transduction. *Science*, 225:1365–1370.

Nishizuka, Y., Kikkawa, U., Kishimoto, A., Nakanishi, H. and Nishiyama. K. (1985) Possible roles of inositol phospholipids in cell surface signal transduction in neuronal tissues. In L.A. Horrocks, G. Toffano and L. Freysz (Eds.), *Phospholipids in the Nervous System*. Liviana Press, Padova, in press.

Orellana, S.A., Solski, P.A. and Brown, J.H. (1985) Phorbol ester inhibits phosphoinositide hydrolysis and calcium mobilization in cultured astrocytoma cells. *J. Biol. Chem.*, 260:5236–5239.

Routtenberg, A. (1985) Protein kinase C and substrate protein F1 (47 kDa, 4.5 p*I*): relation to synaptic plasticity and dendritic spine growth. In B. Will and P. Schmitt (Eds.) *Brain Plasticity, Learning and Memory*, Plenum Press, New York, in press.

Sagi-Eisenberg, R., Lieman, H. and Pecht, I. (1985) Protein kinase C regulation of the receptor-coupled calcium signal in histamine-secreting rat basophilic leukaemia cells. *Nature*, 313:59–60.

Starke, K. (1980) Presynaptic receptors and the control of noradrenaline release. *Trends Pharmacol. Sci.*, 1:268–271.

Sugden, D., Vanecek, J., Klein, D.C., Thomas, T.P. and Anderson, W.B. (1985) Activation of protein kinase C potentiates isoprenaline-induced cyclic AMP accumulation in rat pinealocytes. *Nature*, 314:359–361.

Swilem, A.F. and Hawthorne, J.N. (1983) Catecholamine secretion by perfused bovine adrenal medulla in response to nicotinic activation is inhibited by muscarinic receptors. *Biochem. Pharmacol.*, 32:3873–3874.

Tamagawa, T., Niki, H. and Niki, A. (1985) Insulin release independent of a rise in cytosolic free Ca^{2+} by forskolin and phorbol ester. *FEBS Lett.*, 183:430–432.

Tanaka, C., Taniyama, K. and Kusunoki, M. (1984) A phorbol ester and A23187 act synergistically to release acetylcholine from the guinea pig ileum. *FEBS Lett.*, 175:165–169.

Tanaka, C., Fujiwara, H. and Fujii, Y. (1986) Acetylcholine release from guinea pig caudate nucleus slices evoked by phorbol ester and calcium. *FEBS Lett.*, 195:129–134.

Tsien, R.Y., Pozzan, T. and Rink, T.J. (1982) T-cell mitogens cause early changes in cytoplasmic free Ca^{2+} and membrane potential in lymphocytes. *Nature*, 295:68–71.

Vicentini, L.M., di Virgilio, F., Ambrosini, A., Pozzan, T. and Meldolesi, J. (1985) Tumor promoter phorbol 12-myristate, 13-acetate inhibits phosphoinositide hydrolysis and cytosolic Ca^{2+} rise induced by the activation of muscarinic receptors in PC12 cells. *Biochem. Biophy. Res. Commun.*, 127:310–317.

Vuilliet, P.R., Woodgett, J.R., Ferrari, S. and Hardie, D.G. (1985) Characterization of the sites phosphorylated on tyrosine hydroxylase by Ca^{2+} and phospholipid-dependent protein kinase, calmodulin-dependent multiprotein kinase and cyclic AMP-dependent protein kinase. *FEBS Lett.*, 182:335–339.

Watson, S.P. and Lapetina, E.G. (1985) 1,2-Diacylglycerol and phorbol ester inhibit agonist-induced formation of inositol phosphates in human platelets: possible implications for negative feedback regulation of inositol phospholipid hydrolysis. *Proc. Natl. Acad. Sci. U.S.A.*, 82:2623–2626.

Wise, B.C., Guidotti, A. and Costa, E. (1983) Phosphorylation induces a decrease in the biological activity of the protein inhibitor (GABA-modulin) of γ-aminobutyric acid binding sites. *Proc. Natl. Acad. Sci. U.S.A.*, 80:886–890.

Wrenn, R.W., Katoh, N., Wise, B.C. and Kuo, J.F. (1980) Stimulation by phosphatidylserine and calmodulin of calcium-dependent phosphorylation of endogenous proteins from cerebral cortex. *J. Biol. Chem.* 255:12042–12046.

Wu, W.C.S., Walaas, S.I., Nairn, A.C. and Greengard, P. (1982) Calcium/phospholipid regulates phosphorylation of a M_r '87k' substrate protein in brain synaptosomes. *Proc. Natl. Acad. Sci. U.S.A.*, 79:5249–5253.

Zavoico, G.B., Halenda, S.P., Sha'afi, R.I. and Feinstein, M.B. (1985) Phorbol myristate acetate inhibits thrombin-stimulated Ca^{2+} mobilization and phosphatidylinositol-4,5-bisphosphate hydrolysis in human platelets. *Proc. Natl. Acad. Sci. U.S.A.*, 82:3859–3862.

Zwiller, J., Revel, M. and Malviya, A.N. (1985) Protein kinase C catalyzes phosphorylation of guanylate cyclase in vitro. *J. Biol. Chem.*, 260:1350–1353.

W.H. Gispen and A. Routtenberg (Eds.)
Progress in Brain Research, Vol. 69
© 1986 Elsevier Science Publishers B.V. (Biomedical Division)

CHAPTER 4

Phosphoprotein B-50: localization and function

P.N.E. De Graan, A.B. Oestreicher, L.H. Schrama and W.H. Gispen

Division of Molecular Neurobiology, Rudolf Magnus Institute for Pharmacology and Institute of Molecular Biology, University of Utrecht, Padualaan 8, 3584 CH Utrecht, The Netherlands

Introduction

An important hypothesis concerning the neurochemical mechanism of the action of behaviorally active neuropeptides is that such peptides might affect synaptic plasticity by influencing the degree of phosphorylation of certain synaptic proteins. This hypothesis was based on two lines of evidence. On the one hand, the work of many investigators (e.g. Heald, Rodnight and Greengard; cf. Weller, 1979) had indicated that covalent modification of synaptic proteins by a cyclic phosphorylation and dephosphorylation process was an important biochemical correlate of neuronal electrical activity and neurotransmission. On the other hand, studies using behavioral paradigms, similar to those used to measure the effect of melanocortins (adrenocorticotropic hormone (ACTH)/melanocyte-stimulating hormone (MSH)), suggested that acquisition of new information was accompanied by changes in the degree of phosphorylation of brain synaptic phosphoproteins (Glassman et al., 1973). The original idea was to test $ACTH_{1-24}$ and its behaviorally active fragments for their effects on the in vitro phosphorylation of synaptosomal membrane proteins. The next step would than be to compare the structural requirements of ACTH for modulating protein phosphorylation with those for modulating extinction of active avoidance behaviour as described by De Wied (Greven and De Wied, 1973). In our first study in this line, we noted that high concentrations of $ACTH_{1-24}$ indeed inhibited the endogenous phosphorylation of a number of phosphoproteins in rat brain synaptic membranes.

The endogenous phosphorylation of these proteins was not affected by cyclic AMP, at that time the most important modulator of protein phosphorylation (Zwiers et al., 1976). These observations prompted us to investigate $ACTH_{1-24}$-induced inhibition of synaptic protein phosphorylation in great detail, focussing on the nature of the substrate proteins and their corresponding kinase. At the first Brain Phosphoprotein Meeting in Utrecht in 1981, we reported on the isolation and characterization of the 48-kDa phosphoprotein B-50 and of its corresponding B-50 kinase, which is similar if not identical to protein kinase C (Zwiers et al., 1982; Aloyo et al., 1982a, 1983). In the present paper we review our current knowledge on this neuron-specific phosphoprotein B-50, with special emphasis on its localization and possible function(s). We discuss the evidence that leads to the formulation of the hypothesis that the degree of phosphorylation of B-50 may modulate receptor-mediated hydrolysis of polyphosphoinositides (Gispen et al., 1985a). We summarize old and new data suggesting that such a modulatory mechanism may underlie ACTH-induced excessive grooming and may be of relevance not only to some behavioral actions of melanocortins, but also to neurotrophic actions.

Isolation and characterization

B-50

In rat brain synaptic plasma membranes (SPM), a great number of phosphoproteins can be identified. In recent years several of these proteins have been characterized and for some proteins a functional role in neurotransmission and membrane function has been documented. Examples are synapsin I (82–80 kDa; see Nestler and Greengard, 1984), calcium/calmodulin-dependent protein kinase II (50 kDa; Goldenring et al., 1983, 1984), the coated vesicle phosphoprotein pp50 (52 kDa; Pauloin et al., 1982, 1984) and B-50. B-50 is an acidic (pI 4.5), 48-kDa protein that is intimately associated with the synaptic membrane, since it can only be solubilized in the presence of detergent (Zwiers et al., 1979, 1980). The purified protein displays microheterogeneity upon isoelectric focussing in a narrow pH gradient (pH 3.5–5.0). Upon two-dimensional polyacrylamide gel electrophoresis, it can be resolved into 4 distinct protein spots (48 kDa) that are in part interconvertible by exhaustive phosphorylation or dephosphorylation. These results, together with data from peptide maps, suggest that B-50 contains at least two phosphorylatable sites (Zwiers et al., 1985). In several chromatographic systems the purified B-50 may form aggregates in the absence of detergents. The significance of this finding to the actual conformation in which B-50 is embedded in the membrane remains to be shown (Schotman et al., 1985). The microheterogeneity of B-50 is not the result of differences in glycomoiety, as B-50 seems to be devoid of sugar residues (Zwiers et al., 1985). Protein B-50 is most likely identical to the 47-kDa protein described by Herschkowitz et al. (1982), to protein γ5 of Rodnight (1982), to protein p54(Ca)p by Mahler et al. (1982) and to protein F_1 characterized by Routtenberg et al. (1982, 1985) (see also Addendum).

Localization of B-50

Antibodies were raised against B-50, which was partially purified from a rat brain membrane extract. Anti-B-50 immunoglobulins (IgGs) were purified by affinity chromatography on a solid immunosorbent conjugated with pure B-50 protein (Oestreicher et al., 1983a). The specificity of these antibodies was ascertained by immunoprecipitation of B-50 from a crude rat brain membrane fraction and immunoblotting. Immunostaining of Western blots with affinity-purified anti-

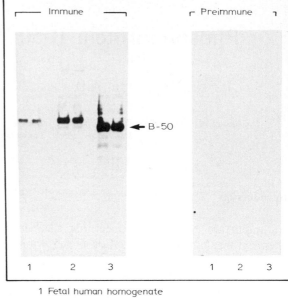

Affinity purified anti B-50 IgG's

1 Fetal human homogenate
2 Adult human SPM
3 Adult rat SPM

Fig. 1. **Western blot showing B-50-like immunoreactivity in** fetal and adult human brain. Fetal human homogenate, adult human and adult rat SPM (30 μg, 10 μg and 10 μg protein, respectively) were separated on 11% SDS-polyacrylamide gels and electrophoretically transferred to nitrocellulose. B-50-like immunoreactivity was assessed with affinity-purified anti-B-50 IgGs or preimmune IgGs.

B-50 IgGs revealed the presence of B-50-like proteins in brain homogenates of various vertebrate species: human, rat, mouse, hamster, rabbit, cow and chick. In fetal human brain homogenate, as well as in adult human brain SPM, a 52-kDa B-50-like protein showed cross-reactivity with the anti-B-50 IgGs (Fig. 1). No B-50 immunoreactivity was detected in homogenates from *Xenopus laevis*, goldfish and trout brain (Oestreicher et al., 1984).

Previous studies using two-dimensional separation techniques and crude B-50-antisera had already revealed that B-50 was present in the particulate fraction of rat brain and spinal cord, and not in subcellular fractions of other rat tissues studied (Kristjansson et al., 1982). Although endogenous B-50 phosphorylation activity was detectable throughout the rat brain, a clear regional distribution pattern was observed. The order of decreasing phosphorylation activity in SPM from the following brain regions is septum > hippocampus and neocortex > thalamus > cerebellum > medulla oblongata > spinal cord (Kristjansson et al., 1982). More recently, a radioimmunoassay (RIA) was developed to measure B-50 levels in different brain regions. The B-50 RIA employs anti-B-50 IgGs and purified ^{32}P-labeled B-50 as tracer. It measures B-50 levels in the range of 0.1–10 ng in small amounts of tissue (5–400 µg wet weight) (Oestreicher et al., 1986). The regional distribution of B-50 in adult rat brain as determined by RIA is as follows: septum > periaqueductal grey > hippocampus and neocortex > cerebellum > medulla spinalis. The septum contains 80 µg B-50/g wet weight tissue. In the cortex cerebrum the amount of B-50 is 0.3 ng/µg total protein and in SPM prepared from this region 3.7 ng/µg total protein (Oestreicher et al., 1986). The content of B-50 in rat cortex cerebrum is roughly 10 times lower than that described for synapsin I (Goelz et al., 1981). The regional distribution pattern obtained by the B-50 RIA is in fair agreement with that previously found by determining the levels of endogenous B-50 phosphorylation activity in SPM (Kristjansson et al., 1982). These data support our earlier suggestions that the regional differences in B-50 phosphorylation in brain SPM reflect differences in the B-50 content rather than in B-50 kinase activity (Kristjansson et al., 1982).

Sörensen et al. (1981) analyzed various subcellular fractions from rat brain for endogenous protein phosphorylation and concluded that B-50 is mainly associated with presynaptic membranes. Indeed, our immunohistochemical studies on adult rat brain indicate that B-50 localization is restricted to the synaptic region (Gispen et al., 1985b). Ultrastructural localization of B-50 in cryosections of adult rat hippocampus revealed that B-50 is predominantly associated with presynaptic terminals (Gispen et al., 1985b). B-50 immunoreactivity was assessed with affinity-purified anti-B-50 IgGs and visualized by a protein A-gold labeling technique. To determine the distribution of the gold particles in a more quantitative manner, 50 randomly chosen areas of 3 cm^2

(magnification 10 000 ×) were analyzed for pre- or postsynaptic localization of B-50. Presynaptic regions contained 15.2 ± 1.4 particles per terminal, whereas in the postsynaptic regions the content of gold particles did not differ significantly from that in control sections (2.5 ± 0.4) (Gispen et al., 1985b). These studies also indicate that B-50 is not present in all hippocampal terminals and synapses, and that B-50 is associated with the inner face of the plasma membrane and possibly with vesicle membranes in the synaptic region (Gispen et al., 1985b).

B-50 kinase and protein kinase C

In the first studies on the effect of ACTH on protein phosphorylation in SPM it was noted that ACTH affected the phosphorylation of substrate proteins other than those modulated by cyclic nucleotides (Zwiers et al., 1976). In addition, we established that the reduction of endogenous B-50 phosphorylation in SPM by ACTH$_{1-24}$ was the result of an inhibition of the protein kinase reaction rather than a stimulation of phosphoprotein phosphatase activity (Zwiers et al., 1978). The B-50 kinase was isolated and purified from rat brain SPM using ACTH-sensitive B-50 phosphorylation to monitor kinase activity (Zwiers et al., 1979, 1980). The purified B-50 kinase has an estimated molecular mass of 70 kDa in sodium dodecylsulfate (SDS) and an isoelectric point (IEP) of 5.5 (Zwiers et al., 1980) and requires both Ca^{2+} and Mg^{2+} for catalyzing the transfer of the γ-phosphate of ATP to B-50 (Gispen et al., 1979).

During our studies on the B-50 kinase, we noted several apparent similarities between B-50 kinase and kinase C. Kinase C is a cyclic nucleotide-insensitive, calcium-requiring protein kinase that was originally isolated from the soluble fraction of rat brain homogenate (Inoue et al., 1977). Later on, however, it was also found in the particulate fraction (Kuo et al., 1980). In fact, evidence is accumulating suggesting that translocation from cytosol to the plasma membrane is a key step in the activation of this enzyme and thus in receptor-mediated transmembrane signal transduction involving polyphosphoinositide (PPI) breakdown (Kraft and Anderson, 1983; Nishizuka, 1984). In a series of experiments we assessed possible similarities between protein kinase C and B-50 kinase. From these studies it was concluded that B-50 kinase is indeed very similar, if not identical, to kinase C (Aloyo et al., 1982a, 1983). This conclusion was based on the following data:

(a) both kinases are cyclic nucleotide-independent;
(b) from a number of kinases tested, only kinase C and B-50 kinase were able to phosphorylate purified B-50;
(c) exogenous kinase C predominantly phosphorylates B-50 in SPM;
(d) the enzymes share marked sensitivity of Ca^{2+}, phospholipids, ACTH, chlorpromazine and Ca^{2+}-dependent protease;
(e) the peptide maps as produced by limited proteolysis with *Staphylococcus aureus* protease V8 are identical (Aloyo et al., 1982a, 1983).

Since kinase C can be activated in many systems by phorbol diesters (Takai et al., 1985), we studied the effects of 4β-phorbol 12,13-dibutyrate (PDB) on B-50 phosphorylation in SPM. B-50 phosphorylation was stimulated in a dose-dependent manner (Fig. 2). A significant increase in B-50 phosphorylation was found at concentrations as low as 10^{-8} M PDB. 4α-Phorbol diesters, which do not stimulate kinase C, were without effect on B-50 phosphorylation in SPM. Our data are in agreement with recent work from Routtenberg and coworkers (Akers and Routtenberg, 1985), who showed that 4β-phorbol 12-myristate-13-acetate (PMA) stimulates the phosphorylation of band F_1 (which is most likely identical to B-50) in a crude mitochondrial/synaptosomal fraction. Moreover, the membrane-permeable, short chain fatty acid-containing diacylglyceride dioctanoylglycerol (DOG) stimulates endogenous B-50 phosphorylation in SPM (Fig. 2). Diacylglycerol (DG), which may be formed by the receptor-mediated hydrolysis of PPI, is also known to stimulate kinase C (Berridge and Irvine, 1984; Nishizuka, 1984a,b).

These data provide additional evidence that the endogenous phosphorylation of B-50 in rat brain SPM is catalyzed by a protein kinase similar, if not identical, to kinase C. One should keep in

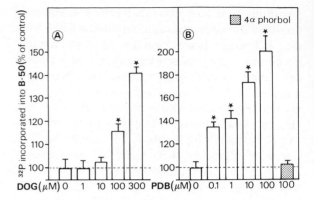

Fig. 2. Concentration-dependent stimulation of B-50 phosphorylation in SPM by 1,2-dioctanoylglycerol (DOG) (A) and 4β-phorbol 12,13-dibutyrate (PDB) (B). SPM (10 μg protein) was phosphorylated with $|\gamma^{-32}P|$-ATP in the presence of different concentrations of DOG, PDB or the inactive 4α-phorbol. Proteins were separated by SDS-PAGE and ^{32}P-incorporation into B-50 was measured by liquid-scintillation counting. Bars denote mean $\pm$ SEM ($n=6$), * significantly different from control ($p<0.001$).

mind, however, that B-50 may not be the only substrate to kinase C in rat brain. In fact, the ubiquitous presence of kinase C (Girard et al., 1985) and the restricted localization of B-50 argue in favor of such a notion. For example, there is increasing evidence that a 87-kDa protein present in brain is a substrate for protein kinase C (Wu et al., 1982).

As B-50 was shown to be a predominant substrate for protein kinase C in SPM, the question arose whether the phosphorylation of B-50 was related to DG stimulation of kinase C occurring during receptor-mediated hydrolysis of PPI.

Polyphosphoinositides (PPI)

During the past several years, an impressive body of information has been accumulating the PPI metabolism plays a central role in cellular signal transduction (Berridge and Irvine, 1984). The prevailing view is that in response to receptor activation by a variety of hormones, neurotransmitters and other external stimuli, a plasma membrane pool of phosphatidylinositol 4,5-bisphosphate (PIP_2) undergoes rapid phosphodiesteratic cleavage to yield two biologically active products: 1,2-diacylglycerol (DG) and inositol 1,4,5-trisphosphate (IP_3). DG is considered to activate the widely distributed Ca^{2+}- and phospholipid-dependent protein kinase C which is capable of phosphorylating many, largely uncharacterized, cellular proteins. IP_3 is believed to trigger the release of sequestered Ca^{2+} from non-mitochondrial stores into the cytosol. The simultaneous processes of protein phosphorylation and Ca^{2+} mobilization are thought to constitute synergistic events, which are integral to a large number of cellular responses (Nishizuka, 1984a,b). While the existence and importance of the receptor-mediated breakdown of PPI is well established, unresolved complications and questions remain, for instance about the significance of IP_4 and isomers of IP_3 like inositol 1,3,4-phosphate which may be generated (Irvine et al., 1985).

The nervous system is characterized not only by a rapid PPI turnover, especially in non-myelin structures (Gonzales-Sastre et al., 1971), but also by the highest known level of protein phosphorylation and dephosphorylation of any tissue (Weller, 1979). These phenomena are particularly prominent in the synaptic regions where mechanisms for dynamic modulation of information transmitted between neurons must be in continual operation. At the molecular level, an interplay between the state of phosphorylation of inositol-containing phospholipids and specific synaptic membrane proteins could contribute to changes in ion permeability or catalytic activity of selected enzymes. Such rapid effects might thus underly short-term adaptation of synaptic function to prevailing environmental conditions.

Modulation of B-50 phosphorylation and phosphatidyl 4-phosphate (PIP) kinase activity by ACTH

Some years ago, we observed that $ACTH_{1-24}$ in concentrations of 10^{-7} to 10^{-4} M inhibited the incorporation of radioactivity into B-50 when preparations of the protein, purified through the DEAE and ammonium sulphate precipitation steps, were incubated with $|\gamma\text{-}^{32}P|$-ATP (Jolles et al., 1980). Using this preparation, which is devoid of PPI phosphodiesterase activity, we found that concentrations of the neuropeptide which inhibited B-50 phosphorylation simultaneously stimulated the conversion of exogenously added PIP to PIP_2. These results prompted us to undertake detailed studies which have convinced us that a reciprocal relationship exists between the extent of B-50 phosphorylation and the degree of PIP kinase activity (Table I). The additional supporting evidence for this conclusion may be summarized as follows:

(a) If partially purified B-50 preparations were exposed to $|\gamma\text{-}^{32}P|$-ATP for increasing periods of time and was PIP then added, progressively more prephosphorylation of the protein decreased the labeling of PIP_2.

(b) The addition of $ACTH_{1-24}$ to SPM prepared from rat or human brain stimulated the incorporation of ^{32}P into endogenous PIP_2 (Table II) (see also Jolles et al., 1981b). The rate of loss of prelabeled PIP_2 in the membranes was unaffected

TABLE I

Summary of the evidence for an inverse relationship between the degree of B-50 phosphorylation and PIP kinase activity in rat brain SPM

Treatment	Date	Phosphorylation of B-50	PIP kinase activity
Prephosphorylation of B-50	1980	increase	decrease
$ACTH_{1-24}$	1980	decrease	increase
Anti-B-50 IgG	1983	decrease	increase
Dopamine (post-hoc)	1984	increase	decrease
B-50 and PIP kinase	1985	increase	increase

TABLE II

Effect of $ACTH_{1-24}$ on ^{32}P incorporation into phosphatidic acid (PA), phosphatidylinositol 4-phosphate (PIP) and phosphatidylinositol 4,5-bisphosphate (PIP_2) in rat and human SPM

SPM	$ACTH_{1-24}$	^{32}P incorporation[a] (fmol P/μg SPM protein):		
		PA	PIP	PIP_2
Rat	–	17.2 ± 2.0	32.8 ± 2.6	20.5 ± 0.5
	10^{-4} M	18.5 ± 0.4 (+7)	25.4 ± 2.1 (−23)	66.2 ± 5.0 (+223)
Human	–	6.1 ± 0.4	17.3 ± 0.2	15.4 ± 1.8
	10^{-4} M	7.0 ± 0.4 (+15)	15.6 ± 1.1 (−9)	47.0 ± 1.0 (+204)

[a]Mean $\pm$ S.E.M. ($n=3$) numbers in parenthesis indicate the percent change relative to incorporation without $ACTH_{1-24}$.

by the peptide, again suggesting that the effect is due to increased PIP_2 synthesis (Jolles et al., 1981a).

(c) Affinity-purified anti-B-50 IgGs added to SPM markedly and specifically inhibited B-50 phosphorylation and simultaneously enhanced PIP_2 labeling several-fold (Oestreicher et al., 1983).

(d) PIP kinase (45 kDa; pI 5.8) has been purified 67-fold and further identified by means of specific immunostaining and accompanying reduction of the enzyme activity due to interaction with affinity-purified anti-45-kDa protein antibodies (Van Dongen et al., 1984, 1986). When the effect of B-50 preparations enriched in either the phosphorylated or dephosphorylated protein was tested on the activity of purified PIP kinase, the dephosphorylated form had no effect, whereas the identical amount of phosphorylated B-50 substantially diminished the formation of PIP_2. To minimize non-specific protein–protein interactions, the experiments were conducted in the presence of bovine serum albumin (Van Dongen et al., 1985).

(e) A similar inverse relationship resulting in decreased B-50 phosphorylation and elevated PIP_2 labeling was obtained when rat hippocampal slices were incubated with 5×10^{-4} M dopamine, SPM prepared and post-hoc phosphorylation then performed. These effects were antagonized by the presence of haloperidol in the incubation medium, consistent with a receptor-mediated process (Jork et al., 1984).

Similar reciprocal effects of $ACTH_{1-24}$ on the phosphorylation of certain proteins and of PIP in subcellular fractions from rabbit iris smooth muscle have been reported by Abdel-Latif et al. (1983). Of relevance also may be the observations by Deshmukh et al. (1984) that in a solubilized myelin preparation containing both myelin basic protein and PIP phosphorylating activities, when exogenously added myelin basic protein and PIP (compounds that easily associate in vitro) are present together, the phosphorylation of each is greatly increased. Such mutual activation may represent another class of interactions involving rapidly reversible phosphorylation of certain proteins and PPI.

These findings have led us to propose that B-50, B-50 kinase and PIP kinase exist together in a multi-molecular complex in the presynaptic plasma membrane and that phosphorylation of B-50 exerts a regulatory effect on PIP kinase. The exact nature of the suggested interaction between these entities in the membrane remains to be elucidated. Possibly direct effects mediated by B-50 binding to PIP kinase are involved or, alternatively, the degree of B-50 phosphorylation could affect membrane topography such that PIP is rendered more or less accessible to the enzyme.

The action of $ACTH_{1-24}$ in this system may ultimately provide important clues as to the precise mechanism involved. So far evidence is lacking that this neuropeptide exerts its effects through binding to a specific membrane receptor

(Witter, 1979). $ACTH_{1-24}$ increases the fluidity of SPM, but not that of liposomes prepared from SPM as judged by fluorescence depolarization experiments using diphenylhexatriene as probe (Hershkowitz et al., 1982; Verhallen et al., 1984). Physicochemical studies have shown that, whereas $ACTH_{1-24}$ penetrates model membranes composed of a mixture of neutral and anionic phospholipids, neither $ACTH_{1-10}$, the hydrophobic portion, nor $ACTH_{11-24}$, the strongly cationic hydrophilic segment, does so, although the latter fragment presumably interacts electrostatically with negatively charged polar head groups on the liposome surface (Gremlich et al., 1983; Gysin and Schwyzer, 1984). Structure–activity studies in our laboratory have revealed that $ACTH_{1-10}$ and $ACTH_{11-24}$ are ineffective in altering either B-50 phosphorylation or PPI metabolism (Zwiers et al., 1978; Jolles et al., 1981c). Moreover, the structural requirements for the ACTH molecule to fluidize SPM correlate with those necessary to alter PPI and protein phosphorylation (Van Dongen et al., 1983). Taken together, these findings indicate that $ACTH_{1-24}$ most likely acts in an amphipathic manner by simultaneously forming complexes with anionic groups at the membrane surface and disrupting the hydrophobic acyl chains in the membrane interior (Verhallen et al., 1984). It is quite reasonable that both phospholipids and proteins should take part in these interactions, but it is unknown whether the primary effect of the neuropeptide is on B-50, either of the kinases or a lipid substrate (Verhallen et al., 1984).

Functional implications

Is B-50 phosphorylation part of a feedback mechanism affecting PIP_2 availability?

Evidence gathered to date indicates that the extent of B-50 phosphorylation influences PIP_2 synthesis in SPM. We suggest that this action of B-50 forms part of a negative feedback loop that contributes to the regulation of the PIP_2 pool available for generation of DG and IP_3 as shown in Fig. 3 (Gispen et al., 1985a; Gispen, 1986). In this scheme, receptor-mediated activation of PIP_2 phosphodiesteratic hydrolysis gives rise to DG

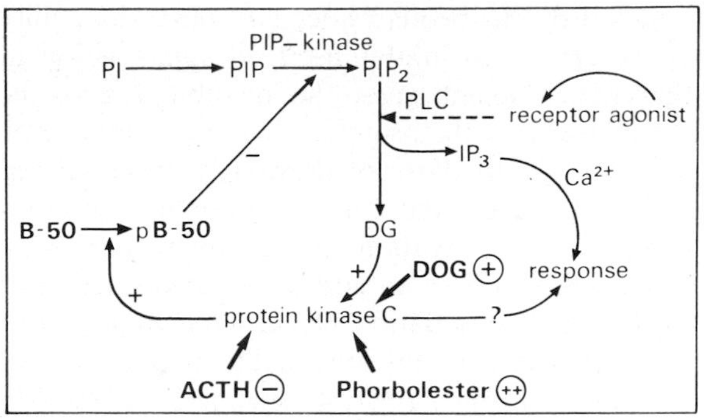

Fig. 3. Model of the regulatory role of B-50 in receptor-mediated polyphosphoinositide hydrolysis in brain.

and this substance in turn stimulates B-50 kinase, thereby tending to decrease PIP kinase activity. The outcome would be to decrease the production of PIP_2 hydrolysis products and their ensuing biological effects when these are no longer needed by the cell. In support of the feedback concept are observations that phorbol diesters, which are known to activate protein kinase C, decrease the carbamylcholine-induced accumulation of inositol phosphates in hippocampal slices and PC12 cells (Labarca et al., 1984; Vicentini et al., 1985). Our model predicts the complementary effect, namely that stimulated PIP_2 breakdown should bring about increased B-50 phosphorylation. In addition, assuming that B-50 phosphorylation plays a role in the 'off' signal for stimulated PIP_2 hydrolysis, we speculate that factors which affect phosphorylation of the protein might do so by interfering with the coupling between receptor–ligand association and the stimulation of PIP_2 hydrolysis. Recent findings support earlier hints (cf. Berridge and Irvine, 1984) that, analogous to the generally accepted mechanism for activation of adenylate cyclase, one or more GTP-binding proteins (N proteins) may be involved in the activation of PPI phosphodiesterase. The presence of GTP analogs has been shown to enhance PPI breakdown in the absence of added Ca^{2+} in plasma membranes from the neutrophils and blowfly salivary gland (Cockcroft and Gomperts, 1985; Litosch et al., 1985). It may be noteworthy that $ACTH_{1-24}$ (10^{-5} M) selectively extracts a 41-kDa protein from SPM (Aloyo et al., 1982b). While the removal of this protein does not affect the ability of $ACTH_{1-24}$ to inhibit B-50 phosphorylation in the treated membranes, the possibility must be considered that the protein, which has a molecular mass similar to those of previously characterized GTP-binding proteins, may be an obligatory component in the activation of PIP_2 hydrolysis. If so, this would point to an additional site of action of ACTH in the regulation of PIP_2 metabolism.

As indicated in the Introduction, our original aim was to explore the neurochemical mechanism of action of behaviorally active melanocortins at the level of the phosphorylation of SPM components. Using this approach we attempted to explain the known effect of these peptides on neurotransmission in certain synapses in the brain (Versteeg, 1980). However, in a variety of studies we have used the peptide $ACTH_{1-24}$ as a tool to modulate the phosphorylation of B-50, irrespective of the question whether such modulation represents a physiological mechanism by which the peptide could affect brain function. The use of broken cell preparations and the relatively high peptide concentrations required to inhibit B-50 phosphorylation (IC_{50} 3×10^{-6} M) have in fact cast some doubt as to the physiological importance of the observed inhibition of protein kinase C activity by $ACTH_{1-24}$ in rat brain SPM. Recent experiments on the sensitivity of endogenous B-50 phosphorylation to $ACTH_{1-24}$ in SPM indicate that under special conditions $ACTH_{1-24}$ significantly inhibits B-50 phosphorylation at concentrations as low as 10^{-7} M (Aloyo et al., in preparation). Indeed, evidence is accumulating to suggest that the proposed mechanism of action of ACTH is of relevance to the induction of excessive grooming behavior (Gispen et al., 1975). First of all, it was observed that intracerebroventricular (icv) administration of $ACTH_{1-24}$ in rats followed by a post-hoc endogenous phosphorylation assay of SPM prepared from the brains of these rats, resulted in a dose- and time-dependent change in the phosphorylation of the same proteins that were affected by ACTH when added to the phosphorylation assay in vitro (Zwiers et al., 1977). Thus, the effect of the peptide can be induced in the intact system, and appears not to be just an artefact in the broken cell preparation.

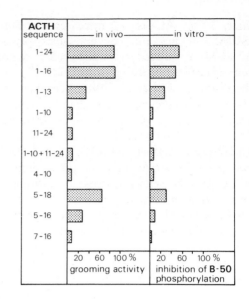

Fig. 4. Comparison of structural requirements of ACTH for inducing excessive grooming and inhibition of B-50 phosphorylation.

Secondly, we have shown that the structural requirements of ACTH for the in vitro inhibition of B-50 kinase in SPM are very similar to those required for ACTH-induced excessive grooming in the rat (Fig. 4) (Zwiers et al., 1978; Gispen et al., 1979). Furthermore, one of the regions which is extremely rich in B-50, the periaqueductal grey, is known to receive peptidergic terminals containing peptides from the proopiomelanocortion (POMC) family (Watson et al., 1978). The periaquaductal grey is the primary target for the induction of excessive grooming behavior by ACTH-like peptides (Spruijt et al., 1986). As icv application of anti-ACTH antibodies has been reported to suppress novelty-induced grooming behavior (Dunn et al., 1979), it seems that at least part of the behavioral effects of ACTH could be mediated through a modulation of the degree of phosphorylation of B-50.

Thirdly, we have recently reported that treatment of rats with DOG or phorbol diesters (icv injection) suppresses $ACTH_{1-24}$-induced grooming (Fig. 5) (Gispen et al., 1985c). These data support the notion that modulation of protein kinase C activity is part of the molecular mechanism underlying ACTH-induced excessive grooming.

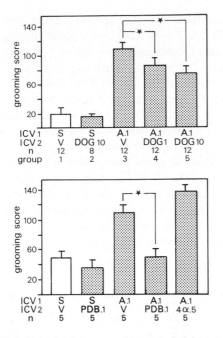

Fig. 5. The effect of 1,2-dioctanoylglycerol (DOG; top panel) and 4β-phorbol 12,13-dibutyrate (PDB; bottom panel) on ACTH-induced excessive grooming. ICV_1 and ICV_2, first and second intracerebroventricular injection; S, saline; V, 0.5% ethanol in saline; A_1, 0.1 µg $ACTH_{1-24}$ in saline; DOG 1 or 10, 1 or 10 µg DOG in 0.5% ethanol in saline; PDB.1, 0.1 µg PDB in 0.5% ethanol in saline; 4α.5, 0.5 µg 4α-phorbol in 0.5% ethanol in saline; n = number of rats. Bars denote mean $\pm$ SEM; * significantly different from group 3 ($p < 0.05$).

Finally, results from recent experiments suggest that in hippocampal slices the inhibition of carbachol-induced hydrolysis of PPI by phorbol diesters can be counteracted by pretreatment with $ACTH_{1-24}$ (Schrama et al., 1986). Again these data show an effect of the peptide on intact tissue in a way that was predicted from the proposed hypothesis on the role of B-50 in receptor-mediated PPI response (see Fig. 3).

Summarizing, we suggest that ACTH may modulate neurotransmission in certain types of synapses at the level of the presynaptic membrane by affecting a complex of protein kinase C, B-50 and PIP kinase. The specificity of such ACTH effects may reside in specific peptidergic projections containing ACTH-like peptides. The precise nature of the interaction between ACTH and the complex (see above) is still an open question.

Development and aging

In view of the restricted localization of B-50 in hippocampal neurons in adult rats, the question arose whether B-50 localization differed as a function of age. Previously, we had demonstrated that after intracranial injection of radiolabeled orthophosphate (Oestreicher et al., 1982) in 8-day-old rats, B-50 was one of the prominent phosphoproteins in neural membranes. Employing affinity-purified anti-B-50 antibodies (Oestreicher et al., 1983a), we showed in a comparative immunocytochemical study of brain regions in the 8-day-old and adult rat (Oestreicher et al., 1983b) that B-50 immunoreactivity (BIR) is distributed in regions rich in synaptic contacts throughout the rat brain (Oestreicher and Gispen, 1986).

After finding that the site of localization of B-50 is dependent on the stage of differentiation and growth of neurons in various brain regions (Oestreicher and Gispen, 1986), we started to compare the immunochemical localization of B-50 in the hippocampus of young, adult and senescent rats in more detail (Oestreicher et al., 1986). The BIR seems rather similarly distributed in the neuropil areas of the stratum oriens and the stratum moleculare-lacunosum of CA. However, a conspicuous difference was revealed in the hippocampus of the 28-month-old rat, in which BIR appeared to be present in 'aggregates' (deposits) near the periphery of the cell body or as 'particulate' material with an uneven distribution in the cytosol of the pyramidal CA3 neurons. The same BIR deposits were seen to a lesser extent in the pyramidal neurons of CA1, CA2 and CA4. Such a distribution of BIR was much less prominent in sections of the hippocampus of the 4-week-old rat. As an immunocytochemical control we compared parallel sections of adult and aged rat hippocampus with antisera against the structural markers myelin and astrocytes. The immunostaining did not display marked qualitative differences in contrast to that of B-50 (Oestreicher et al., 1986). At present it is unclear what the significance of this age-related change in cellular B-50 localization is. It is tempting to speculate that it relates to the decrease in synaptic plasticity seen in the hippocampus of aged rats. Further work is in progress to gain insight in the nature and precise subcellular localization of these BIR deposits around pyramidal cells in the CA3 layer of the hippocampus of old rats.

Holmes and Rodnight (1981) reported on the ontogeny of substrate proteins for protein kinases in rat brain membrane fractions. They found that maximal phosphorylation of their 48-kDa, $\gamma5$ protein (B-50), was reached 15 days after birth and from then on decreased to adult level. We observed that the B-50 content in total rat brain, as measured by RIA, was indeed highest immediately after birth and decreased to lower levels during further postnatal development (Oestreicher et al., 1986). Studying age-related changes in the brain

regional B-50 content in more detail, we found that the level of B-50 in the septum, hippocampus and cortex cerebrum was 40–50% lower in 28-month-old than in 2-month-old rats. Surprisingly, the content of the cerebellum did not undergo notable changes with age (Oestreicher et al., 1986).

The only other data available on the fate of B-50 during aging are those reported by Hershkowitz et al. (1982; Hershkowitz, 1983). He reported that the basal endogenous phosphorylation of his 47-kDa (B-50) protein in membranes prepared from brains from old mice was higher than in membranes from young animals. In fact, this 47-kDa protein was the only protein which showed an increase in phosphorylation in the

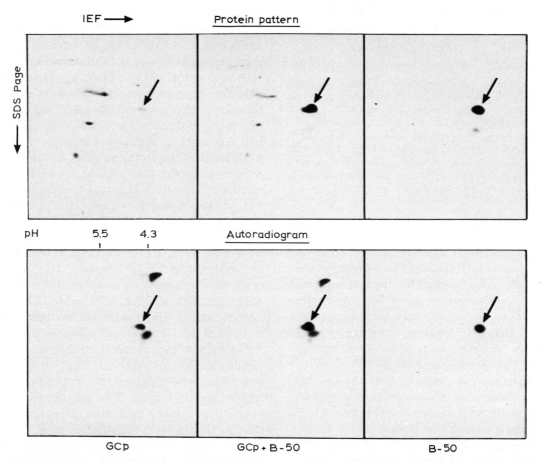

Fig. 6. Comigration of the 48-kDa protein in the growth cone particulate fraction (GCp) and purified B-50 after two-dimensional electrophoresis. Protein-staining pattern and autoradiogram of endogenous phosphorylated GCp is shown in the absence (GCp) and presence (GCp + B-50) of purified ^{32}P-labeled B-50 (B-50). Arrow denotes position of B-50. Only the 120–25 kDa molecular mass region of the gels is shown.

more viscous membranes of aged mice. Interestingly, this increase in basal endogenous phosphorylation could be counteracted by in vivo treatment of the mice with the membrane fluidizer AL721, a special lipid mixture from egg yolk (Hershkowitz et al., 1982). Hence, the authors suggested that the increased phosphorylation of the 47-kDa protein is related to a diminished lipid fluidity of the brain membranes in old rats.

Since B-50 is a predominant phosphoprotein in 8-day-old rats (Oestreicher et al., 1982) and appears to be localized in outgrowing neurites (Oestreicher et al., 1986), it was investigated whether B-50 was present in the growth cones of these neurites. Nerve growth cones were isolated from fetal rat brain essentially according to the method of Pfenninger et al. (1983). Morphological inspection of growth cone-enriched fractions revealed a relatively homogenous population of vesicular structures, enclosing various cellular organelles, primarily smooth endoplasmic reticulum and large clear polymorph vesicles (De Graan et al., 1985). Thus, the ultrastructural appearance closely resembles that described by Pfenninger et al. (1983) and Gordon-Weeks and Lockerbie (1984). The particulate material isolated from this growth cone-enriched fraction (GCp) was subjected to in vitro endogenous protein phosphorylation with or without the addition of 3×10^{-6} M ACTH$_{1-24}$. In the GCp fraction we found a phosphoprotein band which was sensitive to ACTH$_{1-24}$ with a relative migration identical to that of B-50 protein in adult rat brain SPM (De Graan et al., 1985). In addition, the GCp phosphoprotein comigrated with radiolabeled purified B-50 after two-dimensional separation (IEF, SDS-PAGE; Fig. 6) and cross-reacted on Western blots with affinity-purified anti-B-50 IgGs (Fig. 7). The B-50 protein in growth cone particulate material is a substrate to protein kinase C, since exogenous purified protein kinase C phosphorylates the protein in heat inactivated GCp fractions (Van Hooff et al., in preparation). The presence of a protein kinase C-like enzyme in growth cone material has also been shown by Pfenninger c.s. (Katz et al., 1985). We found that the addition of active phorbol diesters, known to stimulate kinase C, stimulates B-50 phosphorylation in GCp. In-

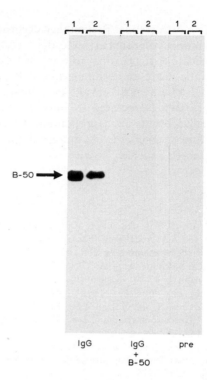

Fig. 7. Cross-reactivity of affinity-purified anti-B-50 IgGs (from antiserum number 8103) with the 48-kDa protein in GCp (1) and SPM (2) as shown by immunoblotting. IgG, anti-B-50 IgG (dilution 1:2000); IgG + B-50, anti-B-50 IgGs, preabsorbed with purified B-50; Pre, preimmune IgGs.

active 4α-phorbol diesters do not. In addition to B-50 and protein kinase C, PPI and their major phosphorylating enzymes are also present in the GCp fraction (Van Hooff et al., in preparation). In this fraction the degree of phosphorylation of B-50 is inversely related to the labeling of PIP$_2$ in a similar way as in adult rat brain SPM (see above). Therefore, the full machinery for a feedback role of B-50 phosphorylation in receptor-mediated PIP$_2$ hydrolysis (see Fig. 3) is present in growth cones.

Besides the role of ACTH in inducing excessive grooming, ACTH and related peptides are known for their trophic actions (Edwards and Gispen, 1985). Since we have shown that in growth cones the major components for the PPI metabolism as well as the B-50 feedback system are present, it is tempting to speculate that trophic actions of POMC peptides are mediated through the B-50 system. The hypothesis that B-50 plays an important role in nerve outgrowth and regeneration is certainly worth testing. Preliminary experiments using immunocytochemical detection methods indeed indicate that proximal to a crush lesion in the rat sciatic nerve an accumulation of B-50 can be detected (Verhaagen et al., in preparation). Further research is required to fully understand the molecular events in neuropeptide action on the brain and to assess the physiological relevance of the proposed scheme.

References

Abdel-Latif, A.A. (1983) Metabolism of phosphoinositides. In A. Lajtha and A.A. Abdel-Latif (Eds.), *Handbook of Neurochemistry, Vol. 3*, Plenum, New York, pp. 91–131.

Akers, R.F. and Routtenberg, A. (1985) Protein kinase C phosphorylates a 47 M_r protein (F_1) directly related to synaptic plasticity. *Brain Res.*, 334:147–151.

Aloyo, V.J., Zwiers, H. and Gispen, W.H. (1982a) B-50 protein kinase and kinase C in rat brain. *Prog. Brain Res.*, 56:303–315.

Aloyo, V.J., Zwiers, H. and Gispen, W.H. (1982b) $ACTH_{1-24}$ releases a protein from synaptosomal plasma membranes. *J. Neurochem.*, 38:871–875.

Aloyo, V.J., Zwiers, H. and Gispen, W.H. (1983) Phosphorylation of B-50 protein by calcium-activated phospholipid-dependent protein kinase and B-50 protein kinase. *J. Neurochem.*, 41:649–653.

Berridge, M.J. and Irvine, R.F. (1984) Inositol trisphosphate, a novel second messenger in cellular signal transduction. *Nature*, 312:315–321.

Cockcroft, S. and Gomperts, B.D. (1985) Role of guanine nucleotide-binding protein in the activation of polyphosphoinositide phosphodiesterase. *Nature*, 314:536–543.

De Graan, P.N.E., Van Hooff, C.O.M., Tilly, B.C., Oestreicher, A.B., Schotman, P. and Gispen, W.H. (1985) Phosphoprotein B-50 in nerve growth cones from fetal rat brain. *Neurosci. Lett.*, 61:235–241.

Deshmukh, D.S., Kuizon, S. and Brockerhoff, H. (1984) Mutual stimulation by phosphatidylinositol-4-phosphate and myelin basic protein of their phosphorylation by the kinase solubilized from rat brain myelin. *Life Sci.*, 34:259–264.

Dunn, A.J., Green, E.J. and Isaacson, R.L. (1979) Intracerebral adrenocorticotropic hormone mediates novelty-induced grooming in the rat. *Science*, 203:281–283.

Edwards, P.M. and Gispen, W.H. (1985) Melanocortin peptides and neural plasticity. In J. Traber and W.H. Gispen (Eds.), *Senile Dementia of the Alzheimer Type*, Springer Verlag, Heidelberg, pp. 231–240.

Girard, P.R., Mazzei, G.J., Wood, J.G. and Kuo, J.F. (1985) Polyclonal antibodies to phospholipid/Ca^{2+}-dependent protein kinase and immunocytochemical localization of the enzyme in rat brain. *Proc. Natl. Acad. Sci. U.S.A.*, 82:3030–3034.

Gispen, W.H. (1986) Phosphoprotein B-50 and phosphoinositides in brain plasma membranes: a possible feedback relationship. *Biochem. Soc. Trans.*, 14:163–165.

Gispen, W.H., Wiegant, V.M., Greven, H.M. and De Wied, D. (1975) The induction of excessive grooming in the rat by intraventricular application of peptides derived from ACTH: structure–activity studies. *Life Sci.*, 17:645–652.

Gispen, W.H., Zwiers, H., Wiegant, V.M., Schotman, P. and Wilson, J.E. (1979) The behaviorally active neuropeptide ACTH as neurohormone and neuromodulator: the role of cyclic nucleotides and membrane phosphoproteins. *Adv. Exp. Med. Biol.*, 116:199–224.

Gispen, W.H., Van Dongen, C.J., De Graan, P.N.E., Oestreicher, A.B. and Zwiers, H. (1985a) The role of phosphoprotein B-50 in phosphoinositide metabolism in brain synaptic plasma membranes. In J.E. Bleasdale, G. Hasuer and J. Eichberg (Eds.) *Inositol and Phosphoinositides*, Human Press, NJ, pp. 399–413.

Gispen, W.H., Leunissen, J.L.M., Oestreicher, A.B., Verkleij, A.J. and Zwiers, H. (1985b) Presynaptic localization of B-50 phosphoprotein: the ACTH-sensitive protein kinase substrate involved in rat brain polyphosphoinositide metabolism. *Brain Res.*, 328:381–385.

Gispen, W.H., Schrama, L.H. and Eichberg, J. (1985c) Stimulation of protein kinase C reduces ACTH-induced excessive grooming. *Eur. J. Pharmacol.*, 114:399–400.

Glassman, E., Gispen, W.H., Perumal, R., Machlus, B. and Wilson, J.E. (1973) The effect of short experiences on the incorporation of radioactive phosphate into synaptosomal and non-histone acid-extractable nuclear proteins from rat and mouse brain. In *Proceedings 5th International Congress Pharmacology, San Francisco, 1972, Vol. 4*, pp. 14–17.

Goelz, S.E., Nestler, E.J., Chehrazi, B. and Greengard, P. (1981) Distribution of protein I in mammalian brain as determined by a detergent-based radioimmunoassay. *Proc. Natl. Acad. Sci. U.S.A.*, 78:2130–2134.

Goldenring, J.R., Gonzalez, B., McGuire, J.S. and DeLorenzo, R.J. (1983) Purification and characterization of a calmodulin-dependent kinase from rat brain cytosol able to phosphorylate tubulin and microtubule-associated proteins. *J. Biol. Chem.*, 258:12632–12640.

Goldenring, J.R., Casanova, J.E. and DeLorenzo, R.J. (1984) Tubulin-associated calmodulin-dependent kinase: evidence from endogenous complex of tubulin with a calcium/calmodulin-dependent kinase. *J. Neurochem.*, 43:1669–1679.

Gonzalez-Sastre, F., Eichberg, J. and Hauser, G. (1971) Metabolic pools of polyphosphoinositides in rat brain. *Biochim. Biophys. Acta*, 248:96–104.

Gordon-Weeks, P.R. and Lockerbie, R.O. (1984) Isolation and partial characterization of neuronal growth cones from neonatal rat forebrain. *Neuroscience*, 13:119–136.

Gremlich, H.-U., Fringeli, U.-P. and Schwyzer, R. (1983) Conformational changes of adrenocorticotropin peptides upon interaction with lipid membranes revealed by intrared attenuated total reflection spectroscopy. *Biochemistry*, 22:4251–4263.

Greven, H.M. and De Wied, D. (1973) The influence of peptides derived from corticotropin (ACTH) on performance. Structure–activity studies. *Prog. Brain Res.*, 39:429–442.

Gysin, B. and Schwyzer, R. (1984) Hydrophobic and electrostatic interactions between adrenocorticotropin-1(1–24)-tetracosapeptide and lipid vesicles. Amphiphilic primary structures. *Biochemistry*, 23:1811–1818.

Hershkowitz, M. (1983) Mechanisms of brain aging. The role of membrane fluidity. *Dev. Neurol.*, 7:85–99.

Hershkowitz, M., Zwiers, H. and Gispen, W.H. (1982) The effect of ACTH on rat brain synaptic plasma membrane lipid fluidity. *Biochim. Biophys. Acta*, 692, 495–497.

Holmes, H. and Rodnight, R. (1981) Ontogeny of membrane-bound protein phosphorylating systems in the rat. *Dev. Neurosci.*, 4:79–87.

Inoue, M., Kishimoto, A., Takai, Y. and Nishizuka, Y. (1977) Studies on a cyclic nucleotide-independent protein kinase and its pro-enzyme in mammalian tissues. *J. Biol. Chem.*, 252:7610–7616.

Irvine, R.F., Anggard, E.E., Letcher, A.J. and Downes, C.P. (1985) Metabolism of inositol-1,4,5-trisphosphate and inositol-1,3,4-trisphosphate in rat parotid gland. *Biochem. J.*, 229:505–511.

Jolles, J., Zwiers, H., Van Dongen, C.J., Schotman, P., Wirtz, K.W.A. and Gispen, W.H. (1980) Modulation of brain polyphosphoinositide metabolism by ACTH-sensitive protein phosphorylation. *Nature*, 286:623–625.

Jolles, J., Schrama, L.H. and Gispen, W.H. (1981a) Calcium-dependent turnover of brain polyphosphoinositides in vitro after prelabelling in vivo. *Biochim. Biophys. Acta*, 666:90–98.

Jolles, J., Zwiers, H., Dekker, A., Wirtz, K.W.A. and Gispen, W.H. (1981b) Corticotropin-1(1–24)-tetracosapeptide affects protein phosphorylation and polyphosphoinositide metabolism in rat brain. *Biochem. J.*, 194:283–291.

Jolles, J., Bär, P.R. and Gispen, W.H. (1981c) Modulation of brain polyphosphoinositide metabolism by ACTH and beta-endorphin: structure–activity studies. *Brain Res.*, 224:315–326.

Jork, R., De Graan, P.N.E., **Van Dongen**, C.J., Zwiers, H., Matthies, H. and Gispen, W.H. (1984) Dopamine-induced changes in protein phosphorylation and polyphosphoinositide metabolism in rat hippocampus. *Brain Res.*, 291:73–81.

Katz, F., Ellis, L. and Pfenninger, K.H. (1985) Nerve growth cones isolated from fetal rat brain. III. Calcium-dependent protein phosphorylation. *J. Neurosci.*, 5:1402–1411.

Kraft, A.S. and Anderson, W.B. (1983) Phorbol esters increase the amount of Ca^{2+}, phospholipid-dependent protein kinase associated with plasma membrane. *Nature*, 301:621–623.

Kristjansson, G.I., Zwiers, H., Oestreicher, A.B. and Gispen, W.H. (1982) Evidence that the synaptic phosphoprotein B-50 is localized exclusively in nerve tissue. *J. Neurochem.*, 39:371–378.

Kuo, J.F., Andersson, R.G.G., Wise, B.C., Mackerlova, L., Salomonsson, I., Brackett, M.L., Katoh, N., Shoji, M. and Wrenn, R.W. (1980) Calcium-dependent protein kinase: widespread occurrence in various tissues and phyla of the animal kingdom and comparison of effects of phospholipid,

calmodulin and trifluoperazine. *Proc. Natl. Acad. Sci. U.S.A.*, 77:7039–7043.

Labarca, R., Janowsky, A., Patel, J. and Paul, S.M. (1984) Phorbol esters inhibit agonist-induced [^{3}H]inositol-1-phosphate accumulation in rat hippocampal slices. *Biochem. Biophys. Res. Commun.*, 123:703–709.

Litosch, I., Wallis, C. and Fain, J.N. (1985) 5-Hydroxytryptamine stimulates inositol phosphate production in a cell-free system from blowfly salivary glands. Evidence for a role of GTP in coupling receptor activation to phosphoinositide breakdown. *J. Biol. Chem.*, 260:5464–5471.

Mahler, H.R., Kleine, L.P., Ratner, N. and Sörensen, R.G. (1982) Identification and topography of synaptic phosphoproteins. *Prog. Brain Res.*, 56:27–48.

Nestler, E.J. and Greengard, P. (1984) *Protein phosphorylation in the nervous system*, John Wiley and Sons, New York, 398 pp.

Nishizuka, Y. (1984a) The role of protein kinase C in cell surface signal transduction and tumor promotion. *Nature*, 308:693–697.

Nishizuka, Y. (1984b) Turnover of inositol phospholipids and signal transduction. *Science*, 225:1365–1370.

Oestreicher, A.B. and Gispen, W.H. (1986) Comparison of the immunocytochemical distribution of the phosphoprotein B-50 in the cerebellum and hippocampus of immature and adult rat brain. *Brain Res.*, 375:267–279.

Oestreicher, A.B., Zwiers, H., Gispen, W.H. and Roberts, S. (1982) Characterization of infant rat cerebral cortical membrane proteins phosphorylated in vivo: identification of the ACTH-sensitive phosphoprotein B-50. *J. Neurochem.*, 39:683–692.

Oestreicher, A.B., Van Dongen, C.J., Zwiers, H. and Gispen, W.H. (1983a) Affinity-purified anti-B-50 protein antibody: interference with the function of the phosphoprotein B-50 in synaptic plasma membranes. *J. Neurochem.*, 41:331–340.

Oestreicher, A.B., Zwiers, H., Leunissen, J.L.M., Verkleij, A.J. and Gispen, W.H. (1983b) Localization of B-50 in rat brain studied by immunolight and electron microscopy. *J. Neurochem.*, 41 Suppl.: S95.

Oestreicher, A.B., Van Duin, M., Zwiers, H. and Gispen, W.H. (1984) Cross-reaction of anti-rat B-50: characterization and isolation of a 'B-50-phosphoprotein' from bovine brain. *J. Neurochem.*, 43:935–943.

Oestreicher, A.B., Dekker, L.V. and Gispen, W.H. (1986a) A radioimmunoassay (RIA) for the phosphoprotein B-50: distribution in rat brain. *J. Neurochem.*, 46:1366–1369.

Oestreicher, A.B., De Graan, P.N.E. and Gispen, W.H. (1986b) Neuronal cell membranes and aging. *Prog. Brain Res.*, (in press).

Pauloin, A., Bernier, I. and Jollès, P. (1982) Presence of cyclic nucleotide Ca^{2+}-independent protein kinase in bovine brain coated vesicles. *Nature*, 298:574–576.

Pauloin, A., Loeb, J. and Jollès, P. (1984) Protein kinase(s) in bovine brain coated vesicles. *Biochim. Biophys. Acta*, 799:238–245.

Pearse, B.M.F. and Robinson, M.S. (1984) Purification and properties of 100-kDa proteins from coated vesicles and their reconstruction with clathrin. *EMBO J.*, 3:1951–1957.

Pfenninger, K.H., Ellis, L., Johnson, H.P., Friedman, L. and Somlo, S. (1983) Nerve growth cones isolated from fetal rat brain: subcellular fractionation and characterization. *Cell*, 35:573–584.

Rodnight, R. (1982) Aspects of protein phosphorylation in the nervous system with particular reference to synaptic transmission. *Prog. Brain Res.*, 56:1–25.

Routtenberg, A. (1982) Brain phosphoproteins and behavioral state. *Prog. Brain Res.*, 56:349–374.

Routtenberg, A., Lovinger, D.M. and Steward, P. (1985) Selective increase in phosphorylation state of a 47-kDa protein (F₁) directly related to long-term potentiation. *Behav. Neural Biol.*, 43:3–11.

Schotman, P., Schrama, L.H. and Edwards, P.M. (1985) Peptidergic systems. In A. Lajtha (Ed.), *Handbook of Neurochemistry, Vol. 8*, Plenum Press, New York, pp. 243–279.

Schrama, L.H., DeGraan, P.N.E., Eichberg, J. and Gispen, W.H. (1986) Feedback control of the inositol phospholipid response in rat brain is sensitive to ACTH. *Eur. J. Pharmacol.*, 121:403–404.

Sörensen, R.G., Kleine, L.P. and Mahler, H.R. (1981) Presynaptic localization of phosphoprotein B-50. *Brain Res. Bull.*, 7:57–61.

Spruijt, B.M., Cools, A.R. and Gispen, W.H. (1986) The periaqueductal grey: a prerequisite for ACTH-induced excessive grooming. *Behav. Brain Res.*, 20:19–25.

Takai, Y., Kaibuchi, K., Tsuda, T. and Hoshijima, M. (1985) Role of protein kinase C in transmembrane signalling. *J. Cell. Biochem.*, 29:143–155.

Van Dongen, C.J., Hershkowitz, M., Zwiers, H., De Laat, S. and Gispen, W.H. (1983) Lipid fluidity and phosphoinositide metabolism in rat brain membranes of aged rats: effects of ACTH(1–24). *Dev. Neurol.*, 7:101–114.

Van Dongen, C.J., Zwiers, H. and Gispen, W.H. (1984) Purification and partial characterization of the phosphatidylinositol 4-phosphate kinase from rat brain. *Biochem. J.*, 223:197–203.

Van Dongen, C.J., Zwiers, H., De Graan, P.N.E. and Gispen, W.H. (1985) Modulation of the activity of purified phosphatidylinositol-4-phosphate kinase by phosphorylated and dephosphorylated B-50 protein. *Biochem. Biophys. Res. Commun.*, 128:1219–1227.

Van Dongen, C.J., Kok, J.W., Schrama, L.H., Oestreicher, A.B. and Gispen, W.H. (1986) Immunochemical characterization of phosphatidylinositol-4-phosphate kinase from rat brain. *Biochem. J.*, 233:859–864.

Verhallen, P.J.E., Demel, R.A., Zwiers, H. and Gispen, W.H. (1984) Adrenocorticotropic hormone (ACTH)–lipid interactions. Implications for involvement of amphipathic helix formation. *Biochim. Biophys. Acta*, 775:246–254.

Versteeg, D.H.G. (1980) Interaction of peptides related to ACTH, MSH and β-LPH with neurotransmitters in the brain. *Pharmacol. Ther.*, 11:535–557.

Vicentini, L.M., Di Virgilio, F., Ambrosini, A., Pozzan, T. and Meldolesi, J. (1985) Tumor promotor phorbol 12-myristate, 13-acetate inhibits phosphoinositide hydrolysis and cytosolic Ca²⁺ rise induced by the activation of muscarinic receptors in PC12 cells. *Biochem. Biophys. Res. Commun.*, 127:310–317.

Watson, S.J., Richard III, C.W. and Barchas, J.D. (1978) Adrenocorticotropin in rat brain: immunocytochemical localization in cells and axons. *Science*, 275:226–228 (1978).

Weller, M. (1979) *Protein Phosphorylation. The Nature, Function and Metabolism of Proteins, which Contain Covalently Bound Phosphorus.* PION, London.

Witter, A. (1979) On the presence of receptors for ACTH-neuropeptides in the brain. In G.C. Pepeu, M. Kuhar and L. Enna (Eds.), *Receptors for Neurotransmitters and Peptide Hormones*, Raven Press, New York, pp. 407–414.

Wu, W.C.-S., Walaas, S.I., Nairn, A.C. and Greengard, P. (1982) Calcium-phospholipid regulates phosphorylation of a '87 K' substrate protein in brain synaptosomes. *Proc. Natl. Acad. Sci. U.S.A.*, 79:5249–5253.

Zwiers, H., Veldhuis, D., Schotman, P. and Gispen, W.H. (1976) ACTH, cyclic nucleotides and brain protein phosphorylation in vitro. *Neurochem. Res.*, 1:669–677.

Zwiers, H., Wiegant, V.M., Schotman, P. and Gispen, W.H. (1977) Intraventricular administered ACTH and changes in rat brain protein phosphorylation: a preliminary report. In S. Roberts, A. Lajtha and W.H. Gispen (Eds.), *Mechanism, Regulation and Special Functions of Protein Synthesis in the Brain*, Elsevier/North-Holland Biomedical Press, Amsterdam, pp. 267–272.

Zwiers, H., Wiegant, V.M., Schotman, P. and Gispen, W.H. (1978) ACTH-induced inhibition of endogenous rat brain protein phosphorylation in vitro: structure–activity. *Neurochem. Res.*, 3:455–463.

Zwiers, H., Tonnaer, J., Wiegant, V.M., Schotman, P. and Gispen, W.H. (1979) ACTH-sensitive protein kinase from rat brain membranes. *J. Neurochem.*, 33:247–256.

Zwiers, H., Schotman, P. and Gispen, W.H. (1980) Purification and some characteristics of an ACTH-sensitive protein kinase and its substrate protein in rat brain membranes. *J. Neurochem.*, 34:1689–1699.

Zwiers, H., Jolles, J., Aloyo, V.J., Oestreicher, A.B. and Gispen, W.H. (1982) ACTH and synaptic membrane phosphorylation in rat brain. *Prog. Brain Res.*, 56:405–417.

Zwiers, H., Verhaagen, J., Van Dongen, C.J., De Graan, P.N.E. and Gispen, W.H. (1985) Resolution of rat brain synaptic phosphoprotein B-50 into multiple forms by two-dimensional electrophoresis: evidence for multisite phosphorylation. *J. Neurochem.*, 44:1083–1090.

W.H. Gispen and A. Routtenberg (Eds.)
Progress in Brain Research, Vol. 69
© 1986 Elsevier Science Publishers B.V. (Biomedical Division)

CHAPTER 5

Polyphosphoinositides, phosphoproteins, and receptor function in rabbit iris smooth muscles

A.A. Abdel-Latif, P.H. Howe, and R.A. Akhtar

Department of Cell and Molecular Biology, Medical College of Georgia, Augusta, GA 30912, U.S.A.

Introduction

Several studies have suggested that activation of Ca^{2+}-mobilizing receptors, such as muscarinic cholinergic and α_1-adrenergic, leads to the contraction of smooth muscle through Ca^{2+}-mobilization (for reviews see Bolton, 1979; Grover and Daniel, 1985). The source of activator Ca^{2+} may be intracellular or extracellular and varies with the pharmacological agent or physiological stimulus producing the contraction. Thus, cholinergic stimulation of tracheal smooth muscle is thought to stimulate extracellular Ca^{2+} influx or release from intracellular stores (Farley and Miles, 1978). It is now generally believed that activation of Ca^{2+}-mobilizing receptors in smooth muscle leads to a rise in cytosolic free Ca^{2+} and that this cation exerts its intracellular effects by binding to the Ca^{2+}-dependent regulatory protein calmodulin (Adelstein and Eisenberg, 1980; Askoy et al., 1982; Ruegg, 1982). The Ca^{2+}–calmodulin complex then activates myosin-light chain kinase, which phosphorylates the 20-kDa light chain of myosin (MLC). This phosphorylation of myosin is required for the actin activation of myosin ATPase necessary for muscle contraction. In tracheal smooth muscle muscarinic agonists, such as carbachol (CCh) and methacholine, increased both MLC phosphorylation and contraction in a dose-dependent manner, implying that phosphorylation could regulate muscle contraction (De Lanerolle et al., 1982; Silver and Stull, 1984).

Activation of Ca^{2+}-mobilizing receptors also leads to the phosphodiesteratic cleavage of phosphatidylinositol 4,5-bisphosphate (PIP_2) into inositol 1,4,5-trisphosphate (IP_3) and 1,2-diacylglycerol (DG) in a wide variety of tissues (for the proceedings of a recent symposium on this topic see Bleasdale et al., 1985). There is now growing experimental evidence which suggests that IP_3 and DG synergistically mediate signal transduction in receptor systems linked to Ca^{2+} mobilization (Berridge and Irvine, 1984; Nishizuka, 1984). IP_3 has been shown to be involved in the release of Ca^{2+} from intracellular stores, and DG activates protein kinase C, which phosphorylates specific proteins. Protein kinase C, another type of Ca^{2+}-dependent protein kinase which requires phosphatidylserine and DG as cofactors has also been reported to phosphorylate MLC (Endo et al., 1982; Nishikawa et al., 1983; Ikebe et al., 1985) and MLC kinase (Ikebe et al., 1985). In many cell types the IP_3–Ca^{2+}–calmodulin and DG systems interact synergistically to produce physiological responses, but the mechanisms involved are not yet defined (Exton, 1985).

In our own laboratory for many years we have been interested in elucidating the role of polyphosphoinositides and protein phosphorylation in muscarinic cholinergic and α_1-adrenergic receptor function in the iris of the eye. The iris contains sphincter and dilator muscles and these are innervated by excitatory cholinergic and adrenergic nerves, respectively (Persson and Sonmark, 1971; Van Alphen, 1976). The presence of muscarinic cholinergic and α_1-adrenergic receptors has also been demonstrated through radioligand binding studies (Page and Neufeld, 1978; Taft et al., 1980).

Since our early observations on the link between PIP$_2$ breakdown and the activation of muscarinic cholinergic and α_1-adrenergic receptors in the iris muscle (Abdel-Latif et al., 1977, 1978), we have reported extensively on the molecular mechanism and physiological significance of the receptor-mediated PIP$_2$ breakdown into IP$_3$ and DG in this tissue (Akhtar and Abdel-Latif, 1980, 1984; Abdel-Latif, 1983; Abdel-Latif et al., 1985). Furthermore, the demonstration of a close correlation between agonist-stimulated PIP$_2$ breakdown and agonist-induced muscle contraction led us to conclude that this phenomenon is an early event in the pathway which leads from receptor activation to muscle response (Grimes et al., 1979). Employing adrenocorticotropic hormone (ACTH) as a physiological modulator, we have demonstrated a close relationship between PIP$_2$ metabolism and protein phosphorylation in iris subcellular fractions (Akhtar et al., 1983). More recently we have focussed our efforts on the concept that the agonist-stimulated breakdown of PIP$_2$ in the iris muscle is a primary (initial) event that could couple activated muscarinic cholinergic and α_1-adrenergic receptors, through mobilization of cellular Ca^{2+}, to muscle contraction. To obtain further support for this hypothesis we have conducted correlative studies on the effects of muscarinic cholinergic and α_1-adrenergic agonists on IP$_3$ accumulation, MLC phosphorylation and muscle contraction in the sphincter and dilator muscles of rabbit iris as well as in the sympathetically denervated dilator.

Muscarinic cholinergic and α_1-adrenergic receptor-mediated PIP$_2$ breakdown in the rabbit iris

Previously, we have shown that when iris muscle, prelabeled with ^{32}Pi, was exposed to acetylcholine (ACh) or norepinephrine (NE), there was a significant loss ($\sim 30\%$) of radioactivity from PIP$_2$ and an increase in the labeling of phosphatidic acid (PA) and phosphatidylinositol (PI), (Abdel-Latif et al., 1977, 1978). Since these experiments were conducted under breakdown conditions, i.e. the availability of ATP for biosynthesis of PIP$_2$ was limiting, the loss of ^{32}P from PIP$_2$ was indicative of stimulated breakdown rather than inhibi-

TABLE I

Effects of CCh and NE, in the absence and presence of their respective antagonists, on the accumulation of myo-[^{3}H]inositol phosphates in the rabbit iris

Additions	Radioactivity in myo-[^{3}H]inositol phosphates (% of control)		
	IP	IP$_2$	IP$_3$
CCh (50 µM)	154 ± 7	153 ± 4	160 ± 6
CCh (50 µM) + atropine (10 µM)	104 ± 8	110 ± 5	105 ± 7
NE (50 µM)	173 ± 2	149 ± 19	144 ± 17
NE (50 µM) + prazosin (10 µM)	85 ± 7	96 ± 10	102 ± 2

Irides were incubated for 90 min in 1 ml Krebs–Ringer bicarbonate buffer (pH 7.4) containing 5 µM myo-[^{3}H]inositol (7.3 µCi/ml). At this time atropine and prazosin were added as indicated and incubations continued for 5 min. This was followed by the addition of CCh and NE and incubation continued for an additional 10 min. The incubations were terminated with 10% (w/v) trichloroacetic acid and the radiolabeled myo-inositol phosphates analyzed by anion exchange chromatography (Akhtar and Abdel-Latif, 1984). The average radioactivity (dpn/iris) recovered in IP, IP$_2$, and IP$_3$ fractions from the control iris muscle was 39 900, 7900, and 4000, respectively. The data are mean $\pm$SEM obtained from three separate experiments conducted in triplicate.

tion of biosynthesis of this phospholipid. These studies showed for the first time that activation of Ca^{2+}-mobilizing receptors, such as muscarinic cholinergic and α_1-adrenergic, leads to the breakdown of PIP$_2$. The fact that there was always a good correlation between agonist-stimulated PIP$_2$ breakdown and the labeling of PA (Abdel-Latif et al., 1977; Akhtar and Abdel-Latif, 1978a), suggested to us that PIP$_2$ phosphodiesterase is involved in this phenomenon. Direct evidence to show that agonist-stimulated PIP$_2$ breakdown was indeed mediated through the phosphodiesteratic cleavage of this phospholipid came from our studies in which the accumulation of water-soluble myo-inositol phosphates, the products of phosphoinositide breakdown, was measured following stimulation of iris muscle prelabeled with myo-[^{3}H]inositol (Akhtar and Abdel-Latif, 1980). As shown in Table I, addition of CCh or NE to iris muscle prelabeled with myo-[^{3}H]inositol caused a significant increase (60%) in the accumulation of

IP_3. There was a similar increase in the accumulation of *myo*-inositol 1-phosphate (IP) and *myo*-inositol bisphosphate (IP_2). The stimulatory effects of CCh and NE were blocked by atropine and prazosin, respectively, implying that the agonist-stimulated phosphodiesteratic cleavage of PIP_2 is mediated by muscarinic cholinergic and α_1-adrenergic receptors (Akhtar and Abdel-Latif, 1980, 1984). These studies showed for the first time that activation of muscarinic cholinergic and α_1-adrenergic receptors leads to the phosphodiesteratic cleavage of PIP_2 into IP_3 and DG. These studies and the fact that PIP_2 phosphodiesterase (phosphoinositide-specific phospholipase C) was found to be localized in part in the microsomal fraction of the iris (Akhtar and Abdel-Latif, 1978b) led us to conclude that the phosphodiesteratic cleavage of PIP_2 into IP_3 and DG is the underlying mechanism for the agonist-stimulated breakdown of PIP_2 (Akhtar and Abdel-Latif, 1980).

Muscarinic and α_1-adrenergic agonists cause rapid breakdown of PIP_2 and accumulation of IP_3 in the iris

When prelabeled iris muscle was stimulated with CCh or NE for 10 min there was an increase in the accumulation of IP, IP_2, and IP_3 in the tissue (Table I; Akhtar and Abdel-Latif, 1980). Since PI, phosphatidylinositol 4-phosphate (PIP) and PIP_2 are in metabolic equilibrium in the tissue, the question arose as to whether the agonists provoked hydrolysis of all three phosphoinositides concomitantly or whether there was selective breakdown of one of the phosphoinositides which then affected the levels of the other two phospholipids and their water-soluble metabolic products. Time-course experiments (Fig. 1) revealed that in ^{32}P-labeled irides, CCh caused a significant loss (10%) of radioactivity from PIP_2 within 15 s which increased to about 30% in 5 min (Akhtar and Abdel-Latif, 1984). Concomitant with PIP_2 breakdown there was a progressive increase in the labeling of PA. In contrast, a significant increase in the labeling of PI was not detectable until about 2 min after CCh was added to the incubation medium. In addition, when irides were labeled with *myo*-[^{3}H]inositol and then stimulated with

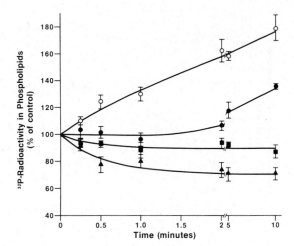

Fig. 1. Time-course for the effect of CCh on the breakdown of ^{32}P-labeled polyphosphoinositides, and accumulation of ^{32}P-labeled PA and PI in the iris muscle. Irides were princubated for 90 min in 1 ml of Krebs–Ringer bicarbonate buffer (pH 7.4) containing 1.5 mM *myo*-inositol and 30 µCi of ^{32}P$_i$. CCh (50 µM) was then added and incubations continued for various time intervals. The incubations were terminated with 10% (w/v) trichloroacetic acid (TCA) and the phospholipids were extracted and analyzed for radioactivity by thin layer chromatography (Akhtar and Abdel-Latif, 1984). Each point is the mean $\pm$ SEM of two separate experiments conducted in triplicate. $\bigcirc$, PA; $\bullet$, PI; $\blacksquare$, PIP; $\blacktriangle$, PIP_2.

CCh, IP_2 and IP_3 began to accumulate immediately (Fig. 2). Thus the increase in IP_2 and IP_3 accumulation could be detected within 15 s and this increased further with time. On the other hand there was a definite delay of about 1 min before the effect of CCh on IP accumulation could be detected. Following this lag period, a steady increase in IP accumulation was observed. Quantitatively, the net increase in IP was more than that of IP_2 and IP_3. This could be due to the fact that the labeling of PI was several times higher than that of PIP and PIP_2, and that some IP could have been formed from the phosphodiesteratic cleavage of PI, in addition to its formation from the stepwise dephosphorylation of IP_3 (Akhtar and Abdel-Latif, 1980, 1984). As with CCh, NE also caused a rapid accumulation of IP_3 in the iris muscle (Akhtar and Abdel-Latif, 1984).

We can conclude from the above studies that in the iris muscle the agonist-stimulated PIP_2 breakdown into IP_3 and DG precedes that of PI break-

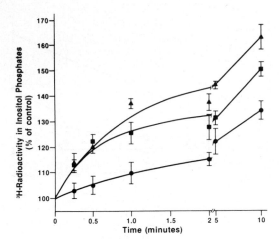

Fig. 2. Time-course for the effect of CCh on the accumulation of myo-[³H]-inositol phosphates in the iris muscle. Irides were preincubated for 90 min in 1 ml of Krebs–Ringer bicarbonate buffer (pH 7.4) containing 5 μM myo-[³H]inositol (pH 7.8 μCi/ml). CCh (50 μM) was then added and incubations continued for various time intervals. The radiolabeled myo-inositol phosphates were analyzed by anion exchange chromatography (Akhtar and Abdel-Latif, 1984). Each point is the mean of values from three separate experiments conducted in triplicate. ●, IP; ■, IP₂; ▲, IP₃.

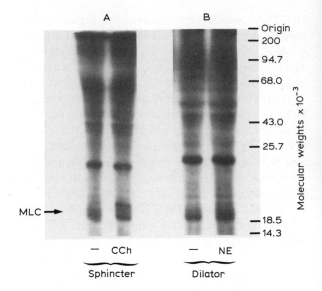

Fig. 3. Autoradiogram, after protein separation by polyacrylamide gel electrophoresis, showing: (A) the effect of CCh (50 μM) on protein phosphorylation in the iris sphincter, and (B) the effect of NE (50μM) on protein phosphorylation in the iris dilator. The muscles were first preincubated in Krebs–Ringer bicarbonate buffer (pH 7.4) containing ³²Pᵢ (50 μCi/ml) at 37°C for 75 min, the muscles were then transferred to fresh Krebs–Ringer buffer containing ³²Pᵢ and preincubation continued for an additional 15 min, to give a total preincubation time of 90 min. Following this incubation, CCh (50 μM) or NE (50 μM) was added to the medium containing the sphincter and dilator, respectively, and incubation continued for 1 min. The reaction was stopped by immersion of the tissue in a methanol–dry ice slurry at -80°C. The dehydrated tissue was homogenized in ice-cold 5% TCA, the insoluble proteins were suspended in an sodium dodecylsulfate (SDS)-containing electrophoresis buffer and solubilized by boiling for 30 min in sealed tubes. Proteins were determined (Lowry et al., 1951) and separated by SDS–polyacrylamide gel electrophoresis (Laemmli, 1970; Goy et al., 1984). Autoradiography was performed and the band corresponding to the 20-kDa MLC was cut from the dried gel and counted in a liquid scintillation counter.

down. Furthermore, the observed rapid accumulation of IP₃ by the agonists strongly suggests that the phosphodiesteratic cleavage of PIP₂ is an early (initial) event in the pathway which links the activation of Ca²⁺-mobilizing receptors to muscle contraction (Akhtar and Abdel-Latif, 1984; Abdel-Latif et al., 1985). A rapid breakdown of PIP₂ has also been demonstrated in a wide variety of tissues in response to various agonists (for reviews see Hawthorne, 1983; Fisher et al., 1984; Berridge and Irvine, 1984; Exton, 1985; Bleasdale et al., 1985).

Muscarinic and α₁-adrenergic agonists stimulate MLC phosphorylation in the iris sphincter and dilator muscles

If MLC phosphorylation is involved in smooth muscle contraction, then activation of muscarinic cholinergic and α₁-adrenergic receptors should increase the extent of MLC phosphorylation in the iris muscles. Fig. 3 shows that several proteins, including 20-kDa protein, identified as MLC, were phosphorylated by endogenous protein kinases in both the sphincter and dilator muscles. Phosphorylation of MLC in the sphincter was enhanced by CCh by about 34%, and in the dilator it was enhanced by NE by about 25%. The CCh- and NE-induced MLC phosphorylation was inhibited by atropine and prazosin, respectively (P.H. Howe, R.A. Akhtar, and A.A. Abdel-Latif, unpublished observations).

CCh induces IP₃ accumulation, MLC phosphorylation, and muscle contraction in the iris sphincter

Since the sphincter and dilator muscles of the iris are enriched in muscarinic cholinergic and α_1-adrenergic receptors, respectively, it was necessary to dissect the muscles from the whole iris and then employ them individually for the correlative studies. Fig. 4 shows the dose-response effect of CCh on IP₃ accumulation, MLC phosphorylation and contraction in the iris sphincter. The agonist increased the accumulation of IP₃, MLC phosphorylation and muscle contraction in a dose-dependent manner, exerting its maximal effects between 20 and 50 μM. Atropine (1 μM), but not D-tubocurarine, significantly inhibited these effects (data not shown), suggesting that the CCh effects on PIP₂ breakdown, MLC phosphorylation and muscle contraction are mediated by muscarinic cholinergic receptors. There is a fairly good correlation between the dose-response curves of IP₃ accumulation and MLC phosphorylation: the EC_{50} for both responses were 2.5 and 4.5 μM, respectively (Fig. 4). However, the dose-response curve for muscle contraction was shifted to the left of that for IP₃ accumulation, with EC_{50} of 0.6 μM. In rabbit aorta, the NE dose-response curve for contraction was also shifted to the left of that for the PI effect (Villalobos-Molina et al., 1982). Such observations can be explained on the assumption that there are 'spare receptors' for the agonists (Michell et al., 1981; Fisher et al., 1983; Aub and Putney, 1985) and that occupancy of a small fraction of the receptors, resulting in only a small increase in IP₃, is sufficient to elicit a maximal contractile response.

Further evidence for a possible correlation between agonist-induced PIP₂ breakdown, MLC phosphorylation and muscle contraction is provided by the time-course experiment given in Fig. 5. CCh induced a rapid increase in IP₃ with a corresponding increase in MLC phosphorylation and muscle contraction. Unlike IP₃ accumulation and MLC phosphorylation, there was a delay of 10–15 s in the initiation of muscle contraction (data not shown). Part of the lag period observed in the contractile response is probably due to the time it

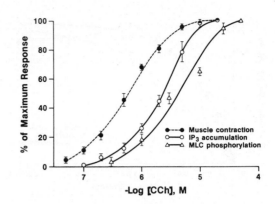

Fig. 4. Effects of different concentrations of CCh on IP₃ accumulation, MLC phosphorylation and muscle contraction in the iris sphincter. For experiments involving IP₃ accumulation, the paired sphincters (from the same rabbit) were incubated in 1 ml of Krebs–Ringer bicarbonate buffer (pH 7.4) containing 10 μCi myo-[³H]inositol for 90 min. At this time the sphincters were washed three times with 4 ml of non-radioactive Krebs–Ringer bicarbonate buffer and then suspended singly (of the paired sphincters, one was used as a control and the other as experimental) in 1 ml of the non-radioactive buffer. 10 mM LiCl was added to each incubation and 10 min later different concentrations of CCh were added and incubations continued for an additional 10 min. The incubations were terminated with 10% (w/v) TCA and the radiolabeled myo-inositol phosphates analyzed by anion exchange chromatography (Akhtar and Abdel-Latif, 1984). The phosphorylation of MLC in the absence and presence of CCh was determined as described in the legend to Fig. 3. For measurement of pharmacological responses (contraction), the sphincter muscles were mounted in 25-ml baths containing Krebs–Ringer bicarbonate buffer which was continously oxygenated (97% O₂/3% CO₂) and maintained at 37°C. The tissues were allowed to equilibrate for 90 min under a resting tension of 50 mg. During this period the muscles were washed with fresh oxygenated Krebs–Ringer buffer (pH 7.4) every 30 min. After equilibration, different concentrations of CCh were added and isometric contractions were recorded using a Grass FT-03 transducer and Grass DC amplifier. In the figure, accumulation of IP₃, MLC phosphorylation and muscle contraction have been expressed as a percentage of the corresponding maximal response to the agonist.

takes for CCh to diffuse in the organ chamber; however, it could also reflect the time it takes for IP₃ to diffuse through the cytoplasm to reach the SR and mobilize Ca^{2+} required for initiation of muscle contraction. Once initiated, however, there was a rapid increase in muscle contraction which paralleled increases in IP₃ accumulation and MLC phosphorylation. The difference in the t1/2 values

56

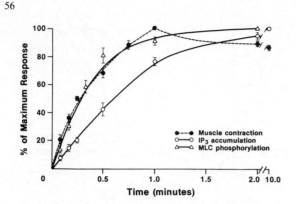

Fig. 5. Time-course of CCh-induced IP$_3$ accumulation, MLC phosphorylation, and muscle contraction in the iris sphincter. The experimental details for determination of IP$_3$ accumulation, MLC phosphorylation, and muscle contraction were the same as given in the legends to Figs. 3 and 4. The concentration of CCh used was 50 µM. The data are means ± SEM of 3 experiments conducted in triplicate.

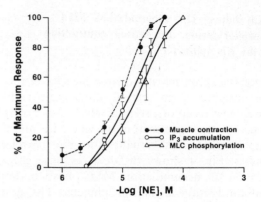

Fig. 6. Effects of different concentrations of NE on IP$_3$ accumulation, MLC phosphorylation and muscle contraction in the iris dilator. The experimental details for determination of IP$_3$ accumulation and MLC phosphorylation were the same as given in the legends to Figs. 3 and 4, except that the paired dilators (from the same rabbit) were used in this experiment. For measurement of contraction response, strips of the iris dilator muscle of about 2 mm width were cut by the method of Kern (1970). The strips were then mounted in 25-ml baths, equilibrated in Krebs–Ringer bicarbonate buffer (pH 7.4) and isometric contraction measured as described in the legend to Fig. 4. The data are means ± SEM of 3 experiments conducted in triplicate.

between the biochemical and physiological responses could also be due to the possibility that cyclic IP$_3$, which is rapidly hydrolyzed, may be involved in muscle contraction. The initial phasic component of muscle contraction was maximum within 1 min of the agonist addition, and this was followed by a slower tonic component which was maintained for several minutes. During the tonic phase of muscle contraction the IP$_3$ level also remained elevated. The initial phasic component of smooth muscle contraction is believed to result from mobilization of intracellular Ca^{2+} whereas the tonic component is dependent on extracellular Ca^{2+} involving increased Ca^{2+} permeability of the plasma membrane (Bolton, 1979; Van Breemen et al., 1982; Weiss, 1982).

NE induces IP$_3$ accumulation, MLC phosphorylation, and muscle contraction in the iris dilator

Dose-response curves for the effects of NE on IP$_3$ accumulation, MLC phosphorylation and muscle contraction in the iris dilator also revealed a close correlation between the three responses with the following EC$_{50}$ values: IP$_3$ accumulation, 14 µM; MLC phosphorylation, 19 µM; and muscle contraction, 10 µM (Fig. 6). These responses were

maximal at agonist concentrations of 50–100 µM. Furthermore, the time-course experiments also revealed a good correlation between NE-induced increase in IP$_3$ accumulation and muscle contraction (Fig. 7). After initial delay of 10–15 s, NE

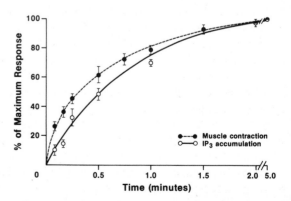

Fig. 7. Time-course of NE-induced IP$_3$ accumulation and muscle contraction in the iris dilator. The experimental details were the same as described in the legends to Figs. 4 and 6. The concentration of NE used was 50 µM. The data are means ± SEM of 6–9 determinations from 3 separate experiments.

induced a rapid increase in muscle contraction which paralleled NE-induced IP_3 accumulation. The muscle developed increased tension as the accumulation of IP_3 increased and the two responses reached their maximum within 2–5 min after the neurotransmitter was added. Time-course experiments of NE-induced MLC phosphorylation in the dilator have not yet been carried out. It can be concluded from the above correlative studies that muscarinic cholinergic and α_1-adrenergic stimulation of the sphincter and dilator muscles, respectively, leads to the breakdown of PIP_2 into IP_3 and DG. Accumulation of IP_3 is very rapid, and could be involved in Ca^{2+} mobilization necessary for MLC phosphorylation and muscle contraction.

Sympathetic denervation increases NE-induced IP_3 accumulation, MLC phosphorylation, and muscle contraction in the iris dilator

Sympathetic denervation of a wide variety of smooth muscles results in a supersensitive response of the tissue to submaximal concentration of NE. Unlike skeletal muscle, denervation supersensitivity in smooth muscle is not due to an increase in density or alteration of receptors controlling contraction (Westfall, 1981; Abel et al., 1985).

Previously, we have reported that after surgical sympathetic denervation of the rabbit iris there is a significant increase in both the NE-induced breakdown of PIP_2 (Abdel-Latif et al., 1979) and in contraction of the iris muscle (Abdel-Latif et al., 1975). These studies led us to conclude that NE-stimulated PIP_2 breakdown is associated with sympathetic denervation supersensitivity. As described in earlier sections, activation of α_1-adrenergic receptors in the dilator smooth muscle leads to PIP_2 breakdown into DG and IP_3, and that IP_3, by mobilizing intracellular Ca^{2+}, could participate in phosphorylation of MLC which is involved in muscle contraction. To shed more light on the hypothesis that an increase in the neurotransmitter-stimulated PIP_2 breakdown could be the underlying mechanism of sympathetic denervation supersensitivity (Abdel-Latif et al., 1979), we have investigated the kinetic inter-

relationships between PIP_2 breakdown, measured as IP_3 accumulation, MLC phosphorylation, and muscle contraction in normal and surgically sympathectomized iris dilator muscle. As shown in Fig. 8 (A–C), the NE dose–response curves for IP_3 accumulation, MLC phosphorylation, and muscle contraction in the denervated dilator were significantly shifted to the left as compared to the control. The EC_{50} values for NE-induced PIP_2 breakdown, PA labeling, IP_3 accumulation, MLC phosphorylation, and muscle contraction for the denervated muscle were significantly lower than those obtained for the normal dilator (see Table II below for summary), implying that all of these responses could be involved in the mechanism of denervation supersensitivity in this tissue. Furthermore, denervation supersensitivity was observed only in response to NE, and not to CCh, and it was inhibited by prazosin, indicating that it is mediated by α_1-adrenergic receptors (Akhtar and Abdel-Latif, 1986). Another interesting finding from this study was that in the denervated dilator, NE induced a more rapid accumulation of IP_3 which was accompanied by an equally rapid development of muscle contraction (Table II).

It has been reported that sympathetic denervation of rat vas deferens resulted in an increase in maximal contraction response to NE (Abel et al., 1985). In the iris dilator, sympathetic denervation did not change the maximal NE-induced IP_3 accumulation, MLC phosphorylation or muscle contraction. However, sympathetic denervation did increase the basal incorporation of myo-[^{3}H]-inositol into phosphoinositides which was also reflected in a corresponding increase in the accumulation of labeled myo-inositol phosphates (Akhtar and Abdel-Latif, 1986). Since the enzymes for phosphoinositide metabolism were not affected by denervation, the exact mechanism underlying increased incorporation of myo-inositol into these lipids remains unclear. It has been reported that sympathetic denervation of rat vas deferens did not increase receptor-mediated polyphosphoinositide breakdown, although the ^{32}P labeling of PA was significantly increased (Takenawa et al., 1983). In another report (Downes et al., 1983) sympathetic denervation decreased the breakdown of polyphosphoinositides in response to substance P

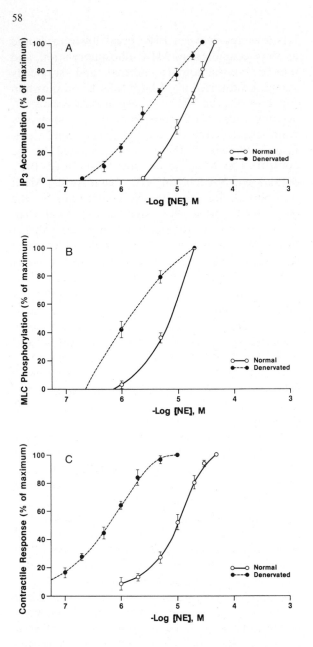

in rat parotid glands. The activities of Ca^{2+}-ATPase and protein kinase C were found to be elevated in the denervated muscle (Akhtar and Abdel-Latif, 1986). However, in contrast to the finding that sympathetic denervation reduced the activity of Na^+-K^+-ATPase in guinea pig vas deferens (Wong et al., 1981), the activity of this enzyme was not affected in the iris dilator following denervation. It has been reported recently that in chemically skinned vas deferens the concentration–response curve for Ca^{2+} in denervated tissue is shifted significantly to the left of the control, suggesting that increased sensitivity of the contractile proteins may contribute to denervation-induced supersensitivity of smooth muscle (Ramos et al., 1986). Our own data suggest that sympathetic denervation renders the coupling between α_1-adrenergic receptors and PIP_2 breakdown into DG and IP_3 more efficient. The NE-stimulated hydrolysis of PIP_2 could bring about Ca^{2+} mobilization, necessary for MLC phosphorylation and ultimately muscle contraction, either directly by causing plasma membrane depolarization or indirectly by IP_3 releasing Ca^{2+} from sarcoplasmic reticulum and/or by DG activating protein kinase C.

Effects of ACTH on PIP_2 metabolism and protein phosphorylation in the iris

Further support for the existence of a close relationship between PIP_2 metabolism and protein phosphorylation in the iris was provided by our

Fig. 8. Effect of denervation on NE-stimulated (A) accumulation of IP_3, (B) phosphorylation of MLC, and (C) muscle contraction in the iris dilator. The procedure for surgical sympathetic denervation was the same as previously described (Abdel-Latif et al., 1975). The superior cervical ganglion on one side (the other served as control) was carefully isolated and removed. Two weeks following the surgical procedure the irides were tested with NE for denervation supersensitivity and 3 days later the animals were sacrificed and the dilators used for experimentation. The normal and denervated dilator muscles were halved (of the two halves, one served as control and the other as experimental), then each muscle was equilibrated in 0.5 ml Krebs–Ringer bicarbonate buffer (pH 7.4) that contained 3.5 μCi-myo-[^{3}H]inositol for 75 min; the medium was then replaced with fresh radioactive medium and incubation continued for an additional 15 min (total preincubation time was 90 min). Various concentrations of NE were added and incubation continued for an additional 10 min. The incubations were terminated with 10% (w/v) TCA followed by extraction and analysis of radiolabeled IP_3. For determination of MLC phosphorylation the normal and denervated dilators were also cut into halves as described above and then used for protein phosphorylation experiments as described in the legend to Fig. 3. The contraction studies on normal and denervated dilators were conducted as described in the legend to Fig. 4. The data are means ± SEM of 3 separate experiments conducted in triplicate.

studies on the effect of ACTH on the in vitro phosphorylation of phospholipids and phosphoproteins (Akhtar et al., 1983). As shown in Fig. 9, addition of the peptide to iris microsomal fraction, incubated in the presence of $[\gamma\text{-}^{32}P]$ATP, resulted in increased labeling of PIP_2 and decreased labeling of several phosphoproteins, including one similar to the B-50 protein (48 kDa; Jolles et al., 1981). Gispen and coworkers have reported that the degree of phosphorylation of B-50 protein by B-50 protein kinase (protein kinase C) in the synaptic membranes inversely affected the activity of PIP kinase (Gispen et al., 1985). More recently these authors (Van Dongen et al., 1985) purified PIP kinase from rat brain and showed it to be inhibited appreciably by the phospho B-50, but not by the B-50 protein. Efforts in our laboratory to demonstrate an effect of ACTH on PIP_2 metabolism and protein phosphorylation in the intact

iris muscle were unsuccessful (W.C. Taft and A.A. Abdel-Latif, unpublished observations).

Conclusions and discussions

In this communication we have: (a) reviewed our previous studies on muscarinic cholinergic and α_1-adrenergic stimulation of PIP_2 breakdown in the iris muscle, then summarized more recent kinetic data obtained on the agonist-stimulated PIP_2 breakdown in this tissue; and (b) described correlative studies in which the effects of muscarinic cholinergic and α_1-adrenergic agonists on PIP_2 breakdown (measured as IP_3 accumulation), MLC phosphorylation and muscle contraction were investigated in the iris sphincter and in normal and sympathetically denervated iris dilator. The data presented add further support to the hypothesis that the breakdown of PIP_2 in the iris could function to couple activated muscarinic cholinergic and α_1-adrenergic receptors to muscle response (Akhtar and Abdel-Latif, 1978a, and, for summary, Abdel-Latif et al., 1985). Thus both the concentration-dependent responses and the time-course studies showed a close relationship between the extent of: (a) PIP_2 breakdown, (b) IP_3 accumulation, (c) MLC phosphorylation, and (d) muscle contraction (Table II). The recent demonstration of rapid breakdown of PIP_2 into IP_3 and DG in a wide variety of tissues in response to several agonists (for several reviews see Bleasdale et al., 1985) and the fact that both of these two putative second messengers could be involved in the pathway from receptor activation to muscle response add further support to the developing concept that PIP_2 breakdown is indeed a primary event in the receptor-mediated transduction mechanism in stimulus–contraction coupling. Our thoughts on how PIP_2 breakdown could be involved in muscle contraction in the iris smooth muscle are summarized in Fig. 10. Agonist-induced hydrolysis of PIP_2 at the plasma membrane could bring about the following events, of which one or more could lead to muscle contraction:

(a) Depolarization of the plasma membrane, followed by: Ca^{2+} mobilization, increase in intracel-

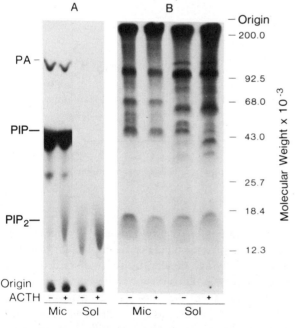

Fig. 9. Autoradiogram (A) after lipid extraction and TLC, and (B) after protein separation by SDS–polyacrylamide gel electrophoresis, showing the effects of ACTH (100 μM) on lipid and protein phosphorylation in iris microsomal (Mic) and 30–50% ammonium sulfate precipitable (Sol) fractions (Akhtar et al., 1983). Incubation of the fractions (50 μg protein) was carried out with $[\gamma\text{-}^{32}P]$ATP for 1 min. The electrophoretic mobility of protein standards is given at the right.

TABLE II

Summary of kinetic parameters of agonist-induced PIP_2 breakdown, IP_3 accumulation, MLC phosphorylation and contraction responses in sphincter and dilator smooth muscles of the iris

| Tissue | Agonist | $EC_{50}^a(\times 10^{-6} M)$ | | | | | $t_{1/2}^b$(seconds) | | |
		PA	PIP_2	IP_3	MLC	Contraction	IP_3	MLC	Contraction
Sphincter	ACh*/CCh	4.4*	5.0*	2.5	4.5	0.6	30	17	17
Normal dilator	NE	12**	10**	14	7.4	10	31	—	19
Denervated dilator	NE	1.9**	1.6**	3	1.4	0.6	11	—	9

[a]Concentration of the agonist required to induce 50% of the maximal response
[b]Time required to achieve 50% of the maximal response
*Taken from Abdel-Latif et al. (1977)
**Taken from Abdel-Latif et al. (1979)

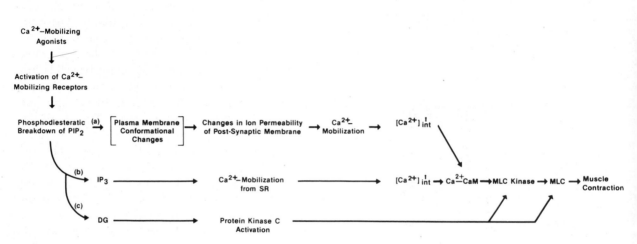

Fig. 10. Scheme of mechanisms by which Ca^{2+}-mobilizing agonists, such as muscarinic cholinergic and α_1-adrenergic, could bring about contraction in smooth muscle.

lular Ca^{2+} concentration, activation of CaM-MLC-kinase to phosphorylate MLC and consequently lead to contraction;
(b) Release of IP_3, followed by: Ca^{2+} mobilization from sarcoplasmic reticulum, increase in cytosolic free Ca^{2+}, activation of CaM-MLC kinase to phosphorylate MLC and consequently lead to contraction; and
(c) Release of DG, followed by: activation of kinase C, phosphorylation of either MLC kinase (Ikebe et al., 1985) or MLC (Endo et al., 1982; Nishikawa et al., 1983; Ikebe et al., 1985), or both, and consequently lead to contraction.

The studies on the sympathetically denervated iris dilator provide a clue to the molecular mechanism underlying denervation supersensitivity in smooth muscle. Thus it is possible that denervation renders the coupling between receptor activation and PIP_2 breakdown more efficient, this could increase the extent of Ca^{2+} mobilization and subsequently muscle contraction (Fig. 10).
Irvine et al. (1985) have recently identified two isomers of IP_3, namely 1,4,5-IP_3 and 1,3,4-IP_3, in parotid glands stimulated by CCh. Wilson et al. (1985) have reported that following hydrolysis of PIP_2 by purified phospholipase C, about 14% of

the total IP_3 was recovered as inositol 1,2 (cyclic)-4,5-trisphosphate. Whether or not these isomers do exist in the iris smooth muscle, and whether one or both are released by the muscarinic cholinergic and α_1-adrenergic agonists in this tissue have not yet been investigated. A functional role for the agonist-induced PIP_2 breakdown and its relationship to protein phosphorylation and consequently to cellular responses has just begun to emerge (Marx, 1984, 1985), and from the papers which I have had the privilege of hearing at this meeting, I am confident that there will be many more important discoveries made in this exciting area of research in the coming years.

Acknowledgements

This research was supported by U.S. Public Health Service Grants EY-04387 and EY-04171 from the National Eye Institute. This is contribution number 0934 from the Department of Cell and Molecular Biology, Medical College of Georgia.

References

Abdel-Latif, A.A. (1983) Metabolism of phosphoinositides. In A. Lajtha (Ed.), Handbook of Neurochemistry, Vol. 3, 2nd Edn., Plenum, New York, pp. 91–131.

Abdel-Latif, A.A., Green, K., Maltheny, J.L., McPherson, J.C. and Smith, J.P. (1975) Effects of norepinephrine and acetylcholine on ^{32}P incorporation into phospholipids of the rabbit iris muscle following unilateral superior cervical ganglionectomy. Life Sci., 17:1821–1826.

Abdel-Latif, A.A., Akhtar, R.A. and Hawthorne, J.N. (1977) Acetylcholine increases the breakdown of triphosphoinositide of rabbit iris muscle prelabeled with [^{32}P]phosphate. Biochem. J., 162:61–73.

Abdel-Latif, A.A., Green, K., Smith, J.P., McPherson, J.C. and Matheny, J.L. (1978) Norepinephrine-stimulated breakdown of triphosphoinositide of rabbit iris smooth muscle: effects of surgical sympathetic denervation and in vivo electrical stimulation of the sympathetic nerve of the eye. J. Neurochem., 30:517–525.

Abdel-Latif, A.A., Green, K. and Smith, J.P. (1979) Sympathetic denervation and the triphosphoinositide effect in the iris smooth muscle: a biochemical method for the determination of α-adrenergic receptor denervation super-sensitivity. J. Neurochem., 32:225–228.

Abdel-Latif, A.A., Smith, J.P. and Akhtar, R.A. (1985) Polyphosphoinositides and muscarinic cholinergic and α_1-adrenergic receptors in the iris smooth muscle. In J.E. Bleasdale, J. Eichberg, and G. Hauser (Eds.), Inositol and Phosphoinositides: Metabolism and Regulation, The Humana Press, Clifton, NJ, pp. 275–298.

Abel, P.W., Johnson, R.D., Tracy, J.M. and Minneman, K.P. (1985) Sympathetic denervation does not alter the density or properties of α_1 adrenergic receptors in rat vas deferens. J. Pharmacol. Exp. Ther., 233:570–577.

Adelstein, R.S. and Eisenberg, E. (1980) Regulation and kinetics of the actin–myosin–ATP interaction. Annu. Rev. Biochem., 49:921–956.

Akhtar, R.A. and Abdel-Latif, A.A (1978a) Calcium ion requirement for acetylcholine-stimulated breakdown of triphosphoinositide in rabbit iris smooth muscle. J. Pharmacol. Exp. Ther., 204:655–668.

Akhtar, R.A. and Abdel-Latif, A.A. (1978b) Studies on the properties of triphosphoinositide phosphomonoesterase and phosphodiesterase of rabbit iris smooth muscle. Biochim. Biophys. Acta, 527:159–170.

Akhtar, R.A. and Abdel-Latif, A.A. (1980) Requirement for calcium ions in acetylcholine stimulated phosphodiesteratic cleavage of phospatidyl-myo-inositol 4,5-bisphosphate in rabbit iris smooth muscle. Biochem. J., 192:783–791.

Akhtar, R.A. and Abdel-Latif, A.A. (1984) Carbachol causes rapid phosphodiesteratic cleavage of phosphatidylinositol 4,5-bisphosphate and accumulation of inositol phosphates in rabbit iris muscle; prazosin inhibits noradrenaline- and ionophore A23187-stimulated accumulation of inositol phosphates. Biochem. J., 224:291–300.

Akhtar, R.A. and Abdel-Latif, A.A. (1986) Surgical sympathetic denervation increases α_1-adrenoceptor-mediated accumulation of myo-inositol trisphosphate and muscle contraction in rabbit iris dilator smooth muscle. J. Neurochem., 46:96–104.

Akhtar, R.A., Taft, W.C. and Abdel-Latif, A.A. (1983) Effects of ACTH on polyphosphoinositide metabolism and protein phosphorylation in rabbit iris subcellular fractions. J. Neurochem., 41:1460–1468.

Askoy, M.O., Murphy, R.A. and Kamm, K.E. (1982) Role of Ca^{2+} and myosin light chain phosphorylation in regulation of smooth muscle. Am. J. Physiol., 242:C109–C116.

Aub, D.L. and Putney, J.W. (1985) Properties of receptor-controlled inositol trisphosphate formation in parotid acinar cells. Biochem. J., 225:263–266.

Berridge, M.J. and Irvine, R.F. (1984) Inositol trisphosphate, a novel second messenger in cellular signal transduction. Nature, 312:316–321.

Bleasdale, J.E., Eichberg, J. and Hauser, G. (Eds.) (1985) Inositol and Phosphoinositides: Metabolism and Regulation. The Humana Press, Clifton, NJ.

Bolton, T.B. (1979) Mechanisms of action of transmitters and other substances on smooth muscle. Physiol. Rev., 59:606–718.

De Lanerolle, P., Condit, J.R., Tanenbaum, M. and Adelstein, R.S. (1982) Myosin phosphorylation, agonist concentration and contraction of tracheal smooth muscle. Nature, 298:871–872.

Downes, C.P., Dibner, M.D. and Hanley, M.R. (1983) Sympathetic denervation impairs agonist-stimulated phosphatidylinositol metabolism in rat parotid glands. *Biochem. J.*, 214:865–870.

Endo, T., Naka, M. and Hidaka, H. (1982) Ca^{2+}-phospholipid-dependent phosphorylation of smooth muscle myosin. *Biochem. Biophys. Res. Commun.*, 105: 942–948.

Exton, J.H. (1985) Mechanisms involved in α_1-adrenergic phenomena. *Am. J. Physiol.*, 248:E633–E647.

Farley, J.M. and Miles, P.R. (1978) The sources of calcium for acetylcholine-induced contractions of dog tracheal smooth muscle. *J. Pharmacol. Exp. Ther.*, 207:340–346.

Fisher, S.K., Klinger, P.D. and Agranoff, B.W. (1983) Muscarinic agonists binding and phospholipid turnover in brain. *J. Biol. Chem.*, 258:7358–7363.

Fisher, S.K., Rooijen, L.A.A. and Agranoff, B.W. (1984) Renewed interest in the polyphosphoinositides. *Trends Biochem. Sci.*, 9:53–56.

Gispen, W.H., Van Dongen, C.J., De Graan, P.N.E., Oestreicher, A.B. and Zwiers, H. (1985) The role of phosphoprotein B-50 in phosphoinositide metabolism in brain synaptic plasma membranes. In J.E. Bleasdale, J. Eichberg and G. Hauser (Eds.), *Inositol and Phosphoinositides: Metabolism and Regulation*, Humana Press, Clifton, NJ, pp. 399–414.

Goy, M.F., Schwarz, T.L. and Kravitz, E.A. (1984) Serotonin-induced protein phosphorylation in a lobster neuromuscular preparation. *J. Neurosci.*, 4:611–626.

Grimes, M.J., Abdel-Latif, A.A. and Carrier, G.O. (1979) Kinetic studies on dose–triphosphoinositide responses and dose–contraction responses in rabbit iris. *Biochem. Pharmacol.*, 28:3213–3219.

Grover, A.K. and Daniel, E.E. (Eds.) (1985) *Calcium and Contractility*, Humana Press, Clifton, NJ.

Hawthorne, J.N. (1983) Polyphosphoinositide metabolism in excitable membranes. *Biosci. Rep.*, 3:887–904.

Ikebe, M., Inagaki, M., Kanamaru, K. and Hidaka, H. (1985) Phosphorylation of smooth muscle light chain kinase by Ca^{2+}-activated, phospholipid-dependent protein kinase. *J. Biol. Chem.*, 260:4547–4550.

Irvine, R.F., Auggard, E.E., Letcher, A.J. and Downes, C.P. (1985) Metabolism of inositol 1,4,5-trisphosphate and inositol 1,3,4-trisphosphate in rat parotid glands. *Biochem. J.*, 229:505–511.

Jolles, J., Zwiers, H., Dekker, A., Wirtz, K.W.A. and Gispen, W.H. (1981) Corticotropin-(1-24)-tetracosapeptide affects protein phosphorylation and polyphosphoinositide metabolism in rat brain. *Biochem. J.*, 194:283–291.

Kern, R. (1970) Die adrenergischen receptoren der intraocularen muskeln des menschen. *Albrecht V. Graefes Arch. Klin. Exp. Ophthalmol.*, 180:231–248.

Laemmli, U.K. (1970) Cleavage of structural proteins during the assembly of the head of bacteriophage T_4. *Nature*, 227:680–685.

Lowry, O.H., Rosebrough, N.J., Farr, A.L. and Randall, R.J. (1951) Protein measurement with the Folin phenol reagent. *J. Biol. Chem.*, 193:265–275.

Marx, J.L. (1984) A new view of receptor action. *Science*, 224:271–274.

Marx, J.L. (1985) The polyphosphoinositides revisited. *Science*, 228:312–313.

Michell, R.H., Kirk, C.J., Jones, L.M., Downes, C.P. and Creba, J.A. (1981) Stimulation of inositol lipid metabolism that accompanies calcium mobilization in stimulated cells: defined characteristics and unanswered questions. *Phil. Trans. R. Soc. London Ser. B*, 296:132–137.

Nishikawa, M., Hidaka, H. and Adelstein, R.S. (1983) Phosphorylation of smooth muscle heavy meromyosin by Ca^{2+}-activated, phospholipid-dependent protein kinase. *J. Biol. Chem.*, 258:14069–14072.

Nishizuka, Y. (1984) Turnover of inositol phospholipids and signal transduction. *Science*, 225:1365–1370.

Page, E.D. and Neufeld, A.H. (1978) Characterization of alpha- and beta-adrenergic receptors in membranes prepared from the rabbit iris before and after development of supersensitivity. *Biochem. Pharmacol.*, 27:953–958.

Persson, H. and Sonmark, B. (1971) Adrenoceptors and cholinoceptors in the rabbit iris. *Eur. J. Pharmacol.*, 15:240–244.

Ramos, K., Gerthoffer, W.T. and Westfall, D.P. (1986) Denervation-induced supersensitivity to calcium of chemically skinned smooth muscle of the guinea-pig vas deferens. *J. Pharmacol. Exp. Ther.*, 236:80–84.

Ruegg, J.C. (1982) Vascular smooth muscle: intracellular aspects of adrenergic receptor contraction coupling. *Experientia*, 38:1400–1404.

Silver, P.J. and Stull, J.T. (1984) Phosphorylation of myosin light chain and phosphorylase in tracheal smooth muscle in response to KCl and carbachol. *Mol. Pharmacol.*, 25:267–274.

Taft, W.C., Abdel-Latif, A.A. and Akhtar, R.A. (1980) [^{3}H]Quinuclidinyl benzilate binding to muscarinic receptors and [^{3}H]-WB-4101 binding to alpha-adrenergic receptors in rabbit iris. *Biochem. Pharmacol.*, 29:2713–2720.

Takenawa, T., Masaki, T. and Goto, K. (1983) Increase in norepinephrine-induced formation of phosphatidic acid in rat vas deferens after denervation. *J. Biochem.*, 92:303–306.

Van Alphen, G.W.H.M. (1976) The adrenergic receptors of the interocular muscles of the human eye. *Invest. Ophthalmol.*, 15:502–505.

Van Breemen, C., Aaronson, P., Cauvin, C., Loutzenhiser, R., Mangel, A. and Saida, K. (1982) Plasmalemmal calcium movements and the calcium cycle in arterial smooth muscle. In S.F. Flain and R. Zelis (Eds.), *Calcium Blockers – Mechanism of Action and Clinical Applications*, Urban and Schwarzenberg, Baltimore, MD, pp. 53–63.

Van Dongen, C.J., Zwiers, H., De Graan, P.N.E. and Gispen, W.H. (1985) Modulation of the activity of purified PIP kinase by phosphorylated and dephosphorylated B-50 protein. *Biochem. Biophys. Res. Commun.*, 128:1219–1227.

Villalobos-Molina, R., Mirna, U.C., Hong, E. and Garcia-Sainz, J.A. (1982) Correlation between phosphatidylinositol labeling and contraction in rabbit aorta: effect of alpha-1 adrenergic activation. *J. Pharmacol. Exp. Ther.*, 222: 258–261.

Weiss, G.B. (1982) Calcium release and accumulation at

cellular sites and compartments in vascular smooth muscle. In S.F. Flain and R. Zelis (Eds.), *Calcium Blockers – Mechanism of Action and Clinical Applications*, Urban and Schwarzenberg, Baltimore, MD, pp. 65–76.

Westfall, D.P. (1981) Supersensitivity of smooth muscle. In E. Bulbring, A.F. Brading, A.W. Jones and T. Tomita (Eds.), *Smooth Muscle – An Assessment of Current Knowledge*, University of Texas Press, Austin, TX, pp. 285–309.

Wilson, D.B., Bross, T.E., Sherman, W.R., Berger, R.A. and Majerus, P.W. (1985) Inositol cyclic phosphates are pro-duced by cleavage of phosphatidylinositols (polyphos-phoinositides) with purified sheep seminal vesicle phos-pholipase C enzymes. *Proc. Natl. Acad. Sci. USA*, 82:4013–4017.

Wong, S.K., Westfall, D.P., Fedan, J.S. and Fleming, W.W. (1981) The involvement of the sodium-potassium pump in post-junctional supersensitivity and the guinea-pig vas deferens as assessed by [^{3}H]ouabain binding. *J. Pharmacol. Exp. Ther.* 219:163–69.

W.H. Gispen and A. Routtenberg (Eds.)
Progress in Brain Research, Vol. 69
© 1986 Elsevier Science Publishers B.V. (Biomedical Division)

CHAPTER 6

Pharmacological aspects of the inositide response in the central nervous system: the muscarinic acetylcholine receptor

Lucio A.A. Van Rooijen, Wolfgang U. Dompert, Ervin Horváth, David G. Spencer Jr. and Jörg Traber

Neurobiology Department, Troponwerke GmbH & Co. KG, Neurather Ring 1, 5000 Cologne 80, F.R.G.

Introduction

Receptor-sensitive operation of the inositide cycle (Fig. 1) constitutes a second messenger system with rapidly growing experimental support and physiological implications. Inositide turnover is involved in the release of free fatty acids (mainly arachidonate), intracellular mobilization of Ca^{2+}, and activation of protein kinase C (for reviews: Irvine, 1982; Abdel-Latif, 1983; Fisher et al., 1984a; Berridge, 1984; Nishizuka, 1984).

Several neurotransmitter receptors have been investigated in the central nervous system in regard to their linkage to the inositide cycle (Table I). For most neurotransmitters different receptor types or subtypes can be identified pharmacologically. Since fairly selective antagonists and agonists are available for the definition of adrenergic and histaminergic receptor subtypes, it was shown that α_1- and H_1-receptors, respectively, mediate the enhancement of inositide turnover (see Table I for references). In two other receptor systems, serotonin (5-HT) and acetylcholine (ACh), contradictory results have been reported. The $5-HT_1$-selective agonists 8-hydroxy-2-(di-*n*-propylamino-tetralin) (Kendall and Nahorski, 1985) and RU 24969 (Godfrey et al., 1985) appeared not to be effective in enhancing inositide turnover in cerebral cortex slices, whereas the $5-HT_2$-selective antagonist ketanserin potently inhibited the

inositide response to serotonin (Conn and Sanders-Bush, 1984; Kendall and Nahorski, 1985). However, no close correlation of the potency of various antagonists to inhibit this inositide response and high affinity [³H]ketanserin binding

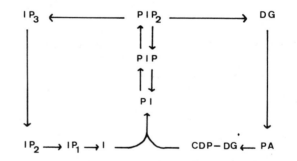

Fig. 1. Receptor-sensitive inositide cycle. Phosphatidylinositol 4,5-bisphosphate (PIP_2) is phosphodiesteratically degraded to yield diacylglycerol (DG) and *myo*-inositol 1,4,5-trisphosphate (IP_3). This step is presumed to be activated by appropriate receptor–ligand interaction. DG is phosphorylated to phosphatidic acid (PA) which is then converted through cytidine diphosphodiacylglycerol (CDP-DG) to phosphatidylinositol (PI). PI can be phosphorylated twice to phosphatidylinositol 4-phosphate (PIP) and PIP_2 sequentially. On the other hand IP_3 is degraded by specific phosphatases, through *myo*-inositol 1,4-bisphosphate (IP_2) and *myo*-inositol 1-monophosphate (IP_1) to *myo*-inositol (I). I is then exchanged with cytidine monophosphate in the conversion of CDP-DG to PI. Only the conversions which are essential for the cycling have been shown. For discussion of the other enzymic events and implications we refer to reviews mentioned in the text.

TABLE I

Neurotransmitter receptor coupled to the inositide cycle in preparations of the central nervous system

Receptor type	Reference
Adrenergic (α_1)	Hokin, 1969; Brown et al., 1984; Janowsky, 1984a, 1984b; Kendall et al., 1984; Minneman and Johnson, 1984; Schoepp et al., 1984
Acetylcholine	Hokin and Hokin, 1953; Durell et al., 1968; Schacht and Agranoff, 1972; Abdel-Latif et al., 1977; Miller, 1977; Griffin et al., 1979; Yandrasitz and Segal, 1979; Fisher and Agranoff, 1980, 1981; Aly and Abdel-Latif, 1982; Berridge et al., 1982; Downes, 1982; Brown et al., 1984; Janowsky et al., 1984b; Kendall and Nahorski, 1984; Labarca et al., 1984; Van Rooijen et al., 1985
M_1 or M_2	Fisher et al., 1983, 1984b; Gonzales and Crews, 1984; Brown et al., 1985; Gil and Wolfe, 1985; Jacobsen et al., 1985; Lazareno et al. 1985
Histamine (H_1)	Daum et al., 1983; Brown et al., 1984; Daum et al., 1984; Kendall and Nahorski, 1984
Serotonin	Berridge et al., 1982; Brown et al., 1984; Kendall and Nahorski, 1984
$5\text{-}HT_1$ or $5\text{-}HT_2$	Berridge et al., 1982; Conn and Sanders-Bush, 1984; Janowsky et al., 1984b; Kendall and Nahorski, 1985; Godfrey et al., 1985

could be found (Kendall and Nahorski, 1985). At present it is not clear which 5-HT receptor type mediates the inositide response to serotonin.

The inositide-response to ACh is mediated through the muscarinic and not the nicotinic receptor type. Of all neurotransmitter receptors, the muscarinic ACh receptor (mAChR) has been most intensively studied for its coupling to the inositide cycle. Already in 1953 Hokin and Hokin (1953) reported that carbamylcholine (CCh) enhanced the incorporation of ^{32}P into the lipid-fraction (selectively phosphatidic acid (PA) and phosphatidylinositol (PI)) from pancreas slices. This finding initiated research into the inositide response. Later

it was postulated that the observations reflected receptor-mediated enhancement of the operation of an inositide cycle (Hokin and Hokin, 1964; Durell et al., 1969). Only recently however, have the polyphosphoinositides become implicated in the inositide response (Abdel-Latif et al., 1977; Fisher and Agranoff, 1980, 1981). In 1975, Michell (1975) described the correlation between the inositide response to receptor activation, and several Ca^{2+}-dependent events, such as smooth muscle contraction or vesicular secretion. Discoveries of the past four years (Castagna et al., 1982; Berridge et al., 1982; Berridge, 1983; Streb et al., 1983) have particularly facilitated the understanding of the role of the inositide cycle in the cellular response to receptor activation as alluded to in the first paragraph. In the central nervous system, the inositide response forms one of the few known biochemical responses to receptor activation.

The mAChR is heterogenous (for review: Hirshowitz et al., 1983; Sokolovski et al., 1983). First, competition experiments with [^{3}H]antagonists and unlabeled ligands and experiments with [^{3}H]agonists revealed different affinity sites of the mAChR. For instance, Birdsall and Hulme (1983) found three separate receptor affinities for CCh, which were termed superhigh, high and low affinity sites. The second mAChR-classification originated in studies on the opossum lower esophageal spincter (Goyal et al., 1978; Gilbert et al., 1984). The mAChR agonist McNeil A 343 (McN) caused relaxation of the muscle through activation of a neuronal mAChR, termed M_1AChR. The mAChR agonist bethanechol caused contraction through activation of a smooth muscle mAChR, termed the M_2AChR. The mAChR antagonist pirenzepine (PZ) selectively inhibited the response to McN. The third line of evidence indicating heterogeneity of the mAChR consists of observations that, in contrast to the mAChR-affinities for non-selective antagonists such as N-methyl-scopolamine, quinuclidinyl benzilate, and atropine, the mAChR-affinities for PZ differ between different tissues and brain structures (Hammer et al., 1980; Birdsall and Hulme, 1983; Garvey et al., 1984; Wamsley et al., 1984; Spencer et al., 1985).

Recently several studies have focussed on the

determination of which mAChR subtype is coupled to the inositide cycle. Analysis of an inositide response to CCh in different brain regions showed that the magnitude of the response was qualitatively related to the putative occurrence of M_1AChR rather than of M_2AChR (Gonzales and Crews, 1984; Jacobson et al., 1985; Lazareno et al., 1985). However, as Downes and colleagues concluded (Jacobson et al., 1985), this approach is not without difficulties, since we know little about the metabolic properties and the receptor–inositide coupling in different brain areas. Another approach employs ligands with differential selectivities for the mAChR subtypes. In this respect, both PZ (M_1AChR; Gonzales and Crews, 1984; Brown et al., 1985; Gil and Wolfe, 1985; Lazareno et al., 1985) and oxotremorine (M_2AChR; Fisher et al., 1983, 1984b; Jacobson et al., 1985) have been shown to alter inositide turnover. Interestingly, oxotremorine and its analog oxotremorine-M (OXO-M) acted as a partial agonist–antagonist and a full agonist respectively. Unfortunately, most mAChR ligands have only a relatively small preference for one of the two receptor subtypes. It is therefore necessary that the relative potencies and efficacies of several ligands on inositide turnover are evaluated and compared with their affinities to mAChR subtypes. Such analysis has, however, not been done to date. It was the aim of the current study to quantitatively compare M_1AChR and M_2AChR affinity for various agonists and antagonists with their potency and efficacy in the inositide response. It was hoped that this approach would provide insight in the mAChR subtype coupling to the inositide cycle.

Methodology

Preparation of neuronal process endings

Neuronal process endings (NPE) were prepared by differential and sucrose gradient centrifugation. Briefly, following decapitation, rat (male Wistar, 180–250 g; Winkelmann, Borchen, F.R.G.) forebrain was rapidly removed and placed in 9 vol of 0.32 M sucrose. Following homogenization (10 strokes, 1200 rpm, Potter–Elvehjem) the material

was centrifuged for 10 min at $1000 \times g$ (Sorvall, SS-34 rotor). The supernatant was collected and the pellet was centrifuged again after rehomogenization (4 strokes) in 5 vol of 0.32 M sucrose. The combined supernatants were centrifuged for 20 min at $10\,000 \times g$ (Sorvall, SS-34 rotor). The resulting supernatant was discarded and the pellet, resuspended in 0.32 M sucrose, was layered on top of a discontinuous gradient consisting of 15 ml 1.2 M and 15 ml 0.8 M sucrose. Following centrifugation at 23 500 rpm (Beckman SW 28 rotor) the 0.8:1.2 M interface was collected.

After dilution of the interface with 1 vol of 0.16 M sucrose, NPE were pelleted by centrifugation for 45 min at $27\,000 \times g$ (Sorvall SS-34) and resuspended in buffer A (30 mM HEPES, 142 mM NaCl, 5.6 mM KCl, 1.0 mM $MgCl_2$, 2.2 mM $CaCl_2$, 3.6 mM $NaHCO_3$, 5.6 mM glucose; pH 7.4). All treatments were carried out at 0–4°C.

For analysis of ligand-binding, NPE were frozen in liquid nitrogen and stored (less than 2 weeks) until use. For analysis of the phospholipid labeling effect, freshly prepared NPE were used.

Binding of [³H]pirenzepine or [³H]oxotremorine-M

Following storage in liquid nitrogen, NPE were thawed and diluted about 10-fold with buffer B (50 mM sodium, potassium, phosphate buffer, pH 7.4) for [³H]PZ or buffer C (20 mM HEPES/Tris, pH 7.4; 10 mM $MgCl_2$) for [³H]OXO-M binding. Following homogenization, the material was centrifuged for 30 min at $20\,000 \times g$ (Sorvall, SS-34 rotor). The supernatant was discarded and the pellet resuspended in the same buffer. For [³H]PZ binding, 200–250 µg of protein was incubated for 60 min in a final volume of 0.5 ml of buffer B in the presence of 0.9–1.0 nM [³H]PZ and various compounds as indicated. The incubations were terminated by the addition of 5 ml of buffer B, followed by rapid filtration through Whatman GF/C filters (Kontron, Eching, F.R.G.) under suction. Tube and filter were rinsed with another 5 ml of buffer B. For [³H]OXO-M binding, 200–250 µg of protein was preincubated for 30 min at 30°C. Then ligands were added and the incubation was continued for an additional 30 min at 30°C in a final volume of

0.5 ml of buffer C in the presence of 2.3–2.7 nM [³H]OXO-M and various compounds as indicated. The incubations were terminated by the addition of 3 ml of buffer C followed by rapid filtration through Whatman GF/C filters under suction. The tube and filter was rinsed twice with 3 ml of buffer C. The radiotracer retained on the filters was quantified by scintillation counting in 3 ml Quickszint 402 (Zinsser Analytic, Frankfurt, F.R.G.) in a Beckman LS 9000 scintillation counter (counting efficiency 45%).

Phospholipid labeling effect

NPE (about 0.7 mg of protein) were incubated in a final volume of 0.5 ml buffer A for 30 min at 37°C in a water bath with shaking. During the incubation, various ligands and 10–20 µCi of $^{32}P_i$ (carrier free) were also present. The incubation was terminated by the addition of 1.5 ml of chloroform:methanol (1:2, v/v) and tubes were placed on ice.

Phospholipids were extracted under acidic conditions. Material was allowed to remain on ice for 15 min–15 h, after which it was brought to room temperature. 1 ml of chloroform and 0.5 ml of 2.4 N HCl were added, material thoroughly mixed, and phases were allowed to separate. The lower, organic phase was transferred to a separate tube containing 1 ml of chloroform:methanol:0.6 N HCl (3:48:47, v/v). After mixing and separation of the phases, the upper aqueous layer was aspirated and the organic layer washed one more time with 1 ml of the chloroform:methanol:0.6 N HCl. An aliquot was taken from the organic phase to establish recovery and tubes were dried under nitrogen at 40–45°C. The remaining material was taken up in 60 µl of chloroform:methanol:H_2O (75:25:2, v/v) and spotted on 1.2% K-oxalate-impregnated thin-layer chromatography plates (Merck, Darmstadt, F.R.G.; silica gel 60, 20 × 20 × 0.025 cm). Phospholipids were separated using the solvent chloroform:acetone:methanol:acetic acid:H_2O (40:15:13:12:7, v/v). Following localization by iodine staining and autoradiography, labeled bands were scraped off, and radiotracer was quantitated by scintillation counting in Quickszint 501 in a Beckman LS 9000 scintillation counter.

Other assays and chemicals

Protein content was determined spectrophotometrically (Bradford, 1976) using bovine serum albumin as standard. EC_{50} and IC_{50} values were determined geometrically.

OXO-M was a generous gift of Dr. B. Ringdahl (UCLA, Los Angeles, CA, U.S.A.). McN was a generous gift of McNeil Pharmaceutical (Spring House, PA, U.S.A.). $^{32}P_i$ (carrier free; Amersham, Braunschweig, F.R.G.), [³H]PZ, [³H]OXO-M (New England Nuclear, Dreieich, F.R.G.), PZ (diHCl; Thomae, Biberach an der Riss, F.R.G.), SCOP (HCl), CCh (Cl) (Sigma, Taufkirchen, F.R.G.) and all other chemicals were at least reagent grade and obtained through commercial sources.

Agonist binding and inositide response

Analysis of mAChR binding of M_1- and M_2-selective ligands was developed for rat forebrain NPE. Scatchard analysis revealed a K_D of 11.7 ± 1.2 (SEM, $n = 3$ experiments) and 5.15 (4.9 and 5.4, $n = 2$) nM for [³H]PZ and [³H]OXO-M binding, respectively. The total amount of binding sites for [³H]PZ was 1.1 ± 0.01 (SEM, $n = 3$) pmol/mg protein. For [³H]OXO-M a smaller B_{max} was found, being 0.44 (0.37 and 0.50, $n = 2$) pmol/mg protein. These values correspond to previously reported data on other cerebral preparations (Yamamura et al., 1983; Bevan, 1984; Luthin and Wolfe, 1984a; 1984b).

Three agonists were selectively chosen for analysis and comparison of binding to the M_1- and M_2AChR with the enhancement of inositide turnover. The metabolism-resistant ACh-analog CCh was selected since, next to ACh it is the most extensively documented mAChR agonist employed for studies on inositide turnover. McN and OXO-M were selected as M_1- and M_2AChR selective agonists, respectively.

Competition of the three agonists for high affinity binding of [³H]PZ (M_1AChR) and

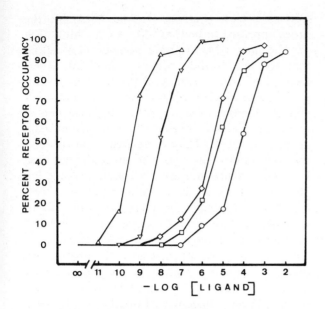

Fig. 2. Ligand affinity of M₁AChR. Displacement by various ligands of high affinity-binding of [³H]PZ to NPE was analyzed as described in the methodology. Data represent means (SEM < 5%) derived from two or three independent experiments each performed in triplicate. Various ligands used were: SCOP (△), PZ (▽), McN (◇), OXO-M (□) and CCh (○).

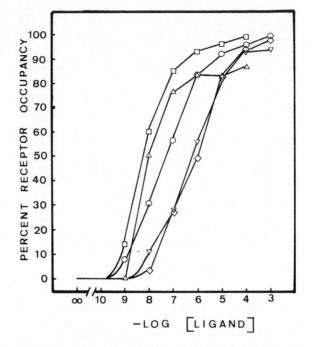

Fig. 3. Ligand affinity of the M₂AChR. Displacement by various ligands of high affinity binding of [³H]OXO-M to NPE was analyzed as described in the methodology. Data represent means (range < 10%) derived from two independent experiments each performed in triplicate. Various ligands used were: OXO-M (□), SCOP (△), CCh (○), PZ (▽) and McN (◇).

[³H]OXO-M (M₂AChR) is shown in Figs. 2 and 3, respectively. 50% inhibition of [³H]PZ-binding by OXO-M, CCh and McN was obtained at 6.3, 79 and 3.2 μM concentration, respectively. Similar values have previously been reported for CCh (Luthin and Wolfe, 1984; Yamamura et al., 1985) and for McN (Luthin and Wolfe, 1984). Higher affinities have been reported for oxotremorine (Luthin and Wolfe, 1984; Yamamura et al., 1985) than for OXO-M which is not surprising since oxotremorine was also more potent than OXO-M to displace [³H]quinuclidinyl benzylate binding to NPE (Fisher et al., 1984b; 1985). 50% inhibition of [³H]OXO-M binding by OXO-M, CCh and McN was reached with 6, 50 and 1000 nM concentrations, respectively. Similar values have been found for displacement of high affinity [³H]OXO-M binding by CCh and oxotremorine (Bevan, 1984). Unfortunately, we know of no comparable data for McN. The agonist OXO-M is clearly selective for M₂AChR as it was about 1000× as potent in inhibiting [³H]OXO-M-binding than that of

[³H]PZ. CCh also showed preference for the M₂AChR with about 1000-fold higher potency. Interestingly these data indicate that McN is not selective for binding to the M₁- or M₂AChR.

Addition of OXO-M, CCh and McN to an incubation of NPE with ³²Pᵢ resulted in a dose-dependent stimulation of the labeling of PA and PI. Stimulation of the labeling of PA was used as a parameter for the effect of mAChR-activation of the inositide cycle, since it is directly subsequent to the generation of DG (cf. Fig. 1). For OXO-M and CCh, which could almost double the radiotracer in PA, EC₅₀ values of 1×10^{-5} M and 7.1×10^{-5} M (Fig. 4), respectively, were determined. These data are in full accordance with other reports of studies in which slices or NPE, derived from rat or guinea pig forebrain or cerebral cortex, were stimulated with CCh and OXO-

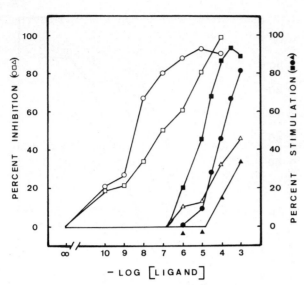

Fig. 4. Agonism and antagonism on the inositide response. Various ligands were tested for their agonistic and antagonistic properties on the inositide response. NPE were incubated in the presence of $^{32}P_i$ and various concentrations of ligands indicated, and phospholipid labeling was analyzed as described in methodology. The results on the labeling of PA are shown. Data represent means (SEM <10%) of values from two independent experiments each performed in duplicate or triplicate. As agonists OXO-M (■), CCh (●) and McN (▲) were analyzed. Antagonists analyzed in the presence of 1 mM CCh, were SCOP (○), PZ (□) and McN (△). In the absence of CCh. SCOP and PZ were ineffective.

M, using either [^{32}P]PA or [^{3}H]inositol phosphates as the measure (Downes, 1982; Fisher et al., 1983; 1984a; 1984b; Gonzales and Crews, 1984; Jacobson et al., 1985). McN also stimulated labeling but appeared much less potent and efficacious. At 10^{-3} M, only a 33% stimulation was seen as compared to the more than 80% stimulation elicited by OXO-M and CCh at this concentration. 50% of the maximal effect (at 10^{-3} M) was reached at about 1.3×10^{-4} M McN (Fig. 4). In the parotid gland a similar small effect of McN was also reported for [^{3}H]inositol phosphate production (Gil and Wolfe, 1985).

With different methods of analysis of receptor properties employed, it is difficult to compare absolute potencies. We have therefore analyzed the potencies of the three agonists relative to each other. Displacement of high affinity [^{3}H]PZ binding (M_1) established a potency order of McN ≃

OXO-M > CCh (Fig. 2). On the M_2AChR this order appeared to be OXO-M > CCh > McN (Fig. 3). The latter (M_2) relative potency best reflects that for an inositide response analyzed as enhancement of the labeling of PA (Fig. 4).

Fisher et al. (1983) identified a high and a low affinity binding site for the displacement of [^{3}H]quinuclidinyl benzilate by various mAChR agonists in NPE. They correlated occupation of the low affinity site with the inositide response. Further evidence indicating a coupling of the low affinity mAChR to the inositide cycle is indirect. Guanine nucleotides convert a high affinity mAChR binding site into a low affinity mAChR binding site (Sokolovski et al., 1980; Hulme et al., 1983; Bevan, 1984). Furthermore, the involvement of a GTP-binding protein in the receptor-mediated enhancement of inositide turnover has recently been suggested (Litosch et al., 1985; Verghese et al., 1985). While the guanine nucleotide effect was studied mostly with M_2AChR and non-selective mAChR ligands, alteration of the M_1AChR affinity seems unlikely (Ehlert et al., 1980; Aronstam et al., 1985). Covalent modification of the mAChR in brain with the alkylating agent N-ethylmaleimide (NEM) has just been shown to decrease the affinity for the M_2AChR-agonist OXO-M but not that for the M_1AChR-selective PZ (Flynn and Potter, 1985). In accordance, we have observed that concurrent exposure to NEM decreases the high affinity binding of [^{3}H]OXO-M but not of [^{3}H]PZ to cerebral brain slices, analyzed by autoradiography (Horvath et al., 1986). When NEM was employed with inositide response to CCh, we found that a low concentration of NEM caused a vast enhancement of the CCh-induced stimulation of labeling of PA (Table II). The NEM effects on mAChR binding (above) and on CCh-induced enhancement PA labeling (Table II) suggest coupling of the low affinity M_2AChR to the inositide response. Further experimental data are obviously required to test this notion.

Antagonist binding and inositide response

Three antagonists were analyzed for comparison of binding to the M_1- and M_2AChR with the

TABLE II

Effect of NEM on the enhancement of labeling of PA by CCh

NEM (M)	CCh (M)		
	10^{-5}	10^{-4}	10^{-3}
0	106	152	176
3×10^{-5}	129	176	216

NPE were incubated in the presence of $^{32}P_i$ and various concentrations of NEM and CCh indicated, and phospholipid labeling was analyzed as described in methodology. The results on the labeling of PA are shown and are expressed as % of control without CCh (100%). NEM alone only slightly (7%) decreased the basal labeling. Data are from one experiment in duplicate. Similar results were obtained in two other independent experiments.

inhibition of the inosamide response to CCh. Scopolamine (SCOP) and PZ were chosen as nonselective and M_1-specific antagonists, respectively. In addition, since the putative M_1AChR agonist McN appeared to also have antagonistic properties on the inosamide response to CCh (Fig. 4), it was also taken up in the comparison here. PZ indeed appeared more selective for M_1-sites as compared to M_2-sites (Fig. 2, 3). 50% inhibition of [^{3}H]PZ binding by SCOP and PZ was reached at 0.4 and 9 nM, respectively. These values correspond closely to those previously reported (Luthin and Wolfe, 1984; Yamamura et al., 1985). [^{3}H]OXO-M binding was 50% inhibited by 10 and 560 nM concentrations of SCOP and PZ, respectively, which is in accordance with the values reported by Bevan (1984). Comparing the potencies of SCOP, PZ and McN revealed the following ranking order: SCOP > PZ ≫ McN at the M_1AChR and SCOP > PZ = McN at the M_2AChR.

SCOP, PZ and McN were also tested for inhibition of the enhancement of inosamide turnover by 1 mM CCh (Fig. 4). Both SCOP and PZ could fully inhibit the CCh effect. 50% inhibition was reached at 3.5 and 100 nM concentration of SCOP and PZ, respectively. McN caused an almost 50% inhibition at the highest concentration (10^{-3} M) tested (Fig. 4). 50% of the maximal inhibitory effect was reached at about 4×10^{-5} M McN. A potency ranking order can be established as SCOP > PZ ≫ McN. Our data closely correspond to previously reported potencies of PZ to inhibit the inosamide response to CCh in cerebral preparations (Gonzales and Crews, 1984; Gil and Wolfe, 1985; Lazareno et al., 1985). In cerebral cortex slices 1 µM SCOP also fully inhibited the response to CCh (Gonzales and Crews, 1984). To our knowledge, a potency of SCOP and McN to inhibit the muscarinic inosamide effect in a cerebral preparation has until now not been established. In parotid glands (Gil and Wolfe, 1985), the CCh-stimulated production of [^{3}H]inositol phosphates was reported to be inhibited by SCOP, PZ and McN at potencies comparable to those observed in the present study. We attempted to relate the potencies of mAChR-antagonists to inhibit the inosamide response to CCh with the apparent M_1- and M_2AChR affinities. A CCh equi-affinity was estimated by dividing the IC_{50} values for the antagonist and CCh on mAChR binding and multiplying this fraction with the concentration of CCh used to stimulate labeling of PA. For SCOP, PZ and McN these values are 5, 114 and 40 000 nM, respectively, when the data from the [^{3}H]PZ-binding experiments were used. Using the data from the [^{3}H]OXO-M-binding experiments, these values are 0.2, 11.2 and 20 mM respectively. When the IC_{50} values of these antagonists to inhibit the CCh-stimulated labeling of PA are compared with the above values, it is apparent that the CCh equi-affinity estimates at the M_1AChR give the best fit. Interestingly, when such calculations were made for oxotremorine, using data reported for [^{3}H]PZ-binding ($IC_{50} = 237$ and 33 000 nM for oxotremorine and CCh, respectively; Yamamura et al., 1985) and for [^{3}H]OXO-M-binding ($K_i = 4$ and 170 nM for oxotremorine and CCh, respectively; Bevan, 1984), values of about 7200 and 23 500 nM were obtained through the M_1- and M_2AChR, respectively. The IC_{50} for oxotremorine on CCh-stimulated PA labeling in NPE is about 3000 nM (Fisher et al., 1984b). Taken together, these data indicate that antagonism of the inositide response to CCh most likely corresponds with occupation of the M_1AChR.

Conclusions

Affinities of various mAChR ligands to the M_1- and M_2AChR were compared with their potency to either evoke or inhibit an inositide response in rat forebrain NPE. Potencies of mAChR antagonist to inhibit the inositide response to CCh corresponded best with ligand affinities for the M_1AChR. Potencies of mAChR agonists to evoke an inositide response corresponded best with ligand affinities for the M_2AChR. The latter was further supported by the fact that NEM, which specifically lowers the affinity of the M_2AChR, enhances the inositide effect to CCh. Further study is required to elucidate unequivocal determination of which mAChR subtype is preferentially coupled to the inositide cycle, and in which manner.

Acknowledgements

We wish to thank Ms. C. Duchstein, W. Scheip, M. Schwiertz and M. Wiertellorz for their technical assistance and Ms. H. Wodarz for typing the manuscript.

References

Abdel-Latif, A. (1983) Metabolism of phosphoinositides. In Lajtha, A. (ed.) *Handbook of Neurochemistry, Vol. 3,* Plenum Press, New York, pp. 91–131.

Abdel-Latif, A.A., Akhtar, R.A. and Hawthorne, J.N. (1977) Acetylcholine increases the breakdown of triphosphoinositide of rabbit iris muscle prelabeled with [^{32}P]-phosphate. *Biochem. J.,* 161:61–73.

Aly, M.I. and Abdel-Latif, A.A. (1982) Studies on the effects of acetylcholine and antiepileptic drugs on ^{32}P$_i$ incorporation into phospholipids of rat brain synaptosomes. *Neurochem. Res.,* 7:159–169.

Aronstam, R.S., Kirby, M.I. and Smith, M.D. (1985) Muscarinic acetylcholine receptors in chick heart: influence of heat and N-etylmaleimide on receptor conformations and interactions with guanine nucleotide-dependent regulatory proteins. *Neurosci. Lett.,* 54:289–294.

Berridge, M.J. (1983) Rapid accumulation of inositol trisphosphate reveals that agonists hydrolyze polyphosphoinositides instead of phosphatidylinositol. *Biochem. J.,* 212:849–858.

Berridge, M.J. (1984) Inositol trisphosphate and diacylglycerol as second messenger. *Biochem. J.,* 220:345–360.

Berridge, M.J., Downes, C.P. and Hanley, M.R. (1982) Lithium amplifies agonist-dependent phosphatidylinositol responses in brain and salivary glands. *Biochem. J.,* 206:587–595.

Bevan, P. (1984) [^{3}H]-Oxotremorine-M binding to membranes prepared from rat brain and heart: evidence for subtypes of muscarinic receptors. *Eur. J. Pharmacol.,* 101:101–110.

Birdsall, N.J.M. and Hulme, E.C. (1983) Muscarinic receptor subclasses. *Trends Pharmacol. Sci.,* 4:459–463.

Bradford, M. (1976) A rapid and sensitive method for the quantitation of microgram quantities of protein utilizing the principle of protein–dye binding. *Anal. Biochem.,* 72:248–254.

Brown, E., Kendall, D.A. and Nahorski, S.R. (1984) Inositol phospholipid hydrolysis in rat cerebral cortical slices. I. Receptor characterisation. *J. Neurochem.,* 42:1379–1387.

Brown, J.H., Goldstein, D. and Brown-Masters, S. (1985) The putative M_1 muscarinic receptor does not regulate phosphoinositide hydrolysis. *Mol. Pharmacol.,* 27:525–531.

Castagna, M., Takai, Y., Kaibuchi, K., Sano, K., Kikkawa, U. and Nishizuka, Y. (1982) Direct activation of calcium-activated, phospholipid-dependent protein kinase by tumor promoting phorbol esters. *J. Biol. Chem.,* 257:7847–7851.

Conn, P.J. and Sanders-Bush, E. (1984) Selective 5HT-2 antagonists inhibit serotonin stimulated phosphatidylinositol metabolism in cerebral cortex. *Neuropharmacology,* 23:993–996.

Daum, P.R., Downes, C.P. and Young, J.M. (1983) Histamine-induced inositol phospholipid breakdown mirrors H_1-receptor density in brain. *Eur. J. Pharmacol.,* 87:497–498.

Daum, P.R., Downes, C.P. and Young, J.M. (1984) Histamine stimulation of inositol 1-phosphate accumulation in lithium-treated slices from regions of guinea pig brain. *J. Neurochem.,* 43:25–32.

Downes, C.P. (1982) Receptor-stimulated inositol phospholipid metabolism in the central nervous system. *Cell Calcium,* 3:413–428.

Durell, J., Sodd, M.A. and Friedel, R.O. (1968) Acetylcholine stimulation of the phosphodiesteratic cleavage of guinea pig brain phosphoinositides. *Life Sci.,* 7:363–368.

Durell, J., Garland, J.T. and Friedel, R.O. (1969) Acetylcholine action: biochemical aspects. *Science,* 165:862–866.

Ehlert, F.J., Roeske, W.R. and Yamamura, H.I. (1980) Regulation of muscarinic receptor binding by guanine nucleotides and N-ethylmaleimide. *J. Supramol. Struct.,* 14:149–162.

Fisher, S.K. and Agranoff, B.W. (1980) Calcium and the muscarinic phospholipid labeling effect. *J. Neurochem.,* 34:1231–1240.

Fisher, S.K. and Agranoff, B.W. (1981) Enhancement of the muscarinic synaptosomal phospholipid labeling effect by the ionophore A23187. *J. Neurochem.,* 37:968–977.

Fisher, S.K., Klinger, P.D. and Agranoff, B.W. (1983) Muscarinic agonist binding and phospholipid turnover in brain. *J. Biol. Chem.,* 258:7358–7363.

Fisher, S.K., Van Rooijen, L.A.A. and Agranoff, B.W. (1984a) Renewed interest in the polyphosphoinositides. *Trends Biochem. Sci.,* 9:53–56.

Fisher, S.K., Figueiredo, J.C. and Bartus, R.T. (1984b) Differential stimulation of inositol phospholipid turnover in brain by analogs of oxotremorine. *J. Neurochem.*, 43:1171–1179.

Flynn, D.D. and Potter, L.T. (1985) Different effects of N-ethylmaleimide on M1 and M2 muscarinic receptors in rat brain. *Proc. Natl. Acad. Sci. U.S.A.*, 82:580–583.

Garvey, J.M., Rossor, M. and Iversen, L.L. (1984) Evidence for multiple muscarinic receptor subtypes in human brain. *J. Neurochem.*, 43:299–302.

Gil, D.W. and Wolfe, B.B. (1985) Pirenzepine distinguishes between muscarinic receptor-mediated phosphoinositide breakdown and inhibition of adenylate cyclase. *J. Pharmacol. Exp. Ther.*, 232:608–616.

Gilbert, R., Rattan, S. and Goyal, R.K. (1984) Pharmacologic identification, activation and antagonism of two muscarinic receptors in the lower esophageal sphincter. *J. Pharmacol. Exp. Ther.*, 230:284–291.

Godfrey, P.P., McClue, S.J., Minchin, M.C.W. and Young, M. (1985) Ru 24969, a 5-HT$_1$ agonist, stimulates inositol phospholipid breakdown in rat brain slices. *Br. J. Pharmacol.*, 84:112.

Gonzales, R.A. and Crews, F.T. (1984) Characterization of the cholinergic stimulation of phosphoinositide hydrolysis in rat brain slices. *J. Neurosci.*, 4, 12:3120–3127.

Goyal, R.K. and Rattan, S. (1978) Neurohumoral, hormonal and drug receptors for the lower esophageal sphincter. *Gastroenterology*, 74:598–619.

Griffin, H.D., Hawthorne, J.N. and Sykes, M. (1979) A calcium requirement for the phosphatidylinositol response following activation of presynaptic muscarinic receptors. *Biochem. Pharmacol.*, 28:1143–1147.

Hammer, R., Berrie, C.P., Birdsall, N.J.M., Burgen, A.S.V. and Hulme, E.C. (1980) Pirenzepine distinguishes between different subclasses of muscarinic receptors. *Nature*, 283:90–92.

Hirshowitz, B.I., Hammer, R., Giachetti, A., Keirns, J.J. and Levine, R.R. (Eds.) (1983) Subtypes of muscarinic receptors. *Trends Pharmacol. Sci.*, (special issue) Elsevier, Amsterdam.

Hokin, M.R. (1969) Effect of norepinephrine on ^{32}P incorporation into individual phosphatides in slices from different areas of the guinea pig brain. *J. Neurochem.*, 16:127–134.

Hokin, M.R. and Hokin, L.E. (1953) Enzyme secretion and the incorporation of ^{32}P into phospholipids of pancreas slices. *J. Biol. Chem.*, 203:967–977.

Hokin, M.R. and Hokin, L.E. (1964) Interconversions of phosphatidylinositol and phosphatidic acid involved in the response to acetylcholine in the salt gland. In Dawson, R.M.C. and Rhodes, D.N. (Eds.) *Metabolism and Physiological Significance of Lipids*. John Wiley and Sons, New York, pp. 423–434.

Horváth, E., Van Rooijen, L.A.A., Traber, J. and Spencer, D.G. (1986) Effects of N-ethylmaleimide on muscarinic acetylcholine receptors subtype autoradiography and inositide response in rat brain. *Life Sci.* (in press).

Hulme, E.C., Berrie, C.P., Birdsall, N.J.M., Jameson, M. and Stockton, J.M. (1983) Regulation of muscarinic agonist binding by cations and guanine nucleotides. *Eur. J. Pharmacol.*, 94:59–72.

Irvine, R.F. (1982) How is the level of free arachidonic acid controlled in mammalian cells? *Biochem. J.*, 204:3–16.

Jacobson, M.D., Wüsteman, M. and Downes, C.P. (1985) Muscarinic receptors and hydrolysis of inositol phospholipids in rat cerebral cortex and parotid gland. *J. Neurochem.*, 44:465–472.

Janowsky, A., Labarca, R. and Paul, S.M. (1984a) Noradrenergic denervation increases α_1-adrenoreceptor-mediated inositol-phosphate accumulation in the hippocampus. *Eur. J. Pharmacol.*, 102:193–194.

Janowsky, A., Labarca, R. and Paul, S.M. (1984b) Characterization of neurotransmitter receptor-mediated phosphatidylinositol hydrolysis in the rat hippocampus. *Life Sci.*, 35: 1953–1961.

Kendall, D.A. and Nahorski, S.R. (1984) Inositol phospholipid hydrolysis in rat cerebral cortical slices. II. Calcium requirement. *J. Neurochem.*, 42:1388–1394.

Kendall, D.A. and Nahorski, S.R. (1985) 5-Hydroxytryptamine-stimulated inositol phospholipid hydrolysis in rat cerebral cortex slices: pharmacological characterization and effects of antidepressants. *J. Pharmacol. Exp. Ther.*, 233:473–479.

Labarca, R., Janowsky, A., Patel, J. and Paul, S.M. (1984) Phorbol esters inhibit agonist-induced ^{3}H-inositol-1-phosphate accumulation in rat hippocampus slices. *Biochem. Biophys. Res. Commun.*, 123:703–709.

Lazareno, S., Kendall, D.A. and Nahorski, S.R. (1985) Pirenzepine indicates heterogeneity of muscarinic receptors linked to cerebral inositol phospholipid metabolism. *Neuropharmacology*, 24:593–595.

Litosch, I., Wallis, C. and Fain, J.N. (1985) 5-Hydroxytryptamine stimulates inositol phosphate production in a cell free system from blowfly salivary glands. *J. Biol. Chem.*, 260:5464–5471.

Luthin, G.R. and Wolfe, B.B. (1984a) Comparison of [^{3}H]pirenzepine and [^{3}H]quinuclidinylbenzilate binding to muscarinic cholinergic receptors in rat brain. *J. Pharmacol. Exp. Ther.*, 228:648–655.

Luthin, G.R. and Wolfe, B.B. (1984b) [^{3}H]Pirenzepine and [^{3}H]quinuclidinylbenzilate binding to brain muscarinic cholinergic receptors. *Mol. Pharmacol.*, 26:164–169.

Michell, R.H. (1975) Inositol phospholipids and cell surface receptor function. *Biochim. Biophys. Acta*, 415:81–147.

Miller, J.C. (1977) A study of the kinetics of the muscarinic effect on phosphatidylinositol and phosphatidic acid metabolism in rat brain synaptosomes. *Biochem. J.*, 168:549–555.

Minneman, K.P. and Johnson, R.D. (1984) Characterization of alpha-1 adrenergic receptors linked to [^{3}H]inositol metabolism in rat cerebral cortex. *J. Pharmacol. Exp. Ther.*, 230:317–323.

Nishizuka, Y. (1984) Turnover of inositol phospholipids and signal transduction. *Science*, 225:1365–1370.

Schacht, J. and Agranoff, B.W. (1972) Effects of acetylcholine on labeling of phosphatidate and phosphoinositides by [^{32}P]orthophosphate in nerve ending fractions of guinea pig cortex. *J. Biol. Chem.*, 247:771–777.

Schoepp, D.D., Knepper, S.M. and Rutledge, C.O. (1984)

74

Norepinephrine stimulation of phosphoinositide hydrolysis in rat cerebral cortex is associated with the alpha$_1$-adrenoceptor. *J. Neurochem.*, 43:1758–1761.

Sokolovsky, M., Gurwitz, D. and Galron, R. (1980) Muscarinic binding in mouse brain: regulation by guanine nucleotides. *Biochem. Biophys. Res. Commun.*, 94:487–492.

Sokolovsky, M., Gurwitz, D. and Kloog, J. (1983) Biochemical characterization of the muscarinic receptors. *Adv. Enzymol.*, 55:137–196.

Spencer, D.G., Horvath, E., Luiten, P., Schuurman, T. and Traber, J. (1985) Novel approaches in the study of brain acetylcholine function: Neuropharmacology, neuroanatomy and behavior. In J. Traber and W.H. Gispen (Eds.), *Senile Dementia of the Alzheimer Type, Advances in Applied Neurological Sciences, Vol. 2*, Springer Verlag, Berlin, pp. 325–354.

Streb, H., Irvine, R.F., Berridge, M.J. and Schulz, I. (1983) Release of Ca^{2+} from non-mitochondrial intracellular store in pancreatic acinar cells by inositol 1,4,5-trisphosphate. *Nature*, 306:67–69.

Van Rooijen, L.A.A., Hajra, A.K. and Agranoff, B.W. (1985) Tetraenoic species are conserved in muscarinically enhanced inositide turnover. *J. Neurochem.*, 44:540–543.

Verghese, M.W., Smith, C.D. and Snyderman, R. (1985) Potential role for a guanine nucleotide regulatory protein in chemoattractant receptor-mediated polyphosphoinositide metabolism, Ca^{2+} mobilization and cellular responses by leukocytes. *Biochem. Biophys. Res. Commun.*, 127:450–457.

Wamsley, J.K., Gehlert, D.R., Roeske, W.R. and Yamamura, H.I. (1984) Muscarinic antagonist binding site heterogeneity as evidenced by autoradiography after direct labeling with ^{3}H-QNB and ^{3}H-pirenzepine. *Life Sci.*, 34:1395–1402.

Yandrasitz, J.R. and Segal, S. (1979) The effect of MnCl$_2$ on the basal and acetylcholine-stimulated turnover of phosphatidylinositol in synaptosomes. *FEBS Lett.*, 108:270–282.

Yamamura, H.I., Watson, M. and Roeske, W.R. (1983) ^{3}H-Pirenzepine specifically labels a high affinity muscarinic receptor in the rat cerebral cortex. In P. Mandel and F.V. DeFeudis (Eds.), *CNS receptors – From Molecular Pharmacology in Behavior*, Raven Press, New York, pp. 331–336.

SECTION II
Ion Channels

W.H. Gispen and A. Routtenberg (Eds.)
Progress in Brain Research, Vol. 69
© 1986 Elsevier Science Publishers B.V. (Biomedical Division)

CHAPTER 7

The role of protein kinases in the control of prolonged changes in neuronal excitability

L.K. Kaczmarek, J.A. Strong and J.A. Kauer

Departments of Pharmacology and Physiology, Yale University School of Medicine, New Haven, CT 06510, U.S.A.

Introduction

Long-lasting changes in the pattern of behavior of a mature animal may be divided into at least two general classes: (*a*) the onset of long-lasting, relatively fixed, patterns of activity, such as feeding and reproductive behaviors, which can be triggered by internal or external stimuli and (*b*) modifications of behavior that can be attributed to learning. In cases in which the neuronal basis of such modifications in behavior have been investigated, it has become clear that changes occur in the electrical properties of neurons in the networks that control the behaviors. There is accumulating evidence that the activation of protein kinases, under the control of cellular second messenger systems, contributes to these changes in excitability. One direct mechanism which has now been shown to modulate excitability is the alteration of the amplitudes and kinetics of specific ionic conductances in the plasma membrane of neurons by protein kinases (Kaczmarek et al., 1980; Castellucci et al., 1980; Adams and Levitan, 1982; DePeyer et al., 1982; Alkon et al., 1983; for review see Levitan, 1985).

In addition to the modulation of ionic conductances, there exist, at least in theory, several other ways to modulate excitability. These include, for example, modulation of the diverse mechanisms that influence the amount or type of neurotransmitter that the cells release. One feature of second messenger systems is that, when activated, they may act on several different cellular targets and can therefore coordinate changes in ionic conduct-

ances with, for example, changes in peptide metabolism. The way that such different cellular mechanisms are, in fact, coordinated within neurons to control or modulate any specific behavior is, however, not yet fully understood for any one type of neuron.

One particularly tractable experimental preparation in which the mechanisms that modulate neuronal activity may be investigated is that of the peptidergic bag cell neurons of *Aplysia*. These neurons undergo a sequence of changes in their cellular and electrical properties and, in so doing, control the onset of a sequence of behaviors that comprise egg-laying in this species. This review gives an account of the properties of these neurons, with a major focus on the modulation of potassium and calcium currents by different second messenger systems linked to activation of protein kinases. A brief account is also given of the evidence that peptide synthesis may be modulated in these neurons and that their excitability can be modulated by the cell's own released peptides. Finally, a description is given of the way in which a change in the nature of the response to a second messenger system is associated with a prolonged modification of excitability.

The bag cell neurons

Within the abdominal ganglion of *Aplysia*, one finds two clusters, of 200–400 neurons each, situated at the junctions of the pleuroabdominal connective nerves with the remainder of the ganglion (Frazier et al., 1967). These neurons have been termed the bag cell neurons. The morphology of these neurons is typically multipolar with elaborate neuritic branching patterns that extend out of the clusters into the surrounding connective tissue and up along the connective nerves as well as into the neuropil of the abdominal ganglion. Transmission electron micrographs reveal the processes to contain numerous 200-nm moderately electron-dense core granules. Freeze-fracture replicas have shown that the processes of these neurons are joined by gap junctions (Kaczmarek et al., 1979).

The bag cell neurons usually show no spontaneous activity. On brief electrical stimulation of one of the pleuroabdominal connective nerves, however, the cells depolarize and start to fire repetitively (Kupfermann and Kandel, 1970). The onset of this afterdischarge can also be induced by

peptides that have been purified from the reproductive tract and triggers a sequence of changes in the properties of these neurons which serve to initiate egg-laying behavior (Heller et al., 1980; Schlesinger et al., 1981) (Fig. 1). The afterdischarge begins with a period of rapid (3–6 Hz) firing, lasting about one minute. After one minute the action potentials of the bag cell neurons begin to increase in height and width and the firing frequency falls to a lower level (<1 Hz) (Fig. 2). This steady rate of discharge is then usually maintained for about thirty minutes (Kaczmarek et al., 1982).

During the discharge the bag cell neurons release several neuroactive peptides which act on other neurons in the abdominal ganglion and on peripheral targets to coordinate egg-laying behavior (Kupfermann, 1970; Branton et al., 1978; Dudek et

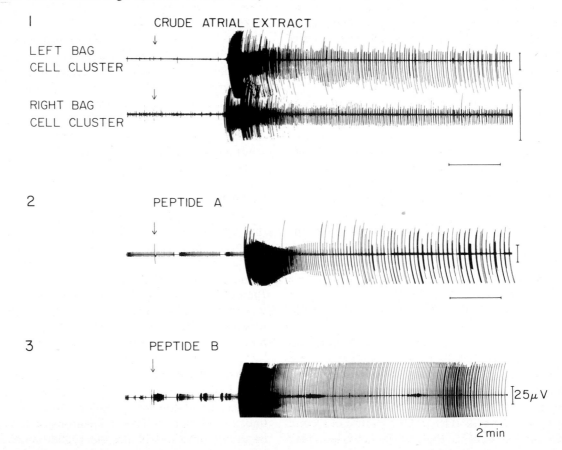

Fig. 1. Extracellular recordings of the onset of afterdischarges in the bag cell neurons on exposure of abdominal ganglia to crude extracts of the atrial gland of the reproductive tract or to purified reproductive tract peptides A and B (Heller et al., 1980).

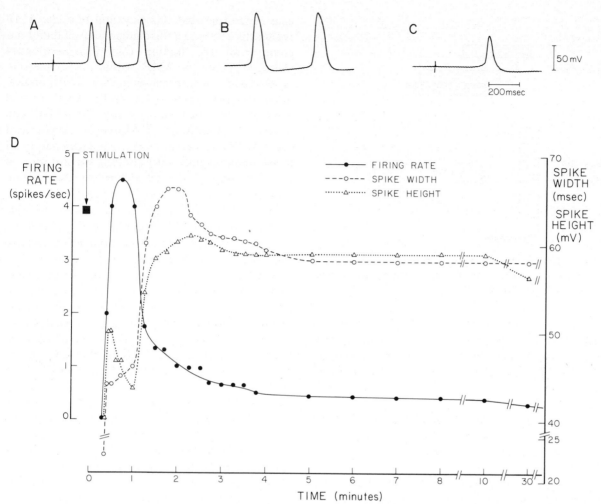

Fig. 2. Onset of an afterdischarge in the bag cell neurons. A: Intracellularly recorded action potentials during stimulation of afterdischarge. B: Enhanced action potentials 10 min after the onset of afterdischarge. C: Stimulated action potentials after the end of an afterdischarge. D: A plot of firing rate and action potential height and width during the afterdischarge (Kaczmarek et al., 1980).

al., 1979; Pinkser and Dudek, 1979; Stuart et al., 1980). The behaviors comprise a sequence of individual components which includes the cessation of feeding, locomotion to a vertical substrate, a characteristic set of head movements and the deposition of the egg mass. This entire behavioral sequence may take the animal several hours to carry out, and considerably outlasts the duration of the afterdischarge in the bag cell neurons (Fig. 3). Following the termination of the afterdischarge the bag cell neurons enter a state in which further stimulation fails to generate a long lasting afterdis-

charge, although intense stimulation can sometimes generate a short, low-frequency discharge. This relatively inexcitable state lasts for many hours and therefore is the state that these neurons are in during the majority of the ongoing behaviors that have been triggered by the discharge. The ability to generate full length afterdischarges recovers gradually over 10–20 hours. This long-lasting inhibited state has been termed the refractory period of the bag cell neurons and it is believed that it serves to prevent major release of neuroactive peptides from these neurons after the

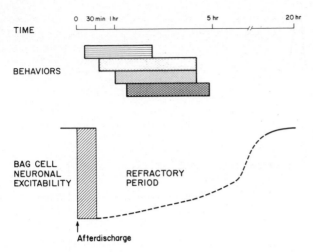

Fig. 3. Diagram showing the time scale of changes in excitability of the bag cell neurons and of the behaviors triggered by afterdischarge in these neurons.

ence suggesting that this elevation of cyclic AMP is causally related to the change in excitability has come from the finding that pharmacological elevation of cyclic AMP within these neurons, using either membrane-permeant phosphodiesterase-resistant analogs of cyclic AMP or the activator of adenylate cyclase, forskolin, can trigger the afterdischarge. Moreover, elevation of cyclic AMP levels at the end of an afterdischarge can reinstate and significantly prolong the duration of the afterdischarge (Kauer and Kaczmarek, 1985a; Table I).

To analyse the ionic conductances that are sensitive to cyclic AMP in the bag cell neurons, experiments have been carried out using isolated bag cell neurons maintained in cell culture. Such isolated neurons retain many of the characteristics of bag cell neurons in intact abdominal ganglia. They retain their multipolar morphology and extend elaborate neuritic branches. Physical contact between the neurites or somata of adjacent neurons in cell culture leads to the re-establishment of electrical contacts (Kaczmarek et al., 1979). After microelectrode impalement, intracellular stimulation of action potentials in these isolated neurons does not normally lead to afterdischarge. Exposure to cyclic AMP analogs such as 8-benzyl-thio-cyclic AMP, however, leads to a significant change their electrical properties (Kaczmarek and Strumwasser, 1981). The three most striking changes observed are a marked enhancement of the width of evoked action potentials, the onset of

behaviors have been initiated (Kaczmarek and Kauer, 1983). The different states of excitability that the bag cell neurons display are summarized in Table I.

The role of cyclic AMP-dependent protein phosphorylation in the control of potassium conductances in the bag cell neurons

The onset of afterdischarge in the bag cell neurons is associated with an increase in the levels of cyclic AMP in these cells (Kaczmarek et al., 1978). Evid-

TABLE 1

Excitability states of the bag cell neurons

State	Typical duration	Characteristic features
Resting	Many days if cells are not stimulated.	High resting potentials. No spontaneous activity.
Afterdischarge (phase 1)	~1 min	Firing rate 3–6 Hz. Relatively narrow action potentials.
Afterdischarge (phase 2)	~30 min	Firing rate 1 Hz. Action potentials increased in height and width.
Post-afterdischarge	~30 min	Electrical stimulation fails to trigger long-lasting discharges but afterdischarge can be restored by an elevation of cellular cyclic AMP levels.
Refractory state	~18 h	Electrical stimulation fails to trigger long-lasting discharges. Discharge cannot be induced or prolonged by elevations of cyclic AMP.

oscillations in membrane potential which can lead to repetitive discharge and a significant increase in input resistance. Similar effects are seen with the adenylate cyclase activator, forskolin (Kaczmarek and Kauer, 1983).

The ionic currents that are sensitive to cyclic AMP have been investigated using both a two-microelectrode voltage clamp and the whole-cell patch clamp technique in isolated bag cell neurons (Kaczmarek and Strumwasser, 1984; Strong, 1984; Strong and Kaczmarek, 1985). In the latter technique the internal ionic composition of the cells is exchanged with that in the recording pipette to provide complete control over both the external and internal ionic composition of the cells. These studies have found that the properties of three distinct components of potassium current are modulated by elevations in cellular cyclic AMP concentrations:

(a) the delayed voltage-dependent potassium current (I_{K1}; sometimes termed the delayed rectifier),
(b) an apparently independent component of potassium current whose voltage dependence resembles that of the delayed rectifier but which inactivates much more rapidly on depolarization (I_{K2}), and
(c) the transient inactivating potassium current (I_A) (A-current).

The effect of an elevation of cyclic AMP on the delayed potassium current, I_{K1}, is to produce a diminution in its amplitude with no apparent change in its kinetics, whereas its effect on the more rapidly inactivating component (I_{K2}) is to produce an increase in its rate of inactivation (Strong and Kaczmarek, 1984, 1985) (Fig. 4). These two components of potassium current both contribute to the repolarization of action potentials and the effects of cyclic AMP on these components is consistent with the enhancement of action potential width that is produced by cyclic AMP.

The A-current is activated in a voltage range that is subthreshold for the generation of action potentials and is believed to play an important role in regulating the firing rate of neurons (Connor and Stevens, 1971). Experimentally this current can be observed, in relative isolation from

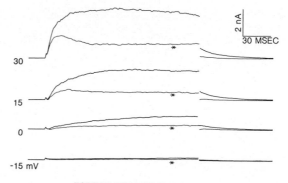

* FORSKOLIN/THEOPHYLLINE

Fig. 4. Depression of delayed potassium currents by elevation of cyclic AMP in an isolated bag cell neuron. The neuron was dialyzed internally with a medium containing 20 nM EGTA to eliminate calcium-activated conductances. Currents we recorded on stepping the membrane potential from −60 mV to the potentials indicated. The upper trace in each case is the control and the lower trace that recorded after elevation of cellular cyclic AMP levels using forskolin (50 μM) and theophylline 1 mM). Strong and Kaczmarek, 1985).

other potassium currents, on depolarization of the membrane from a negative potential (−95mV) to potentials between −50 and −30mV. Elevations of cyclic AMP produce an increase in the rate at which this current inactivates following its activation by such depolarizations (Fig. 5) (Strong, 1984; Kaczmarek and Strumwasser, 1984). Such an increase in inactivation rate would be expected to allow the cell to fire more rapidly on depolarization and is consistant with the onset of spontaneous activity and increased firing rate in response to depolarization that is seen in cells exposed to cyclic AMP analogs or to forskolin.

Although the alterations in these three voltage-dependent potassium currents may account for a major part of the effects of cyclic AMP on the electrical characteristics of these neurons, they probably do not account for all of the changes seen in either the intact clusters of neurons or the isolated cells. In particular, two characteristics whose ionic bases are not, as yet, clearly defined are the increase in input resistance seen in current-clamped cells (Kaczmarek and Strumwasser, 1981) and the emergence of a region of negative slope resistance in the steady-state current voltage relations in cells voltage-clamped using micro-

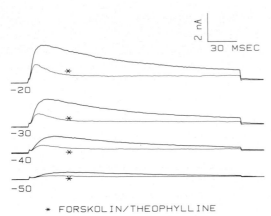

2 nA

30 MSEC

−20

−30

−40

−50

* FORSKOLIN/THEOPHYLLINE

Fig. 5. Depression and increase in rate of inactivation of A-current by elevation of cyclic AMP in an isolated bag cell neuron. The cell was dialyzed internally as described in the legend to Fig. 4. Currents were recorded on stepping the membrane potential from −90 mV to the potentials indicated at the left side of the traces (Strong, 1984).

electrodes (Kaczmarek and Strumwasser, 1984). The latter phenomenon has not been observed using the internally dialyzed cells and is therefore probably sensitive to dialysis. These findings suggest that additional components of ion conductance that are modified by elevations of cyclic AMP will be found in these neurons.

The only way by which cyclic AMP is known to act in eukaryotic cells is by activating a cyclic AMP-dependent protein kinase (Nestler and Greengard, 1984). Evidence that the effects of cyclic AMP on ionic conductances are also mediated by this enzyme has come primarily through experiments which have investigated the electrical effects of exogenous kinases and related proteins. Injection of the catalytic subunit of cyclic AMP-dependent protein kinase into isolated bag cell neurons has been shown to enhance their action potentials, increase input resistance and generate subthreshold oscillations in membrane potential (Kaczmarek et al., 1980). Moreover, microinjection of the protein kinase inhibitor protein, which binds to endogenous catalytic subunit and prevents the catalysis of protein phosphorylation (Ashby and Walsh, 1972), both prevents and reverses the effects of cyclic AMP elevations on the action potentials of cultured bag cell neurons

(Kaczmarek et al. 1984). Ongoing work also indicates that this protein can reverse the specific effects of elevations of cyclic AMP on the kinetics and amplitudes of the voltage-dependent potassium currents in internally dialyzed bag cell neurons (unpublished results). These results are consistant with the hypothesis that cyclic AMP exerts its electrical effects through the agency of the cyclic AMP-dependent protein kinase.

In other types of neurons that have been subjected to internal dialysis the catalytic subunit of cyclic AMP-dependent protein kinase has been shown to enhance the calcium current and to help prevent the loss of calcium current during dialysis (Doroshenko et al. 1984; Chad and Eckert, 1984). Elevations of cyclic AMP over resting levels using forskolin or cyclic AMP analogs have not been found to have a significant effect on peak calcium current in isolated bag cell neurons (Kaczmarek and Strumwasser, 1984). It is not known, however, whether the maintenance of calcium current in dialyzed bag cell neurons is sensitive to the catalytic subunit.

Protein kinase C and the modulation of calcium current

In addition to the cyclic AMP-dependent protein kinase, the bag cell neurons contain several types of calcium-dependent protein kinases. The major form is a calcium/calmodulin-dependent protein kinase that by immunoreactivity, substrate specificity and peptide mapping resembles the enzyme calmodulin kinase II isolated from mammalian nervous tissue (DeRiemer et al., 1984). The function of this enzyme in the activity of the bag cell neurons is not yet known. These neurons also contain the calcium/phospholipid-dependent protein kinase that has been called protein kinase C and that requires phosphatidylserine and diacylglycerol for its activation (Fig. 6) (DeRiemer et al., 1983, 1985a). Under physiological conditions, the activity of this enzyme is believed to be enhanced by stimuli that activate a phosphodiesterase which hydrolyzes membrane phosphoinositides to inositol polyphosphates and to diacylglycerol (Nishizuka, 1984). Recent work has indicated that stimulation of the pleuroabdominal connective

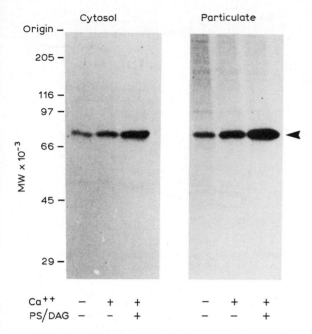

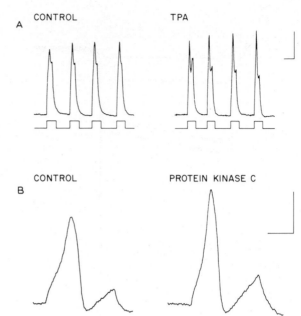

Fig. 6. Protein kinase C activity in cytosolic and particulate fractions prepared from the bag cell neurons. Enzyme activity was stimulated by addition of Ca^{2+} and phosphatidylserine with diacylglycerol (PS/DAG) and was measured on this autoradiogram by the degree of incorporation of ^{31}P from [γ-^{32}P]ATP into an exogenous protein substrate which is specific for protein kinase C (De Riemer et al., 1985a).

Fig. 7. Enhancement of action potentials of bag cell neurons by phorbol ester and by protein kinase C. A: Action potentials evoked in an isolated bag cell neuron by a train of depolarizing current pulses before and after exposure to TPA. B: Action potentials evoked by a single depolarizing current pulse before and after microinjection of protein kinase C. Scale bars 20 mV, 200 ms (De Riemer et al., 1985a).

nerve to trigger afterdischarges in the bag cell neurons results in the activation of such a polyphosphoinositide phosphodiesterase (Milburn and Kaczmarek, unpublished results) and suggests that protein kinase C could play a role in the transformations of the properties of the bag cell neurons.

As has been described in other tissues, the activity of protein kinase C in the bag cell neurons may be stimulated by phorbol esters such as 12-O-tetradecanoyl-13-phorbol acetate (TPA) at concentrations of 10–100 nM (DeRiemer et al., 1985a). Exposure of isolated bag cell neurons to these concentrations of TPA results in a significant enhancement of the height of their action potentials (Fig. 7). This effect differs from that of elevations in cyclic AMP in that no significant broadening of the action potentials or change in input resistance is observed. Voltage clamp experiments using isolated, internally dialyzed neurons

have shown that this effect results from an increase in the amplitude of the calcium current in these cells (Fig. 8) (DeRiemer et al., 1985b). TPA has no effect on the voltage-dependent potassium currents whose properties are modulated by the cyclic AMP-dependent protein kinase.

Data to support the idea that these actions of TPA are caused by the activation of protein kinase C have come from experiments in which this enzyme was directly microinjected into isolated bag cell neurons in cell culture (DeRiemer et al., 1985b). This was shown to enhance the height of action potentials evoked by depolarizing current pulses in a manner similar to that produced by TPA (Fig. 7). These data are consistent with the notion that TPA acts to enhance calcium current via the activation of protein kinase C, although voltage clamp studies using the enzyme have yet to be carried out.

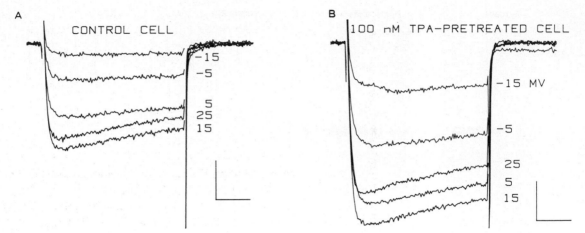

Fig. 8. Enhancement of calcium current in bag cell neurons by TPA. Isolated bag cell neurons in cell culture were dialyzed internally with a solution containing tetraethylammonium and cesium ions and containing no potassium ions to eliminate potassium current. Inward calcium currents, evoked by stepping from −60 mV to the indicated potentials, are shown for a control and a TPA-treated cell. Scale bars 0.25 mA, 20 ms (De Riemer et al., 1985b).

Protein phosphorylation, peptide synthesis and peptide processing during neuronal discharge

Studies using ^{32}P-radiolabeled clusters of bag cell neurons have shown that at least two bag cell phosphoproteins undergo a change in phosphorylation state on stimulation of an afterdischarge (Jennings et al., 1982). These proteins were visualized on autoradiograms of one-dimensional sodium dodecylsulfate (SDS) gels and it is certain that changes in minor phosphoprotein components, such as those that might regulate the activity of ion channels, escaped detection. Current evidence indicates that these two proteins have roles related to the synthesis and processing of the neuroactive peptides of the bag cell neurons.

One of the phosphoproteins whose phosphorylation state is enhanced on stimulation of afterdischarge has an apparent molecular weight of 33 000 and has been shown to be a substrate for cyclic AMP-dependent protein kinase in vitro. This protein is not specific to the bag cell neurons, being found in all regions of the nervous system (Jennings et al., 1982). Preliminary work, using two-dimensional gel electrophoresis, supports the hypothesis that this protein is S6, a protein component of the small subunit of ribosomes (Kaczmarek, Jahn, DeRiemer and Knorr, unpub-

lished results). In the bag cell neurons, depolarization and elevation of cyclic AMP levels have been shown to increase the rate of synthesis of the precursor to the neuroactive peptides released during an afterdischarge (Berry and Arch, 1981; Bruehl and Berry, 1985). It is therefore possible that changes in the phosphorylation state of S6 within the bag cell neurons are related to this stimulation of peptide synthesis, although the full details of mechanisms that coordinate electrical activity with alterations in protein synthesis remain to be explored.

The second protein into which a change in the rate of incorporation of ^{32}P can be observed on stimulation of an afterdischarge has a molecular weight of 21 000 and is specific to, or very much enriched in, the bag cell neurons (Jennings et al., 1982). This protein is a major component in bag cell neuronal membrane fractions prepared from large mature *Aplysia*. This protein was eluted from one-dimensional SDS gels of membrane fractions from such animals and a partial amino acid sequence of the N terminus was determined. This sequence was subsequently found to match a region within the cloned sequence for the precursor to the bag cell peptides (Scheller et al., 1983), suggesting that this protein is part of, or closely related to, this precursor (Azhderian et al.,

1984). The precursors to a number of other biologically active peptides have been shown to undergo phosphorylation within cells although the physiological significance of such modifications to the precursors is not yet known (Bennett et al., 1981; Eipper and Mains, 1982; Bhargava et al., 1983).

An elevation in cyclic AMP, in addition to influencing the synthesis of the precursor to the secreted peptides may also promote the processing of the protein precursor. The precursor to the bag cell peptides and its processing intermediates may readily be labeled using [^{3}H]amino acids (Arch et al., 1981). Current work indicates that elevation of cyclic AMP levels and electrical stimulation of afterdischarge each promote the conversion of labeled precursor intermediates to lower molecular weight forms (Azhderian and Kaczmarek, unpublished results). It is not yet known if this effect is in any way related to direct phosphorylation of components of the precursor. A similar effect of cyclic AMP has been proposed for the processing of opioid peptide precursors (Wilson et al., 1984).

Feedback actions of neuropeptides released during neuronal discharge

Is there any link between the amount of peptide stored and released by these neurons and the mechanisms that regulate their electrical properties? Evidence is accumulating for one such link: the regulation of changes in excitability by one of the peptides released during the afterdischarge.

The bag cell neurons release several peptides including a 36-amino acid peptide, egg laying hormone (ELH) (Chiu et al. 1979), and α-BCP, a 9-amino acid peptide (Rothman et al. 1983). The sequence of the precursor to these peptides suggests that two other short peptides, β-BCP and γ-BCP, which have sequences that are similar to α-BCP, may also be synthesized in these cells (Scheller et al., 1983). There is an interesting homology between α-BCP and the peptides from the reproductive tract that can trigger an afterdischarge in the bag cell neurons (Table II). Rothman et al. (1983) have found that α-BCP can act on certain other neurons in the abdominal ganglion to modify their properties during a bag cell afterdischarge. In addition, they found the effects of α-BCP$_{1-8}$ and α-BCP$_{1-7}$ to be more potent than those of the complete 9-amino acid sequence.

α-BCP can also be shown to exert a potent influence on the bag cell neurons themselves. When 1 μM α-BCP$_{(1-9)}$, α-BCP$_{(1-8)}$ or α-BCP$_{(1-7)}$ is applied to the bag cell neurons shortly after the onset of an afterdischarge they prematurely terminate the afterdischarge (Fig. 9) (Kaczmarek and Kauer, 1985b). A likely explanation for this effect is that α-BCP attenuates the production of cyclic AMP. Brief exposure to 1 μM α-BCP$_{(1-7)}$ results in a potent inhibition of the ability of forskolin to elevate cyclic AMP levels in clusters of bag cell neurons. A similar inhibition of forskolin stimula-

TABLE II

N-Terminal sequences of reproductive tract and bag cell peptides

Peptide	Sequence	Reference[a]
Reproductive tract peptides		
Peptide A	- -Thr-Pro-Arg-Leu-Arg-Phe-Tyr-Pro-Ile	1
Peptide B	- -Thr-Pro-Arg-Leu-Arg-Phe-Tyr-Pro-Ile	1
ERH	- -Thr-Pro-Arg-Leu-Arg-Phe-Tyr-Pro-Ile	2
Bag cell peptides		
α-BCP	Ala-Pro-Arg-Leu-Arg-Phe-Tyr-Ser-Leu	3
β-BCP	Arg-Leu-Arg-Phe-His	4
γ-BCP	Arg-Leu-Arg-Phe-Asp	4

[a]1, Heller et al. (1980); 2, Schlesinger et al. (1981); 3, Rothman et al. (1983); 4, Scheller et al. (1983).

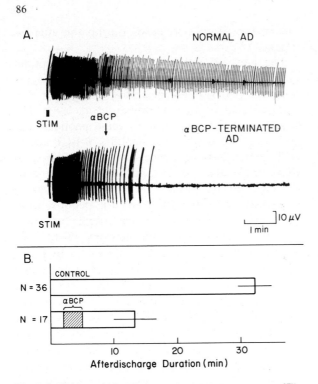

Fig. 9. Inhibition of afterdischarge by α-BCP. A: Extracellular recordings of the onset of a normal afterdischarge and of an afterdischarge terminated by application of 1 μM α-BCP$_{(1-7)}$ 2 min after the onset of discharge. B: Mean durations ($\pm$SEM) of control afterdischarges and of afterdischarges in which α-BCP$_{(1-7)}$ was applied after the onset of afterdischarge (Kauer and Kaczmarek, unpublished results).

tion of cyclic AMP levels is seen at the termination of a normal afterdischarge (Kaczmarek and Kauer, 1985a,b).

In addition to this biochemical effect, α-BCP may have additional effects on ionic conductances in the bag cell neurons. Rothman et al. (1983) have provided data that α-BCP$_{(1-7)}$, when applied to intact abdominal ganglia at concentrations of 1 μM to 1 mM, may depolarize the bag cell neurons and occasionally trigger an afterdischarge. This depolarizing response appears, however, to be very labile and to desensitize rapidly. On the other hand, studies with isolated bag cell neurons in cell culture have shown that α-BCP can hyperpolarize these cells directly through a mechanism that is probably an increase in a potassium conductance (Kaczmarek and Kauer, 1985b).

In summary, there is evidence that α-BCP may act to modify the electrical characteristics of the bag cell neurons. The physiological mechanisms by which such feedback occurs, whether they all act through autoreceptors or through other neurons, and the way they influence parameters such as pattern of firing, duration of afterdischarge and onset of the refractory period have yet to be investigated fully. Such feedback mechanisms are of particular significance because they provide a direct link between the states of peptide synthesis, processing and storage and the excitability of these peptidergic neurons.

Loss of response to cyclic AMP after the onset of the prolonged refractory period

For several hours after the termination of a normal afterdischarge, electrical stimulation, comparable to that which triggered the afterdischarge, is relatively ineffective in triggering subsequent discharges. More intense repetitive stimulation, however, can often result in shorter, lower-frequency discharges. As described above, this period of relative inexcitability may serve to allow the behaviors released by the bag cell peptides to proceed to completion.

There is evidence that the onset of the refractory period depends on calcium entry during the afterdischarge. If either sodium or calcium ions are omitted from the external medium, afterdischarges can still be evoked if tetraethylammonium ions are present in the medium to block some of the potassium conductance. In such media lacking calcium, multiple high-frequency afterdischarges may be stimulated with no evidence of a refractory period. On the other hand, in media containing calcium, but lacking sodium, only a single afterdischarge can be evoked after which the cells become refractory to further stimulation (Kaczmarek et al., 1982). Moreover, in normal media, a prolonged refractory period may be triggered by treatments which elevate intracellular calcium levels without triggering afterdischarge (Kaczmarek and Kauer, 1983).

This change in the electrical properties of these neurons during the refractory period is associated with an alteration in their sensitivity to elevations of cyclic AMP by forskolin. When cyclic AMP levels are increased in the bag cell neurons either before stimulation of a first afterdischarge or within 10 min of the termination of afterdischarge, the duration of subsequent discharge can be prolonged significantly over that induced by stimulation alone. Moreover, elevations of cyclic AMP frequently trigger discharges at these times without additional stimulation. Within one hour of the termination of a normal afterdischarge, however, elevations of cyclic AMP are without effect on duration of evoked discharges (Fig. 10). Intracellular recordings have been carried out using forskolin-treated bag cell neurons within clusters of cells that were isolated from abdominal ganglia after the onset of the refractory period. These experiments have shown that these cells still display enhanced action potentials and changes in excitability which suggest that the effects of cyclic AMP on the delayed potassium currents and the

A-current are, at least qualitatively, unchanged in the refractory period (Kaczmarek and Kauer, 1985a). The ionic or biochemical basis for this inability to trigger or prolong discharge is therefore not yet known. One attractive possibility, which would perhaps not be apparent in a straightforward analysis of ionic currents, is that the concentrations of releasable peptides, with autoreceptor actions which influence discharge, are altered in the prolonged refractory period.

Summary

The bag cell neurons have proved to be a model system for the investigation of mechanisms regulating changes in neuronal excitability that result in alterations in animal behavior. The phosphorylation of proteins, coordinated through the activation of second messenger systems, results in alterations of the properties of ionic currents which regulate the excitability of these neurons and in changes in the synthesis of peptides to be released during neuronal activity.

The changes that occur in the properties of specific ionic conductances following the activation of the cyclic AMP-dependent protein kinase or protein kinase C fall into two classes: changes in the amplitude of currents with no apparent change in their macroscopic kinetics (I_{K1} and I_{Ca}), and changes that are caused by significant alterations in kinetic behavior (I_{K2} and I_A). It should be noted that although specific second messenger-related protein kinases have been shown to modulate the properties of these ionic currents, neurons may possess additional, as yet uncharacterized, protein kinases which may also be able to modulate the activity of ion channels and which may induce changes similar to those of the characterized second messenger-related protein kinases. The way in which such modifications of ion channel activity are brought about are a major task for future research and may only be fully understood after the biochemical identity of these channels has been clarified. General possibilities are (a) that the channel proteins themselves undergo phosphorylation, (b) that the modification occurs via some other cytoplasmic or membrane component which is the direct substrate for

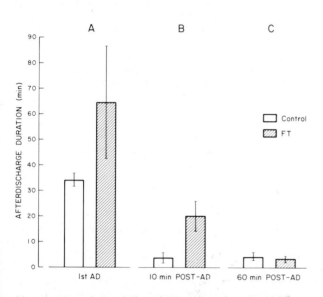

Fig. 10. Loss of the ability of elevations of cyclic AMP to prolong afterdischarge in the refractory period. Mean durations ($\pm$SEM) are shown for afterdischarges stimulated in the presence or absence of forskolin (50 μM) and theophylline (1 mM) (FT) to elevate cellular cyclic AMP levels. Forskolin prolongs afterdischarges stimulated in the resting state (1st AD) and those stimulated within 10 min of the end of a first afterdischarge. In the refractory period (60 min post AD), however, forskolin fails to prolong or initiate discharge, even though its ability to elevate cyclic AMP levels is unimpaired at this time (Kauer and Kaczmarek, 1985a).

the protein kinase and which modulates the activity of the ion channel, and (c) that changes in the activity of certain ion channels are the result of a more general cellular changes, perhaps involving altered interactions with the cytoskeleton or endocytosis and exocytosis of associated plasma membrane. The first of these hypotheses is the simplest and evidence in favor of such a direct action of phosphorylation has been adduced for one class of potassium channel from *Helix* (Ewald et al., 1985). Biochemical evidence also exists for the phosphorylation of one class of calcium channel which is known to be modulated by cyclic AMP (Curtis and Catterall, 1985). There exists, however, suggestive evidence for a role for cytoplasmic factors in the regulation of some ion channel responses to second messenger systems (Schuster et al., 1985). Moreover mechanisms such as (c) have been demonstrated for some non-neuronal cells (Lewis and de Moura, 1982) and may be able to produce longer-lasting modifications of excitability.

A parallel role for second messenger-induced protein phosphorylation is the modulation of the intracellular synthesis and handling of the neuroactive peptides that are released during neuronal activity. On stimulation of neurons these processes presumably occur relatively independently of the changes in properties of specific ionic conductances. Once released, however, the peptides may directly influence the excitability of the neurons. Investigation of the range of biochemical and electrical effects that specific bag cell peptides may have on these neurons, and the degree to which the releasable pool of such peptides can be modulated, has only begun. Modifications in the releasable pool of peptides that act through autoreceptors could, however, constitute a powerful mechanism for the induction of long-lasting changes in the excitability of a neuron.

References

Adams, W.B. and Levitan, I.B. (1982) Intracellular injection of protein kinase inhibitor blocks the serotonin induced increase in K$^+$ conductance in *Aplysia* neuron R15. *Proc. Natl. Acad. Sci. U.S.A.*, 79:3877–3880.

Alkon, D.L., Acosta-Urquidi, J., Olds, J., Kuzma, G. and Neary, J. (1983) Protein kinase injection reduces voltage dependent potassium currents. *Science*, 219:303–306.

Arch, S., Smock, T. and Earley, P. (1976) Precursor and product processing in the bag cell neurons of *Aplysia californica*. *J. Gen. Physiol.*, 68:211–225.

Ashby, C.D. and Walsh, D.A. (1972) Characterization of the interaction of a protein inhibitor with adenosine 3′,5′-monophosphate-dependent protein kinases. *J. Biol. Chem.*, 247:6637–6642.

Azhderian, E., DeRiemer, S.A., Casnellie, J., Greengard, P. and Kaczmarek, L.K. (1984) Antisera to a peptide fragment from a bag cell phosphoprotein specifically stains bag cell neurons. *Soc. Neurosci. Abstr.*, 10:895.

Bennett, H.P.J., Browne, C.A. and Solomon, S. (1981) Biosynthesis of phosphorylated forms of corticotropin-related peptides. *Proc. Natl. Acad. Ssi. U.S.A.*, 78:4713–4717.

Berry, R.W. (1981) Proteolytic processing in the biogenesis of the neurosecretory egg-laying hormone in *Aplysia*. I. Precursors, intermediates and products. *Biochemistry*, 20:6200–6205.

Berry, R.W. and Arch, S. (1918) Activation of neurosecretory cells enhances their synthesis of secretory protein. *Brain Res.*, 215:115–123.

Bhargava, G., Russell, J. and Sherwood, L. (1983) Phosphorylation of parathyroid secretory protein. *Proc. Natl. Acad. Sci. U.S.A.*, 86:878–881.

Branton, W.D., Mayeri, E., Brownell, P. and Simon, S.B. (1978) Evidence for local hormonal communication between neurones in *Aplysia*. *Nature*, 274:70–72.

Bruehl, C.L. and Berry, R.W. (1985) Regulation of synthesis of the neurosecretory egg-laying hormone of *Aplysia*: Antagonistic roles of calcium and cyclic adenosine 3′,5′-monophosphate. *J. Neurosci.*, 5:1233–1238.

Castellucci, V.F., Kandel, E.R., Schwartz, J.H., Wilson, F., Nairn, A.C. and Greengard, P. (1980) Intracellular injection of the catalytic subunit of cyclic AMP-dependent protein kinase simulates facilitation of transmitter release underlying behavioural sensitization in *Aplysia*. *Proc. Natl. Acad. Sci. U.S.A.*, 77:7492–7496.

Chad, J.E. and Eckert, R. (1984) Stimulation of cAMP-dependent protein phosphorylation retards both inactivation and 'washout' of Ca current in dialysed *Helix* neurons. *Soc. Neurosci. Abstr.*, 10:866.

Chiu, A.Y., Hunkapiller, M.W., Heller, E., Stuart, D.K., Hood, L.E. and Strumwasser, F. (1979) Purification and primary structure of neuroactive egg-laying hormone of *Aplysia californica*. *Proc. Natl. Acad. Sci. U.S.A.*, 76:6656–6660.

Connor, J.A. and Stevens, C.F. (1971) Predictions of repetitive firing behaviour from voltage clamp data on an isolated neurone soma. *J. Physiol.*, 213:31–53.

Curtis, B.M. and Catterall, W.A. (1985) Phosphorylation of the calcium antagonist receptor of the voltage-sensitive calcium channel by cyclic AMP-dependent protein kinase. *Proc. Natl. Acad. Sci. U.S.A.*, 82:2528–2532.

DePeyer, J.E., Cachelin, A.B., Levitan, I.B. and Reuter, H. (1982) Ca^{2+}-activated K$^+$ conductance in internally perfused snail neurons is enhanced by protein phosphorylation. *Proc. Natl. Acad. Sci. U.S.A.*, 79:4207:4211.

DeRiemer, S.A., Kaczmarek, L.K., Albert, K.A. and Greengard, P. (1983) Calcium/phospholipid-dependent protein phosphorylation in *Aplysia* neurons. *Soc. Neurosci. Abstr.*, 9.77.

DeRiemer, S.A., Kaczmarek, L.K., Lai, Y., McGuinness, T.L. and Greengard, P. (1984) Calcium/calmodulin-dependent protein phosphorylation in the nervous system of *Aplysia. J. Neurosci.*, 4:1618–1625.

DeRiemer, S.A., Greengard, P. and Kaczmarek, L.K. (1985a) Calcium/phosphatidylserine/diacylglycerol-dependent protein phosphorylation in the *Aplysia* nervous system. *J. Neurosci.*, 5:2672–2676.

DeRiemer, S.A., Strong, J.A., Albert, K.A., Greengard, P. and Kaczmarek, L.K. (1985b) Enhancement of calcium current in *Aplysia* neurones by phorbol ester and protein kinase C. *Nature*, 313:313–316.

Doroshenko, P.A., Kostyuk, P.G., Martynyuk, A.E., Kursky, M.D. and Vorobetz, Z.D. (1984) Intracellular protein kinase and calcium currents in perfused neurones of the snail *Helix pomatia. Neuroscience*, 11:263.

Dudek, F.E., Cobbs, J.S. and Pinsker, H.M. (1979) Bag cell electrical activity underlying spontaneous egg laying in freely behaving *Aplysia brasiliana. J. Neurophysiol.*, 42:804–817.

Eipper, B.A. and Mains, R.E. (1982) Phosphorylation of pro-adrenocorticotropin/endorphin-derived peptides. *J. Biol. Chem.*, 257:4907–4915.

Ewald, D.A., Williams, A. and Levitan, I.B. (1985) Modulation of single Ca^{2+}-dependent K^+-channel activity by protein phosphorylation. *Nature*, 315:503–506.

Frazier, W.T., Kandel, E.R., Kupfermann, I., Waziri, R. and Coggeshall, R.E. (1967) Morphological and functional properties of identified neurons in the abdominal ganglion of *Aplysia californica. J. Neurophysiol.*, 30:1288–1351.

Heller, L.K., Kaczmarek, L.K., Hunkapiller, M.W., Hood, L.E. and Strumwasser, F. (1980) Purification and primary structure of two neuroactive peptides that cause bag cell afterdischarge and egg-laying in *Aplysia. Proc. Natl. Acad. Sci. U.S.A.*, 77:2328–2332.

Jennings, K.R., Kaczmarek, L.K., Hewick, R.M., Dreyer, W.J. and Strumwasser, F. (1982) Protein phosphorylation during afterdischarge in peptidergic neurons of *Aplysia. J. Neurosci.*, 2:158–168.

Kaczmarek, L.K. and Kauer, J.A. (1983) Calcium entry causes a prolonged refractory period in peptidergic neurons of *Aplysia. J. Neurosci.*, 3:2230–2239.

Kaczmarek, L.K. and Strumwasser, F. (1981) The expression of long-lasting afterdischarge by isolated *Aplysia* bag cell neurons. *J. Neurosci.*, 1:626–634.

Kaczmarek, L.K. and Strumwasser, F. (1984) A voltage-clamp analysis of currents underlying cyclic-AMP-induced membrane modulation in isolated peptidergic neurons of *Aplysia. J. Neurophysiol.*, 52:340–349.

Kaczmarek, L.K., Jennings, K. and Strumwasser, F. (1978) Neurotransmitter modulation, phosphodiesterase inhibitor effects, and cAMP correlates of afterdischarge in peptidergic neurites. *Proc. Natl. Acad. Sci. U.S.A.*, 75:5200–5204.

Kaczmarek, L.K., Finbow, M., Revel, J.P. and Strumwasser, F. (1979) The morphology and coupling of *Aplysia* bag cells within the abdominal ganglion and in cell culture. *J. Neurobiol.*, 10:535–550.

Kaczmarek, L.K., Jennings, K.R., Strumwasser, F., Nairn, A.C., Walter, U., Wilson, F.D. and Greengard, P. (1980) Microinjection of catalytic subunit of cyclic AMP-dependent protein kinase enhances calcium action potentials of bag cell neurons in cell culture. *Proc. Natl. Acad. Sci. U.S.A.*, 77:7427–7491.

Kaczmarek, L.K., Jennings, K.R. and Strumwasser, F. (1982) An early sodium and a late calcium phase in the afterdischarge of peptide secreting neurons of *Aplysia. Brain Res.*, 238:105–115.

Kaczmarek, L.K., Nairn, A.C. and Greengard, P. (1984) Microinjection of protein kinase inhibitor prevents enhancement of action potentials in peptidergic neurons of *Aplysia. Soc. Neurosci. Abstr.*, 10:895.

Kauer, J.A. and Kaczmarek, L.K. (1985a) Peptidergic neurons of *Aplysia* lose their response to cyclic adenosine 3′,5′-monophosphate during a prolonged refractory period. *J. Neurosci.*, 5:1339–1345.

Kauer, J.A. and Kaczmarek, L.K. (1985b) A neuropeptide autoreceptor mediates changes in neuronal excitability. *Soc. Neurosci. Abstr.*, 11:710.

Kupfermann, I. (1970) Stimulation of egg laying by extracts of neuroendocrine cells (bag cells) of abdominal ganglion of *Aplysia, J. Neurophysiol.*, 33:877–881.

Kupfermann, I. and Kandel, E.R. (1970) Electrophysiological properties and functional interconnections of two symmetrical neurosecretory clusters (bag cells) in abdominal ganglion of *Aplysia. J. Neurophysiol.*, 33:865–876.

Levitan, I.B. (1986) Phosphorylation of ion channels. *J. Membr. Biol.*, 87:177–190.

Lewis, S.A. and de Moura, J.L.C. (1982) Incorporation of cytoplasmic vesicles into apical membrane of mammalian urinary bladder epithelium. *Nature*, 297:685–688.

Nestler, E.J. and Greengard, P. (1984) Protein phosphorylation in the nervous system, John Wiely & Sons, New York.

Nishizuka, Y. (1984b) Turnover of inositol phospholipids and signal transduction. *Science*, 225:1365–1370.

Pinsker, H.M. and Dudek, F.E. (1977) Bag cell control of egg laying in freely-behaving *Aplysia. Science*, 197:490–493.

Rothman, B.S., Mayeri, E., Brown, R.O., Yuan, P. and Shively, J. (1983) Primary structure and neuronal effects of α-bag cell peptide, a second candidate neurotransmitter encoded by a single gene in bag cell neurons of *Aplysia. Proc. Natl. Acad. Sci. U.S.A.*, 80:5733–5757.

Scheller, R.H., Jackson, J.F., McAllister, L.B., Rothman, B., Mayeri, E. and Axel, R. (1983) A single gene encodes multiple neuropeptides mediating a stereotyped behavior. *Cell*, 32:7–22.

Schlesinger, D.H., Babirack, S.P. and Blankenship, J.E. (1981) In Schlesinger, D.H. (Ed.), *Symposium on Neurohypophyseal Peptide Hormones and Other Biologically Active Peptides*, Elsevier North-Holland, New York, pp. 137–150.

Schuster, M.J., Camarado, J.S., Siegelbaum, S.A. and Kandel,

E.R. (1985) Cyclic AMP-dependent protein kinase closes the serotonin-sensitive channels of *Aplysia* sensory neurons in cell-free membrane patches. *Nature*, 313:392–394.

Strong, J. (1984) Modulation of potassium current kinetics in bag cell neurons of *Aplysia* by an activator of adenylate cyclase. *J. Neurosci.*, 4:2772–2783.

Strong, J.A. and Kaczmarek, L.K. (1984) Modulation of multiple potassium currents in dialysed bag cell neurons of *Aplysia*. *Soc. Neurosci. Abstr.*, 10:1101.

Strong, J.A. and Kaczmarek, L.K. (1985) Multiple components of delayed potassium current in peptidergic neurons of *Aplysia*: Modulation by an activator of adenylate cyclase. *J. Neurosci.*, 6:814–822.

Stuart, D.K., Chiu, A.Y. and Strumwasser, F. (1980) Neurosecretion of egg-laying hormone and other peptides from electrically active bag cell neurons of *Aplysia*. *J. Neurophysiol.*, 43:488–498.

Wilson, S.P., Unsworth, C.D. and Viveros, O.H. (1984) Regulation of opioid peptide synthesis and processing in adrenal chromaffin cells by catecholamines and cyclic adenosine 3',5'-monophosphate. *J. Neurosci.* 4:2993-3001.

W.H. Gispen and A. Routtenberg (Eds.)
Progress in Brain Research, Vol. 69
© 1986 Elsevier Science Publishers B.V. (Biomedical Division)

CHAPTER 8

Modulation of ion channels by Ca²⁺-activated protein phosphorylation: a biochemical mechanism for associative learning

Joseph T. Neary

Section on Neural Systems, Laboratory of Biophysics, IRP, National Institute of Neurological and Communicative Disorders and Stroke, National Institutes of Health at the Marine Biological Laboratory, Woods Hole, MA 02543, U.S.A. (Current address: Departments of Pathology and Biochemistry, University of Miami, School of Medicine, P.O. Box 016960, Miami, FL 33101, U.S.A.

Introduction

Protein phosphorylation has been implicated in the regulation of many neural functions (for recent reviews, see Nestler and Greengard, 1984; Browning et al., 1985). Neural tissue contains high levels of protein phosphorylating systems, i.e. protein kinases, phosphatases, and substrates (Rodnight, 1982). Several types of protein kinases are activated by second messengers (Krebs, 1983). Three of the major kinases and their second messenger activators are diagrammed in Fig. 1. Following stimulation of ligand- or voltage-sensing receptors by neurotransmitters, neurohormones, or electrical impulses, second messenger systems are activated which stimulate distinct protein kinases, which in turn catalyze protein phosphorylation. This process gives rise to phosphoproteins which, either directly or through a series of subsequent phosphorylations, lead to the appropriate biological response to the extracellular signal.

In the past five years, major advances have been made in our understanding of the structure and function of ion channels. It is now well established that the activity of ion channels can be altered by protein phosphorylation. This finding comes from a number of studies in both invertebrate and vertebrate neurons in which the effects of protein kinases or inhibitors on properties of ionic currents in whole and perfused cells, membrane patches, and reconstituted bilayers have been recorded (e.g. see Chapters 7, 9 and 11).

This chapter contains a discussion of the hypothesis that modulation of ion channel activity by Ca²⁺-dependent protein phosphorylation may be part of the biological processes that underlie associative learning. Evidence from a series of studies on the nudibranch mollusc, *Hermissenda crassicornis*, indicates that intracellular Ca²⁺ increases during the presentation of paired stimuli, that elevated Ca²⁺ can inactivate K⁺ currents that are reduced following conditioning, and that intracellular injection of protein kinases can mimic, at least in part, the effects of associative learning on K⁺ currents (for recent review, see Alkon, 1984).

Another topic discussed here concerns a comparison of catalytic properties of the *Hermissenda* neural protein kinases with their mammalian counterparts. In electrophysiological studies, mammalian protein kinases have been injected into *Hermissenda* neurons to study the effects of protein phosphorylation on the K⁺ currents that are modified following associative learning. It therefore becomes important to characterize the *Hermissenda* neuronal protein kinases to determine if they function in a manner similar to the mammalian protein kinases.

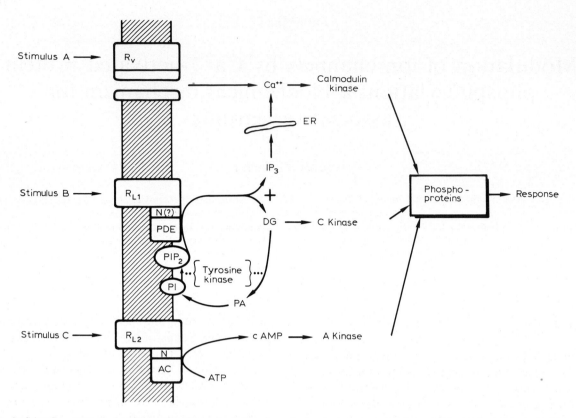

Fig. 1. Stimulus–response coupling of voltage- and ligand-sensing receptors to second messenger activated protein kinases. Phosphorylations may occur on the same or different protein substrates. Abbreviations: R_V and R_I, voltage- and ligand-sensing receptors; AC, adenylate cyclase; N, GTP-binding regulatory proteins; PA, phosphatidic acid; PI, phosphatidylinositol; PIP_2, polyphosphatidylinositols; PDE, phosphodiesterase (phospholipase C); DG, diacylglycerol; IP_3, inositol trisphosphate; C kinase, Ca^{2+}/diacylglycerol-activated, phospholipid-dependent protein kinase (protein kinase C); A kinase, cAMP-dependent protein kinase; ER, endoplasmic reticulum.

Changes in K^+ currents and protein phosphorylation observed following associative learning in *Hermissenda*

A model of associative learning in *Hermissenda* has been developed which results in a modification of the phototactic response, i.e. animals can be conditioned to take significantly longer times to locomote from a region of dim illumination to a region of bright light. Repeated presentations of light and rotation were shown in an early study to result in modification of the phototactic response (Alkon, 1974a). The increase in latency to move toward a light spot is produced by the temporal pairing of two stimuli, light and rotation (Crow and Alkon, 1978). Conditioning with paired light and rotation results in a much greater latency than the presentation of random or unpaired light and rotation. In brief, training consists of 50 trials of paired light and rotation per day for 3 days. The duration of each trial is 30 s with a variable inter-trial interval of 1 to 3 min. Details of the automated training and testing procedure and apparatus have been published previously (Crow and Alkon, 1978; Tyndale and Crow, 1979). A non-associative component of the response to paired light and rotation is present immediately after training but decreases rapidly during the first hour following training (Alkon, 1974a; Crow, 1983).

During stimulation with light and rotation, photoreceptors receive synaptic input from hair cells in the gravity-sensing organ, the statocyst

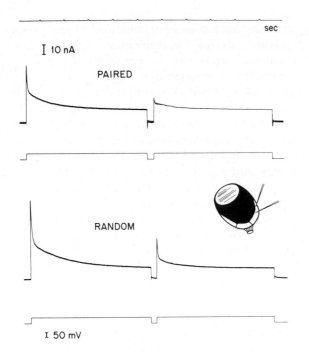

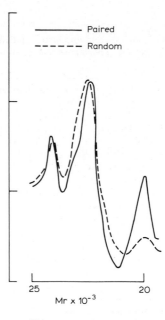

Fig. 2. Reduction of rapidly inactivating K^+ current (I_A) in type B photoreceptors of animals whose phototactic behavior had been modified by conditioning with paired light and rotation, as compared to the random control. (From Alkon et al., 1982a).

Fig. 3. Increase in ^{32}P incorporation in M_r 20 000 in eyes of animals whose phototactic behavior had been modified by conditioning with paired light and rotation (solid line), as compared to the random control (dashed line). A densitometric scan of the M_r 25 000 to 20 000 region is shown here; see Table I for data on other phosphoproteins. (From Neary et al., 1981.)

(Alkon, 1973a,b, 1974b, 1975; Akaike and Alkon, 1980). A number of electrophysiological correlates of the modified behavioral response have been found in the type B photoreceptors of conditioned animals (Crow and Alkon, 1980; West et al., 1982; Alkon et al., 1982a; Crow, 1982, 1985; Forman et al., 1984). (The eye of *Hermissenda* consists of five photoreceptors: two type A and three type B cells; the type A and B photoreceptors are distinguished by their electrophysiological properties.) The effects of conditioning that are most pertinent to the discussion here are those revealed by voltage-clamp studies. Alkon et al. (1982a) found that the early K^+ current (I_A) was reduced by 25–30% in type B photoreceptors in animals whose phototactic behavior had been modified by conditioning with paired light and rotation, as compared to those that received random light and rotation (see Fig. 2). Further studies suggest that other membrane currents in type B photoreceptors also change following conditioning, as has recently

been proposed (Alkon, 1982–1983; Crow, 1983). For example, a late Ca^{2+}-dependent K^+ current (I_C) is also reduced following conditioning (Farley and Alkon, 1983; Forman et al., 1984; Alkon et al., 1985).

A biochemical correlate of associative learning in *Hermissenda* has also been found (Neary et al., 1981). Several hours following acquisition, there was a significant increase in ^{32}P incorporation in a phosphoprotein with an apparent molecular weight (M_r) of 20 000 in the eyes of animals whose phototactic behavior had been modified by pairing light and rotation (Fig. 3). No significant difference in ^{32}P incorporation in M_r 20 000 was found in eyes from animals receiving random or unpaired stimuli. The specificity of this effect was further indicated by the lack of significant changes in ^{32}P incorporation in ten other phosphoprotein bands that were present in the eyes of all animals studied (Table I). As the eye of *Hermissenda* consists of only five photoreceptors, a lens, and pigment and epithelial cells, a biochemical change

TABLE I

Effect of paired, random, and unpaired stimulation on ^{32}P incorporation in specific phosphoprotein bands in *Hermissenda* eyes[a]

Phosphoprotein band	Ratio of experimental/untreated (Mean + S.E.M.)		
(M_r)	Paired ($N = 16$)	Random ($N = 12$)	Unpaired ($N = 5$)
72 000	0.83 ± 0.08	1.05 ± 0.23	1.30 ± 0.38
55 000	1.02 ± 0.04	1.04 ± 0.09	0.88 ± 0.07
44 000	0.88 ± 0.12	1.35 ± 0.10	1.04 ± 0.44
42 000	1.27 ± 0.14	1.18 ± 0.08	1.08 ± 0.13
38 000	1.11 ± 0.07	0.87 ± 0.10	1.23 ± 0.14
34 000	1.55 ± 0.21	1.22 ± 0.20	1.56 ± 0.32
31 000	1.12 ± 0.14	1.23 ± 0.18	0.91 ± 0.16
29 000	0.89 ± 0.11	1.24 ± 0.17	1.15 ± 0.41
24 000	1.12 ± 0.17	0.90 ± 0.15	1.10 ± 0.18
22 000	1.04 ± 0.10	1.16 ± 0.14	0.76 ± 0.07
20 000	[b]2.16 ± 0.28	1.13 ± 0.10	1.18 ± 0.14

[a]For experimental details, see Neary et al. (1981).
[b]$F_{2,30} = 6.49$; $p < 0.01$.

correlated with associative learning has been localized to a few cells within a nervous system.

Thus, several studies in animals whose phototactic response has been modified by temporal pairing of stimuli indicate that changes in K^+ currents and protein phosphorylation occur following associative learning. These studies on conditioned animals provide the basis for detailed investigations of the mechanisms involved in associative learning in *Hermissenda* and how these mechanisms are regulated.

Ca^{2+}-mediated regulation of K^+ currents and protein kinases

A key feature in a recently proposed hypothesis of biophysical and biochemical mechanisms underlying associative learning in *Hermissenda* involves an increase in intracellular Ca^{2+} in type B photoreceptors, an increase which results from the pairing of stimuli (for recent review, see Alkon, 1984). During paired stimulation with light and rotation, hair cells in the gravity-sensing organ, the statocyst, cause brief inhibitory, followed by prolonged excitatory synaptic input in the type B photoreceptors. This synaptic input, when coupled

with the light-induced stimulation of the photoreceptors during the repetition of paired conditioning, leads to a persistent increase in membrane depolarization (Crow and Alkon, 1980; Alkon, 1986). (When stimulation of hair cells and photoreceptors are uncoupled in time, no such persistent increase occurs). The increase in membrane depolarization can then give rise to an increase in intracellular Ca^{2+}. (See sequence of events outlined in Fig. 4). A rise in intracellular Ca^{2+}, as detected by an increase in Arsenazo dye signal, is enhanced in axotomized type B photoreceptors by pairing light with depolarization (Connor and Alkon, 1984). (The depolarization current delivered to the axotomized photoreceptor simulates the excitatory input of the hair cells during rotation.) The paired stimuli-induced rise in intracellular Ca^{2+} can, in turn, affect the early and late K^+ currents shown to change following modification of the phototactic response. Investigations of the properties of the early and late K^+ currents have shown that Ca^{2+} increases the rate of inactivation of both I_A and I_C (Alkon et al., 1982b; Alkon and Sakakibara, 1984, 1985). The change in K^+ conductance in the type B photoreceptors would then result in an altered electrical signal to the follower cells in the neural network that underlies phototaxis in *Hermissenda*, thereby giving rise to a change in the animals' locomotor behavior.

These studies suggest that the observed reductions of I_A and I_C following conditioning with paired light and rotation are brought about by a rise in intracellular Ca^{2+}. One type of biochemical mechanism that could underlie a Ca^{2+}-induced

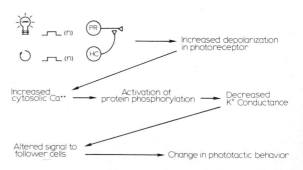

Fig. 4. Proposed sequence of events underlying pairing-specific change in *Hermissenda* phototactic behavior.

inactivation of K^+ currents is Ca^{2+}-dependent protein phosphorylation. Two general kinds of Ca^{2+}-dependent protein kinases, Ca^{2+}/calmodulin-dependent protein kinase (Ca^{2+}/CaMdPK) and Ca^{2+}/phospholipid-dependent protein kinase (protein kinase C; see Chapter 3), are present in relatively high concentrations in mammalian brain tissue, and a Ca^{2+}/calmodulin-dependent protein phosphatase (calcineurin) has also been discovered (Stewart et al., 1982). An increase in intracellular Ca^{2+} could activate protein phosphorylation/dephosphorylation directly by acting on Ca^2-dependent protein kinases and phosphatases or indirectly by acting on Ca^{2+}-activated adenylate cyclase which in turn could activate cAMP-dependent protein kinase (cAMPdPK). In order to test the effects of protein phosphorylation on K^+ currents, we have injected Ca^{2+}/CaMdPK and cAMPdPK into type B photoreceptors and measured their effects on K^+ currents under voltage clamp conditions. In addition, we have stimulated the endogenous Ca^{2+}-dependent protein kinases with a phorbol ester or 1-oleoyl-2-acetylglycerol (to activate protein kinase C) and with a transient Ca^{2+} signal (to activate Ca^{2+}/CaMdPK) in an attempt to investigate possible synergistic effects of these two Ca^{2+}-dependent protein kinases on K^+ currents (Neary et al., 1985; Alkon et al., 1986). As described below, the results of these studies show that intracellular injection of Ca^{2+}/CaMdPK and cAMPdPK can mimic the biophysical effects of conditioning on *Hermissenda* photoreceptors. Furthermore, our preliminary experiments suggest that long-lasting reductions in K^+ currents may require the combined activation of Ca^{2+}/CaMdPK and protein kinase C.

Our initial study on the effects of Ca^{2+}/CaMdPK on K^+ currents involved the use of phosphorylase kinase, as suggested by Dr. Howard Rasmussen and purified from rabbit muscle by Dr. E.G. Krebs and associates. Phosphorylase kinase is composed of two sets of four subunits, one of which is calmodulin (Cohen, 1982). Two of the other subunits are substrates for cAMPdPK, and phosphorylation of one of these subunits activates the enzyme 15–20 fold at saturating levels of Ca^{2+} and increases the affinity for Ca^{2+} about 15 fold (Cohen, 1980). The major

substrate for this enzyme is phosphorylase *b*; glycogen synthase (Embi et al., 1979), synapsin I (Kennedy and Greengard, 1981) and endogenous proteins of *Hermissenda* ganglia (Neary, unpublished observations) can also be phosphorylated by the enzyme.

Intracellular injection of phosphorylase kinase into *Hermissenda* type B photoreceptors leads to an increase in input resistance and to reductions in early and late K^+ currents (Acosta-Urquidi et al., 1984a; see footnote). These effects are dependent on Ca^{2+}: (*a*) omission of Ca^{2+} from the bathing medium prevents the phosphorylase kinase-mediated increase in input resistance, and (*b*) under voltage clamp, injection of phosphorylase kinase was effective in reducing K^+ currents only when a Ca^{2+} load was delivered to the cell by pairing light and depolarization (Fig. 5). Intracellular injection of phosphorylase kinase into giant neurons in *Hermissenda* also reduces the amplitude of I_A and I_C, and the enzyme has been shown to increase the Ca^{2+}-mediated inactivation of K^+ currents (Acosta-Urquidi et al., 1983). In these studies, as well as studies using other protein kinases, injection of inactivated enzymes did not have a significant effect on the ionic currents under investigation.

In the kinase experiments described here, the enzymes were injected into *Hermissenda* neurons by means of iontophoresis, i.e. an enzyme was placed in a buffer solution at an alkaline pH to obtain negatively charged molecules, the solution was loaded into a microelectrode, and negatively charged molecules were ejected by passing negative current through the electrode. With this technique, small ions are ejected more readily than larger, less densely charged protein molecules. Because the transference number of the kinases were not known, it was necessary to demonstrate that enzyme could be ejected from the electrode. This was done by attempting to assay, under conditions of iontophoresis, the amount of kinase ejected into 10-μl microwells. For all three enzymes studied, small amounts of enzyme activities above controls (carrier solution) could be measured in the microwells. It should be noted that in the iontophoretic technique, as well as in the pressure injection technique used in other kinase studies, non-physiological amounts of kinases may be introduced into neurons. Hence, it is important to conduct parallel experiments designed to stimulate the endogenous kinases under physiologically relevant conditions.

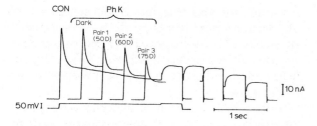

Fig. 5. Reduction of K$^+$ currents in type B photoreceptors by intracellular injection of phosphorylase kinase (PhK), a type of Ca^{2+}/calmodulin-dependent protein kinase. CON: control, before injection of phosphorylase kinase. PAIR refers to pairings of light and depolarization (D, mV). Records of late K$^+$ currents on right are from the same experiment as on left, and are displaced for purposes of comparison. (From Acosta-Urquidi et al., 1984.)

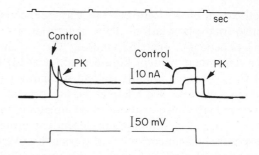

Fig. 6. Reduction of early and late K$^+$ currents in type B photoreceptors by intracellular injection of the catalytic subunit (PK) of cAMP-dependent protein kinase. (From Alkon et al., 1983.)

These early studies employed phosphorylase kinase as a model type of Ca^{2+}/CaMdPK because of the wealth of information known about its properties and because of the initial difficulty of obtaining a highly purified neuronal CaM kinase in a stable form. Since then, however, several laboratories have succeeded in preparing a purified, relatively stable form of neuronal CaM kinase (Fukunaga et al., 1982; Bennett et al., 1983; Goldenring et al., 1983; Yamauchi and Fugisawa, 1983; Kuret and Schulman, 1984; McGuinness et al., 1985). In collaboration with Drs. DeLorenzo and Goldenring, we have found that injection of the rat brain CaM kinase II into giant neurons (Acosta-Urquidi et al., 1984b) and type B photoreceptors (Sakakibara et al., manuscript in preparation) in *Hermissenda* also leads to reductions in I_A and I_C, although its effects appear to be more complex than phosphorylase kinase and depend on the particular neuron under study (Acosta-Urquidi et al., manuscript in preparation). Thus, the results of these experiments using two different kinds of Ca^{2+}/CaMdPK suggest a role for Ca^{2+}/CaM-dependent protein phosphorylation in mediating the effects of Ca^{2+} on K$^+$ currents.

Addition of an inhibitor of Ca^{2+}/CaMdPK, trifluoperazine (TFP; 5 µM), to the bathing medium results in an increase in I_A and I_C in type B photoreceptors (Sakakibara et al., manuscript in preparation). Because TFP can also inhibit protein kinase C (e.g. DeRiemer et al., 1985), the site

of action of TFP cannot be stated with certainty. Nonetheless, it is interesting to note that TFP causes an increase in I_A and I_C whereas the Ca^{2+}-dependent protein kinases bring about a decrease in these K$^+$ currents. An increase in I_A and I_C would be expected if TFP were inhibiting a Ca^{2+}-dependent protein kinase.

A different type of protein kinase, cAMPdPK, also affects input resistance and early and late K$^+$ currents in type B photoreceptors. Injection of the catalytic subunit of bovine brain cAMPdPK (again kindly supplied by Dr. E. Krebs and associates) also reduced the early and late K$^+$ currents (Fig. 6) and increased input resistance (Alkon et al., 1983). In addition, we found that the catalytic subunit of bovine heart cAMPdPK phosphorylates the same *Hermissenda* neural proteins that are phosphorylated by the endogenous cAMPdPK (Neary et al., 1984).

The results of these studies indicate that both CaM kinase and cAMPdPK can reduce the amplitude of the early and late K$^+$ currents that are decreased by associative learning. An increase in intracellular Ca^{2+} could affect these currents directly via CaM kinase or indirectly via CaM-sensitive adenylate cyclase and cAMPdPK, as illustrated in Fig. 7. While these mechanisms may be related to an early phase of stimulus–response coupling, it is likely that additional mechanisms(s) are involved in long-lasting physiological and behavioral responses because the rise in intracellular Ca^{2+} is brief whereas the behavioral response in *Hermissenda* lasts for several days. One mech-

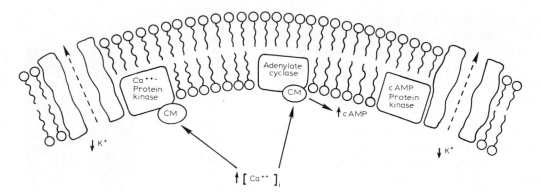

Fig. 7. Cartoon for reduction of K$^+$ currents by an increase in cytosolic Ca^{2+}, as mediated directly by CaM kinase or indirectly by CaM-sensitive adenylate cyclase, which results in increased cAMP and activation of cAMPdPK.

anism that appears to underlie sustained responses to the transient Ca^{2+} signal in mammalian systems involves the activation of two branches of the Ca^{2+} messenger system, CaM kinase and protein kinase C and, as well as the cycling of Ca^{2+} across the plasma membrane (Rasmussen et al., 1984). From studies in platelets, Nishizuka and co-workers have found that an increase in intracellular Ca^{2+}, as induced by a Ca^{2+} ionophore, brings about phosphorylation of M_r 20 000 presumably catalyzed by CaM kinase, whereas activation of protein kinase C leads to phosphorylation of M_r 40 000 (Kaibuchi et al., 1983). Based on an extensive series of experiments in adrenal glomerulosa cells, Rasmussen and colleagues have proposed that integrated Ca^{2+}-mediated mechanisms which give rise to responses that outlast the transient Ca^{2+} signal involve the transient activation of a calmodulin-regulated system, such as CaM kinase, coupled temporally with the activation of protein kinase C, which is regulated by cycling Ca^{2+} across the plasma membrane (Kojima et al., 1984). Activation of the CaM system gives rise to a prompt but brief response, and activation of protein kinase C leads to a sustained, but submaximal response. When both systems are activated, the sustained, maximum response is obtained. This suggests that sustained physiological and behavioral responses may require multi-substrate and/or multi-site phosphorylation, catalyzed by at least two different protein kinases.

Could the temporal requirement of activation of protein kinase systems described above be related to the temporal specificity of paired stimuli-induced associative learning in *Hermissenda*? In order to test this possibility, a series of experiments were conducted in *Hermissenda* type B photoreceptors in which (*a*) a short term increase in intracellular Ca^{2+} was produced by stimulating the cell with light and depolarization, which by analogy with the above systems would activate endogenous CaM kinase, and (*b*) activation of endogenous protein kinase C obtained by addition of a phorbol ester or 1-oleoyl-2-acetylglycerol (OAG) to the bathing solution. The working hypothesis was that the increased Ca^{2+} would be sufficient to stimulate the endogenous CaM kinase but not protein kinase C because both Ca^{2+} and phospholipids are required to activate the latter enzyme, both in mammalian (Takai et al., 1979; Kaibuchi et al., 1981) and in molluscan nervous systems (DeRiemer et al., 1985; Neary et al., 1985). The phorbol ester or OAG was added to stimulate protein kinase C, perhaps by promoting the translocation of cytosolic protein kinase C to the plasma membrane (Kraft and Anderson, 1983) where it would be in position to be activated by membrane phospholipids. In addition, the protein kinase C activators may serve to increase the sensitivity of *Hermissenda* protein kinase C to Ca^{2+} (Kishimoto et al., 1980), thereby converting it to a form which is active at resting or near resting levels of Ca^{2+}.

Recent experiments have shown that combined treatment of type B photoreceptors with a Ca^{2+} load and a protein kinase C activator leads to reductions in I_A and I_C which persist longer than when either treatment is given separately (Alkon et al., 1986). The Ca^{2+} load alone results in a transient reduction in I_A or I_C (1 to 5 min). No significant effect on I_A or I_C is seen with the protein kinase C activator alone. Combined treatment with both Ca^{2+} load and protein kinase C activator results in reductions which last as long as the recording period (up to 3 h). Moreover, the reductions in K^+ currents persist following the removal of the protein kinase C activator. When the Ca^{2+} load is paired with inactive analogs of diacylglycerol or phorbol esters, the sustained effect is not observed. The Ca^{2+} load alone does not appear to be sufficient to activate protein kinase C because addition of a protein kinase C activator is necessary to bring about the long-lasting effects on I_A and I_C.

These results suggest a possible model for the retention of associative memory which involves the activation of two or more protein kinases. However, many questions need to be addressed before a valid analogy can be made between these results and the temporally dependent, synergistic model Rasmussen and colleagues have proposed to explain how the transient Ca^{2+} signal is converted into a long-lasting physiological response. For example, does the pairing of light and rotation bring about activation of two different protein kinases? If so, which stimulus activates CaM kinase and which one activates protein kinase C? Are different sets of proteins phosphorylated by CaM kinase and protein kinase C as in the platelet system, or are multiple sites on the same protein phosphorylated by the different kinases? Do the paired stimuli activate polyphosphoinositide hydrolysis to bring about increases in diacylglycerol and inositol 1,4,5-trisphosphate? Is cAMPdPK activated during the combined treatment paradigm? Although it is tempting to speculate that the mechanism that underlies the temporal pairing of light and rotation to bring about a change in phototactic behavior involves the combined activation of two or more protein kinases, further studies are needed to explore this hypothesis.

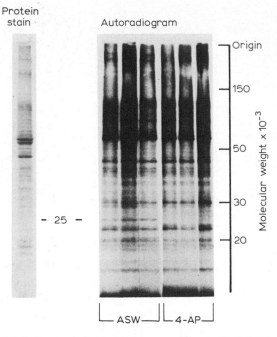

Fig. 8. Reduction in level of ^{32}P incorporation in M_r 25 000 by 4-AP. Three different samples from controls (artificial seawater, ASW) and 4-AP experiments are shown to indicate sample-to-sample variations in the relative intensities of the phosphoprotein bands. Decreased ^{32}P incorporation in M_r 25 000 can be observed in all 4-AP-treated samples. (From Neary and Alkon, 1983.)

Another approach to studying the biochemical mechanisms that underlie the regulation of voltage-dependent ionic currents and their role in associative learning involves (a) the use of channel blockers which preferentially block specific types of ionic currents in molluscan neurons (for review, see Adams et al., 1980) and (b) the use of high external K^+ to inactivate voltage-dependent K^+ currents. Application of 4-aminopyridine (4-AP), which blocks I_A in molluscan neurons (Thompson, 1977, 1982; Byrne et al., 1979; Alkon et al., 1984), to *Hermissenda* CNS that were previously labeled with $^{32}P_i$ leads to a marked reduction ($\geqslant 85\%$, Fig. 8) of ^{32}P incorporation in a M_r 25 000 in eyes and ganglia (Neary and Alkon, 1983). This effect occurred over a concentration range (1–10 mM) and time course (5–30 min) that are similar to those required to block I_A by 4-AP when the presence of the sheath surrounding the ganglia is

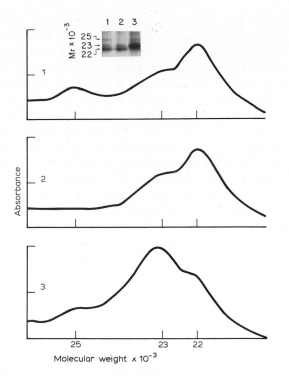

Fig. 9. Reversibility of 4-AP effect on M_r 25 000. Autoradiograms (inset) and densitometric scans are from experiments in which ^{32}P-labeled CNS were incubated (1) in ASW alone, (2) in 10 mM 4-AP for 30 min, or (3) in ASW (30 min) following a 30 min incubation in 10 mM 4-AP. (From Neary and Alkon, 1983.)

taken into consideration. In addition, the effect of 4-AP is reversible; removal of 4-AP leads to an increase in ^{32}P incorporation in M_r 25 000 and also in M_r 23 000 (Fig. 9).

The effect of 4-AP on the level of ^{32}P in M_r 25 000 does not appear to be the result of a 4-AP-induced increase in impulse activity which can occur during 4-AP treatment (for review of effects of aminopyridines on synaptic transmission, see Thesleff, 1980). Neurons in the eye were isolated from the site of initiation of impulse activity and synaptic inputs by a lesion made in the optic tract between the eye and optic ganglia (Alkon, 1979). Eyes from the lesioned preparations still exhibited the 4-AP effect on M_r 25 000, thereby suggesting that this effect cannot be explained by an indirect effect of 4-AP on impulse activity.

Since depolarization and increased intracellular Ca^{2+} are key steps in the proposed sequence of events leading to a conditioning-induced change in phototaxis (see Fig. 4), we have also used high external K^+ to bring about sustained depolarization of *Hermissenda* neurons, increased Ca^{2+} uptake, and inactivation of voltage-dependent K^+ currents. We have found that M_r 25 000 which is reduced by 4-AP is also reduced by sustained depolarization with 100 mM K^+ (Neary and Alkon, 1983). This effect persists even after the nervous systems are returned to artificial seawater (ASW) containing normal K^+ (Naito et al., 1985). High $[K^+]$ increases ^{32}P incorporation in M_r 56 000, which, as discussed later, is a substrate for protein kinase C and cAMPdPK. However, the effect of high $[K^+]$ on this phosphoprotein is reversed by returning the nervous systems to normal ASW. The sustained exposure to high K^+, followed by return to normal ASW, may provide a useful biochemical model to investigate some of the effects of conditioning in *Hermissenda*.

Protein kinases and substrates in the *Hermissenda* nervous system: comparison of molluscan and mammalian enzymes

In order to study the regulation of phosphorylation of the proteins that appear to be related to associative learning and K^+ conductance, we have investigated the activation of endogenous protein kinases by cAMP, Ca^{2+}, CaM, phospholipids, and diacylglycerol (DG). In addition, because experiments on the regulation of ionic currents in molluscan neurons have utilized mammalian protein kinases, it is important to characterize the molluscan enzymes to determine if their properties are similar to those of their mammalian counterparts.

As shown in Fig. 10, cAMPdPK, Ca^{2+}/CaMdPK, and protein kinase C activities can be readily demonstrated in subcellular fractions from *Hermissenda* nervous systems. The region of the electrophoresis gel containing the major substrates is shown here, but many other proteins are also phosphorylated (Neary et al., 1984). For example, addition of cAMP to CNS homogenates leads to phosphorylation of at least 15 protein bands, and addition of Ca^{2+} to CNS homogenates gives rise to increased labeling in at

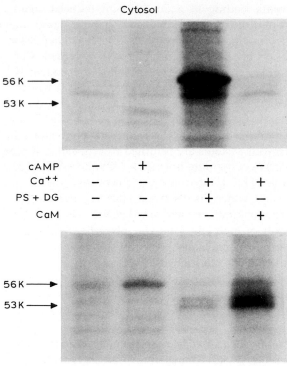

Cytosol

56 K ⟶

53 K ⟶

cAMP	−	+	−	−
Ca⁺⁺	−	−	+	+
PS + DG	−	−	+	−
CaM	−	−	−	+

56 K ⟶

53 K ⟶

Membrane

Fig. 10. cAMPdPK, Ca^{2+}/CaMdPK, and protein kinase C activities and protein substrates in the *Hermissenda* nervous system. Autoradiograms are shown from the portion of the gel containing the major substrates, but many other substrates can be detected with longer exposure and in other regions of the gel (Neary et al., 1984). Nervous systems were homogenized in Ca^{2+}-free buffer containing 50 mM Tris, pH 7.0, 2 mM EGTA, and 2 mM dithiothreitol, and supernatant and particulate fractions were prepared by centrifugation at $23\,000 \times g$ for 30 min at 5°C. The kinases were stimulated with 20 μM 8-bromo-cAMP, 20 μM free Ca^{2+} (1 mM $CaCl_2$, 1 mM EGTA, pH 7.0), 10 μM CaM, 50 μg/ml PS and 5 μg/ml DG, as indicated, for 2 min at 20°C.

least 10 protein bands. As shown in Fig. 10, M_r 56 000 is the major substrate for cAMPdPK in the membrane fraction. This protein is also the major substrate for cytosolic protein kinase C, which is activated by addition of Ca^{2+}, phosphatidylserine (PS), and DG. As measured by two-dimensional gel electrophoresis, the major substrate for both cAMPdPK and protein kinase C has a $pI = 5.1$. The similarity in M_r and pI suggest that M_r 56 000, which is present in the supernatant and pellet fractions, is a substrate for both cAMPdPK and protein kinase C. At least seven other protein

bands are substrates for protein kinase C, and some of these proteins also appear to be substrates for cAMPdPK. Centrifugation of the homogenate at $23\,000 \times g$ results in good separation of CaM kinase and protein kinase C; most of the CaM kinase activity is in the pellet while about 80% of protein kinase C activity is in the supernatant. Addition of Ca^{2+} and CaM to the membrane fraction results in phosphorylation of at least five protein bands, some of which also appear to be substrates for cAMPdPK and protein kinase C. M_r 53 000 is the major substrate for Ca^{2+}/CaMdPK; as discussed later, this protein band appears to be autophosphorylated CaM kinase. Although not shown in this figure, Ca^{2+} alone is not effective in stimulating the membrane CaM kinase or the cytosolic protein kinase C (Neary et al., 1984, 1985).

Our preliminary results indicate that M_r 20 000, which is increased by associative learning, is a substrate for both protein kinase C and cAMPdPK, and M_r 25 000, which is affected by agents that reduce voltage dependent K^+ currents, is a substrate for cAMPdPK and Ca^{2+}-dependent protein kinase(s). However, two-dimensional gel electrophoresis (O'Farrell, 1975; Neary, 1984) and proteolytic peptide maps (Cleveland et al., 1977) are needed to confirm these preliminary observations concerning the comparison of protein bands from in vivo labeling (incubation of whole cell preparations with ^{32}P) with in vitro labeling studies (incubation of cell-free homogenates with $[\gamma-^{32}P]ATP$).

Time course studies during in vitro labeling of homogenates suggest the presence of protein phosphatases, some of which may be Ca^{2+} dependent. When phosphorylation is stimulated by either cAMP or Ca^{2+}, two markedly different time courses of ^{32}P incorporation into specific protein bands are observed. In one group, ^{32}P incorporation increases gradually and then remains relatively constant during the remainder of the incubation, whereas in the second group, which includes M_r 56 000 and 53 000, phosphorylation peaks in 1–2 min and then rapidly declines. This suggests that some *Hermissenda* CNS phosphoproteins are more susceptible to phosphatases than others.

The physiological relevance of the Ca^{2+}-dependent protein kinases has been investigated by measuring CaM kinase and protein kinase C activities over a range of free Ca^{2+} concentrations. Ca^{2+}-stimulated incorporation in M_r 53 000 can be detected at 0.5 µM free Ca^{2+} and approaches a plateau in the range of 2–20 µM. Most substrates for protein kinase C activity can be phosphorylated, in the presence of lipids, at <0.5 µM free Ca^{2+}, but two substrates (M_r 56 000 and 71 000) require higher free Ca^{2+} (2–5 µM). Extracellular stimulation of many systems leads to increases in cytosolic Ca^{2+} from 0.1 to 2 µM (for recent review, see Rasmussen and Barrett, 1984). Thus, the Ca^{2+}-stimulated protein kinases in the *Hermissenda* nervous system are capable of activation in response to extracellular signals and may play a role in stimulus–response coupling in *Hermissenda*.

A key feature of mammalian protein kinase C, in terms of its role in sustained physiological response mechanisms, is the ability of DG to increase its sensitivity for Ca^{2+} (Nishizuka, 1984). Accordingly, the effect of DG on *Hermissenda* protein kinase C has been investigated. As with the mammalian enzyme, addition of DG, in the presence of phosphatidylserine, increases the activity of *Hermissenda* neural protein kinase C. DG and OAG are more effective than triacylglycerol. These studies suggest that the affinity of the *Hermissenda* protein kinase C can be increased by diacylglycerols, but further experiments are needed to establish the Ca^{2+} concentration range over which this effects takes place.

From these studies and from studies on protein kinases in *Aplysia*, it is clear that the molluscan protein kinases have many properties in common with the mammalian cAMPdPK, Ca^{2+}/CaMdPK, and protein kinase C. The mammalian cAMPdPK phosphorylates many of the same *Hermissenda* neural proteins that are phosphorylated by the endogenous cAMPdPK. Mammalian cAMPdPK has also been shown to phosphorylate *Aplysia* nervous system proteins (Jennings et al., 1982; Novak-Hofer and Levitan, 1983). Kaczmarek and colleagues have presented evidence that CaM kinase in *Aplysia* ganglia cross-reacts with antibodies to mammalian CaM kinase II, and that its peptide fragments co-migrate with those of the mammalian

enzyme (DeRiemer et al. 1984). The *Hermissenda* protein kinase C can phosphorylate lysine-rich histone, a substrate for mammalian protein kinase C, and DG increases the activity of the *Hermissenda* enzyme. Phosphatidylethanolamine is not as effective as PS in stimulating the mammalian protein kinase C (Takai et al., 1979; Kaibuchi et al., 1981); similar observations have been made with the *Hermissenda* enzyme. The *Aplysia* protein kinase C can be activated by a phorbol ester and can phosphorylate M_r 87 000 from bovine brain, a substrate for mammalian protein kinase C (DeRiemer et al., 1985). Thus, these studies provide evidence that molluscan cAMPdPK, Ca^{2+}/CaMdPK, and protein kinase C have properties that are similar to those of the mammalian enzymes. These findings justify the use of purified mammalian protein kinases in studies designed to elucidate the role of protein phosphorylation in the regulation of ionic currents in molluscan neurons.

A role for protein kinase C in mammalian learning and memory has been proposed (Routtenberg, 1985; Chapter 18). Electrical stimulation of neuronal pathways in the hippocampus leads to long-lasting changes in synaptic transmission, and this system has been used as a model for mechanisms underlying neural plasticity. Changes in phosphoproteins have previously been observed following electrical stimulation of hippocampal slices (Browning et al., 1979; Bar et al., 1980). Routtenberg et al. (1985) have now found that long-term potentiation in the intact hippocampus leads to a selective increase in phosphorylation of M_r 47 000, a substrate for protein kinase C (Akers and Routtenberg, 1985; Nelson and Routtenberg, 1985). This protein may be identical to B-50, a brain-specific, synaptically enriched phosphoprotein that has been studied in detail by Gispen and colleagues and that is known to be a substrate for protein kinase C (Aloyo et al., 1983). In addition, proteins (M_r 24 000, 21 000 and 19 000) whose level of phosphorylation is altered by active avoidance training appear to be substrates for protein kinase C (Lyn-Cook et al., 1985). It is also of interest to note that phorbol esters reduce the slow Ca^{2+}-dependent K^+ component of afterhyperpolarization in hippocampal pyramidal neurons (Baraban et al., 1985) and that afterhyperpolarization is reduced in hippocampal neurons following classical conditioning (Disterhoft et al., 1984). These findings, together with the *Hermissenda* results, support the concept that protein kinase C plays a role in both molluscan and mammalian associative learning.

Concluding remarks

The results of the *Hermissenda* studies summarized here indicate that cAMPdPK and CaMdPK decrease the amplitudes of I_A and I_C, K^+ currents that are reduced in photoreceptors following associative learning. In addition, we have found that cAMPdPK, CaM kinase, and protein kinase C in the *Hermissenda* nervous system have catalytic properties that are similar to the mammalian protein kinases. Of particular interest are the findings that the Ca^{2+}-dependent protein kinases can be activated by physiologically relevant concentrations of Ca^{2+} and that DG can increase the activity of the *Hermissenda* protein kinase C. Taken together, our biophysical and biochemical observations to date indicate that Ca^{2+}-stimulated protein phosphorylation can alter the activity of K^+ currents and that these phosphorylation mechanisms may be related to associative learning in *Hermissenda*. Second messenger systems, protein phosphorylation, and K^+ currents have also been implicated as mechanisms of learning and behavior in other invertebrates, such as *Aplysia* (Abrams et al., 1984; Occur et al., 1984) and *Drosophila* (Byers et al., 1981; Shotwell, 1983; Dudai and Zvi, 1984; Devay et al., 1984; Livingstone et al. 1984) and, as mentioned in the previous section, evidence has been presented for the involvement of Ca^{2+}-dependent protein phosphorylation and K^+ currents in mammalian learning. Thus, both vertebrates and invertebrates may utilize these mechanisms for learning and behavior.

As described in Chapters 7, 9 and 11, it is now well established that many types of ionic currents can be modulated by protein phosphorylation. This finding raises interesting questions concerning the identification of the proteins that are phosphorylated by the injected kinases, the ability of protein phosphatases to reverse the effects of the kinases, and the interactions between kinases, phosphatases, and their protein substrates that modulate ion channel activity. It is not clear whether the effects of protein kinases on ion channel activity is brought about directly by phosphorylation of the channel or indirectly by phosphorylation of channel-associated proteins. The results of pioneering studies by Shuster et al. (1985) and Ewald et al. (1985), in which the effects of cAMPdPK on channels in membrane patches or in reconstituted membrane bilayers have been investigated, indicate that phosphorylation must occur on the ion channel itself or on intimately associated proteins. While this approach will help to define the minimal elements involved in the effects of enzymes on ion channel activity, other approaches may be necessary to understand in situ modulation. For example, in reconstituted bilayers, the channels are expected to be at infinite dilution, and in the preparation of inside-out patches, detachment of some cytoskeletal elements is likely to occur. A number of cytoskeletal proteins are phosphorylated, and these phosphoproteins may play a role in the flow of information from the cell exterior to interior. Separation of these proteins from communication with the membrane may remove an important element for the control of ion channel activity. Precedent for the involvement of non-integral membrane proteins in ion channel function comes from the studies of Kung and colleagues on the Ca^{2+} current in *Paramecium*. Addition of a cytosolic protein from wild type organisms gives rise to a Ca^{2+} current in a mutant that originally lacked this current (Haga et al., 1984).

While several types of ionic currents can be modulated by protein kinases, the effects have not always been uniform and appear to depend on the particular cell under investigation. Although cAMPdPK and forskolin, an adenylate cyclase activator, increase inactivation of the early K^+ current in *Hermissenda* photoreceptors and *Aplysia* bag cells (Alkon et al., 1983; Strong, 1984; Strong and Kaczmarek, 1984), the effect of the enzyme on I_C has not been consistent. cAMPdPK increases I_C in *Helix* neurons (DePeyer et al., 1982) and decreases I_C in *Hermissenda* photoreceptors (Alkon et al., 1983). Another example of differing effects of the same enzyme in different cells is the finding that CaM kinase increases Ca^{2+} current in two giant neurons whereas the same enzyme reduces the Ca^{2+} current in other large neurons (Acosta-Urquidi et al., manuscript in preparation) and type B photoreceptors (Sakakibara et al., manuscript in preparation). The contrasting effects of a single type of protein kinase on the modulation of a particular channel may reflect differences in the amino acid sequence of the ion channel in different cells, or it may suggest the importance of cell-specific channel associated components.

Several interesting approaches are now available that should help to determine the molecular components that define the functional properties of a particular current. One involves the insertion of purified channels into lipid bilayers (reviewed by Coronado and Labarca, 1984). Purified, phosphorylated subunits of sodium and calcium channels and the acetylcholine receptor have been obtained (Costa and Catterall, 1984; Huganir et al., 1984; Curtis and Catterall, 1985), and it should be feasible to reconstitute the purified channels and putative regulatory proteins, in their phosphorylated and non-phosphorylated forms, into lipid bilayers and measure activation and inactivation properties with patch clamp techniques. Another approach involves the injection of mRNA into cells that lack the particular current under investigation and measurement of effects of the newly synthesized proteins on the ionic properties of the cell (reviewed by Yellen, 1984). In addition, site-directed mutagenesis (Mishina et al., 1985) may yield channel proteins in which the phosphorylation site is lacking, thereby leading to altered function. It can be expected that application of these biochemical, molecular biological, and biophysical methodologies will provide significant advances in our understanding of the mechanisms by which protein phosphorylation modulates ion channel activity.

Acknowledgements

I am grateful to my colleagues Juan Acosta-Urquidi, Dan Alkon, Doug Coulter, Terry Crow, Bob DeLorenzo, Susan DeRiemer, Ann DeWeer, Hal Gainer, Paul Gallant, Jim Goldenring, June Harrigan, Len Kaczmarek, Paul Kandel, Michinori Kubota, Alan Kuzirian, Greg Kuzma, Shigetaka Naito, Jim Olds, Harish Pant, Howard Rasmussen, Manabu Sakakibara, James Stulman, and Leslie Tengelsen for their contributions to the work described here. I also thank Jeanne Kuzirian for secretarial support.

References

Abrams, T.W., Bernier, L., Hawkins, R.D. and Kandel, E.R. (1984) Possible roles of Ca^{2+} and cAMP in activity-dependent facilitation, a mechanism for associative learning in *Aplysia. Soc. Neurosci. Abstr.*, 10:269.

Acosta-Urquidi, J., Alkon, D.R., Connor, J.A. and Neary, J.T. (1983) Intracellular injection of a Ca^{2+}-dependent protein kinase amplifies Ca^{2+}-mediated inactivation of a transient K^+ current (I_A) in *Hermissenda* giant neurons. *Soc. Neurosci. Abstr.*, 9:501.

Acosta-Urquidi, J., Alkon, D.L. and Neary, J.T. (1984a) Ca^{2+}-dependent protein kinase injection in a photoreceptor mimics biophysical effects of associative learning. *Science*, 224:1254–1257.

Acosta-Urquidi, J., Neary, J.T., Goldenring, J.R., Alkon, D.L. and DeLorenzo, R.J. (1984b) Modulation of I_{Ca} and late K currents by intrasomatic injection of Ca-calmodulin-dependent protein kinase in *Hermissenda* giant neurons. *Soc. Neurosci. Abstr.*, 10:1129.

Adams, D.J., Smith, S.J. and Thompson, S.H. (1980) Ionic currents in molluscan soma. *Annu. Rev. Neurosci.*, 3:141–167.

Akaike, T. and Alkon, D.L. (1980) Sensory convergence on central visual neurons in *Hermissenda. J. Neurophysiol.*, 44:501–513.

Akers, R.J. and Routtenberg, A. (1985) Protein kinase C phosphorylates a 47-M_r protein (F_1) directly related to synaptic plasticity. *Brain Res.*, 334:147–151.

Alkon, D.L. (1973a) Neural organization of a molluscan visual system. *J. Gen. Physiol*, 61:444–461.

Alkon, D.L. (1973b) Intersensory interactions in *Hermissenda. J. Gen. Physiol.*, 62:185–202.

Alkon, D.L. (1974a) Associative training of *Hermissenda. J. Gen. Physiol.*, 64:70–84.

Alkon, D.L. (1974b) Sensory interactions in the nudibranch mollusc *Hermissenda crassicornis. Fed. Proc.*, 33:1083–1090.

Alkon, D.L. (1975) A dual synaptic effect on hair cells in *Hermissenda. J. Gen. Physiol.*, 65:385–397.

Alkon, D.L. (1979) Voltage-dependent calcium and potassium ion conductances: A contingency mechanism for an associative learning model. *Sciene*, 205:810–816.

Alkon, D.L. (1980) Membrane depolarization accumulates during acquisition of an associative behavioral change. *Science*, 210:1375–1376.

Alkon, D.L. (1982–1983) Regenerative changes of voltage-dependent Ca^{2+} and K^+ currents encode a learned stimulus association. *J. Physiol. Paris*, 78:700–706.

Alkon, D.L. (1984) Calcium-mediated reduction of ionic currents: A biophysical memory trace. *Science*, 226:1037–1045.

Alkon, D.L. and Sakakibara, M. (1984) Prolonged inactivation of a Ca^{2+}-dependent K^+ current but not Ca^{2+} current by light-induced elevation of intracellular calcium. *Soc. Neurosci. Abstr.*, 10:10.

Alkon, D.L. and Sakakibara, M. (1985) Calcium activates and inactivates a photoreceptor soma K^+ current. *Biophys. J.*, 48:983–985.

Alkon, D.L. Lederhendler, I. and Shoukimas, J.J. (1982a) Primary changes of membrane currents during retention of associative learnings. *Science*, 215:693–695.

Alkon, D.L., Shoukimas, J.J. and Heldman, E. (1982b) Calcium-mediated decrease of a voltage-dependent K^+ current. *Biophys. J.*, 40:245–250.

Alkon, D.L., Acosta-Urquidi, J., Olds, J., Kuzma, G. and Neary, J.T. (1983) Protein kinase injection reduces voltage-dependent potassium currents. *Science*, 219:303–306.

Alkon, D.L., Farley, J., Sakakibara, M. and Hay, B. (1984) Voltage-dependent calcium and calcium-activated potassium currents of a molluscan photoreceptor. *Biophys. J.*, 46:605–614.

Alkon, D.L., Sakakibara, M., Forman, R., Harrigan, J., Lederhendler, I. and Farley, J. (1985) Reduction of two voltage-dependent K^+ currents mediates retention of a learned association. *Behav. Neural Biol.*, 44:278–300.

Alkon, D.L., Kubota, M., Neary, J.T., Naito, S., Coulter, D. and Rasmussen, H. (1986) C-Kinase activation prolongs Ca^{2+}-dependent inactivation of K^+ currents. *Biochem. Biophys. Res. Commun.*, 134:245–1253.

Aloyo, V.J., Zwiers, H. and Gispen, W.H. (1983) Phosphorylation of B-50 protein by calcium-activated, phospholipid-dependent protein kinase and B-50 protein kinase. *J. Neurochem.*, 41:649–653.

Bar, P.R., Schotman, P., Gispen, W.H., Tielen, A.M. and Lopes da Silva, F.H. (1980) Changes in synaptic membrane phosphorylation after tetanic stimulation in the dentate area of the rat hippocampal slice. *Brain Res.*, 198:478–484.

Baraban, J.M., Synder, S.H. and Alger, B.E. (1985) Protein kinase C regulates ionic conductance in hippocampal pyramidal neurons: electrophysiological effects of phorbol esters. *Proc. Nat. Acad. Sci. U.S.A.*, 82:2538–2542.

Bennett, M.K., Erondu, N.E. and Kennedy, M.B. (1983) Purification and characterization of a calmodulin-dependent protein kinase that is highly concentrated in brain. *J. Biol. Chem.*, 258:12735–12744.

Browning, M., Dunwiddie, T., Bennett, W., Gispen, W. and Lynch, G. (1979) Synaptic phosphoproteins: specific changes after repetitive stimulation of the hippocampal slice. *Science*, 203:60–62.

Browning, M.D., Huganir, R. and Greengard, P. (1985) Protein phosphorylation and neuronal function. *J. Neurochem.*, 45:11–23.

Byers, D., Davis, R.L. and Kiger, J.A. (1981) Defect in cyclic AMP phosphodiesterase due to the *dunce* mutation of learning in *Drosophila melanogaster*. *Nature*, 289:79–81.

Byrne, J.H., Shapiro, E., Dieringer, N. and Koester, J. (1979) Biophysical mechanisms contributing to inking behavior in *Aplysia*. *J. Neurophysiol.*, 42:1233–1250.

Cleveland, D.W., Fischer, S.G., Kirschner, M.W. and Laemmli, U.K. (1977) Peptide mapping by limited proteolysis in sodium dodecyl sulfate and analysis by gel electrophoresis. *J. Biol. Chem.*, 252:1102–1106.

Cohen, P. (1980) The role of calcium ions, calmodulin and troponin in the regulation of phosphorylase kinase from rabbit skeletal muscle. *Eur. J. Biochem.*, 111:563–574.

Cohen, P. (1982) The role of protein phosphorylation in neural and hormonal control of cellular activity. *Nature*, 296:613–620.

Connor, J. and Alkon, D.L. (1984) Light- and voltage-dependent increases of calcium ion concentration in molluscan photoreceptors. *J. Neurophysiol.*, 51:745–752.

Coronado, R. and Labarca, P.P. (1984) Reconstitution of single ion channel molecules. *Trends Neurosci.*, 7:155–160.

Costa, M.R.C. and Catterall, W.A. (1984) Phosphorylation of the α subunit of the sodium channel by protein kinase C. *Cell Mol. Neurobiol.*, 4:291–297.

Crow, T. (1982) Sensory neuronal correlates of associative learning in *Hermissenda*. *Soc. Neurosci. Abstr.*, 8:824.

Crow, T. (1983) Conditioned modification of locomotion in *Hermissenda crassicornis*: Analysis of time-dependent associative and non-associative components. *J. Neurosci.*, 3:2621–2628.

Crow, T. (1985) Conditioned modification of phototactic behavior in *Hermissenda*. II. Differential adaptation of B photoreceptors. *J. Neurosci.*, 5:215–223.

Crow, T.J. and Alkon, D.L. (1978) Retention of an associative behavioral change in *Hermissenda*. *Science*, 201:1239–1241.

Crow, T.J. and Alkon, D.L. (1980) Associative behavioral modification in *Hermissenda*: Cellular correlates. *Science*, 209:412–414.

Curtis, B.M. and Catterall, W.A. (1985) Phosphorylation of the calcium antagonist receptor of the voltage-sensitive calcium channel by cAMP-dependent protein kinase. *Proc. Natl. Acad. Sci. U.S.A.*, 82:2528–2532.

DePeyer, J.E., Cachelin, A.B., Levitan, I.B. and Reuter, H. (1982) Ca^{2+}-activated K^+ conductance in internally perfused snail neurons is enhanced by protein phosphorylation. *Proc. Natl. Acad. Sci. U.S.A.*, 79:4207–4211.

DeRiemer, S.A., Kaczmarek, L.K., Lai, Y., McGuinness, T.L. and Greengard, P. (1984) Calcium/calmodulin-dependent protein phosphorylation in the nervous system of *Aplysia*. *J. Neurosci.*, 4:1618–1625.

DeRiemer, S.A., Greengard, P. and Kaczmarek, L.K. (1985) Calcium/phosphatidylserine/diacylglycerol-dependent protein kinase in the *Aplysia* nervous system. *J. Neurosci.* 5:2672–2676.

Devay, P., Solti, M., Kiss, I., Dombradi, V. and Friedrich, P. (1984) Differences in protein phosphorylation in vivo and in vitro between wild type and dunce mutant strains of *Drosophila melanogaster*. *Int. J. Biochem.*, 16:1401–1408.

Disterhoft, J., Coulter, D.A. and Alkon, D.L. (1984) Conditioning causes intrinsic changes of rabbit hippocampal neurons in vitro. *Biol. Bull.*, 167:526.

Dudai, Y. and Zvi, S. (1984) Adenylate cyclase in the *Drosphila* memory mutant rutabaga displays an altered Ca^{2+}-sensitivity. *Neurosci. Lett.*, 47:119–124.

Embi, N., Rylatt, D.B. and Cohen, P. (1979) Glycogen synthase kinase 2 and phosphorylase kinase are the same enzyme. *Eur. J. Biochem.*, 100:339–347.

Ewald, D.A., Williams, A. and Levitan, I.B. (1985) Modulation of single Ca^{2+}-dependent K^+ channel activity by protein phosphorylation. *Nature*, 315:503–506.

Farley, J. and Alkon, D.L. (1983) Changes in *Hermissenda* type B photoreceptors involving a voltage-dependent Ca^{2+} current and a Ca^{2+}-dependent K^+ current during retention of associative learning. *Soc. Neurosci. Abstr.*, 9:167.

Forman, R., Alkon, D.L., Sakakibara, M., Harrigan, J., Lederhendler, I. and Farley, J. (1984) Changes in I_A and I_C but not I_{Na} accompany retention of conditioned behavior in *Hermissenda. Soc. Neurosci. Abstr.*, 10:121.

Fukunaga, K., Yamamoto, H., Matsui, K., Higashi, K. and Miyamoto, E. (1982) Purification and characterization of a Ca^{2+}- and calmodulin-dependent protein kinase from rat brain. *J. Neurochem.*, 39:1607–1617.

Goldenring, J.R., Gonzalez, B., McGuire, J.S. Jr. and DeLorenzo, R.J. (1983) Purification and characterization of a calmodulin-dependent kinase from rat brain cytosol able to phosphorylate tubulin and microtubule-associated proteins. *J. Biol. Chem.*, 258:12632–12640.

Haga, N., Forte, M., Ramanathan, R., Hennessey, T., Takahashi, M. and Kung, C. (1984) Characterization and purification of a soluble protein controlling Ca^{2+} channel activity in *Paramecium. Cell*, 39:71–78.

Huganir, R.L., Miles, K. and Greengard, P. (1984) Phosphorylation of the nicotinic receptor by an endogenous tyrosine-specific protein kinase. *Proc. Natl. Acad. Sci. U.S.A.*, 81:6968–6972.

Jennings, K.R., Kaczmarek, L.K., Hewick, R.M., Dreyer, W.J. and Strumwasser, F. (1982) Protein phosphorylation during afterdischarge in peptidergic neurons of *Aplysia. J. Neurosci.*, 2:158–168.

Kaibuchi, K., Takai, Y. and Nishizuka, Y. (1981) Cooperative roles of various membrane phospholipids in the activation of calcium-activated, phospholipid-dependent protein kinase. *J. Biol. Chem.*, 256:7146–7149.

Kaibuchi, K., Takai, Y., Sawamura, M., Hoshijima, M., Fujikura, T. and Nishizuka, Y. (1983) Synergistic functions of protein phosphorylation and calcium mobilization in platelet activation. *J. Biol. Chem.*, 258:6701–6704.

Kennedy, M.B. and Greengard, P. (1981) Two calcium/calmodulin-dependent protein kinases, which are highly concentrated in brain, phosphorylate protein I at distinct sites. *Proc. Natl. Acad. Sci. U.S.A.*, 78:1293–1297.

Kojima, I., Kojima, K., Kreutter, D. and Rasmussen, H. (1984) The temporal integration of the aldosterone secretory response to angiontensin occurs via two intracellular pathways. *J. Biol. Chem.*, 259:14448–14457.

Kraft, A.S. and Anderson, W.B. (1983) Phorbol esters increase the amount of Ca^{2+}, phospholipid-dependent protein kinase associated with plasma membrane. *Nature*, 301:621–623.

Krebs, E.G. (1983) Historical perspectives on protein phosphorylation and a classification system for protein kinases. *Phil. Trans. R. Soc. Lond. Ser. B.* 302:3–11.

Kuret, J. and Schulman, H. (1984) Purification and characterization of a Ca^{2+}/calmodulin-dependent protein kinase from rat brain. *Biochemistry*, 23:5495–5504.

Livingstone, M.S., Sziber, P.P. and Quinn, W.G. (1984) Loss of calcium/calmodulin responsiveness in adenylate cyclase of rutabaga, a *Drosophila* learning mutant. *Cell*, 37:205–215.

Lyn-Cook, B.D., Ruder, F.J. and Wilson, J.R. (1985) Regulation of phosphate incorporation into four brain phosphoproteins that are affected by experience. *J. Neurochem.*, 44:552–559.

McGuinness, T.L., Lai, T. and Greengard, P. (1985) Ca^{2+}/calmodulin-dependent protein kinase. II. Isozymic forms from rat forebrain and cerebellum. *J. Biol. Chem.*, 260:1696–1704.

Mishima, M., Tobimatsu, T., Imoto, K., Tanaka, K., Fujita, Y., Fukuda, K., Kurasaki, M., Takahashi, H., Morimoto, Y., Hirose, T., Inayama, S., Takahashi, T., Kuno, M. and Numa, S. (1985) Location of functional regions of acetylcholine receptor α-subunit by site-directed mutagenesis. *Nature*, 313:364–369.

Naito, S., Neary, J.T., Sakakibara, M. and Alkon, D.L. (1985) Elevated external potassium causes persistent change of specific protein phosphorylation in *Hermissenda* nervous system. *Soc. Neurosci. Abstr.* 11:746.

Neary, J.T. (1984) Biochemical correlates of associative learning: Protein phosphorylation in *Hermissenda crassicornis*, a nudibranch mollusc, In (D.L. Alkon and J. Farley (Eds.), *Primary Substrates of Learning and Behavioral Change*, Cambridge University Press, New York, pp. 325–336.

Neary, J.T. and Alkon, D.L. (1983) Protein phosphorylation/dephosphorylation and the transient, voltage-dependent potassium conductance in *Hermissenda crassicornis. J. Biol. Chem.*, 258:8979–8983.

Neary, J.T., Crow, T. and Alkon, D.L. (1981) Change in a specific phosphoprotein band following associative learning in *Hermissenda. Nature*, 293:658–660.

Neary, J.T., DeRiemer, S.A., Kaczmarek, L.K. and Alkon, D.L. (1984) Ca^{2+} and cyclic AMP regulation of protein phosphorylation in the *Hermissenda* nervous system. *Soc. Neurosci. Abstr.*, 10:805.

Neary, J.T., Naito, S. and Alkon, D.L. (1985) Ca^{2+}-activated, phospholipid-dependent protein kinase (C-kinase) activity in the *Hermissenda* nervous system. *Soc. Neurosci. Abst.* 11:746.

Nelson, R.B. and Routtenberg, A. (1985) Characterization of protein F1 (47 kDa, 4.5 p*I*): a kinase C substrate directly related to neural plasticity. *Exp. Neurol.*, 89:213–224.

Nestler, E.J. and Greengard, P. (1984) *Protein phosphorylation in the nervous system*, John Wiley and Sons, New York.

Nishizuka, Y. (1984) Turnover of inositol phospholipids and signal transduction. *Science*, 225:1365–1370.

Novak-Hofer, I. and Levitan, I.B. (1983) Ca^{2+}/calmodulin-regulated protein phosphorylation in the *Aplysia* nervous system. *J. Neurosci.*, 3:473–481.

Ocorr, K.A., Walters, E.T. and Byrne, J.H. (1985) Associative conditioning analog selectively increases cAMP levels of tail sensory neurons in *Aplysia*. *Proc. Natl. Acad. Sci. U.S.A.*, 82:2548–2552.

O'Farrell, P.H. (1975) High resolution two-dimensional electrophoresis of proteins. *J. Biol. Chem.*, 250:4007–4021.

Rasmussen, H. and Barrett, P.Q. (1984) Calcium messenger system: an integrated view. *Physiol. Rev.*, 64:938–984.

Rasmussen, H., Kojima, I., Kojima, K., Zawalich, W. and Apfeldorf, W. (1984) Calcium as intracellular messenger: sensitivity modulation, C-kinase pathway, and sustained cellular response. *Adv. Cyclic Nucleotide Protein Phos. Res.*, 18:159–193.

Rodnight, R. (1982) Aspects of protein phosphorylation in the nervous system with particular reference to synaptic transmission. *Prog. Brain Res.*, 56:1–25.

Routtenberg, A. (1984) Brain phosphoproteins, kinase C and protein F1: protagonists of plasticity in particular pathways, In G. Lynch, J. McGaugh, and N. Weinberger (Eds.), *Memory Neurobiology*, Guilford Press, New York, pp. 479–490.

Routtenberg, A., Lovinger, D.M. and Steward, O. (1985) Selective increase in phosphorylation of a 47-kDa protein (F1) directly related to long-term potentiation. *Behav. Neural Biol.*, 43:3–11.

Shotwell, S. (1983) Cyclic adenosine 3',5'-monophosphate phosphodiesterase and its role in learning in *Drosphila*. *J. Neurosci.*, 3:739–747.

Shuster, M.J., Camardo, J.S., Siegelbaum, S.A. and Kandel, E.R. (1985) Cyclic AMP-dependent protein kinase closes the serotonin-sensitive K^+ channels of *Aplysia* sensory neurons

in cell-free membrane patches. *Nature*, 313:392–395.

Stewart, A.A., Ingebritsen, T.S., Manalan, A., Klee, C.B. and Cohen, P. (1982) Discovery of a Ca^{2+}- and calmodulin-dependent protein phosphatase. *FEBS Lett.*, 137:80–84.

Strong, J.A. (1984) Modulation of potassium current kinetics in bag cell neurons of *Aplysia* by an activator of adenylate cyclase. *J. Neurosci.*, 4:2772–2783.

Strong, J.A. and Kaczmarek, L.K. (1984) Modulation of multiple potassium currents in dialyzed bag cell neurons of *Aplysia*. *Soc. Neurosci. Abstr.*, 10:1101.

Takai, Y., Kishimoto, A., Iwasa, Y., Kawahara, Y., Mori, T. and Nishizuka, Y. (1979) Calcium-dependent activation of a multifunctional protein kinase by membrane phospholipids. *J. Biol. Chem.*, 254:3692–3695.

Thesleff, S. (1980) Aminopyridines and synaptic transmission. *Neuroscience*, 5:1413–1419.

Thompson, S.H. (1977) Three pharmacologically distinct potassium channels in molluscan neurons. *J. Physiol. London*, 265:465–488.

Thompson, S.H. (1982) Aminopyridine block of transient potassium current. *J. Gen. Physiol.*, 80:1–18.

Tyndale, C.L. and Crow, T. (1979) An IC control unit for generating random and nonrandom events. *IEEE Trans. Biomed. Eng.*, 26:649–655.

West, A., Barnes, E. and Alkon, D.L. (1982) Primary changes of voltage responses during retention of associative learning. *J. Neurophysiol.*, 48:1243–1255.

Yamauchi, T. and Fujisawa, H. (1983) Purification and characterization of the brain calmodulin-dependent protein kinase II, which is involved in the activation of tryptophan 5-monooxygenase. *Eur. J. Biochem.* 132:15–21.

Yellen, G. (1984) Channels from genes: The oocyte as an expression system. *Trends. Neurosci.*, 7:457–458.

W.H. Gispen and A. Routtenberg (Eds.)
Progress in Brain Research, Vol. 69
© 1986 Elsevier Science Publishers B.V. (Biomedical Division)

CHAPTER 9

Regulation of ion channel activity by protein phosphorylation

José R. Lemos[1], Ilse Novak-Hofer[2] and Irwin B. Levitan[3]

[1]*Worcester Foundation for Experimental Biology, Shrewsbury, MA 01545, U.S.A.,* [2]*Zentrum für Lehre und Forschung, Kantonspital, CH-4002 Basel, Switzerland and* [3]*Graduate Dept. of Biochemistry, Brandeis University. Waltham, MA 02254, U.S.A.*

Introduction

During the last thirty years a great deal of progress has been made in our understanding of how neurotransmitters can regulate the activity of excitable cells. More recently, *long-lasting* modulation of the activity of ion channels, and hence of the electrical activity of the cell, has begun to be investigated in detail. One can think of such long-lasting changes in terms of a scheme such as that described in Fig. 1: here the changes in ion channel properties are not dependent on the continued occupation of a receptor by a transmitter, but rather result from some long-lasting metabolic modification (for example, phosphorylation) of an ion channel. This scheme suggests that the receptor and channel need not necessarily be intimately associated in a single macromolecular complex, but may communicate via some intracellular second messenger which is produced upon occupancy of the receptor by agonist. The second messenger sets in motion a series of steps, culminating in some covalent modification of the channel which alters its activity, and the functional change persists until the covalent modification has been reversed (again this may require a series of steps).

The large size and ready identifiability of many molluscan neurons makes them particularly convenient for combined biochemical and electrophysiological studies on individual nerve cells. A number of laboratories have taken advantage of these favorable properties to investigate the role of intracellular second messengers in neurotransmitter actions, and have implicated cAMP and cAMP-dependent protein phosphorylation in the regulation of potassium channels in several different molluscan neurons (reviewed in Siegelbaum and Tsien, 1983). Our studies have focused on the identified neuron R15, in the abdominal ganglion of the marine mollusc *Aplysia californica*. R15 is an endogenous burster; it exhibits a pattern of spontaneous activity consisting of bursts of action potentials separated by interburst hyperpolarizations (Fig. 2A). We have found that serotonin (5-HT) causes R15 to hyperpolarize and stop bursting (Fig. 2B–E). This is also true if dopamine, another putative neurotransmitter, is applied to R15 (Ascher, 1972). Both these responses are prolonged ones, and long outlast the initial stimulus (application of the neurotransmitter). Furthermore, stimulation of the branchial nerve of the abdominal ganglion leads to a long-lasting synaptic hyperpolarization of neuron R15 (Adams et al., 1980). In this paper we review our current understanding of the molecular mechanisms underlying such long-lasting modulation of the electrical properties of this nerve cell.

Results and discussion

Mechanism of the 5-HT response

We have studied the mechanism underlying the hyperpolarization of R15 by 5-HT using voltage clamp techniques. The membrane potential was

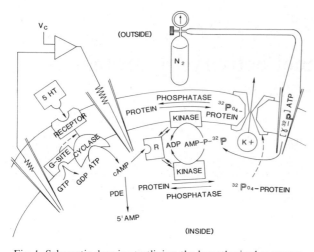

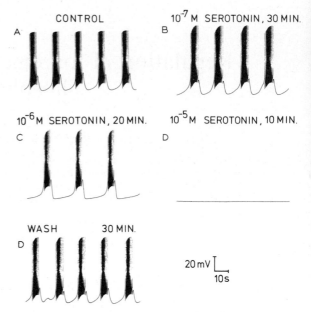

Fig. 1. Schematic drawing outlining the hypothesized sequence of events underlying the response of neuron R15 to 5-HT, and the experimental paradigm used to measure single-cell phosphorylation. Beginning at the left of the diagram: when 5-HT binds to its receptor on the plasma membrane of neuron R15 it activates the membrane-bound enzyme adenylate cyclase (CYCLASE) by displacing GDP from the GTP-binding protein (G-SITE) and allowing GTP to bind. This leads to the production of 3′,5′-adenosine monophosphate (cAMP) from ATP by the CYCLASE. This elevation in intracellular cAMP leads to the activation of either membrane-bound or cytosolic cAMP-dependent protein kinases by binding to the regulatory (R) subunit of the protein kinase and releasing the active catalytic subunit (KINASE). These KINASES can then phosphorylate specific proteins (PROTEIN), either in the membrane or cytosol, by transfering the terminal phosphate (P) from ATP to the protein. This reaction can be monitored by pressure injecting (γ-^{32}P]ATP (AMP-P-^{32}P) into the cell via a microelectrode. The resulting radioactive phosphoproteins (^{32}PO$_4$-PROTEIN), which can be resolved using two-dimensional polyacrylamide gel electrophoresis followed by autoradiography (see Fig. 6), may regulate, either directly or via intermediaries (indicated by the dashed line), the conductance of the anomalously rectifying potassium channel (K$^+$). The activity of this channel can be monitored by placing two microelectrodes into the cell and voltage clamping the R15 membrane. The sequence of events is reversed by phosphoprotein phosphatases (PHOSPHATASE) which remove the phosphate from the phosphoproteins, and by phosphodiesterases (PDE) which hydrolyze cAMP to 5′-AMP. OUTSIDE and INSIDE refer to the extracellular and intracellular space, respectively, of *Aplysia* neuron R15.

swept between -120 and -40 mV (dV/d$t =$ 4 mV/s) and the total membrane current was measured. This rate of change is slow compared to the time constant of the cell's membrane, but

Fig. 2. Voltage response of R15 to 5-HT. The normal rhythmic activity of this neuron is a series of action potentials (burst) separated by an interburst hyperpolarization (A). When the abdominal ganglion is perfused with increasing concentrations of 5-HT (B–D) there is first a decrease in burst rate and an increase in the depth of the interburst hyperpolarization and, in the presence of 10^{-5} M 5-HT, the cell becomes silent with its voltage stable near -80 mV. These effects reverse within about 30 min after removal of 5-HT (E). The effects of 100 µM dopamine on the voltage of R15 (not shown) are very similar to those of 10^{-5} M 5-HT but, as shown in Fig. 4, the two neurotransmitters act via different ionic mechanisms. (Modified from Drummond et al., 1980a.)

is rapid compared to the response to 5-HT. A plot of the membrane potential versus the total membrane current (Fig. 3A) yields a steady-state current–voltage (I–V) relationship. The slope of such an I–V relationship is a measure of the ionic conductance of the cell membrane.

If the abdominal ganglion is perfused with 5 µM 5HT, there is an increase in conductance which reverses sign (compared to the resting conductance) at around -80 mV (Fig. 3B). This reversal at the potassium equilibrium potential suggests that 5-HT increases a potassium conductance. A variety of pharmacological treatments, and the pronounced inward rectification of the 5-HT-evoked current, indicate that it is an anomalously rectifying potassium conductance (Benson

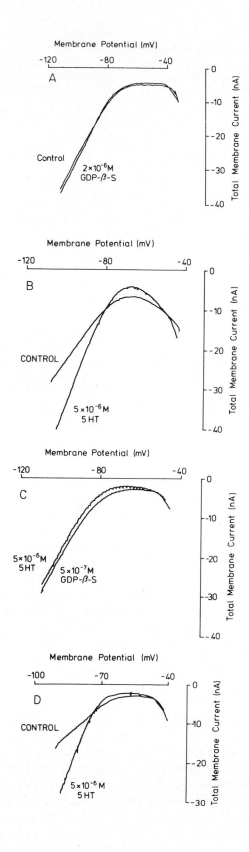

and Levitan, 1983). Although this is the predominant effect of 5-HT, other currents also appear to be affected by 5-HT in this cell (Eckert and Ewald, 1983; Lotshaw et al., 1986).

Intracellular messenger

A series of biochemical and pharmacological experiments have satisfied all of the criteria (Greengard, 1976) necessary to establish that cAMP mediates this response to serotonin: for example,

(*a*) injection of cAMP derivatives into R15 elicits the same potassium conductance increase as 5-HT (Drummond et al, 1980a);
(*b*) phosphodiesterase inhibitors enhance the response to low concentrations of 5-HT (Drummond et al., 1980a);
(*c*) serotonin causes cAMP to accumulate within cell R15 (Levitan and Drummond, 1980);
(*d*) 5-HT stimulates adenylate cyclase activity in membranes prepared from R15 somata (Levitan, 1978); and
(*e*) the serotonin receptors mediating adenylate cyclase stimulation and R15 hyperpolarization are pharmacologically very similar (Drummond et al., 1980b).

Is the stimulation of adenylate cyclase, and the subsequent elevation of cAMP intracellularly,

Fig. 3. Effect of GDPβS on the 5-HT response. The membrane potential was swept between -120 and -40 mV ($dV/dt = 4$ mV/s) and the total membrane current was measured in nanoamperes (nA). A: Lack of effect of GDPβS injection into neuron R15 on the steady state *I–V* relationship. *I–V* curves from cell before (Control) and after injection with 2 μM GDPβS. B: Normal response to 5-HT in cell R15. Steady-state *I–V* curves from an uninjected neuron before (Control) and 20 min after perfusion of 5 μM 5-HT. Notice the reversal of the response of about -80 mV, near the potassium equilibrium potential for this neuron. C: The same cell after intraneuronal injection of 0.5 μM GDPβS. GDPβS has no direct effect on the *I–V* characteristics of the cell (see A), but completely blocks the cell's response to 5-HT (compare to B). GDPβS is a non-phosphorylatable and slowly hydrolyzed analog of GDP which inhibits adenylate cyclase. D: After 24 h the cell is able to respond normally to 5-HT, indicating breakdown of GDPβS. (Reproduced from Lemos and Levitan, 1984, by copyright permission of the Rockefeller University Press.)

110

necessary for the response to 5-HT to occur in neuron R15? GDPβS, a slowly hydrolyzable analog of GDP (Eckstein et al, 1979), is a specific inhibitor of adenylate cyclase (Cassel et al. 1979). At μM concentrations this GDP analog inhibits the stimulation of adenylate cyclase by 5-HT in membranes prepared from *Aplysia* nervous system (Lemos and Levitan, 1984). If GDPβS is injected by pressure (see Fig. 1) into a voltage-clamped R15 to a final intracellular concentration of about 1 μM, then the increase in potassium conductance normally elicited by 5-HT (Fig. 3B) is blocked (Fig. 3C). The cell can recover from the GDPβS block after many hours (Fig. 3D), presumably after the GDP analog has been broken down. Dopamine, on the other hand, can still hyperpolarize R15 in the presence of GDPβS, confirming that its response is not mediated by cAMP (Lemos and Levitan, 1984). Furthermore, derivatives of cAMP can still evoke an increase in potassium conductance in GDPβS-injected cells, pinpointing the block of the 5-HT response at the adenylate cyclase (Lemos and Levitan, 1984). Thus the stimulation of adenylate cyclase is indeed a *necessary* step in the activation of the anomalously rectifying potassium conductance by 5-HT in this cell.

Protein phosphorylation – physiological studies

Is protein phosphorylation involved in the activation of the anomalously rectifying potassium channel? Protein kinase inhibitor (PKI) is a 10-kDa protein which binds with high affinity to the active catalytic subunit of cAMP-dependent protein kinase and inhibits its activity (Walsh et al., 1971). We have found that PKI, purified to homogeneity from rabbit skeletal muscle (Demaille et al., 1977), is a potent inhibitor of cAMP-dependent protein kinase from *Aplysia* (Adams and Levitan, 1982). When PKI is pressure-injected via a microelectrode directly into neuron R15 (see Fig. 1), the increase in potassium conductance normally elicited by 5-HT (Fig. 4A) is completely blocked (Fig. 4B). Furthermore, the cell's response to cAMP analogs also is blocked by PKI (Lemos and Adams, unpublished observations). To test the selectivity of this inhibition by PKI, R15's res-

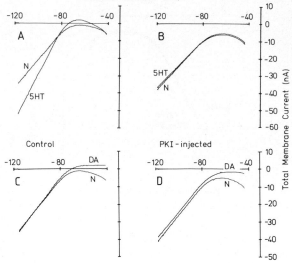

Fig. 4. Protein Kinase Inhibitor (PKI) effects on R15. A: Normal R15 response to 5 μM 5-HT. B: After intraneuronal injection of PKI, the same concentration of 5-HT elicits no increase in potassium conductance. C: Normal response of R15 to 100 μM dopamine (DA). Note the decrease in voltage-dependent inward current as compared to control (N). D: The cell still responds normally to DA after injection of PKI. Labeling as in Fig. 3. (Modified from Adams and Levitan, 1983.)

ponse to dopamine was examined. As shown in Fig. 4C, dopamine causes a decrease in voltage-dependent inward current (Wilson and Wachtel, 1978), which is *not* dependent on cAMP (Lemos and Levitan, 1984). A comparison of Figs. 4C and D demonstrates that PKI injection does not affect this dopamine response. Thus the blocking by PKI of the neurotransmitter effect appears to be selective for the 5-HT-induced, cAMP-mediated increase in potassium conductance (Adams and Levitan, 1982). Therefore cAMP-dependent protein phosphorylation is also a *necessary* step in this 5-HT-induced modulation of electrical activity in neuron R15.

Protein phosphorylation – biochemical studies

Having implicated protein phosphorylation in the control of potassium conductance in R15, it is important to identify the phosphoproteins which may be involved in this regulation. Previous attempts to measure protein phosphorylation in individual nerve cells have involved incubating ganglia with $^{32}P_i$, followed by isolation of individual nerve cell somata and analysis of radioactive phosphoproteins (Levitan et al., 1974; Paris et al., 1981; Jennings et al., 1982; Neary and Alkon, 1983). Although this approach has provided useful information, it suffers from several disadvantages. First, the cell body can never be isolated totally free of glia and portions of neighboring cell bodies, which will contribute to the labeling pattern; and second, the neuropil processes of the cell, which

are the sites at which most synaptic contacts occur (Frazier et al., 1967), are not sampled by this procedure. To circumvent these problems we have developed methods (Lemos et al., 1982) to inject $[\gamma-^{32}P]ATP$ directly into R15 (see Fig. 1), in amounts sufficient to label phosphoproteins. We can confirm, by autoradiography of sections of the abdominal ganglion, that virtually all the radio-activity remains within neuron R15 following such injections (compare Figs. 5C and D). Thus we can process the entire abdominal ganglion, including the neuropil region, for gel electrophoresis with

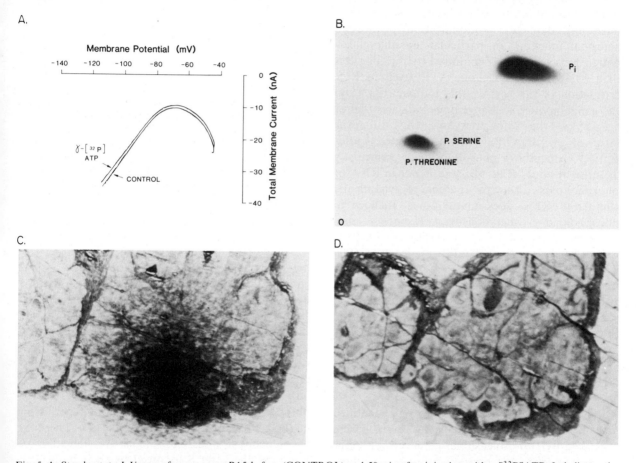

Fig. 5. A: Steady-state *I–V* curve from neuron R15 before (CONTROL) and 50 min after injection with $\gamma-[^{32}P]ATP$. Labeling as in Fig. 3. B: Phosphoamino acids from phosphoproteins from R15 after treatment with 5HT: separation by two-dimensional high-voltage paper electrophoresis. Most of the ^{32}P incorporation appears at phosphoserine (P.SERINE) residues, with some labeling of phosphothreonine (P.THREONINE), but none is detectable at phosphotyrosine. C: Localization of the injected radioactivity. Autoradiogram of an abdominal ganglion section which includes part of the soma of neuron R15. The cell had been injected with $[\gamma-^{32}P]ATP$ 50 min prior to fixation. D: Autoradiogram of the section adjacent to the one shown in C, but which does not include any part of the soma or processes of R15. Note that there are no silver grains, indicating that the radioactivity remains confined to neuron R15.

the confidence that virtually all the *radioactive* phosphoproteins observed originate from within R15. An important feature is that the physiological properties of the cell are monitored under voltage clamp with intracellular microelectrodes throughout the labeling period (Fig. 1), so changes in the phosphoprotein labeling pattern may be related directly to changes in membrane conductance. In addition, voltage clamping assures that phosphorylation changes result directly from the effects of the neurotransmitter, rather than indirectly from changes in the cell's spontaneous activity induced by the transmitter.

The injection protocol has been chosen to minimize any damage or modification of normal neuronal function. In particular possible metabolic effects have been minimized by injecting less than 1% of the endogenous ATP levels in R15. Extraction of the acid-soluble radioactivity from the ganglion after such injections indicates that at least 85% of the radioactivity injected is still in the form of $[\gamma\text{-}^{32}P]$ATP. The incorporated radioactivity is mainly in phosphoproteins, principally at serine residues (Fig. 5B), and is not in RNA or phospholipids, although analysis of synaptically stimulated R15s does reveal some changes in phospholipid metabolism (Lemos and Drummond, unpublished observations). Furthermore, by using $[\gamma\text{-}^{32}P]$ATP of high (> 5000 Ci/mmol) specific activity, we are able to keep our injection volumes to less than 5% of the soma volume. This protocol has minimized any injection artifacts and produces no perceptible alteration of the *I–V* characteristics of the injected neuron (Fig. 5A).

5-HT effects on protein phosphorylation

Proteins phosphorylated within a single identified neuron during a 50-min labeling period were separated by two-dimensional gel electrophoresis. Fig. 6 is a schematic representation of the phosphoprotein pattern from an R15 perfused with normal *Aplysia* medium for 30 min, and then with 5-HT for an additional 20 min after injection with $[\gamma\text{-}^{32}P]$ATP; more than 70 phosphoproteins can be detected, although not all are represented here. It is important to note that most of these are not

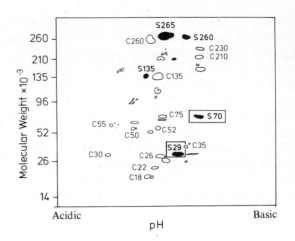

Fig. 6. Summary of 5-HT effects on protein phosphorylation pattern in neuron R15. This is a schematic representation of an autoradiograph of a two-dimensional gel electrophoretic separation of phosphoproteins. The outlined spots correspond to phosphoproteins seen in normal or control R15s, and some of them are marked with a C and their apparent molecular weight $\times 10^{-3}$. The filled in spots (marked with an S and their apparent molecular weight $\times 10^{-3}$) correspond to phosphoproteins whose appearance or disappearance is dependent on 5-HT (S29, S70, S135, S260, and S265). We have been unable, using a variety of pharmacological treatments, to dissociate the phosphoproteins enclosed in boxes (S29 and S70) from the increase in potassium conductance. The numbers on the left side of the gel are apparent molecular weights $\times 10^{-3}$ and the acidic and basic extremes of the isoelectric focussing dimension are marked at the bottom (Modified from Lemos et al., 1985).

major proteins in neuron R15 (or the abdominal ganglion), and thus this phosphorylation pattern does not merely reflect labeling of major substrates in the cell. Some of the phosphoproteins that are detectable in control cells are designated by a C followed by their molecular weight $\times 10^{-3}$. Concomitant with the potassium conductance increase, 5-HT alters the amount of ^{32}P incorporated into at least a dozen proteins (Table I). Five phosphoproteins are detected only after perfusion of the abdominal ganglion with 5-HT. These 5-HT-dependent phosphoproteins are indicated in Fig. 6 by the letter S followed by their molecular weight $\times 10^{-3}$, and by double arrows in Table I. In addition to causing the appearance of the 5-HT-dependent phosphoproteins, 5-HT also alters the phosphorylation of a number of other proteins which can be observed in control cells (Table I; Lemos et al., 1984).

TABLE I

Summary of the effects of various pharmacological probes on phosphoproteins from neuron R15

Phosphoproteins	5-HT	cAMP	5-HT + GDPβS
S265	↑↑	0	−
C260	−	0	−
S260	↑↑	0	↑↑
C230	↓	↓	−
S135	↑↑	−	↑↑
C135	↑	↑	↑
C75	−	−	−
*S70	↑↑	↑↑	−
C55	↓	↑	−
C52	↑	−	−
C35	↑	↑	↑
C30	↑	↑	−
*S29	↑↑	↑↑	−
C26	↑	↑	↑
C22	↓	↑	↓

A single upward arrow indicates an increase and a downward arrow a decrease in phosphorylation. Double arrows indicate the appearance or disappearance of phosphoproteins as a result of 5-HT, GDPβS, or cAMP treatment, 0 indicates phosphoproteins which did not enter gel. Phosphoproteins which could not be dissociated from the 5-HT-induced increase in potassium conductance are indicated with an asterisk. (Modified from Lemos et al., 1984, 1985.)

Phosphoproteins associated with the increase in the anomalously rectifying potassium conductance

We have focussed attention on those phosphoproteins which show the largest and most consistent changes in response to 5-HT (see Table I). In order to determine whether any of these phosphoproteins is involved in the regulation of the potassium channel, we have utilized a variety of agents to probe specific sites in the sequence of events hypothesized to occur in neuron R15 as a result of 5-HT application (see Fig. 1).

Whenever an agonist or partial agonist which interacts with the 5-HT receptor elicits an increase in the inwardly rectifying potassium conductance in R15, it also evokes the appearance of most of the 5-HT-dependent phosphoproteins (Lemos et al., 1985). When 5-HT does not elicit this increase in the anomalously rectifying current (this occurs on very rare occasions), the above phosphorylation changes do *not* appear (Fig. 7A). Thus, the

appearance of most of the 5-HT-dependent phosphoproteins and the increase in potassium conductance seem to be closely associated.

Intraneuronal injection or perfusion with an analog of cAMP, 8-benzylthio cAMP, mimics some, but not all, of the changes in phosphoprotein pattern elicited by 5-HT (Fig. 8B). Since stimulation of adenylate cyclase (Lemos and Levitan, 1984) and the subsequent elevation of cAMP levels (Drummond et al., 1980a) are necessary for the increase in potassium conductance to be elicited by 5-HT, it would appear that only those phosphoproteins which respond to both 5-HT and cAMP (see Table I) can be involved in the regulation of the anomalously rectifying potassium channel. Another way to examine the role of cAMP is by using the adenylate cyclase inhibitor GDPβS. Low concentrations (μM intracellularly) of GDPβS completely block the conductance increase (Fig. 4B), and also block many of the phosphorylation changes normally elicited by 5-HT (Fig. 8C). It is significant that some of the changes in the phosphorylation pattern are *not* blocked, thus effectively dissociating these phosphoproteins from the increase in potassium conductance (see Table I).

One would expect that phosphoprotein changes involved in the regulation of channel properties must necessarily accompany the change in potassium conductance. Although for technical reasons it is difficult to do a rigorous kinetic analysis of the phosphorylation response, experiments designed to answer this question reveal that the phosphoproteins S265, S70, and S29 are most closely associated, in time, with the increase in potassium conductance (Lemos et al., 1985). These experiments, together with the pharmacological approaches described above, have demonstrated that it is possible to dissociate many of the phosphorylation changes from the physiological response. However, we have been unable to dissociate the phosphorylation of S70 and S29 from the potassium conductance increase (Fig. 6 and Table I), and thus these phosphoproteins remain candidates for ion channel regulatory components (Lemos et al., 1985).

The turnover of the proteins phosphorylated in response to 5-HT appears to be quite rapid. If R15

114

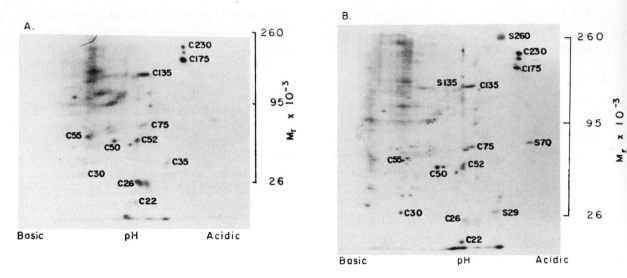

Fig. 7. A: lack of effect of 5-HT on protein phosphorylation pattern of R15. This cell was injected with [γ-³²P]ATP 30 min prior to start of perfusion with 5 μM 5-HT, and then was frozen after 20 min of 5-HT perfusion when conductance changes are normally maximal. This is a rare case in which this concentration of 5-HT *failed* to elicit any increase in potassium conductance. Autoradiogram of a two-dimensional gel electrophoretic separation of phosphoproteins. Note that the 5-HT-dependent phosphoproteins (Fig. 6) are not evident. B: Turnover of phosphoproteins in R15. This cell was perfused with 5 μM 5-HT until a maximal increase in potassium conductance was elicited. The cell was then injected with [γ-³²P]ATP and frozen 30 min after continued perfusion with the same concentration of 5-HT. The maximal conductance response to 5-HT was maintained during this period. Autoradiogram of a two-dimensional gel electrophoretic separation of phosphoproteins. Labeling as in Fig. 6.

is injected with labeled ATP *after* the conductance response to 5-HT is already maximal (and the proteins presumably are already labeled with cold, endogenous phosphate), one can see incorporation of ³²P into the same proteins as in normally 5-HT-treated cells (Fig. 7B), indicating that the phosphate is turning over in these phosphoproteins, even in the continued presence of 5-HT. One can see the same 5-HT-dependent phosphoprotein pattern even after only 3 min of labeling (the fastest we could measure) in such experiments. This is consistent with results in *Aplysia* sensory neurons (Castellucci et al., 1982), which indicate that it is the continued elevation of cAMP, and continued stimulation of phosphorylation, which is important for a persistent change in another potassium conductance.

Although it might be thought that membrane phosphoproteins are more likely candidates to be channel regulatory components, the only 5-HT-dependent phosphoprotein found associated with the membrane, at least in vitro, is S70 (Lemos et

al., 1985). There is no a priori reason, however, to limit such regulatory proteins to either a membrane or cytosolic localization. It is even conceivable that the relevant phosphoprotein(s) is not the last or even near the last component in the cascade of events leading from occupancy of the receptor by 5-HT to the gating of the anomalously rectifying potassium channel. Calculations based on channel density in the membrane, and sensitivity limits to radioactivity, reveal that if the anomalously rectifying channel were being phosphorylated directly as a result of 5-HT treatment, it would be detectable using our techniques (Lemos et al., 1985). Single-channel recording of this channel from R15 could help to determine whether the channel is indeed phosphorylated directly.

Single-channel phosphorylation

Although such single-channel experiments have not yet been done with the anomalously rectifying

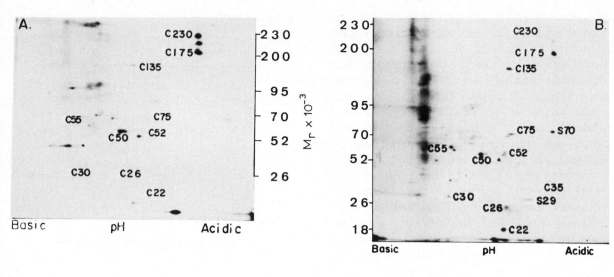

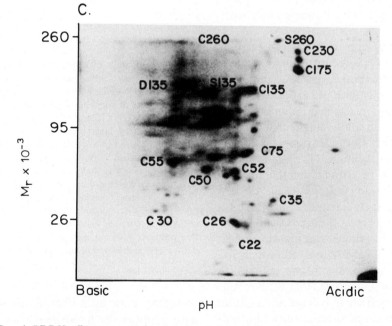

Fig. 8. Cyclic AMP and GDPβS effects on protein phosphorylation. A: Control protein phosphorylation pattern from an R15 neuron which had been perfused with normal *Aplysia* medium for 50 min after injection with [γ-^{32}P]ATP. Autoradiograph of a two-dimensional gel electrophoretic separation of phosphoproteins. B: Effects of 8-benzylthio cAMP, a non-hydrolyzable analog of cyclic AMP, on the protein phosphorylation pattern of R15. Injection protocol as in Fig. 7A, but 300 µM 8-benzylthio cAMP was perfused for the last 20 min of the labeling period. This concentration of 8-benzylthio cAMP evokes an increase in potassium conductance identical to that elicited by 5-HT (Drummond et al., 1980). Autoradiograph of a two-dimensional gel electrophoretic separation of phosphoproteins. Note the appearance of S70 and S29. C: Effect of 1 µM GDPβS on protein phosphorylation in R15. The neuron was first injected with GDPβS to a final intracellular concentration of 1 µM, and then was injected with [γ-^{32}P]ATP. 30 min later the cell was perfused with 5 µM 5-HT. Under these conditions 5-HT did not evoke any increase in potassium conductance (as in Fig. 3). After 20 min the ganglion was frozen and processed for gel electrophoresis. Autoradiograph of a two-dimensional gel electrophoretic separation of phosphoproteins. Labeling as in Fig. 6 (Modified from Lemos, et al., 1985).

116

potassium channel in neuron R15, there are several other ion channels whose activity has been shown to be regulated directly by phosphorylation. Using patch recording techniques, the catalytic subunit of cAMP-dependent protein kinase has been applied directly to the cytoplasmic membrane surface of an isolated membrane patch, while the activity of single ion channels in the patch was recorded. Such experiments have demonstrated that potassium channels from *Aplysia* sensory neurons can be closed (Shuster et al., 1985), and the activity of calcium-dependent potassium channels from *Helix* neurons can be enhanced (Ewald et al., 1985), by catalytic subunit. Thus the phosphorylated protein(s) responsible for altering ion channel activity must come away with the membrane patch when it is isolated from the cell. The relevant phosphoprotein might be the ion channel itself, or some other protein, for example a cytoskeleton component, which comes away with the patch.

A complementary approach is to examine single-channel activity in a reconstituted system. It is possible to fuse membrane vesicles, containing functional ion channels, with an artificial bilayer membrane consisting of added phospholipids, under conditions which allow single-channel currents to be measured (for a review see Miller, 1983). A recent modification of this technique allows the bilayer to be formed on the tip of a patch recording electrode (Wilmsen et al., 1983), a configuration particularly favorable for high-resolution single-channel recordings. Ewald et al. (1985) have observed single calcium-dependent potassium channels (Fig. 9A and B), which are similar to those in native membrane patches, in such 'tip-dip' bilayers. The probability of the channel being open, at a particular voltage and calcium concentration, is increased dramatically after addition of catalytic subunit to the side of the bilayer corresponding to the cytoplasmic membrane surface (Fig. 9C; Ewald et al., 1985). These results indicate that the phosphorylation target is either the potassium channel itself, or some regulatory component so intimately associated with the channel that it travels with it in the artificial bilayer. Although it is not clear to what extent these findings can be extrapolated to the anomalously

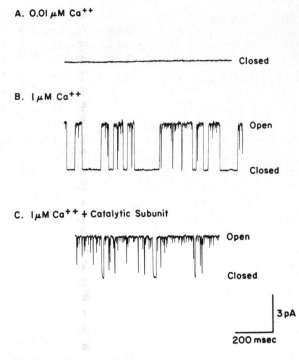

Fig. 9. Modulation of single ion channel activity by protein phosphorylation. Crude membrane vesicles, prepared from *Helix* neurons by differential centrifugation, were reconstituted with a mixture of phosphatidylethanolamine and phosphatidylserine (PE/PS, 3/1). Using techniques introduced by Wilmsen et al. (1983), a bilayer was formed from these reconstituted vesicles on the tip of a patch recording electrode. This bilayer contains a single potassium selective channel, which at $+40$ mV is closed virtually all the time in 0.01 μM calcium (A), but can open in the presence of 1 μM calcium (B). The activity of this calcium-dependent potassium channel is increased dramatically after phosphorylation with the catalytic subunit of cAMP-dependent protein kinase (C). Unpublished data of D. Ewald, A. Williams and I.B. Levitan; for details of methodology and similar results see Ewald et al. (1985).

rectifying potassium channel in neuron R15, the data support the hypothesis that one or more of the phosphoprotein spots, identified in the R15 labeling experiments, might be an ion channel regulatory component.

Summary

Studies from a number of laboratories have demonstrated that the electrical activity of some nerve cells can be modulated by intracellular second messengers such as cAMP. Furthermore the injection of protein kinases and inhibitors of protein kinases into individual nerve cells has provided evidence that some of these modulatory effects are mediated by cAMP-dependent protein phosphorylation. We have taken two approaches to examine the molecular mechanisms of such neuromodulation. On the one hand techniques have been developed for measuring protein phosphorylation in individual living nerve cells, following the intracellular injection of radioactive ATP. This approach has allowed the identification of several proteins in *Aplysia* neuron R15 whose phosphorylation is closely associated with the modulation by serotonin of an anomalously rectifying potassium current, and it seems possible that these phosphoproteins are ion channel regulatory components. The second approach has been to investigate the effects of protein kinases on the activity of individual ion channels, using either patch recording or reconstitution techniques. We have identified a calcium-dependent potassium channel in detached membrane patches from *Helix* neurons, and have found that its activity can be modulated by treatment with the catalytic subunit of cAMP-dependent protein kinase. Furthermore we have been able to reconstitute a calcium-dependent potassium channel from *Helix* membrane vesicles in an artificial phospholipid bilayer, under conditions which allow single-channel currents to be measured. Addition of catalytic subunit and ATP to the bilayer chamber results in a marked increase in the activity of the channel. The results indicate that the phosphorylation target is either the ion channel protein itself, or some regulatory component which is intimately associated with the channel.

Acknowledgements

A number of colleagues including Drs. William B. Adams, Jack A. Benson, Alan H. Drummond, Douglas A. Ewald and Alan Williams participated in many of the experiments described here. Supported by Grant NS17910 to Irwin B. Levitan from the National Institute of Neurological and Communicative Disorders and Stroke.

References

Adams, W.B. and Levitan, I.B. (1982) Intracellular injection of protein kinase inhibitor blocks the serotonin-induced increase in K+ conductance in *Aplysia* neuron R15. *Proc. Natl. Acad. Sci. U.S.A.*, 79:3877–3880.

Alkon, D.L., Acosta-Urquidi, J., Olds, J., Kuzma, G. and Neary, J.T. (1983) Protein kinase injection reduces voltage-dependent potassium currents. *Science*, 219:303–306.

Ascher, P. (1972) Inhibitory and excitatory effects of dopamine on *Aplysia* neurons. *J. Physiol. London*, 225:173–209.

Benson, J.A. and Levitan, I.B. (1983) Serotonin increases an anomalously rectifying K+ current in the *Aplysia* neuron R15. *Proc. Natl. Acad. Sci. U.S.A.*, 80:3522–3525.

Cassel, D., Eckstein, F., Lowe, M. and Selinger, Z. (1979) Determination of the turn-off reaction for the hormone-activated adenylate cyclase. *J. Biol. Chem.*, 254:9835–9838.

Demaille, J., Peters, K. and Fisher, E. (1977) Isolation and properties of the rabbit skeletal muscle protein inhibitor of cAMP-dependent protein kinases, *Biochemistry*, 16:3080–3086.

Deterre, P., Paupardin-Tritsch, D., Bockaert, J. and Gerschenfeld, H.M. (1981) Role of cAMP in the serotonin-evoked slow inward current in snail neurons. *Nature*, 290:783–785.

Drummond, A., Benson, J. and Levitan, I.B. (1980a) Serotonin-induced hyperpolarization of an identified *Aplysia* neuron is mediated by cyclic AMP. *Proc. Natl. Acad. Sci. U.S.A.*, 77:5013–5017.

Drummond, A., Bucher, F. and Levitan, I.B. (1980b) Distribution of serotonin and dopamine receptors in *Aplysia* tissues: analysis by ³H-LSD binding and adenylate cyclase stimulation. *Brain Res.*, 184:163–177.

Eckstein, F., Cassel, D., Lefkowitz, H., Lowe, M. and Selinger, Z. (1979) Guanosine 5′-O-2-thiodiphosphate: an inhibitor of adenylate cyclase stimulation by guanine nucleotides and fluoride ions. *J. Biol. Chem.*, 254:9829–9834.

Ewald, D., Williams, A. and Levitan, I.B. (1985) Modulation of single Ca++-dependent K+ channel activity by protein phosphorylation. *Nature*, 315:503–506.

Frazier, W., Kandel, E., Kupfermann, I., Waziri, R. and Coggeshall, R. (1967) Morphological and functional properties of identified neurons in the abdominal ganglion of *Aplysia californica*. *J. Neurophysiol.*, 30:1288–1351.

Greengard, P. (1976) Possible role of cyclic nucleotides and phosphorylated membrane proteins in postsynaptic actions of neurotransmitters. *Nature*, 260:101–108.

Jennings, K., Kaczmarek, L., Hewick, R., Dreyer, W. and Strumwasser, F. (1982) Protein phosphorylation during afterdischarge in peptidergic neurons of *Aplysia*. *J. Neurosci.*, 2:158–168.

Klein, M., Camardo, J. and Kandel, E. (1982) Serotonin modulates a specific K+ current in the sensory neurons that show presynaptic facilitation in *Aplysia*. *Proc. Natl. Acad. Sci. U.S.A.*, 79:5713–5717.

Lemos, J.R. and Levitan, I.B. (1984) Intracellular injection of guanyl nucleotides alters the serotonin-induced increase in

118

potassium conductance in *Aplysia* neuron R15. *J. Gen. Physiol.*, 83:269–285.

Lemos, J.R., Novak-Hofer, I. and Levitan, I.B. (1982) Serotonin alters the phosphorylation of specific proteins inside a single living nerve cell. *Nature*, 298:64–65.

Lemos, J.R., Novak-Hofer, I. and Levitan, I.B. (1984) Synaptic stimulation alters protein phosphorylation in vivo in a single *Aplysia* neuron. *Proc. Natl. Acad. Sci. U.S.A.*, 81:3233–3237.

Lemos, J.R., Novak-Hofer, I. and Levitan, I.B. (1985) Phosphoproteins associated with the regulation of a specific potassium channel in the identified *Aplysia* neuron R15. *J. Biol. Chem.*, 260:3207–3214.

Levitan, I.B. (1978) Adenylate cyclase in isolated *Helix* and *Aplysia* neuronal cell bodies: stimulation by serotonin and peptide-containing extract. *Brain Res.*, 154:404–408.

Levitan, I.B. and Drummond, A.H. (1980) Neuronal serotonin receptors and cAMP: biochemical, pharmacological and electrophysiological analysis. In U. Littauer et al. (eds.), *Neurotransmitters and their Receptors*, John Wiley and sons, London, pp. 163–176.

Levitan, I.B., Madsen, C. and Barondes, S. (1974) Cyclic AMP and amine effects on phosphorylation of specific protein in abdominal ganglion of *Aplysia californica*; localization and kinetic analysis. *J. Neurobiol.*, 5:511–525.

Lotshaw, D.P., Levitan, E.S. and Levitan, I.B. (1986) Fine tuning of neuronal electrical activity: modulation of several ion channels by intracellular messengers in a single identified nerve cell. *J. Exp. Biol.*, in press.

Miller, C. (1983) Integral membrane channels: Studies in model membranes. *Physiol. Rev.*, 63:1209–1242.

Neary, J.T. and Alkon, D.L. (1983) Protein phosphorylation/dephosphorylation and the transient, voltage-dependent potassium conductance in *Hermissenda crassicornis*. *J. Biol. Chem.*, 258:8979–8993.

Novak-Hofer, I., Lemos, J.R., Villermain, M. and Levitan, I.B. (1985) Calcium and cyclic nucleotide dependent protein kinases and their substrates in the *Aplysia* nervous system. *J. Neurosci.*, 5:151–159.

Paris, C., Castellucci, V., Kandel, E. and Schwartz, J.H. (1981) Protein phosphorylation, presynaptic facilitation, and behavioral sensitization in *Aplysia*. *Cold Spring Harbor Conf. Cell Prolif.*, 8:1361–1375.

Shuster, M., Camardo, J., Siegelbaum, S. and Kandel, E. (1985) Cyclic AMP-dependent protein kinase closes the serotonin-sensitive K^+ channels of *Aplysia* sensory neurones in cell-free membrane patches. *Nature*, 313:392–395.

Siegelbaum, S. and Tsien, R.W. (1983) Modulation of gated ion channels as a mode of transmitter action. *Trends Neurosci.*, 6:307–313.

Walsh, D.A., Ashby, C.D., Gonzales, C., Calkins, D., Fischer, E.H. and Krebs, E.G. (1971) Purification and characterization of a protein inhibitor of cAMP-dependent kinases. *J. Biol. Chem.*, 246:1977–1985.

Wilmsen, U., Methfessel, C., Hanke, W. and Boheim, G. (1983) Channel current fluctuation studies with solvent-free lipid bilayers using Neher-Sakmann pipettes. In *Physical Chemistry of Transmembrane Ion Motions*, Elsevier, Amsterdam, pp. 479–485.

Wilson, W.A. and Wachtel, H. (1978) Prolonged inhibition in burst firing neurons: synaptic inactivation of the slow regenerative inward current. *Science*, 202:772–775.

W.H. Gispen and A. Routtenberg (Eds.)
Progress in Brain Research, Vol. 69
© 1986 Elsevier Science Publishers B.V. (Biomedical Division)

CHAPTER 10

Modulation of the 'S' K^+ channel by cAMP-dependent protein phosphorylation in cell-free membrane patches

Michael J. Shuster, Joseph S. Camardo,
Steven A. Siegelbaum and Eric R. Kandel

Center for Neurobiology and Behavior, Departments of Physiology and Pharmacology, College of Physicians & Surgeons, Columbia University and Howard Hughes Medical Institute, 722 West 168th Street, New York, NY 10032, U.S.A.

Introduction

Post-synaptic effects of neurotransmitters are broadly divisible into mediatory and modulatory modes of action. Mediatory actions can be illustrated by the vertebrate neuromuscular junction where acetylcholine binds to a receptor–ionophore complex and directly mediates the flow of current throug a transmitter-gated ion channel (see Karlin, 1980; Colquhoun and Sakmann, 1983; Hille, 1984 for reviews of biochemistry and function of the nicotinic acetylcholine receptor). This direct link between transmitter binding and ion channel gating causes the membrane permeability changes accompanying conventional transmission to be brief and localized to subsynaptic regions of the cell where they move the membrane potential toward or away from threshold. These properties make this mode of transmission well suited to signals which change rapidly. In contrast to mediatory forms of transmission, in modulatory forms transmitter binding does not directly result in the opening of an ion channel (see Kupfermann, 1979 for review of modulatory actions of transmitters). One modulatory mechanism which has been the object of considerable study is second messenger-mediated transmission. This form differs from mediatory transmission in several respects:

(*a*) The receptor for the transmitter and the ion channel it affects are separate molecules which communicate through a receptor-mediated change in the concentration of small second messenger molecules inside the cell.

(*b*) The ion channels affected by second messengers can be gated by voltage and thus play key roles in determining action potential threshold, duration, and size (see Siegelbaum and Tsien, 1983 for review of transmitter modulation of gated channels).

(*c*) Second messenger-mediated synaptic actions tend to be longer lasting than conventional actions (see Kupfermann, 1980), and the small size of the second messenger allows it in principle to diffuse throughout the cell and globally affect target ion channels.

These differences make this form of transmission well suited for producing long-lasting changes in the electrical behavior of post-synaptic cells (see Kupfermann, 1979).

One of the best characterized second messenger systems is the cAMP (cyclic 5′,3′-adenosine monophosphate) cascade (for reviews see Krebs, 1979; Kupfermann, 1980; Nestler and Greengard, 1983) which results in the activation of cAMP-dependent protein kinase (cAMPdPK) according to the following scheme (see Fig. 1): Neurotransmitter (the first messenger), binds to a receptor coupled to the enzyme adenylate cyclase, and leads to a rise in intracellular levels of cAMP (the second messenger). cAMP binds to the regulatory subunit

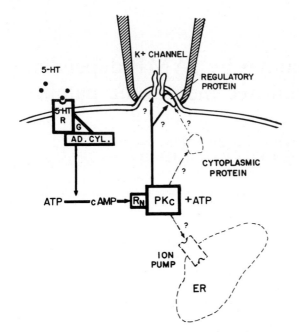

Fig. 1. The 5-HT–cAMP cascade and several possible substrates (indicated with question marks) for protein phosphorylation. 5-HT binds to membrane receptors which activate adenylate cyclase. The cyclase catalyzes the conversion of ATP to cAMP (the intracellular second messenger). Elevated intracellular levels of cAMP result in the activation of cAMP-dependent protein kinase (cAMPdPK), which phosphorylates many substrate proteins. Phosphorylation could alter the activity of an ion pump in the endoplasmic reticulum, which could modulate the channel indirectly. Other possible substrates include cytoplasmic regulatory proteins, membrane-associated regulatory proteins, or the channel itself. Cell-free patch experiments, in which the cytoplasm is washed away and the ionic composition of the medium can be controlled, are helpful in distinguishing between these possibilities. (Taken with permission from Camardo et al., 1983.)

a variety of ways (for review of neuronal protein phosphorylation see Kennedy, 1983; Levitan et al., 1983). These include the demonstration that a neurotransmitter's effect is mimicked by intracellular injection of cAMP, or bath application of membrane-permeable analogs of cAMP (for examples see Levittan and Adams, 1981; Madison and Nicoll, 1982; Siegelbaum et al., 1982; Kaczmarek and Strumwasser, 1984; Brum et al., 1984), by application of drugs which stimulate adenylate cyclase (Strong, 1984), or by direct injection of the catalytic subunit of cAMPdPK (Castellucci et al., 1980; Kaczmarek et al., 1980; DePeyer et al., 1982; Alkon et al., 1983). Blockade of cAMP effects have also been demonstrated using a specific protein inhibitor of the catalytic subunit of cAMPdPK (Castellucci et al., 1982; Adams and Levitan, 1982).

In *Aplysia* sensory cells, serotonin (5-HT) produces a slow excitatory post-synaptic potential mediated by cAMP, that contributes to presynaptic facilitation and behavioral sensitization of the animal's gill withdrawal reflex (Kandel and Schwartz, 1982). Work by Klein, Camardo, and Kandel (1982) led to the identification of a K^+ current whose magnitude is reduced by 5-HT. They named this the 'S' (for serotonin-sensitive) current, by analogy to the 'M' current, a voltage-dependent K^+ current found in bullfrog sympathetic neurons, which is reduced by muscarine (Brown and Adams, 1980). The S current is non-inactivating, is active at the resting potential, and is independent of (Ca_i^{2+}). It is therefore a resting background conductance, and its modulation by cAMP-dependent protein phosphorylation can alter the sensory neurons's action potential threshold, height, and duration (Klein et al., 1982).

Using the patch clamp technique to record single-channel currents from cell-attached patches (Hamill et al., 1981), Siegelbaum, Camardo, and Kandel (1982) found a K^+ channel whose properties closely matched those of the S current. Like the current, the S channel is open at the resting potential, it does not inactivate with prolonged depolarization, and its gating is independent of (Ca_i^{2+}) (see Camardo et al., 1983). Serotonin application and cAMP injection cause prolonged all-or-none closure of this channel and thereby reduce the magnitude of the S current by reducing the

of cAMPdPK, and activates the enzyme by causing the dissociation of the regulatory from the catalytic subunit. Free catalytic subunit then phosphorylates target substrate proteins. cAMP-dependent protein phosphorylation has been shown to affect several voltage gated conductances in neurons and heart muscle (for reviews see Siegelbaum and Tsien, 1983; Nestler and Greengard, 1983; Reuter, 1983). Evidence for the role of cAMP in neurotransmission has been obtained in

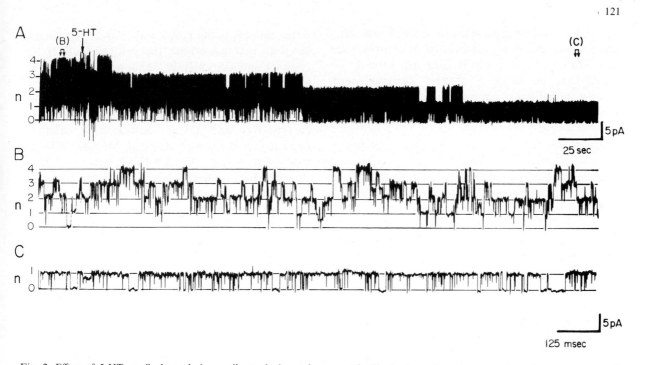

Fig. 2. Effect of 5-HT on S channels in a cell-attached membrane patch. Single-channel current recordings from a sensory cell membrane patch which contained 4 active S channels. A: Patch current shown on a compressed time base. Left hand ordinate (n) shows the current level associated with 0 to 4 open channels. Before bath application of 5-HT the patch contains 4 active channels and the current level fluctuates between $n=0$ and $n=4$ due to random superpositioning of channel openings. At the arrow, a concentrated drop of 5-HT is added to the bath to achieve a final concentration of $100\,\mu M$. Several moments later a stepwise decrease appears in the current level as one channel enters and remains in a prolonged closed state. Several minutes later a second and a third drop appear in the current level as two more channels close. B: Expanded time current record taken from control period indicated by bracketed (B) in panel A. Sweep shows random fluctuations in current level due to rapid superposition of channel openings and closings. Notice n fluctuates between 0 and 4. C: Expanded time current record following addition of 5-HT. Sweep taken from bracketed area of panel A labeled (C), following closure of 3 of the four S channels initially active in the patch. Current level now fluctuates between 0 and 1 open channel. The small change seen in unit current amplitude following the addition of 5-HT is due to an increased driving force for K^+ ions as the cell depolarized in response to 5-HT, changing the membrane potential across the patch from 0 mV in the beginning of the experiment to $+4$ mV at the end. Current records filtered at 500 Hz in A and 1 kHz in B and C. (Figure taken with permission from Camardo et al., 1983.)

number of S channels which are functionally available to carry the outward current. This effect is illustrated in Fig. 2. In this experiment, serotonin is added to the bath solution and a few seconds later there is a characteristic step-wise decrease in the current flowing across the patch as S channels enter into periods of prolonged closure. Because serotonin is physically prevented from coming in contact with the S channels under the patch electrode by the tight seal between the electrode and the membrane, this experiment provides independent corroboration of serotonin's second messenger mode of action in the LE sensory cells.

While these results provided a molecular description of the action of cAMPdPK at the molecular level of S channel gating the identity and subcellular localization of the phosphoproteins that control channel activity were unknown. In principle, cAMPdPK could exert its effects through phosphorylation of a number of possible substrates, including cytoplasmic regulatory proteins, ion pumps, membrane-associated regulatory proteins, and perhaps even by direct phosphorylation of the ion channel itself. These various possibilities are illustrated in Fig. 1. As a first step toward localizing the site of kinase action, and, in particular, to determine whether critical substrate proteins are membrane-associated or cytoplasmic, the actions of the purified catalytic subunit of cAMPdPK on single S channel currents were studied in cell-free membrane patches from *Aplysia* sensory neurons.

Methods

Abdominal ganglia were dissected from 100–220-g *Aplysia*, pinned ventral side up in a Sylgard-lined dish, and the left hemi-ganglion was desheathed to expose the LE sensory neuron cluster. For some experiments cell surfaces were cleaned by exposing the ganglion to 0.1–0.2% trypsin (Sigma type IX) for 10–20 min at room temperature (approx. 22°C). For the initial part of the experiment the bath was continuously superfused with artificial sea water (ASW; composition: 460 mM NaCl, 10 mM KCl, 11 mM $CaCl_2$, 55 mM $MgCl_2$, and 10 mM Tris buffer, pH 7.5. Final pH of solution adjusted to 7.5 with NaOH.) All solutions were filtered through 0.2 µM pore size Millipore filter immediately prior to their use. Patch electrodes were pulled according to methods outlined in Hamill et al. (1981), and were filled with ASW. Electrodes had resistances between 1 and 2 MΩ. Inside-out membrane patches were obtained from identified LE cells according to methods described in Hamill et al. (1981). The technique is diagrammed in Fig. 3. Briefly, the tip of a fire-polished patch electrode was brought into contact with an LE cell body. Gentle suction was then applied to form a high resistance seal between the cell membrane and the electrode. Seal resistances were typically between 10 and 100 GΩ. At this point, the bath solution was switched to a high K^+, low Ca^{2+} intracellular-like medium (composition: 360 mM KCl, 2 mM $MgCl_2$, 20 mM Na-HEPES pH 7.5, 1 mM $CaCl_2$, 1.5 mM EGTA, 272 mM sucrose), and inside-out cell-free membrane patches were formed by backing the tip of the electrode away from the cell. In this patch orientation, the cytoplasmic side of the membrane faces into the bath, and is readily accessible to bath-applied agents.

For experiments examining the effects of protein kinase on S channel currents, the membrane potential across the patch was held at depolarized levels to inactivate both the delayed rectifier K^+ channel and the early K^+ channel (Adams et al., 1980). Under these conditions, the two types of channel currents observed in the cell-free patch corresponded to the non-inactivating S channel current (I_S), and a Ca^{2+}-activated K^+ channel current (I_C) (Adams et al., 1980; Meech, 1978). To study the action of cAMPdPK on S channel currents in isolation, the bath concentration of Ca^{2+} was kept at 0.2 µM, a concentration which does not activate the Ca^{2+}-activated K^+ channel in *Aplysia* at potentials below 100 mV (M.J. Shuster, unpublished data). The catalytic subunit of cAMPdPK was purified from bovine heart according to methods of Beavo et al. (1974). Purified enzyme was stored at −70°C in a buffer containing 2 M glycerol, and 50 mM KH_2PO_4, pH 7.2. 1–7 days before use an aliquot (50–500 µl) of kinase was dialyzed against the 'intracellular' solution to remove the glycerol and raise the K^+ concentration. Specific activity of the enzyme was determined by measuring the rate of ^{32}P incorporation into a synthetic peptide substrate (Kemptide) using the assay method of Maller et al. (1978). In experiments with cAMPdPK, S channel currents were first identified in the inside-out patch on the basis of their Ca^{2+}-insensitivity, relative voltage independence and characteristic unit current amplitude (about 3.5 pA at 0 mV). The patch pipette was then moved to a small well which was superfused with the intracellular medium solution, and channel currents were recorded for 5–15 min to obtain a stable baseline of S channel activity. Purified catalytic subunit of cAMPdPK (0.1–1 µM) was then added to the bath either with or without Mg-ATP. (See Fig. 3.)

Membrane-associated phosphatase activity was determined as follows. Soluble and particulate fractions from *Aplysia* central nervous system (CNS) were prepared by homogenizing CNS ganglia (abdominal, cerebral, buccal, pleural, and pedal ganglia) from 2 adult animals in 250 µl of ice-cold buffer containing 1 M sucrose, 10 mM K-HEPES pH 7.5, 50 mM KCl, 0.2% saponin, 1 mM EGTA, and 1 mM phenylmethylsulfonylfluoride (final pH adjusted to 7.5 with KOH) using a ground glass homogenizer. The homogenate was

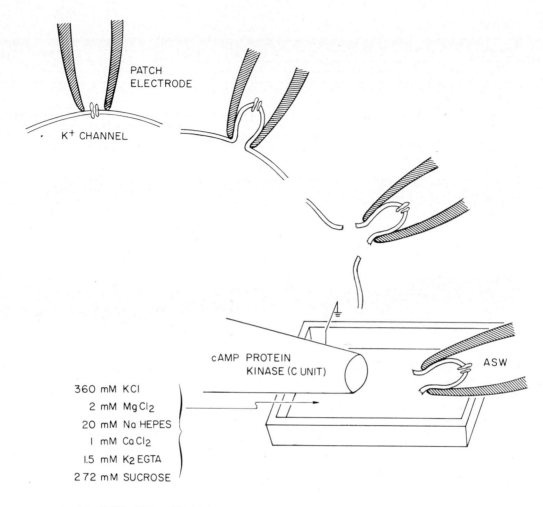

PATCH
ELECTRODE

· K⁺ CHANNEL

cAMP PROTEIN
KINASE (C UNIT)

ASW

360 mM KCl
2 mM MgCl₂
20 mM Na HEPES
1 mM CaCl₂
1.5 mM K₂ EGTA
272 mM SUCROSE

ISOLATED WELL (200 λ)

Fig. 3. Design of the cell-free experiment. A patch is obtained on the cell, the pipette is withdrawn; separating membrane-associated from cytoplasmic proteins, and the patch is isolated in a 200-μl well containing a high K⁺, low Ca²⁺ solution. The catalytic subunit of cAMPdPK and Mg-ATP are then injected directly into the bath. (Taken with permission from Camardo et al., 1983.)

centrifuged at $10\,000 \times g$ for 15 min to pellet sheath and unhomogenized tissue. The supernatant (S1) was removed, and the pellet was washed with 125 μl of buffer and was spun again at $10\,000 \times g$ for 15 min. The supernatant from this spin was combined with S1, and the combined supernatants were diluted with an appropriate volume of a buffer identical in composition to the homogenization buffer, except for the omission of sucrose, to obtain a final sucrose concentration of 0.25 M. The combined supernatants were then spun at $10\,000 \times g$ for 60 min to pellet the particulate fraction. This pellet was assayed

for phosphatase activity by measuring release of ³²PO₄ from labeled phosphorylase A according to methods described in Hemmings et al. (1984). Protein content of the membrane pellet was determined using a modification of the methods of Lowry (1951).

Results

An example of the effect of cAMPdPK on S channels in an inside-out membrane patch is shown in Fig. 4. The bottom panel shows a com-

124

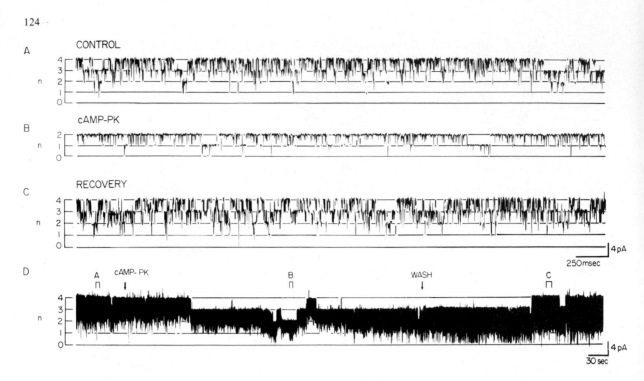

Fig. 4. cAMPdPK closes S channels in an inside-out membrane patch. A, B, and C: Expanded record of channel currents before, during and after application of cAMPdPK. 1 mM Mg-ATP present initially. Left hand ordinate shows number of open channels (n). A: Before addition of kinase, patch contained four active channels open for a large fraction of time. Current record fluctuates from four to one channel open simultaneously due to superimposition of random openings and closings of individual channels. The patch contained a fifth channel which opened occasionally throughout the experiment (seen as brief upward spikes in D) and was not analyzed further. B: 7 min after addition of cAMPdPK (0.1 μM, final concentration) plus 1 mM Mg-ATP (2.0 mM, final concentration) two channels are closed. Current level now fluctuates between 0 and 2 channels open; however, unit current amplitude and open probability of remaining active channels are unchanged from control. C: After recovery, channels again fluctuate between four levels. D: Closure and reopening of same channels illustrated in A, B, and C, but on a slower time sweep. Channel currents were recorded for over 8 min before addition of cAMPdPK, during which time there were no closures longer than 10 s. At arrow, cAMPdPK was added to the bath. After a latency of 3 min, one channel closed (downward step in maximal current level), and after another 4 min a second channel closed. The two closed channels then reopened (upward step changes in maximal current level in D, followed by a final prolonged closure. During washout of the enzyme, the remaining closed channel reopened after 5 min. Mean duration of cAMPdPK-produced closures in this experiment was 3 min. All expanded records were taken from the areas indicated by brackets lettered A, B, and C on panel D. In tabulating this experiment for Table I and Fig. 5, 2 out of 5 active channels were counted as closed by cAMPdPK. Channel probability fluctuated between 0.5 and 0.7 throughout the experiment. Fluctuations were uncorrelated with the addition of kinase or Mg-ATP. Bath Ca^{2+} concentration was 0.2 μM. Specific activity of cAMPdPK was 4.8×10^6 units/mg protein (1 unit = 1 pmole PO_4^{-3} transferred/min. Current records filtered at 500 Hz in D, and 1 kHz in A, B, and C. Membrane potential held at 0 mV throughout. (Taken with permission from Shuster et al., 1985).

pressed time record of current flowing across an inside-out membrane patch with 4 active S channels. At the arrow the purified catalytic subunit of cAMPdPK was added to the bath along with Mg-ATP. A few minutes later, a stepwise decrease can be seen in the current record as one channel enters a period of prolonged all-or-none closure. Several minutes later a second channel closes, then one channel reopens briefly and closes again. In the

maintained presence of kinase there are repeated cycles of long closures and reopenings. After the kinase is washed out of the bath, the patch current returns to its control level with 4 active channels.

In the presence of Mg-ATP, cAMPdPK produced prolonged periods of all-or-none channel closure in 73% of all experiments (n = 42) (see Fig. 5). Such prolonged closures (lasting for over 20 s; see below) were seldom observed during control

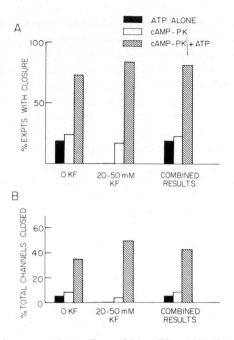

Fig. 5. Summary of the effects of Mg-ATP, cAMPdPK, and cAMPdPK plus Mg-ATP on S channel currents. Data were obtained in the presence and absence of potassium fluoride as indicated. A: Percent of experiments in which a given treatment produced prolonged closures of the S channel. Graph shows results of applications of ATP alone (filled bars), cAMPdPK alone (open bars), and cAMPdPK in the presence of Mg-ATP (shaded bars). cAMPdPK concentrations were in the range of 0.1 to 1.0 µM. The data have been grouped according to whether treatments were applied in the absence of KF (0 KF), or in the presence of 20–50 mM KF in the bath solution (see Results section). In addition, combined results pooled from both sets of experiments are also shown. In tabulating combined results, only those results from treatments in the presence of fluoride were used whenever a given treatment was applied to a patch in both the absence and presence of fluoride. B: Percent of total channels closed by same treatments as in A. KF treatment results in a statistically significant increase in the percent of channels closed by cAMPdPK + Mg-ATP (paired *t*-test, $p < 0.05$). The percentage was obtained by dividing the maximum number of channels closed simultaneously with a given agent by the number of channels initially active in the patch. In determining percent experiments with prolonged closure and percent channels closed, a 20-s closed period was used as a threshold for considering a prolonged closure significant (see Results section). Note that if a channel reopens after 20 s, it is still counted as a closure. The average reduction in patch current has not been calculated, and it would be somewhat less than the percentage of channels closed. Numbers of experiments with Mg-ATP, cAMPdPK, and cAMPdPK + Mg-ATP were respectively: 26, 17, and 40 in 0 KF; 2, 6, and 12 in presence of KF; and 27, 18, and 42 for combined results. (Figure taken with permission from Shuster et al., 1985.)

recordings before the addition of kinase, or after the kinase was washed out of the bath.

Several criteria were set for counting a channel closure as prolonged:

(*a*) Channel closure had to last for at least 20 s, as this was found to be longer on average than spontaneous channel closures which sometimes occurred in the absence of cAMPdPK + Mg-ATP, yet shorter on average than closures which followed the addition of cAMPdPK + Mg-ATP. (Similar results were obtained when analyzing the data using closed time thresholds between 10 and 30 s.)

(*b*) No prolonged closures (lasting > 20 s) could take place during a control period extending back from the time an agent was added to the bath whose duration was set at twice the latency between the addition of that agent and the first prolonged closure.

These criteria were chosen to provide a way to distinguish closures mediated by cAMPdPK from spontaneous closures which sometimes occurred in the absence of any experimental manipulation. Using these criteria for analyzing the data, it was found that protein kinase closed an average of 1.3 ± 1.0 (mean $\pm$ S.D.) channels out of an average of 3.8 ± 1.9 channels initially active per patch. Thus, the kinase closed 34% of all channels in all patches, including channels from those patches where kinase failed to produce any significant closure (see Fig. 5). To control for any non-specific effects of cAMPdPK not mediated by phosphorylation (as well as any bias introduced by the criteria for significant closure), the effects of catalytic subunit of the cAMPdPK were tested in the absence of Mg-ATP. Without this source of high-energy phosphate, kinase was much less effective, producing channel closures in less than 24% of all experiments and closing only 8% of all channels. Similarly, Mg-ATP by itself (in concentrations up to 10 mM) had little effect on S channel activity. The results of these controls are summarized in Fig. 5. In addition to these controls, experiments were done using heat-inactivated cAMPdPK. It was found that the heat-inactivated enzyme (in the presence of 1.0 mM Mg-ATP) never produced the all-or-none closures produced by the active kinase

($n = 8$). However, in some experiments the denatured enzyme caused a slight decrease in the probability of a channel being open. Such changes in probability were not seen with active kinase, either in the presence or absence of Mg-ATP.

Several possible explanations have been considered for the prolonged closures which sometimes occur with cAMPdPK in the absence of Mg-ATP, or with Mg-ATP alone. One possibility is that these closures reflect a low spontaneous closure rate of the channel that is independent of cAMPdPK or Mg-ATP. Another possibility is that the closures result from the action of endogenous kinase or Mg-ATP which might sometimes remain associated with the patch. If membrane-associated kinase or ATP were present in the patch, bath application of Mg-ATP or cAMPdPK might combine with the membrane-associated factor and catalyze protein phosphorylation. Because the cell-free patch has not yet been well characterized biochemically, it is difficult to determine whether this is a likely explanation for the closures which sometimes occur in the absence of combined application of cAMPdPK and Mg-ATP. Nevertheless, the marked stimulation of channel closure by cAMPdPK in the presence of Mg-ATP argues that these closures represent a phosphorylation reaction mediated by the kinase. The mean latency between addition of cAMPdPK and the first channel closure was 4.5 ± 4.0 min. (range 30 s to 15 min). Some of this latency may have resulted from inadequate mixing of the cAMPdPK when the small volume of enzyme (40 µl) was added to the 200-µl isolation well. In the 10 most recent experiments where care was taken to ensure adequate mixing of the bath, the mean latency was reduced to <2.5 min.

A detailed comparison was made between the modulation seen in cell-free and cell-attached patches to highlight their similarities and differences (see Table I). Extracellular application of serotonin and intracellular injection of cAMP produce prolonged all-or-none closures of the S channel without affecting either the elementary conductance of the channel or its gating (Siegelbaum et al., 1982; Fig. 1). The effects of cAMPdPK on the cell-free patch resemble the physiological effects of extracellular application of 5-HT and cAMP injection in that the cell-free closures are long lasting and occur without any accompanying change in the unit current amplitude or the gating of the remaining open channels. There is also good quantitative agreement among the cell-attached and cell-free experiments in both the percentage of experiments with channel closure and the percentage of channels closed. This supports the idea that the effects of cAMPdPK in the cell-free patch play a physiological role in the modulation of the S channel by 5-HT. However, there are two important differences between the action of cAMPdPK in the isolated patch and of serotonin and cAMP in the intact cell. First, although in 25% of the experiments cAMPdPK produced closures that persisted for over 10 min, in most experiments the channels closed for a mean duration of 2–3 min and then reopened, even in the presence of the kinase. 5-HT, on the other hand, caused closures that persisted for the entire dura-

TABLE I

Comparison of modulatory effects in cell-attached and cell-free membrane patches

Patch type	Treatment	n	Experiments with closures (%)	channels closed (%)	Latency to first closure (min)	Closed time[a] (min)
Cell-attached	Serotonin	33	76.5	45.8	1.7 ± 1.3	>5
	cAMP	7	71.4	52.2	4.5 ± 1.6	>5
Cell-free	cAMPdPK + ATP[b]	42	81.0	42.0	4.5 ± 4.6	3.0 ± 2.7

[a]Closed times in serotonin and cAMP generally outlasted the experiment so 5 min is a lower limit. Average closed time with cAMPdPK was calculated using data from experiments where channels showed recovery from closure ($n = 18$).
[b]Results are combined ($\pm$) fluoride results from Fig. 5.

tion of transmitter application (>5 min; see Fig. 2 and Table I). Second, cAMPdPK closed fewer channels than serotonin (34% as opposed to 46%; see Table I and Fig. 5).

One possible explanation for these differences is that the cell-free patch contains an endogenous protein phosphatase that limits the action of the kinase by cleaving the phosphate from the phosphoprotein (see Ingebritsen and Cohen, 1983). The lack of any specific phosphatase inhibitor for molluscan cells prevents direct testing of this hypothesis. However, evidence consistent with the presence of membrane-associated phosphatase in the patch comes from two sources:

(a) Preliminary experiments by Shuster, Hemmings and Nairn show that a membrane fraction isolated from *Aplysia* central nervous system contains phosphoprotein phosphatase activity. This activity is inhibited by potassium fluoride, a non-

specific phosphatase inhibitor (Revel, 1963). The phosphatase inhibitor protein, inhibitor 2 (see Ingebritsen and Cohen, 1983) appears to inhibit some of this activity in a dose-dependent manner.

(b) Based on these findings, experiments were done in which KF was added to the solution bathing the inside of the patch. KF (20–50 mM) slightly increased the percentage of experiments in which cAMPdPK produced channel closure, and significantly increased the fraction of channels closed (paired t-test; $p < 0.05$; see Fig. 5). An example of KF converting a non-responsive to a responsive patch is shown in Fig. 6. In the absence of KF cAMPdPK + Mg-ATP had no effect on channel gating. After KF was washed into the bath, cAMPdPK + Mg-ATP produced prolonged channel closures. In three experiments in which kinase produced only brief closures (<20 sec long) in the absence of a phosphatase inhibitor, the

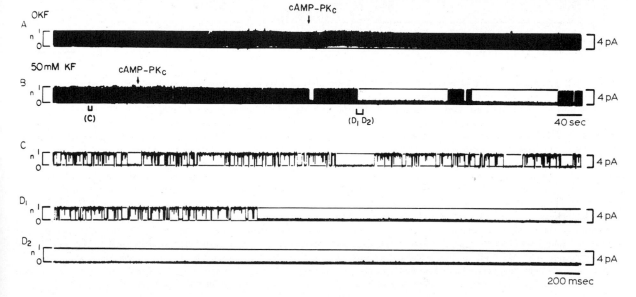

Fig. 6. KF increases percent of experiments with channel closure. Current from an inside-out patch of membrane containing one S channel. A: In the absence of KF, cAMPdPK (0.1 μM, final concentration; specific activity = 5.9×10^6 units/mg protein) and Mg-ATP (1.0 mM) have no effect on single channel activity measured for 11 mins after kinase application. B: Single channel current recorded in the presence of 50 mM KF. Addition of cAMPdPK (0.1 μM) and Mg-ATP (1.0 mM) now produces prolonged periods of channel closure (mean closed time = 2 min). C: Expanded time record of single-channel current showing the normal channel gating process taken in the presence of 50 mM KF before the addition of kinase and Mg-ATP to the bath. D1, D2: Continuous sweeps showing transition from the normal gating process to a period of prolonged closure after the addition of kinase + Mg-ATP to the bath. The channel exhibits normal gating behavior up to the time it enters a prolonged closed state. Bracketed areas in panel B labeled C, and D1, D2 indicate areas of record from which the fast time sweep records were taken. Membrane potential held at 0 mV throughout experiment. Current record filtered at 250 Hz in A, and B, and 1 K Hz in C, and D (Figure taken with permission from Shuster et al., 1985.)

128

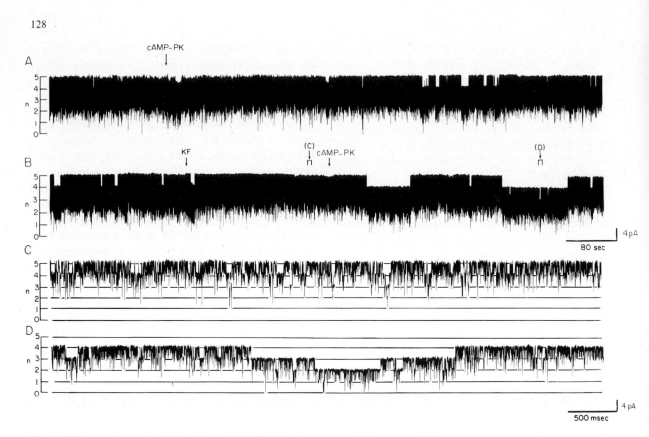

Fig. 7. KF potentiates threshold effects of cAMPdPK. Current record from an inside-out patch of membrane containing 5 S channels. Left-hand ordinate (n) shows current level associated with 0–5 simultaneously open channels. A: Compressed time record taken in absence of KF showing modest effects of cAMPdPK with Mg-ATP. Purified catalytic subunit (0.1 μM final concentration; specific activity $= 6.1 \times 10^5$ units/mg protein) along with Mg-ATP (1.0 mM, final concentration) was added to the bath at the arrow. After a 6-min latency, brief stepwise decreases appear in current record as one channel enters and exits prolonged closed state. B: Compressed time record continuous with A showing repeated cycling of channel closure and reopening in presence of cAMPdPK + Mg-ATP. At the arrow, the bath solution was changed for one containing 50 mM KF. The long closures cease as the protein kinase is washed out of the bath. After a 3.5-min control period, purified catalytic subunit and Mg-ATP are added to the bath in the same concentrations as in panel A. In less than 1 min, the record shows a stepwise decrease in maximal current level as one channel enters a prolonged closed state. Notice the potentiation of the time spent in prolonged closed state in the presence of KF. Mean closed time was 5 s without, and 34 s with 50 mM KF. C: Expanded sweep taken from bracketed area in panel B showing normal channel gating in the presence of 50 mM KF before addition of protein kinase and Mg-ATP. The current level fluctuates between 1 and 5 simultaneously open channels. D: Expanded sweep taken from the bracketed area in panel B after addition of protein kinase and Mg-ATP during prolonged closure of one channel. The current level now fluctuates between 0 and 4 simultaneously open channels. Channels remaining open gate normally. Membrane potential held at 0 mV throughout experiment. Current records filtered at 500 Hz in panels A, and B, and 1 kHz in C and D. (Unpublished experiment from M. Shuster.)

duration of channel closure was prolonged 5 to 10-fold in the presence of inhibitor (two experiments with fluoride and one with a different inhibitor, 2 mM p-nitrophenylphosphate, see Fig. 7). KF alone had no effect on channel activity nor did it potentiate the effects of cAMPdPK in the absence of Mg-ATP or the effects of Mg-ATP alone, results that suggest that fluoride's effect on the patch is specifically related to protein phos-

phorylation (see Fig. 5). As fluoride stimulates adenylate cyclase (Rall and Sutherland, 1958), controls were done in which cAMP was added directly to the patch to test whether the effects of KF are mediated by cAMP production. In the presence of Mg-ATP, but without cAMPdPK, cAMP (0.1–1.0 mM) had no significant effect on channel activity ($n = 6$), nor did it significantly potentiate the effects of cAMPdPK.

Discussion

It is now clear that a wide variety of ionic currents are specifically modulated by cAMPdPK (see Introduction). The recent work of Acosta-Urquidi et al. (1984) and DeRiemer et al. (1985) demonstrates that other protein kinases can also produce modulatory effects on ionic currents. Several tasks must be completed before it is understood how protein phosphorylation alters ion channel function. These include the identification and characterization of the relevant kinases, phosphatases, and their substrates. One attractive hypothesis suggests that direct phosphorylation of ion channel proteins results in modulation of their function. Work done by Catterall and colleagues on sodium channels purified from rat brain (Costa et al., 1982), and by Huganir and Greengard on nicotinic acetylcholine receptors from *Torpedo californica* (Huganir and Greengard, 1983) has shown that both of these proteins are phosphorylated by cAMPdPK. In addition, the acetylcholine receptor is phosphorylated by at least two other kinases (Huganir et al., 1984). So far, no clear physiological function has been associated with the phosphorylation of these purified ion channels.

Work with the S channel, and with a Ca^{2+}-activated K^+ channel from *Helix* neurons (Shuster et al., 1985; Ewald et al., 1985) demonstrates that ion channel modulation takes place in cell-free patches. This suggests that phosphorylation occurs either on the ion channel itself, or on a closely associated membrane protein. The results presented here indicate that cAMPdPK can produce prolonged all-or-none closures of single S channels in cell-free membrane patches. The similarities in the actions of cAMPdPK in cell-free patches with those of 5-HT and cAMP acting through a complicated cellular system support the view that the closures produced by kinase in the cell-free patches are physiologically relevant. Moreover, these actions are produced by concentrations of enzyme (0.1–1.0 µM) that are in a physiological range and represent less than the total concentration of cAMPdPK in the sensory neuron (estimated from data of Bernier (1984) to be approximately 3.5 µM). The effects of cAMPdPK do not completely mimic those of 5-

HT. and cAMP in the intact cell. In the cell-free patch the kinase tends to close somewhat fewer channels and the closures are briefer, suggesting that either the cell-free patches lack adequate amounts of some component necessary for complete channel modulation, or the patches contain a phosphoprotein phosphatase which terminates the kinase-induced closures. The finding that KF, a non-specific phosphatase inhibitor, potentiates the effects of cAMPdPK provides indirect evidence for the involvement of a phosphatase in terminating the cAMPdPK-induced closures of the S channel.

Phosphoprotein phosphatase activity has been found in post-synaptic *Torpedo* membrane acetylcholine receptors. This phosphatase activity was capable of dephosphorylating membrane-bound receptors and was inhibited by fluoride ions (Gordon et al., 1979). Some of the difference in the duration of channel closure between cell-attached and cell-free patches might be explained if the sensory neurons contain a cytoplasmic protein, similar to phosphatase inhibitor proteins found in other tissues, which is capable of regulating phosphatase activity. Some of these inhibitor proteins have been shown to inhibit specific mammalian phosphatase activities only after being phosphorylated by cAMPdPK (Hemmings and Greengard 1984; Ingebritsen and Cohen 1983). This scheme could provide coordinated regulation of kinase and phosphatase activities and serve to fine tune the steady state level of protein phosphorylation in the cell. If *Aplysia* has such cytoplasmic inhibitor proteins, coordinated regulation of kinase and phosphatase activities would be lost in the cell-free patch since the cell-free patch separates membrane associated and cytoplasmic constituents. Preliminary evidence for the existance of such inhibition comes from the result of one experiment in which the effects of dilution on phosphatase activity from *Aplysia* CNS were examined. It was found that the specific activity of the membrane fraction (units phosphatase/mg protein) increased and then stabilized as the fraction was diluted from 5 to 0.05 mg protein/ml. This result suggests the presence of an endogenous inhibitor protein in the membrane preparation whose concentration falls below its dissociation constant for binding phosphatase as the membrane preparation is

130

diluted (Shuster, Hemmings, and Nairn, unpublished observations). It is interesting to note that in some experiments done on cell-attached patches with low doses of 5-HT, S channel modulation more closely resembles the modulation seen with cAMPdPK in the cell-free patch. Instead of the usual sustained prolonged closure (> 5 min), channels are seen to cycle between prolonged closures and normal gating, in a manner similar to channels in cell-free patches in the presence of kinase and Mg-ATP (see Fig. 8). This behavior is consistent with the notion that repeated cycling of prolonged channel closure and reopening may reflect repeated phosphorylation and dephosphorylation events which could occur during threshold stimulation of cAMPdPK (low dose of transmitter), or in the presence of a poorly regulated phosphatase activity. In the future, it will be important to determine to what extent specific phosphatase inhibitor proteins potentiate cAMPdPK-produced closures in the cell-free patch. Finally, although it cannot be determined whether the kinase phosphorylates the S channel itself, these results suggest that the isolated membrane contains at least some of the phosphoproteins necessary for producing prolonged channel closure.

Note added in proof

It has recently been shown that phosphrylation of the nicotinic acetylcholine receptor by cAMPdPK increases its rate of desensitization (Huganir et al., 1986). This result provides the first confirmation of the hypothesis that direct phosphorylation of an ion channel modulates channel function.

Acknowledgements

We thank Mark Eppler for collaborating on the early stages of this work; E.G. Krebs, Charles Rubin, Deepak Bhatnagar and Robert Roskoski for making available the purified catalytic subunit of cAMP-dependent protein kinase; Richard W. Tsien, James H. Schwartz, John Koester and Francesco Belardetti for comments on an earlier version of this manuscript; Harriet Ayers for typing this manuscript; and Kathrin Hilten and Louise Katz for preparing the figures. This work was supported by USPHS Grant R01 NS19569-02 to S.A.S. and NIH Grant 5 P01 GM32099-03 to E.R.K.

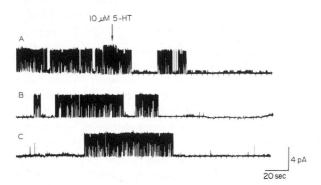

Fig. 8. Effect of low dose of 5-HT on a single S channel in a cell-attached patch. Current record from cell-attached patch showing effects of low dose of 5-HT on S channel gating. A, B, and C are continuous sweeps. The beginning of panel A shows the current record from the control period in the absence of 5-HT. At the arrow a concentrated drop of 5-HT was added to the bath to achieve a final concentration of 10 μM. Before addition of 5-HT, the channel was open for about 70% of the time. In the presence of 5-HT, the channel displays prolonged closures alternating with bursts of apparently normal opening activity. A channel that carries a small outward current is also visible in these traces. Current records filtered at 1 KHz, membrane potential across patch was 0 mV. (Figure taken with permission from Camardo and Siegelbaum, 1983.)

References

Acosta-Urquidi, J., Alkon, D. and Neary, J. (1984) Ca^{2+}-dependent protein kinase injection in a photoreceptor mimics biophysical effects of associative learning. *Science*, 224:1254–1257.

Adams, W. and Levitan, I.B. (1982) Intracellular injection of protein kinase inhibitor blocks the serotonin-induced increase in K^+ conductance in *Aplysia* neuron R15. *Proc. Natl. Acad. Sci. U.S.A.*, 79:3877–3880.

Adams, D.J., Smith, S.J. and Thompson, S.H. (1980) Ionic currents in molluscan soma. *Annu. Rev. Neurosci.*, 3:141–167.

Alkon, D., Acosta-Urquidi, J., Olds, J., Kuzma, G. and Neary, J. (1983) Protein kinase injection reduces voltage-dependent potassium currents. *Science*, 219:303–306.

Beavo, J.A., Bechtel, P.J. and Krebs, E.G. (1974) Preparation of homogenous cyclic-AMP-dependent protein kinase(s) and its subunits from rabbit skeletal muscle. *Meth. Enzymol.*, 38:299–308.

Bernier, L. (1984) *The Role of Cyclic Nucleotides in Synaptic Plasticity in Aplysia californica*. Ph.D. Thesis, Columbia University.

Brown, D.A. and Adams, P.R. (1980) Muscarinic suppression

of a novel voltage-sensitive K$^+$-current in a vertebrate neuron. *Nature*, 283:673–676.

Brum, G., Osterrieder, W. and Trautwein, W. (1984) β-Adrenergic increase in the calcium conductance of cardiac myocytes studied with the patch clamp. *Pfluegers Arch.*, 401:111–118.

Camardo, J.S. and Siegelbaum, S.A. (1983) Single-channel analysis in *Aplysia* neurons. In B. Sakmann and E. Neher (Eds.), *Single-Channel Recording*, Plenum Press, New York, pp. 409–423.

Camardo, J.S., Shuster, M.J., Siegelbaum, S.A. and Kandel, E.R. (1983) Modulation of a specific potassium channel in sensory neurons of *Aplysia* by serotonin and cAMP-dependent protein phosphorylation. In *Cold Spring Harbor Symposia on Quantitative Biology, Vol. 48*, The Cold Spring Harbor Laboratory, New York, pp. 213–220.

Colquhoun, D. and Sakmann, B. (1983) Bursts of openings in transmitter-activated ion channels. In B. Sakmann and E. Neher (Eds.), *Single-Channel Recording*, Plenum Press, New York, pp. 345–364.

Castellucci, V.F., Kandel, E.R., Schwartz, J.H., Wilson, F.D., Nairn, A.C. and Greengard, P. (1980) Intracellular injection of the catalytic subunit of cyclic AMP-dependent protein kinase simulates facilitation of transmitter release underlying behavioral sensitization in *Aplysia*. *Proc. Natl. Acad. Sci. U.S.A.*, 77:7492–7496.

Castellucci, V.F., Nairn, A., Greengard, P., Schwartz, J.H. and Kandel, E.R. (1982) Inhibition of adenosine 3′,5′-monophosphate-dependent protein kinase blocks presynaptic facilitation in *Aplysia*. *J. Neurosci.*, 12:1673–1681.

Costa, M.R., Casnellie, J.E. and Catterall, W.A. (1982) Selective phosphorylation of the α subunit of the sodium channel by cAMP-dependent protein kinase. *J. Biol. Chem.*, 14:7918–7921.

DePeyer, J.E., Cachelin, A.B., Levitan, I.B. and Reuter, H. (1982) Ca^{2+}-activated K+ conductance in internally perfused snail neurons is enhanced by protein phosphorylation. *Proc. Natl. Acad. Sci. U.S.A.*, 79:4207–4211.

DeRiemer, S.A., Strong, J.A., Albert, K.A., Greengard, P. and Kaczmarek, L.K. (1985) Enhancement of calcium current in *Aplysia* neurons by phorbol ester and protein kinase C. *Nature*, 313:313–316.

Ewald, D.A., Williams, A. and Levitan, I.B. (1985) Modulation of single Ca^{2+}-dependent K$^+$-channel activity by protein phosphorylation. *Nature*, 315:503–506.

Gordon, A.S., Milfay, D., Davis, C.G. and Diamond, I. (1979) Protein phosphatase activity in acetylcholine receptor-enriched membranes. *Biochem. Biophys. Res. Commun.*, 87:876–883.

Hamill, O.P., Marty, A., Neher, E., Sakmann, B. and Sigworth, F.J. (1981) Improved patch-clamp techniques for high-resolution current recording from cells and cell-free membrane patches. *Pfluegers Arch.*, 391:85–100.

Hille, B. (1984) *Ionic Channels of Excitable Membranes*, Sinauer, Sunderland, pp. 117–147.

Huganir, R.L. and Greengard, P. (1983) cAMP-dependent protein kinase phosphorylates the nicotinic acetylcholine receptor. *Proc. Natl. Acad. Sci. U.S.A.*, 80:1130–1134.

Huganir, R.L., Miles, K. and Greengard, P. (1984) Phosphorylation of the nicotinic acetylcholine receptor by an endogenous tyrosine-specific protein kinase. *Proc. Natl. Acad. Sci. U.S.A.*, 81:6968–6972.

Huganir, R.L., Delcour, A.H., Greengard, P. and Hess, G.P. (1986) Phosphorylation of the nicotinic acetylcholine receptor regulates its rate of desensitization. *Nature*, 321:774–776.

Hemmings, H.C. Jr. and Greengard, P. (1984) DARP-32, a dopamine-regulated neuronal phosphoprotein, is a potent inhibitor of protein phosphatase-1. *Nature*, 310:503–505.

Ingebritsen, T.S. and Cohen, P. (1983) Protein phosphatases: properties and role in cellular regulation. *Science*, 221:331–338.

Karlin, A. (1980) Molecular properties of nicotinic acetylcholine receptors. In C.W. Cotman, G. Poste, and G.L. Nicolson (Eds.), *Cell Surface Reviews: The Cell Surface and Neuronal Recognition, Vol. 6*, North-Holland, Amsterdam, pp. 191–250.

Kaczmarek, L.K. and Strumwasser, F. (1984) A voltage-clamp analysis of currents underlying cyclic AMP-induced membrane modulation in isolated peptidergic neurons of *Aplysia*. *J. Neurophys.*, 52:340–349.

Kaczmarek, L.K., Jennings, K.R., Strumwasser, F., Nairn, A.C., Walter, U., Wilson, F.D. and Greengard, P. (1980) Microinjection of catalytic subunit of cyclic AMP-dependent protein kinase enhances calcium action potentials of bag cell neurons in cell culture. *Proc. Natl. Acad. Sci. U.S.A.*, 77:7487–7491.

Kandel, E.R. and Schwartz, J.H. (1982) Molecular biology of learning: modulation of transmitter release. *Science*, 218:433–443.

Kennedy, M.B. (1983) Experimental approaches to understanding the role of protein phosphorylation in the regulation of neuronal function. *Annu. Rev. Neurosci.*, 6:493–525.

Klein, M., Camardo, J. and Kandel, E.R. (1982) Serotonin modulates a specific potassium current in the sensory neurons that show presynaptic facilitation in *Aplysia*. *Proc. Natl. Acad. Sci. U.S.A.*, 79:5713–5717.

Krebs, E.G. and Beavo, J.A. (1979) Phosphorylation-dephosphorylation of enzymes. *Annu. Rev. Biochem.*, 48:923–959.

Kupfermann, I. (1979) Modulatory actions of neurotransmitters. *Annu. Rev. Neurosci.*, 2:447–465.

Kupfermann, I. (1980) Role of cyclic nucleotides in excitable cells. *Annu. Rev. Physiol.*, 42:629–641.

Levitan, I.B. and Adams, W.B. (1981) Cyclic AMP modulation of a specific ion channel in an identified nerve cell: possible role for protein phosphorylation. *Adv. Cyc. Nuc. Res.*, 14:647–653.

Levitan, I.B., Lemos, J.R. and Novak-Hofer, I. (1983) Protein phosphorylation and the regulation of ion channels. *Trends neurosci.*, 6:496–499.

Lowry, O.H., Rosebrough, N.J., Farr, A.L. and Randall, R.J. (1951) Protein measurement with the Folin phenol reagent. *J. Biol. Chem.*, 193:265–275.

Madison, D.V. and Nicoll, R.A. (1982) Noradrenaline blocks accomodation of pyramidal cell discharge in the hippocampus. *Nature*, 299:636–638.

132

Maller, J.L., Kemp, B.E. and Krebs, E.G. (1978) In vivo phosphorylation of a synthetic peptide substrate of cyclic AMP-dependent protein kinase. *Proc. Natl. Acad. Sci. U.S.A.*, 75:248–251.

Meech, R.W. (1978) Calcium-dependent potassium activation in nervous tissues. *Annu. Rev. Biophys. Bioeng.*, 7:1–18.

Nestler, E.J. and Greengard, P. (1983) Protein phosphorylation in the brain. *Nature*, 305:583–588.

Rall, W.T. and Sutherland, E.W. (1958) Formation of a cyclic adenine ribonucleotide by tissue particles. *J. Biol. Chem.*, 232:1065–1076.

Reuter, H. (1983) Calcium channel modulation by neurotransmitters, enzymes and drugs. *Nature*, 301:569–574.

Revel. H.R. (1963) Phosphoprotein phosphatase. *Meth. Enzymol.*, 6:211–214.

Shuster, M.J., Camardo, J.S., Siegelbaum, S.A. and Kandel, E.R. (1985) Cyclic AMP-dependent protein kinase closes the serotonin-sensitive K^+ channels of *Aplysia* sensory neurons in cell-free membrane patches. *Nature*, 313:392–395.

Siegelbaum, S.A. and Tsien, R.W. (1983) Modulation of gated ion channels as a mode of transmitter action. *Trends neurosci.*, 6:307–313.

Siegelbaum, S.A., Camardo, J.S. and Kandel, E.R. (1982) Serotonin and cyclic AMP close single K^+ channels in *Aplysia* sensory neurons. *Nature*, 299:413–417.

Strong, J.A. (1984) Modulation of potassium current kinetics in bag cell neurons of *Aplysia* by an activator of adenylate cyclase. *J. Neurosci.*, 4:2772–2783.

W.H. Gispen and A. Routtenberg (Eds.)
Progress in Brain Research, Vol. 69
© 1986 Elsevier Science Publishers B.V. (Biomedical Division)

CHAPTER 11

Cyclic nucleotides as modulators and activators of ionic channels in the nerve cell membrane

Platon G. Kostyuk

Bogomoletz Institute of Physiology, Ukrainian Academy of Sciences, 252601 Kiev, U.S.S.R.

Introduction

According to a general scheme of excitable membrane functioning widely recognized at present, ionic channels and cell metabolism represent two operationally independent systems involved in the mechanism maintaining cellular reactivity. Metabolism only creates the necessary prerequisites for generation of ionic currents forming transmembrane electrochemical gradients by active ion transport. This scheme seemed universal for a long time; but now more and more experimental data are available indicating that in certain cases the function of ionic channels may be directly influenced by intracellular metabolic processes. This paper presents a survey of such data and discusses their significance for the understanding of integrative functions of the cell.

Electrically operated calcium channels

For the first time the suggestion that the function of electrically operated channels can be under direct metabolic control was stated proceeding from the studies of calcium inward currents in cardiac muscle fibers. These currents are known to be largely potentiated by catecholamines. In parallel to such potentiation, an increase in 3,5-cAMP content takes place inside the fibers (Reuter, 1974). Direct introduction of cAMP into cardiac muscle fibers is accompanied by the analogous effect. Considering modern ideas about the role of cyclic nucleotides and phosphorylation of functional cell proteins catalyzed by cyclic nucleotides, it was suggested that involvement of additional calcium channels in the activity is mediated through cAMP synthesis by membrane adenylate cyclase activated, in turn, by catecholamines. Protein phosphorylation of calcium channels is a factor maintaining the ability of the channels to be activated, as if they have an additional gating mechanism directly operated by cellular biochemical processes (Reuter, 1983).

Calcium channels of the somatic membrane of nerve cells possess a property which served a convenient basis for the study of metabolic dependence of their function. In the course of intracellular perfusion by saline solution, the calcium currents of the somatic membrane rapidly decline – for several minutes in large snail neurons and for several tens of seconds in smaller mammalian neurons (Kostyuk and Krishtal, 1977; Fedulova et al., 1981; Byerly and Hagiwara, 1982). The speed of calcium current decline decelerates considerably with decreasing temperature, implying the participation in normal function of just calcium channels of some cytoplasmic factor(s) washed out or destroyed during cell perfusion by saline solution. In the absence of these factors the channels are rendered inactive ('sleeping').

The intracellular perfusion technique extremely facilitated the search of such factors. Introduction of cAMP together with ATP and Mg^{2+} ions into the perfusing solution not only prevented the further decline of calcium conductance but largely restored it, sometimes to its initial level. Separate introduction of either ingredient into the cell could exert some stabilizing effect, yet it was weak. In perfused snail neurons the maximum effect was observed at about 10^{-4} M cAMP, though restoration was also seen even at micromolar concentrations (Doroshenko et al., 1982). Similar concentration dependences have been obtained for restoration of the calcium conductance in rat neurons (Fedulova et al., 1981). Intracellular administration of cGMP had no effect on the calcium conductance decline.

Evidence that the activity of membrane-bound enzymes, which can be potentiated by introduction of corresponding substrates, is preserved during intracellular perfusion was obtained in experiments with addition of fluoride ions to the perfusate in quantities necessary to activate adenylate cyclase (several millimoles). In combination with ATP and Mg^{2+} ions, such introduction also induced restoration of the calcium conductance. On the contrary, addition of small amounts of Cu^{2+} ions (blockers of adenylate cyclase) interrupted this restoring effect (Doroshenko et al., 1982).

The activation of cell phosphodiesterase and the corresponding reduction in cAMP level during perfusion is likely to be an essential (if not principal) factor underlying the suppression of calcium conductance. Intracellular administration of theophylline also slowed down the decline of calcium currents, though less effectively than the introduction of cAMP. The participation of calmodulin in the described process triggered by elevation of the intracellular free Ca^{2+} level is corroborated by data about the effect of calmodulin blockers (trifluoperazine and R24571) on the rate of calcium conductance decline. Introduction of these substances into the perfused neuron considerably reduced the rate of calcium conductance decline (Doroshenko and Martynyuk, 1984).

These experimental findings do not confirm directly the idea that intracellular cAMP has its effect on calcium conductance through the change in the activity of membrane phosphoprotein kinases phosphorylating membrane proteins essential for the function of calcium channels, though such a possibility is most likely. It is known that catalytic subunit (CS) can be obtained as a homogenous protein; the properties of the enzyme isolated from various tissues and different

animal species are practically identical. These data promoted the studies of the effects of intracellularly introduced CS on calcium current in perfused snail neurons. CS of the cAMP-dependent protein kinase with a molecular weight of 35 000 was obtained from the rabbit myocardium, its specific activity was about 20 nM ^{32}P/mg protein/min. Addition of 0.7 µM CS + ATP to the perfusing solution stopped the decline of calcium conductance and slowly restored it to the initial level (Doroshenko et al., 1984). Removal of ATP from the perfusing solution resulted in fast decline of the calcium conductance.

The opposite effect – inhibition of cAMP-dependent protein kinase – can be achieved by some specific blockers, e.g. tolbutamide. Experiments with tolbutamide introduction into perfused snail neurons have shown that this produces the same effect as the decrease in intracellular cAMP level does, i.e. it accelerates the decline of calcium conductance (Doroshenko and Martynyuk, 1984).

The data from our laboratory have been recently verified in several other laboratories. The 'wash-out' of calcium currents during a high-speed cell perfusion was always observed in experiments made by Yazejian and Byerly (1984); it could be stopped by intracellular introduction of ATP and Mg^{2+}. However, these authors did not observe a specific effect of cAMP in this process. But Chad and Eckert (1984) were able to restore the diminished calcium conductance by intracellular introduction of CS (together with ATP and Mg^{2+}) or by application of forskoline (adenylate cyclase activator). The authors concluded that the 'wash-out' of calcium currents during cell perfusion is due to progressive dephosphorylation of the channel-forming proteins; their phosphorylation is necessary for keeping the channels in an active state. Natural inactivation of calcium channels may also be due to dephosphorylation, as this is slowed down by the indicated factors.

The described experiments give reason to confirm that the function of electrically operated calcium channels does depend on phosphotransferase activity of the cAMP-dependent protein kinase. In cardiomyocytes isolated from the guinea pig heart CS injection induced an increase of slow inward current similar to the effect produced by intracellular cAMP injection (Brum et al., 1983).

Thus, calcium channels represent highly dynamic structures whose normal functioning requires continuous metabolic support; the weakening dephosphorylation of the corresponding proteins by cell phosphatases makes the channels inactive. The question whether this statement can be extended to all types of calcium channels in various excitable membranes is still open. Recently it was reported that two components of calcium currents can be distinguished in the somatic membrane of rat sensory neurons. A slowly developing component has the same characteristics as the above-described calcium currents in the somatic membrane of mollusc neurons; it rapidly decreases in the course of cAMP and ATP depletion. A weaker fast component proves to be more stable to the intracellular perfusion, and intracellularly administered cAMP does not significantly affect its amplitude (Fedulova et al., 1985). It is likely that the corresponding 'fast' calcium channels do not require metabolic support for their function.

Chemically operated ionic channels

It was found in 1975 that intracellular introduction of cAMP into snail neurons produces depolarization of the membrane associated with induction of ionic conductance (Liberman et al., 1975). Further studies of this effect undertaken in our laboratory showed that the reason for membrane depolarization is the development of an inward current (Kononenko, 1980). Addition of theophylline (a phosphodiesterase blocker) to the medium potentiated the effect, while imidazole (activator of phosphodiesterase) produced its inhibition. The action of tolbutamide (protein kinase inhibitor) favors the fact that the cAMP effect is mediated through the activation of cellular protein kinases. At 5 mM concentration it produced a 4-fold reduction of the rate of rise and decline of the cAMP-induced current and the corresponding decrease of its amplitude (Kononenko et al., 1983).

The data obtained confirm the idea that the neuronal membrane has ionic channels opened in a chemical way by the increase in intracellular cAMP level; these channels in their selectivity properties are similar to chemically operated ionic channels activated by chemical factors from the external side of the membrane. The stationary inward current arising during metabolic activation of these channels produces depolarization of the membrane sufficient for the generation (in the absence of voltage clamp) of propagating impulses. Obviously, the described effect of intracellularly injected cAMP represents the final step of some natural cellular reaction(s), in which the initial step is formed by activation of membrane adenylate cyclase; the increased cAMP synthesis is then responsible for the opening of membrane ionic channels (via phosphorylation of their proteins). Further investigations on the same neurons have shown that similar changes in membrane conductance can be produced by extracellular application of serotonin. All influences which change the cyclic nucleotide metabolism and consequently the development of cAMP-induced currents exert the same effect on the development of the serotonin-induced inward current (Shcherbatko, 1985).

The amplitude and duration of the cAMP-induced inward current proved to be largely increased after preliminary elevation of the intracellular Ca^{2+} concentration. The most interesting is the fact that the increase of cAMP-induced current is preserved even if the internal free calcium concentration returned to its initial level. Consequently, this effect is related to some prolonged Ca^{2+}-induced biochemical reactions. From biochemical data one may suppose that the corresponding ionic channels have two centers of phosphorylation – one cAMP-dependent and one Ca^{2+}-calmodulin-dependent – and phosphorylation of both centers is needed to open them (Kononenko and Shcherbatko, 1985).

Conclusion

Thus, cellular enzymatic systems cannot be regarded only as a source of energy for the transmembrane transfer of ions and creation of the corresponding electrochemical gradients. In many cases the function of ionic channels itself is under direct metabolic control via phosphorylation of their protein components. In one case, such phos-

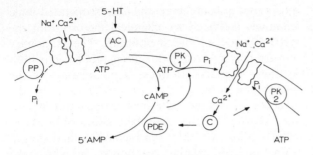

Fig. 1. Scheme of activation of ionic channels in the surface membrane through the system of cAMP-dependent phosphorylation of membrane proteins. AC, adenylate cyclase; PDE, phosphodiesterase; PK_1, cAMP-dependent protein kinase; PK_2, Ca^{2+}-calmodulin-dependent protein kinase; C, calmodulin; PP, protein phosphatase. Dotted line shows presumed influences which have not been studied experimentally.

phorylation appears to play the role of 'gating' mechanism per se, changing the channel from the closed to the open state (see Fig. 1); in another case (Fig. 2) it only creates conditions for normal function of the channels' own gating mechanism.

It should be noted that the presence of direct metabolic control is most characteristic for those ionic channels whose activation or current transfer is determined by calcium ions (calcium and calcium-dependent potassium channels). The role of calcium ions in the regulation of practically all intracellular processes, viz. the synthesis of substances necessary for cellular activity, their intracellular transport and incorporation into the corresponding cellular structures, and their release from the cell, is well known. Therefore, injection of

a certain amount of these ions during every excitatory cycle should be considered mainly as a factor directly coupling the membrane and intracellular activity. Accordingly, to ensure the continuous function of the cell, just such an injection must be, in turn, under recurrent control of the intracellular metabolic systems.

The presence in the nerve cell (like in other excitable cells) of the mechanism mediating external chemical influences via the system of intracellular metabolic intermediates, which alter the function of membrane ionic channels, creates vast possibilities for the regulation of the effects of these influences depending on the current activity of the cell. In particular, the possibility of protein phosphorylation in certain ionic channels not only by cAMP-dependent but also by Ca^{2+}-calmodulin-dependent protein kinase may be especially suitable for the establishment of intracellular interconnection between different systems of ionic channels (electrically and chemically operated). The increase in the intracellular free Ca^{2+} level during spike activity may be accompanied by prolonged changes in the efficacy of chemical (transmitter or hormonal) influences on the same cell that, in turn, may be a basis for prolonged changes in its integrative properties.

References

Brum, G., Flockerzi, V., Hofmann, F., Osterrieder, W. and Trautwein, W. (1983) Injection of catalytic subunit of cAMP-dependent protein kinase into isolated cardiac myocytes. *Pfluegers Arch.*, 398:147–154.

Byerly, L. and Hagiwara, S. (1982) Calcium currents in internally perfused nerve cell bodies in *Limnea stagnalis*. *J. Physiol. (London)*, 322:503–528.

Chad, J.E. and Eckert, R. (1984). Stimulation of cAMP-dependent protein phosphorylation retards both inactivation and 'washout' of Ca current in dialyzed *Helix* neurons. *Soc. Neurosci. Abstr.*, 10:866, part 2.

Doroshenko, P.A. and Martynyuk, A.E. (1984) Effect of calmodulin blockers on inhibition of potential-dependent calcium conductance by intracellular calcium ions in the nerve cell. *Dokl. AN SSSR (Moscow)*, 274:471–473.

Doroshenko, P.A., Kostyuk, P.G. and Martynyuk, A.E. (1982) Intracellular metabolism of adenosine 3′,5′-cyclic monophosphate and calcium inward current in perfused neurones of *Helix pomatia*. *Neuroscience*, 9:2125–2134.

Doroshenko, P.A., Kostyuk, P.G., Martynyuk, A.E., Kursky,

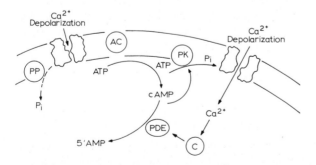

Fig. 2. Scheme of regulation of calcium ionic channels through the system of cAMP-dependent phosphorylation of membrane proteins. For symbols see Fig. 1.

M.D. and Vorobetz, Z.D. (1984) Intracellular protein kinase and calcium inward currents in perfused neurones of the snail *Helix pomatia*. *Neuroscience*, 11:263–267.

Fedulova, S.A., Kostyuk, P.G. and Veselovsky, N.S. (1981) Calcium channels in the somatic membrane of the rat dorsal root ganglion neurons, effect of cAMP. *Brain Res.*, 214:210–214.

Fedulova, S.A., Kostyuk, P.G. and Veselovsky, N.S. (1985) Two types of calcium channels in the somatic membrane of newborn rat dorsal root ganglion neurones. *J. Physiol.* (*London*) 359:431–446.

Kononenko, N.I. (1980) Ionic mechanisms of the transmembrane current evoked by injection of cyclic AMP into identified *Helix* neurons. *Neurophysiology* (*Kiev*), 12:526–532.

Kononenko, N.I., Kostyuk, P.G. and Shcherbatko, A.D. (1983) The effect of intracellular cAMP injections on stationary membrane conductance and voltage- and time-dependent ionic currents in identified snail neurons. *Brain Res.*, 268:321–328.

Kononenko, N.I. and Shcherbatko, A.D. (1985) Effect of elevation of intracellular Ca^{2+} concentration on transmembrane current induced by iontophoretic injection of cAMP in *Helix* neurons. *Neurophysiology* (*Kiev*), 17:78–84.

Kostyuk, P.G. and Krishtal, O.A. (1977) Separation of sodium and calcium currents in the somatic membrane of mollusc neurones. *J. Physiol.* (*London*), 270:545–568.

Liberman, E.A., Minina, S.V. and Golubtsov, K.V. (1975) Study of the metabolic synapse. I. Effect of intracellular 3′,5′-AMP microinjection. *Biofizika* (*Moscow*), 20:451–456.

Reuter, H. (1974) Localization of beta adrenergic receptors and effects of noradrenaline and cyclic nucleotides on action potentials, ionic currents and tension in mammalian cardiac muscle. *J. Physiol.* (*London*), 242:429–451.

Reuter, H. (1983) Calcium channel modulation by neurotransmitters, enzymes and drugs. *Nature*, 301:569–574.

Shcherbatko, A.D. (1985) Possible participation of cyclase system in mediation of serotonin-induced electrical response of the neuron. *Dokl. AN SSSR* (*Moscow*), 281:1014–1016.

Yazejian, B. and Byerly, L. (1984) Temporary reversal of calcium current washout in internally perfused snail neurons. *Biophys. J.*, 45:37a.

SECTION III

Receptors

W.H. Gispen and A. Routtenberg (Eds.)
Progress in Brain Research, Vol. 69
© 1986 Elsevier Science Publishers B.V. (Biomedical Division)

CHAPTER 12

Phosphorylation of the nicotinic acetylcholine receptor

Adrienne S. Gordon and Ivan Diamond

Departments of Neurology, Pediatrics and Pharmacology, University of California, San Francisco, and Ernest Gallo Clinic and Research Center, San Francisco General Hospital, San Francisco, CA 94110, U.S.A.

We have found that the acetylcholine receptor (AChR) of *Torpedo californica* is phosphorylated and dephosphorylated in situ by a membrane-bound protein kinase and phosphatase (Gordon and Diamond, 1979). There is increasing evidence that other neurotransmitters (Stadel et al., 1983), light (Kuhn et al., 1973; Weller et al., 1975a, b; Frank and Buzney, 1975), polypeptide hormones (Smith et al., 1979; Roth and Cassell, 1983), and growth factors (Carpenter et al., 1978, 1979) may act by regulating the level of phosphorylation of their receptors. These observations suggest that membrane protein phosphorylation may be a general regulatory mechanism affecting the response of cells to exogenous metabolic and physical signals.

To understand the role of receptor phosphorylation, we have chosen to study AChR-enriched membranes purified from the electric organ of *T. californica*. This organ is an ideal model system for such studies since it is a rich source of AChR. Membranes can be purified from the electric organ that are enriched in AChR (Duguid and Raftery, 1973) and that show cholinergic agonist-dependent changes in cation flux (Popot et al., 1976). Moreover, the AChR from *T. californica* has been purified (Karlin et al., 1975), biochemically characterized (Michaelson et al., 1974), and used to generate specific antibodies (Patrick and Lindstrom, 1973). Receptor-enriched membranes contain only a few other proteins that are closely associated with the receptor in the postsynaptic membrane. We have taken advantage of these

conditions to study phosphorylation of the membrane-bound AChR in this well-defined homogeneous system.

When the electric organ of *T. californica* is homogenized and the resulting membranes purified by ultracentrifugation through a discontinuous sucrose gradient, one membrane fraction was found to be enriched in the AChR (Gordon et al., 1977a). Sodium dodecylsulfate (SDS) gel electrophoresis of these membranes shows six major polypeptides (Fig. 1, lane 1). Four of these polypeptides are subunits of the AChR with molecular weights of 40 000, 50 000, 58 000 and 65 000 (α, β, γ, and δ, respectively). The other two polypeptides are of molecular weight 43 000 and 90 000. The M_r 90 000 polypeptide is the Na^+/K^+-ATPase present in these membranes and is similar to Na^+/K^+-ATPase from other sources.

If phosphorylation regulates receptor function in the postsynaptic membrane, then receptor-enriched membranes should contain endogenous protein kinase activity. When these membranes were incubated with $[\gamma^{-32}P]ATP$ in the presence of Mg^{2+}, several polypeptides corresponding in molecular weight to subunits of the AChR were found to be phosphorylated (Fig. 1, lane 2). Using 2-dimensional immunoelectrophoresis we showed that the δ subunit of the AChR was phosphorylated in situ in these membranes (Gordon et al., 1977b). This was the first membrane receptor protein to be identified as a substrate for an endogenous membrane protein kinase. The phosphorylated substrate in our studies is a subunit of a

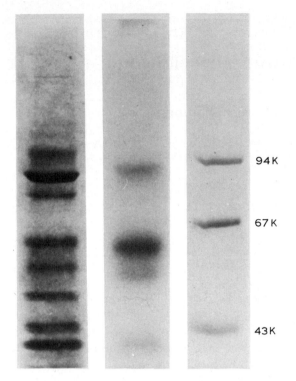

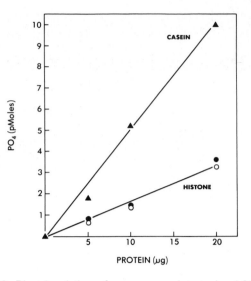

Fig. 2. Phosphorylation of exogenous substrate by AChR-enriched membranes. Assay carried out as described by Gordon et al. (1980). Reported values are corrected for endogenous membrane protein kinase activity in the absence of exogenous substrate. ▲, casein; ○, histone; ●, histone and 10 μm 3′,5′-cAMP.

Fig. 1. Endogenous phosphorylation in AChR-enriched membranes. AChR-enriched membranes were incubated for 1 min at room temperature in 100 μl of 400 mM NaCl, 10 mM Tris-HCl, pH 7.4, 1 mM EDTA, 20 mM MnCl$_2$, 1.6 mM ouabain, 5 μM ATP with 2 μCi of [γ-^{32}P]ATP. Lane 1: Coomassie blue stained SDS gel of membranes. Lane 2: Autoradiography of dried SDS gel of membranes. Lane 3: Molecular weight markers.

postsynaptic membrane protein whose function is known and that has been biochemically characterized. This is an important first step in correlating phosphorylation of membrane proteins with membrane function. These results have since been confirmed by Teichberg et al. (1977) and Huganir and Greengard (1983). All the data on phosphorylation of the AChR, taken together, show that the β, γ and δ subunits of the AChR are phosphorylated by the protein kinase present in these membranes. The α subunit, which contains the acetylcholine binding site, is not phosphorylated under the conditions of our assay.

Our results show that AChR-enriched membranes contain a protein kinase activity that phosphorylates the membrane-bound AChR. The pro-

tein kinase that phosphorylates the AChR is specific for ATP. No phosphorylation occurs with GTP. In our hands, phosphorylation is not affected by Ca^{2+}, cAMP, cGMP or calmodulin. The receptor kinase is also able to phosphorylate casein exogenously with phosphorylation increasing as a function of membrane concentration (Fig. 2) (Gordon et al., 1980).

We have further investigated the specificity and localization of the AChR kinase by comparing the phosphorylation of the receptor in the receptor-enriched membranes (R-E) to that in a sealed right-side-out (S-R) vesicle preparation also prepared from *T. californica* electric organ (Davis et al., 1982). If the kinase which phosphorylates the AChR is located on the external side of the postsynaptic membrane, the receptor should become phosphorylated with ^{32}P after addition of [γ-^{32}P]ATP to intact vesicles. However, if the kinase is on the cytoplasmic side of the membrane, receptor labeling should occur only after the vesicles are made permeable and [γ-^{32}P]ATP becomes available to the inside kinase.

Incubation of intact S-R vesicles with [γ-^{32}P]

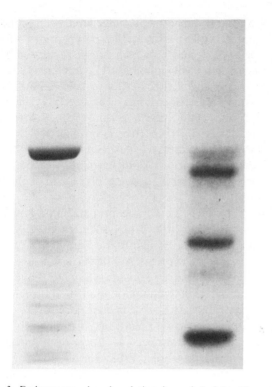

Fig. 3. Endogenous phosphorylation in sealed right-side-out vesicles. Assay carried out as described in Fig. 1. Lane 1: Coomassie blue-stained SDS gel. Lane 2: Autoradiography of Lane 1. Lane 3: Autoradiogram of S-R vesicles hypoosmotically shocked by dilution to 200 mM NaCl.

for 1 min resulted in only trace labeling of polypeptides in the M_r range of AChR subunits (Fig. 3, lane 2). Changing the incubation period to 0.1 min or 20 min did not affect the phosphorylation pattern. To test the possibility that AChR subunits had been rapidly phosphorylated and dephosphorylated, we used a common inhibitor of protein phosphatase activity, sodium fluoride, which we have shown inhibits AChR dephosphorylation (Gordon et al., 1979). If rapid turnover of phosphate were occurring on the external surface of sealed vesicles, the addition of sodium fluoride to the reaction should result in greatly increased labeling. However, we found that 100 mM NaF had virtually no effect on the level of phosphorylation; it increased phosphorylation of low M_r bands by $<5\%$. Therefore, we conclude that the low level of phosphorylation in sealed vesicles is not due to rapid dephosphorylation.

When S-R vesicles were hypotonically lyzed in the presence of 5 µM $[\gamma\text{-}^{32}P]ATP$, phosphorylation of five polypeptides of molecular weights 40 000, 60 000, 65 000, 92 000, and 94 000 was greatly increased (Fig. 3, lane 3). Similar results were obtained with 0.25 mM ATP. In many experiments, increased phosphorylation of an M_r 36 000 polypeptide was also observed. The specificity of the reaction in S-R vesicles was strikingly similar to the phosphorylation pattern of receptor-enriched membranes (cf. Fig. 1, lane 2), even though the S-R preparation had many more proteins than did the R-E preparation. Indeed, with the exception of the M_r 94 000 band, the phosphorylation patterns of the two membrane preparations were identical, despite the fact that the Coomassie blue staining patterns were very different. Whereas the S-R membranes showed more than 30 polypeptides (Fig. 3, lane 1), R-E membranes have only 6–8 major polypeptides (Fig. 1, lane 1), and four are subunits of the AChR.

Control experiments showed that the effect of hypoosmotic shock on phosphorylation was not due to solubilization of the kinase or its substrates. These results strongly suggest that the receptor kinase which phosphorylates the AChR is localized to the cytoplasmic surface of the postsynaptic membrane. Other methods of membrane lysis were also tested to confirm that AChR phosphorylation occurred only when ATP was available to the internal membrane kinase. Triton X-100 at a concentration of 0.02% caused a significant increase in phosphorylation of the same peptides. Digitonin, a detergent specific for cholesterol, had an identical effect at the same concentration. Neither detergent solubilized significant amounts of AChR in these experiments.

Since phosphorylation was not observed in intact S-R vesicles, while three different methods of membrane lysis resulted in greatly increased membrane phosphorylation of AChR subunits, we believe that the AChR kinase is located on the cytoplasmic side of the postsynaptic membrane. Furthermore, the kinase activity in AChR-enriched membranes appears to be highly specific for the AChR.

To identify the receptor kinase in the R-E, we first used a photoaffinity ATP ligand, 8-azido [α-

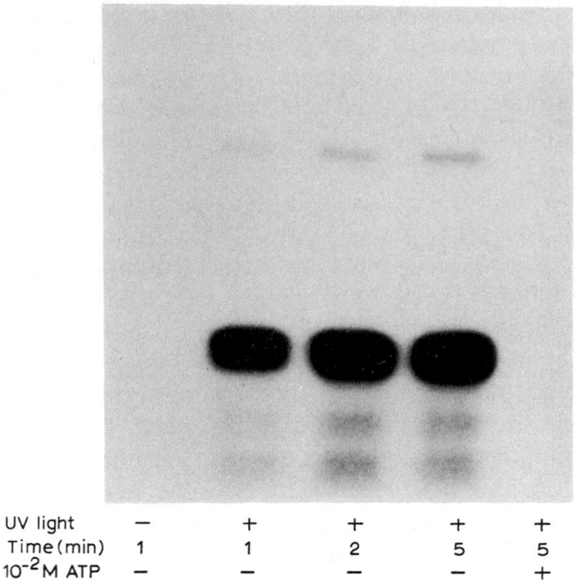

UV light	—	+	+	+	+
Time (min)	1	1	2	5	5
10^{-2} M ATP	—	—	—	—	+

Fig. 4. Autoradiogram of a SDS/polyacrylamide electrophoresis gel of AChR-enriched membranes that had been incubated with 1 μCi of 8-azido-[α-^{32}P]ATP (97 Ci/mmol) in buffer (Fig. 1) containing 0.02% Triton X-100 for 5 min and then irradiated for the indicated times. Where indicated, the membranes were first incubated for 1 min with unlabeled 10 mM ATP. The major band is at M_r 43 000.

^{32}P]ATP (Gordon et al., 1983). Incubation of AChR-enriched membranes with 8-azido[α-^{32}P]ATP and subsequent irradiation with UV light resulted in covalent labeling of a major band of molecular weight 43 000 (Fig. 4). Alkali-stripped membranes that show a selective reduction in the M_r 43 000 polypeptide also show a corresponding reduction in incorporation of photoaffinity label (Fig. 5). In addition, the neutralized alkaline extract also showed one band at M_r 43 000 when labeled with the photoaffinity ligand (Fig. 6). After alkali extraction, endogenous protein kinase activity decreased in the membranes in proportion to the loss of M_r 43 000 peptide although this may have been due to loss of protein kinase activity during incubation at pH 11. However, the alkaline extract was able to phosphorylate casein in an exogenous assay system (Fig. 7) just as the membrane-bound kinase. These results suggest that a M_r 43 000 polypeptide in AChR-enriched membranes in the AChR kinase.

AChR-enriched membranes have been found to contain 3 alkali-extractable polypeptides of M_r 43 000 (v_1, v_2 and v_3) which can be separated by 2-dimensional electrophoresis (Gysin et al., 1981). v_2 (pI 6–6.5) and v_3 (pI 5.6) have been identified as creatine kinase (Barrantes et al., 1983; Gysin et al., 1983) and actin (Gysin et al., 1983; Porter and Froehner, 1983) respectively, both of which have ATP binding sites. v_2 has been reported to be associated with AChR-enriched membrane vesicles in addition to being present at high concentrations in the cytosol (Gysin et al., 1981); highly purified membrane preparations, however, appear to have little v_2 (Nghiem et al., 1983). In contrast, v_1 is only membrane-bound (pI 7.0–7.4) and copurifies with the AChR (Gysin et al., 1981, 1983; Porter and Froehner, 1983). We have used an anti-M_r 43 000 monoclonal antibody (mcAb) to demonstrate that v_1 is a protein kinase.

Antibodies to v_1 react almost exclusively with the innervated surface of Torpedo electrocytes (Porter and Froehner, 1983) and cross-react with a component of the rat neuromuscular junction that is highly concentrated at the synapse (Porter and Froehner, 1983; Froehner et al., 1981). Both v_1 (Froehner et al., 1981), which we believe is a protein kinase, and the AChR receptor kinase (Davis et al., 1982) are localized to the cytoplasmic side of the postsynaptic membrane. In addition, both v_1 and the receptor kinase can be extracted from AChR-enriched membranes by mild alkali treatment (Davis et al., 1982; Neubig et al., 1979; Elliot et al., 1980). Although it is clear that v_1 phosphorylates casein, it remains to be determined if the M_r 43 000 protein kinase is the same enzyme which phosphorylates the AChR in postsynaptic membranes.

Recently Kennedy et al. (1983) and Kelly et al. (1984) have shown that the major 'postsynaptic density' protein of mammalian brain also is a protein kinase. This kinase, in contrast to the acetylcholine receptor kinase (Huganir and Greengard, 1983; Zavoico et al., 1983), is a calmodulin-dependent enzyme. The finding that major postsynaptic membrane proteins in brain and in electric organ are protein kinases suggests that protein phosphorylation may be important for postsynaptic function. In Torpedo, the major substrate in situ

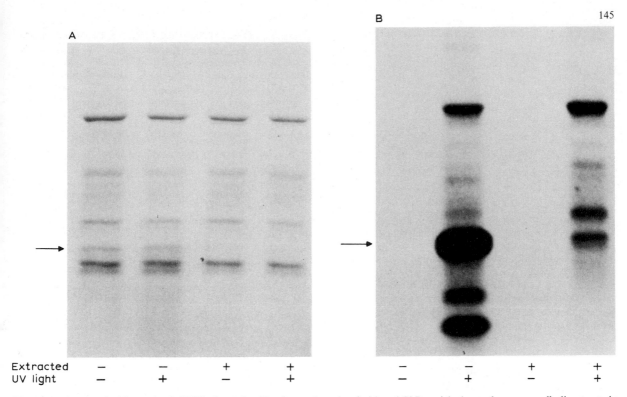

Extracted   −   −   +   +
UV light   −   +   −   +

Fig. 5. A: Coomassie blue-stained SDS/polyacrylamide electrophoresis of either AChR-enriched membranes or alkali-extracted membranes (20 µg of protein) after incubation with 1 µCi of 8-azido-[α-^{32}P]ATP in NTE buffer containing 0.02% Triton for 5 min followed by incubation for 1 min in the presence or absence of UV light. B: Autoradiogram of the gel shown in A. Arrows indicate the M_r 43 000 polypeptide.

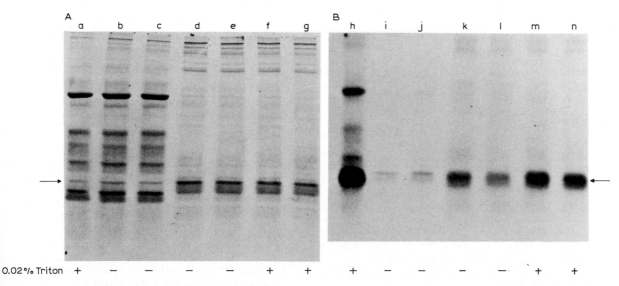

0.02% Triton   +   −   −   −   −   +   +   +   −   −   −   −   +   +

Fig. 6. A: Coomassie blue-stained SDS/polyacrylamide electrophoresis gel of either AChR-enriched membranes (lanes a–c) or alkaline extract (lanes d–g) after incubation with 1 µCi of 8-azido-[α-^{32}P]ATP in buffer in the presence or absence of 0.02% Triton X-100 for 5 min followed by irradiation for 1 min with UV light. Lanes b and c, d and e, and f and g are duplicate samples. B: Autoradiogram of the gel shown in A. Arrows indicate the M_r 43 000 polypeptide.

146

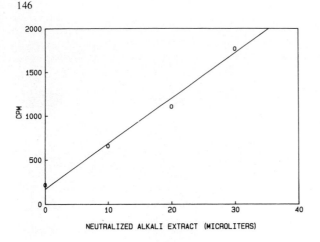

Fig. 7. Exogenous protein kinase activity. Incorporation of $^{32}PO_4$ into casein as a function of the amount of alkaline extract in the incubation medium. The amount of $^{32}PO_4$ incorporated was corrected by subtracting the endogenous phosphorylation of the alkaline extract and the casein blank from the experimental values.

for protein kinases appears to be the AChR. However, alkali extraction of AChR-enriched membranes, which removes v_1, does not affect the binding of cholinergic ligands or agonist-induced changes in binding affinity and ion permeability (Neubig et al., 1979; Elliot et al., 1980). It seems more likely that the M_r 43 000 kinase and AChR phosphorylation play a role in the clustering or stabilization of the AChR at the synapse. Isolation, identification and purification of this post-synaptic membrane protein kinase now make it possible to test this hypothesis.

References

Barrantes, F.J., Mieskes, G. and Wallimann, T. (1983) Creatine kinase activity in the *Torpedo* electrocyte and in the nonreceptor, peripheral v proteins from acetylcholine receptor-rich membranes. *Proc. Natl. Acad. Sci. U.S.A.*, 80:5440–5444.

Carpenter, G., King, L. Jr. and Cohen, S. (1978) Epidermal growth factor stimulates phosphorylation in membrane preparations in vitro. *Nature*, 276:409–410.

Carpenter, G., King, L. Jr. and Cohen, S. (1979) Rapid enhancement of protein phosphorylation in A-431 cell membrane preparations by epidermal growth factor. *J. Biol. Chem.*, 254:4884–4891.

Davis, C.G., Gordon, A.S. and Diamond, I. (1982) Specificity and localization of the acetylcholine receptor kinase. *Proc. Natl. Acad. Sci. U.S.A.*, 79:3666–3670.

Duguid, J.R. and Raftery, M.A., (1973) Fractionation and partial characterization of membrane particles from *Torpedo californica* electroplax. *Biochemistry*, 12:3593–3597.

Elliot, J., Blanchard, S.G., Wu, W., Miller, J., Stader, C.D., Hartig, P., Moore, H.-P., Racs, J. and Raftery, M.A. (1980) Purification of *Torpedo californica* post-synaptic membranes and fractionation of their constituent proteins. *Biochem. J.*, 185:667–677.

Frank, R.N. and Buzney, S.M. (1975) Mechanism and specificity of rhodopsin phosphorylation. *Biochemistry*, 14:5110–5117.

Froehner, S.C., Gulbrandsen, V., Hyman, C., Jeng, A.Y., Neubig, R.R. and Cohen, J.B. (1981) Immunofluorescence localization at the mammalian neuromuscular junction of the MR 43 000 protein of *Torpedo*. *Proc. Natl. Acad. Sci. U.S.A.*, 78:5230–5234.

Gordon, A. and Diamond, I. (1979) Phosphorylation of the acetylcholine receptor. *Adv. Exp. Med. Biol.* 116:175–198.

Gordon, A.S., Davis, C.G. and Diamond, I. (1977a) Phosphorylation of membrane proteins at a cholinergic synapse. *Proc. Natl. Acad. Sci. U.S.A.*, 74:263–267.

Gordon, A.S., Davis, C.G., Milfay, D. and Diamond, I. (1977b) Phosphorylation of acetylcholine receptor by endogenous membrane protein kinase in receptor-enriched membranes of *Torpedo californica*. *Nature*, 267:539–540.

Gordon, A.S., Milfay, D., Davis, C.G. and Diamond, I. (1979) Protein phosphatase activity in acetylcholine receptor-enriched membranes. *Biochem. Biophys. Res. Commun.*, 87:876–883.

Gordon, A.S., Davis, C.G., Milfay, D., Kaur, J. and Diamond, I. (1980) Protein phosphorylation in acetylcholine receptor-enriched membranes. *Biochim. Biophys. Acta*, 600:421–431.

Gordon, A.S., Milfay, D. and Diamond, I. (1983) Identification of molecular weight 43 000 protein kinase in acetylcholine receptor-enriched membranes. *Proc. Natl. Acad. Sci. U.S.A.*, 80:5862–5865.

Gysin, R., Wirth, M. and Flanagan, S.D. (1981) Structural heterogeneity and subcellular distribution of nicotinic synapse-associated proteins. *J. Biol. Chem.*, 256:11373–11376.

Gysin, R., Yost, B. and Flanagan, S.D. (1983) Immunochemical and molecular differentiation of 43 000 molecular weight proteins associated with *Torpedo* neuroelectrocyte synapses. *Biochemistry* 22:5782–5789.

Huganir, R.L. and Greengard, P. (1983) cAMP-dependent protein kinase phosphorylates the nicotinic acetylcholine receptor. *Proc. Natl. Acad. Sci. U.S.A.*, 80:1130–1134.

Karlin, A. McNamee, M.G., Weill, C.L. and Valderrama, R. (1975) Facets of the structures of acetylcholine receptors from *Electrophorus* and *Torpedo*. *Cold Spring Harbor Symp. Quant. Biol.* 40:203.

Kelly, P.T., McGuiness, T.L. and Greengard, P., (1984) Evidence that the major postsynaptic destiny protein is a component of a Ca^{2+}-calmodulin-dependent protein kinase. *Proc. Natl. Acad. Sci. U.S.A.*, 81:945–949.

Kennedy, M.B., Bennett, M.K. and Erondu, N.E. (1983) Biochemical and immunological evidence that the 'major postsynaptic density protein' is a subunit of a calmodulin-dependent protein kinase. *Proc. Natl. Acad. Sci. U.S.A.*, 80:7357–7361.

Kuhn, H., Cook, J.H. and Dreyer, J.W. (1973) Phosphorylation of rhodopsin in bovine photoreceptor membranes: A dark reaction after illumination. *Biochemistry*, 12:2495–2502.

Michaelson, D., Vandlen, R., Bode, J., Moody, T., Schmidt, J. and Raftery, M.A. (1974) Some molecular properties of an isolated acetylcholine receptor ion translocation protein. *Arch. Biochem. Biophys.*, 165:796–804.

Neubig, R.R., Krodel, E.K., Boyd, N.D. and Cohen, J.B. (1979) Acetylcholine and local anesthetic binding of *Torpedo* nicotinic postsynaptic membranes after removal of non-receptor peptides. *Proc. Natl. Acad. Sci. U.S.A.*, 76:690–694.

Nghiem, H.-O., Cartaud, J., Dubreuil, C., Kordeli, C., Buttin, G. and Changeux, J.-P. (1983) Production and characterization of a monoclonal antibody directed against the 43 000 dalton v_1 polypeptide from *Torpedo marmorata* electric organ. *Proc. Natl. Acad. Sci. U.S.A.*, 80:6403–6407.

Patrick, J. and Lindstrom, J. (1973) Autoimmune response to acetylcholine receptor. *Science*, 180:871–872.

Popot, J.-L., Sagiyama, H. and Changeux, J.-P. (1976) Studies on the electrogenic action of acetylcholine with *Torpedo marmorata* electric organ. II. The permeability response of receptor-rich membrane fragments to cholinergic agonists in vitro. *J. Mol. Biol.*, 106:469–483.

Porter, S. and Froehner, S.C. (1983) Characterization and localization of the Mr = 43 000 proteins associated with acetylcholine receptor-rich membranes. *J. Biol. Chem.*, 258:10034–10040.

Roth, R.A. and Cassell, D.J. (1983) Insulin receptor: Evidence that it is a protein kinase. *Science*, 219:299–301.

Smith, C.J., Wejksnora, P.J., Warner, J.R., Rubin, C.S. and Rosen, O.M. (1979) Insulin-stimulated protein phosphorylation in 3T3 Li preadipocytes. *Proc. Natl. Acad. Sci. U.S.A.*, 76:2725–2729.

Stadel, J.M., Nambi, P., Shorr, R.G.L., Sawyer, D.F., Caron, M.G. and Lefkowitz, R.J. (1983) Catecholamine-induced desensitization of turkey erythrocyte adenylate cyclase is associated with phosphorylation of the beta-adrenergic receptor. *Proc. Natl. Acad. Sci. U.S.A.*, 80:3173–3177.

Teichberg, V.I., Sobel, I. and Changeux, J.-P. (1977) In vitro phosphorylation of the acetylcholine receptor. *Nature*, 267:540–542.

Weller, M., Virmaux, N. and Mandel, P. (1975a) Role of light and rhodopsin phosphorylation on control of permeability of retinal rod outer segment disks to Ca^{2+}. *Nature*, 256:68–70.

Weller, M., Virmaux, N. and Mandel, P. (1975b) Light-stimulated phosphorylation of rhodopsin in the retina. *Proc. Natl. Acad. Sci. U.S.A.*, 72:381–385.

Zavoico, G.B., Comerci, C., Subers, E., Egan, J.J., Huang, C.K., Feinstein, M.B. and Smilowitz, H. (1983) cAMP not Ca^{2+}/calmodulin regulates the phosphorylation of acetylcholine in *Torpedo californica* electroplax. *Biochim, Biophys. Acta*, 770:225–229.

W.H. Gispen and A. Routtenberg (Eds.)
Progress in Brain Research, Vol. 69
© 1986 Elsevier Science Publishers B.V. (Biomedical Division)

CHAPTER 13

DARPP-32, a dopamine-regulated phosphoprotein

Hugh C. Hemmings, Jr. and Paul Greengard

Laboratory of Molecular and Cellular Neuroscience, The Rockefeller University, 1230 York Avenue, New York, NY 10021, U.S.A.

Introduction

Protein phosphorylation is a general regulatory mechanism involved in the control of many cellular processes and appears to play a prominent role in intercellular communication (for reviews, see Greengard, 1978; Krebs and Beavo, 1979; Cohen, 1982). The study of protein phosphorylation in the nervous system has resulted in the detection of a great variety of neuronal phosphoproteins, supporting the view that this regulatory mechanism is involved in many aspects of neuronal function (for review, see Nestler and Greengard, 1984). Direct evidence for a role of three major classes of protein kinases in the regulation of neuronal function has recently been obtained by microinjection experiments (for reviews, see Nestler and Greengard, 1983; Hemmings et al., 1986a, 1986b; Nairn et al., 1985). In these experiments, microinjection of purified protein kinases or specific protein kinase inhibitors into single neurons has been used to demonstrate that activation of specific protein kinases is both necessary and sufficient to produce a variety of neurophysiological responses to depolarization, synaptic activation or neurotransmitter stimulation. The results of these studies provide direct evidence for a causal relationship between protein phosphorylation and neurophysiological responses, including neurotransmission. The results also support the view that the identification and characterization of the specific substrate proteins for these protein kinases is of considerable importance in establishing the biochemical mechanisms underlying these responses.

The regulation of protein phosphorylation by dopamine acting at D-1 dopamine receptors has been found to be mediated by the intracellular second messenger cyclic AMP. The levels of cyclic AMP are specifically elevated in appropriate tissues following stimulation of adenylate cyclase by dopamine binding to D-1 dopamine receptors, which leads in turn to activation of cyclic AMP-dependent protein kinase and to phosphorylation of specific substrate proteins (for reviews, see Kebabian and Calne, 1979; Stoof and Kebabian, 1984; Hemmings et al., 1986c). In some cells, the levels of cyclic AMP also appear to be regulated by an inhibitory influence on adenylate cyclase exerted by dopamine binding to D-2 dopamine receptors (Stoof and Kebabian, 1981).

In the central nervous system, dopamine-sensitive adenylate cyclase activity is concentrated in brain regions rich in dopamine innervation (for review, see Miller and McDermed, 1979), for example the neostriatum (Kebabian et al., 1972), nucleus accumbens and olfactory tubercle (Clement-Cormier et al., 1974). Furthermore, dopamine-sensitive adenylate cyclase activity is highly enriched in subcellular fractions containing synaptic structures, consistent with a role in neurotransmission (Clement-Cormier et al., 1975). Considerable evidence supports the hypothesis that dopamine-sensitive adenylate cyclase is involved in mediating some of the neurotransmitter functions of dopamine. Thus, some of the electrophysiological effects of iontophoretically applied dopamine on individual neurons in the rat caudatoputamen (Siggins et al., 1974, 1976), nucleus accumbens (Bunney and Aghajanian 1973) and olfactory tubercle (Bunney and Aghajanian, 1973; Woodruff et al., 1976) can be mimicked by the application of cyclic AMP or cyclic AMP analogs and potentiated by the application of phosphodiesterase inhibitors. Furthermore, pharmacological studies of dopamine-elicited behaviors in the rat have provided evidence for the involvement of D-1 dopamine receptors in a distinct set of behaviors (Rosengarten et al., 1983; Molloy and Waddington, 1984). Taken together, these findings demonstrate an important role for D-1 dopamine receptors and cyclic AMP in mediating some of the neurophysiological and behavioral effects of dopamine. Most, if not all, of the actions of cyclic AMP in eukaryotic cells are mediated by activation of cyclic AMP-dependent protein kinase (Kuo and Greengard, 1969; Greengard, 1978). The detection and characterization of the phosphoproteins regulated by dopamine and cyclic AMP in dopaminoceptive cells is therefore a necessary step in the analysis of the molecular mechanisms of dopamine action.

The phosphoproteins in the mammalian nervous system that have been found to be regulated by dopamine and cyclic AMP can be divided into two general classes, those with widespread anatomical distributions and those with restricted anatomical distributions (Hemmings et al., 1986c). Synapsin I and Protein III are both synaptic vesicle-associated neuronal phosphoproteins which exhibit widespread anatomical distributions. They appear to be concentrated within virtually all axon terminals, and may be involved in the presynaptic regulation of synaptic vesicle function by dopamine (for review, see Hemmings et al., 1986c). The cyclic AMP-dependent phosphorylation of these proteins in certain presynaptic axon terminals can be regulated by dopamine acting on D-1 dopamine receptors (Nestler and Greengard, 1980, 1982; Tsou and Greengard, 1982; Treiman and Greengard, 1985; S.I. Walaas and P. Greengard, unpublished observations). DARPP-32 (**d**opamine- and cyclic **A**MP-**r**egulated **p**hosphoprotein, $M_r = 32\,000$) is the prototypic member of a second class of dopamine- and cyclic AMP-regulated phosphoproteins which exhibit restricted anatomical distributions corresponding to the distribution of dopaminergic axon terminals.

DARPP-32 was originally observed in a study of the regional distributions of cyclic AMP-regulated protein phosphorylation systems in the rat central nervous system (Walaas et al., 1983b, 1983c; for review, see Walaas et al., 1986). Certain of the cyclic AMP-regulated phosphoproteins detected, one of which was DARPP-32, were found to have restricted regional distributions in the brain which paralleled the gross regional distribution of dopaminergic axon terminals. Using slices prepared from rat caudatoputamen, the application of dopamine or an analog of cyclic AMP was found to increase the state of phosphorylation of DARPP-32, while the application of several other neurotransmitters was without effect (Walaas et al., 1983a; Walaas and Greengard, 1984). Furthermore, the effect of dopamine was blocked by the dopamine receptor antagonist fluphenazine. The discovery of DARPP-32, a dopamine-regulated phosphoprotein which is anatomically associated with dopaminergic axon terminals, suggested that the function of DARPP-32 may be related to dopaminergic neurotransmission. Further studies of DARPP-32 were undertaken as an approach to elucidating the molecular bases of dopamine action.

Distribution of DARPP-32

The distribution of DARPP-32 in various brain regions, peripheral tissues, animal species, and neuronal cell types was studied by use of a phosphorylation assay (Walaas and Greengard, 1984), and by use of immunocytochemical (Ouimet et al., 1983, 1984) and radioimmunoassay techniques (Hemmings and Greengard, 1986). In each of these studies, the distribution of DARPP-32 in the rat central nervous system was found to parallel the distribution of dopaminergic synapses. More specifically, the distribution of DARPP-32 was found to be strongly correlated with the distribution of the D-1 subclass of dopamine receptors (dopamine receptors coupled to the stimulation of adenylate cyclase), and showed no apparent correlation with the distribution of D-2 dopamine receptors.

The regional distribution of DARPP-32 in the rat central nervous system determined by radio-immunoassay is shown in Table I. The highest concentrations of immunoreactive DARPP-32 were found in substantia nigra, caudatoputamen and globus pallidus, while slightly lower concentrations were found in olfactory tubercle and nucleus accumbens. The caudatoputamen, nucleus accumbens and olfactory tubercle receive most of the terminals of the nigrostriatal and mesolimbic dopamine system neurons (Lindvall and Björklund, 1978), while the globus pallidus and substantia nigra are the main anatomical targets of these three dopamine-innervated brain regions. By use of immunocytochemical methods, strong DARPP-32 immunoreactivity was observed within cell bodies and dendrites of the caudatoputamen, nucleus accumbens and olfactory tubercle. In contrast, strong DARPP-32 immunoreactivity was observed within axon terminals in the globus pallidus and substantia nigra pars reticulata (Ouimet et al., 1984). In the caudatoputamen and nucleus accumbens, DARPP-32 was localized to the medium-sized

TABLE I

Regional distribution of DARPP-32 in rat central nervous system determined by radioimmunoassay[a]

Region	Immunoreactive DARPP-32 (pmol/mg total protein)
Substantia nigra	133.6 ± 11.0
Caudatoputamen	129.5 ± 9.4
Globus pallidus	112.3 ± 7.0
Olfactory tubercle	77.3 ± 14.6
Nucleus accumbens	60.3 ± 12.4
Thalamus	16.5 ± 3.2
Cerebellum	14.8 ± 2.6
Cerebral cortex	8.0 ± 3.2
Hippocampus	7.4 ± 2.1
Retina	6.3 ± 3.0
Frontal cortex	6.0 ± 1.0
Hypothalamus	5.0 ± 1.0
Amygdala	4.3 ± 1.2
Septum	3.4 ± 0.8
Pons/medulla	2.2 ± 0.6
Olfactory bulb	1.1 ± 0.6
Spinal cord	0.6 ± 0.4

[a]Taken from Hemmings and Greengard (1986).

spiny neurons, which directly receive most of the dopamine input to the caudatoputamen and comprise about 96% of the neurons in this brain region (DiFiglia et al., 1976; Pasik et al., 1979; Dimova et al., 1980; Groves, 1983). DARPP-32 was found to be a cytosolic protein present throughout the cytoplasm of the cell bodies of the medium-sized spiny neurons of the neostriatum, and in their dendrites, axons and axon terminals (Ouimet et al., 1983). DARPP-32 was absent from the nigrostriatal dopaminergic neurons and their axon terminals. From these studies, it appears that DARPP-32 is present in those dopaminoceptive cells that possesses D-1 dopamine receptors, and not in those that possess only D-2 dopamine receptors. The correlation between the anatomical distributions of DARPP-32 and of D-1 dopamine receptors suggests that DARPP-32 may represent a useful molecular marker for dopaminoceptive cells that possess D-1 dopamine receptors within the mammalian central nervous system.

Immunological methods have been used to carry out a phylogenetic survey of DARPP-32 localization (Hemmings and Greengard, 1986). DARPP-32 was found at relatively high concentrations in the turtle basal forebrain and in the canary paleostriatum, but not in central nervous system tissue from carp, frog or members of several invertebrate phyla. In turtle and canary, as in rat, the brain regions that contained the greatest amounts of immunoreactive DARPP-32 are the regions that receive the major dopaminergic inputs, and are thought to be homologous to the neostriatum of mammals (Parent et al., 1984; Reiner et al., 1984). In the canary, the localization of DARPP-32 has been further investigated by use of immunocytochemical methods, which showed that DARPP-32 was contained within dopamine-innervated neurons within the paleostriatum (Burd et al., 1985; G.D. Burd, H.C. Hemmings Jr., F. Nottebohm and P. Greengard, unpublished observations). From these studies, it appears that the regional distribution of DARPP-32 in the central nervous systems of several mammalian and non-mammalian vertebrates corresponds to the distribution of dopamine innervation, and probably reflects the different locations of dopaminoceptive neurons possessing D-1 dopamine receptors in these various species. Immunoreactive DARPP-32 could not be detected in the brains of members of the two anamniote vertebrate classes, the fish or the frog, which lack the hypertrophic mesencephalic dopamine neuron system characteristic of the amniote vertebrate classes.

Recently, the development of DARPP-32 has been investigated in the central nervous system of the prenatal and newborn rat by immunocytochemical methods (Foster et al., 1986). DARPP-32 immunoreactivity first appears in the rat brain at day 14 of gestation in the anlage of the caudatoputamen, with the number of immunoreactive cell bodies increasing rapidly over the next two days. The arrival of tyrosine hydroxylase immunoreactive axon terminals followed the appearance of DARPP-32 immunoreactive cell bodies by at least two days. The development of DARPP-32 is largely complete by the day of birth, and does not appear to depend on the prior appearance of dopaminergic innervation.

Biochemical characterization of DARPP-32

A variety of biochemical techniques has been employed to characterize DARPP-32. DARPP-32 has been purified to homogeneity from bovine caudate nucleus cytosol and its physicochemical properties examined (Hemmings et al., 1984b). Purified DARPP-32 was found to exist in solution as a highly elongated monomer. It exhibited an extremely acidic isoelectric point and remained soluble and phosphorylatable upon either heat or acid treatment. Purified DARPP-32 was phosphorylated in vitro with favourable kinetic parameters by cyclic AMP-dependent protein kinase on a single threonine residue on the carboxy-terminal side of four consecutive arginine residues (Hemmings et al., 1984c, 1984d). It was also phosphorylated by cyclic GMP-dependent protein kinase, but not by calcium/calmodulin-dependent protein kinase I, calcium/calmodulin-dependent protein kinase II or protein kinase C. DARPP-32 was dephosphorylated most efficiently in vitro by protein phosphatase-2B (Hemmings et al., 1984a; King et al., 1984), also known as calcineurin, a calcium/calmodulin-dependent

protein phosphatase. This observation is of particular interest since the substrate specificity of protein phosphatase-2B has been reported to be quite limited (Stewart et al., 1982; Ingebritsen and Cohen, 1983b). Protein phosphatase-2B is concentrated in many of the same brain regions as DARPP-32, including the basal ganglia (Wallace et al., 1980); within the caudatoputamen, calcineurin appears to be contained within medium-sized spiny neurons (Wood et al., 1980), as is DARPP-32.

Enzymological studies have established a biochemical function of DARPP-32. In the initial characterization of DARPP-32 (Hemmings et al., 1984b), several similarities were noted between the physicochemical properties of DARPP-32 and those of protein phosphatase inhibitor-1 (inhibitor-1), a potent inhibitor, in its phosphorylated form, of the catalytic subunit of the enzyme protein phosphatase-1 (Huang and Glinsmann, 1976; Nimmo and Cohen, 1978). The amino acid sequence surrounding the phosphorylatable threonine residue of DARPP-32 exhibits considerable homology with the sequence surrounding the phosphorylatable threonine residue of inhibitor-1 (Table II). By determining the complete amino acid sequence of DARPP-32 (Williams et al., 1986), this homology was found to extend to other regions of inhibitor-1 that may be essential to its ability to inhibit protein phosphatase-1 (Aitken and Cohen, 1982). When the effect of DARPP-32 on protein phosphatase-1 activity was tested in vitro (Fig. 1), phosphorylated, but not dephosphorylated, DARPP-32 was found to act as a potent inhibitor (Hemmings et al., 1984a). Further studies revealed that the potency and specificity of phospho-DARPP-32 as a protein phosphatase inhibitor and as a substrate for the various purified protein phosphatase preparations were very similar to those of phospho-inhibitor-1 (Fig. 1). These studies indicated that the basal ganglia of mammalian brain contain a region-specific neuronal phosphoprotein, namely DARPP-32, that is regulated by dopamine and that is a potent inhibitor, in its phosphorylated form, of protein phosphatase-1. Although the biochemical and functional properties of DARPP-32 and of inhibitor-1 are

TABLE II

Amino acid sequences around the phosphorylatable threonine residues of DARPP-32 and inhibitor-1

Phosphoprotein	Sequence[a]
DARPP-32[b]	**-Ile-Arg-Arg-Arg-Arg-Pro-Thr(P)-Pro-Ala**-Met·Leu-Phe-Arg-
Inhibitor-1[c]	**-Ile-Arg-Arg-Arg-Arg-Pro-Thr(P)-Pro-Ala**-Thr- Leu-Val-Leu-

[a]Sequence homology between DARPP-32 and inhibitor-1 is indicated in bold.
[b]From Hemmings et al. (1984d); Williams et al., 1986.
[c]From Aitken et al. (1982).

very similar, DARPP-32 and inhibitor-1 are clearly distinct proteins that appear to be related by a common ancestral gene (Williams et al., 1986).

Physiological role of DARPP-32

Dopamine acting at D-1 dopamine receptors increases the state of phosphorylation of DARPP-32 in intact nerve cells by elevating cyclic AMP levels and thereby activating cyclic AMP-dependent protein kinase. These observations suggest that DARPP-32, as an intracellular 'third messenger' for dopamine, is involved in the regulation of one or more specific dopamine-regulated physiological processes in dopaminoceptive

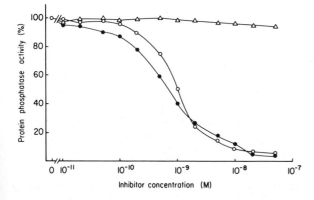

Fig. 1. Inhibition of the catalytic subunit of purified protein phosphatase-1 by various concentrations of phospho-DARPP-32(○), dephospho-DARPP-32 (△) or phospho-inhibitor-1 (●). Protein phosphatase activity was determined by measuring the release of ^{32}P from ^{32}P-labeled phosphorylase a. Both phosphoproteins demonstrate similar potencies in their ability to inhibit protein phosphatase-1. (Taken from Hemmings et al., 1984a.)

cells possessing D-1 dopamine receptors, and may therefore be an important component of the molecular machinery involved in mediating physiological responses to dopamine acting at D-1 dopamine receptors. A mechanism by which DARPP-32 may mediate some of the effects of dopamine has been discovered by studying the effects of DARPP-32 on the activity of purified preparations of protein phosphatases (see above). Thus, dopamine may produce some of its physiological effects by increasing the state of phosphorylation of DARPP-32 and thereby inhibiting the activity of protein phosphatase-1. The inhibition of protein phosphatase-1 by phospho-DARPP-32 would be expected to inhibit the dephosphorylation of other phosphoproteins which are substrates for protein phosphatase-1, and thereby prolong and/or potentiate their own physiological actions. This potentiating effect might pertain not only to proteins phosphorylated by cyclic AMP-dependent protein kinase (a positive feedback mechanism), but also to proteins phosphorylated by other protein kinases (a mechanism allowing the interaction of the cyclic AMP-regulated protein phosphorylation system with other protein phosphorylation systems in dopaminoceptive cells).

Fig. 2 illustrates a mechanism by which the inhibition of protein phosphatase-1 by phospho-DARPP-32 may regulate some of the physiological effects produced by dopamine. Regions of the brain that contain DARPP-32, most notably the basal ganglia, also contain many other substrates for cyclic AMP-dependent protein kinase (Walaas et al., 1983b, 1983c). It is likely that many of these substrates can be dephosphorylated by

154

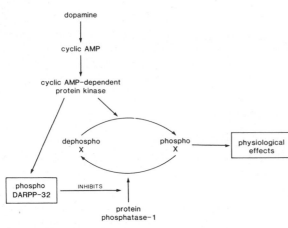

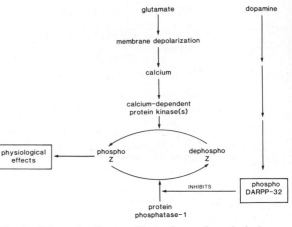

Fig. 2. Schematic diagram illustrating a hypothetical positive feedback mechanism by which DARPP-32 may be involved in regulating some of the physiological effects of dopamine acting on D-1 dopaminoceptive cells. The first messenger dopamine, by interacting with D-1 dopamine receptors, activates adenylate cyclase and thereby elevates intracellular cyclic AMP levels and activates cyclic AMP-dependent protein kinase. Cyclic AMP-dependent protein kinase then stimulates the phosphorylation of DARPP-32 and of various other substrate proteins in target cells. The phosphorylation of DARPP-32 converts it to an active inhibitor of protein phosphatase-1. Phospho-DARPP-32 decreases the dephosphorylation of some of the other proteins (represented by X) that are substrates for both cyclic AMP-dependent protein kinase and protein phosphatase-1. By increasing the state of phosphoryation of X, which is involved in producing the physiological effects of dopamine acting at D-1 dopamine receptors, phospho-DARPP-32 represents a positive feedback signal through which some of the actions of dopamine are amplified.

Fig. 3. Schematic diagram illustrating a hypothetical mechanism by which DARPP-32 may be involved in mediating interactions between dopamine and another neurotransmitter (glutamate in the example given) at the level of protein phosphorylation. Glutamate stimulation produces membrane depolarization which increases intracellular calcium ion levels and leads to the activation of calcium-dependent protein kinase(s) and thereby to the phosphorylation of specific substrate proteins (represented by Z). These proteins are in turn involved in mediating some of the physiological effects of glutamate. By inhibiting protein phosphatase-1 activity and decreasing the dephosphorylation of Z, phospho-DARPP-32 represents an intracellular signal through which dopamine may modulate the action of glutamate. A similar mechanism may allow dopamine to interact with other excitatory neurotransmitters.

protein phosphatase-1, as has been found for other substrates of cyclic AMP-dependent protein kinase, since protein phosphatase-1 has a relatively broad substrate specificity (Ingebritsen and Cohen, 1983b). The phosphorylation and activation of DARPP-32 in these brain regions could therefore inhibit the dephosphorylation of these other substrates for cyclic AMP-dependent protein kinase, and thereby amplify the effects of cyclic AMP by a positive feedback mechanism.

Inhibition of protein phosphatase-1 by phospho-DARPP-32 may also allow interactions between dopamine and other neurotransmitters acting on D-1 dopaminoceptive cells. In addition to phosphoproteins that are substrates for cyclic AMP-dependent protein kinase, protein

phosphatase-1 dephosphorylates phosphoproteins that are substrates for other protein kinases (Ingebritsen and Cohen, 1983a, 1983b). Thus, phosphorylation and activation of DARPP-32 could allow dopamine, acting through cyclic AMP, to modulate the phosphorylation state of substrates for other second messenger-regulated protein kinases. By this mechanism, dopamine and cyclic AMP would be able to interact with other first and second messenger systems at the level of protein phosphorylation by regulating the state of phosphorylation of some of the same substrate proteins. The inhibition by dopamine of the dephosphorylation by protein phosphatase-1 of substrate protein(s) phosphorylated in response to another neurotransmitter, acting through another second messenger and protein kinase, would provide a molecular mechanism for synergistic interactions between dopamine and another neurotransmitter. This effect is illustrated schematically in Fig. 3. for dopamine interacting with glutamate.

In Fig. 3, dopamine is shown to regulate the phosphorylation of DARPP-32 through cyclic AMP, while glutamate is shown as an example of a neurotransmitter that produces some of its effects through the elevation of intracellular calcium ion concentration. The medium-sized spiny neurons of the caudatoputamen are directly innervated by a large dopaminergic projection from the substantia nigra pars compacta (Lindvall and Björklund, 1978; Freund et al., 1984) and by a large projection from the cerebral cortex (Pickel et al., 1981; Bouyer et al., 1984; Freund et al., 1984) which is primarily glutamatergic (Divac et al., 1977; McGeer et al., 1977), as shown schematically in Fig. 4. Changes in intracellular calcium ion concentration due to glutamate-induced membrane depolarization may be involved in producing some of the physiological effects of glutamate (Sonnhof and Bührle, 1981; MacDermott et al., 1986), possibly involving activation of calcium-dependent protein kinase(s). If the putative glutamate-regulated substrates for calcium-dependent protein kinase(s) are substrates for dephosphorylation by protein phosphatase-1, then the dopamine-induced phosphorylation of DARPP-32 and consequent inhibition of protein phosphatase-1 represents one possible mechanism through which dopamine could influence glutamate excitability of these cells.

Electrophysiological studies suggest that dopa-

mine is able to inhibit the activity produced by application of glutamate onto caudate neurons (for review, see Moore and Bloom, 1978). At least two mechanisms for this inhibitory action of dopamine on glutamate excitability are possible at the level of protein phosphorylation. First, a protein phosphorylated in response to a dopamine-induced elevation of cyclic AMP (X in Fig. 2) may have a direct inhibitory effect on glutamate excitability, which would be potentiated by DARPP-32 phosphorylation if this phosphoprotein (phospho-X) were a substrate for protein phosphatase-1. Second, the inhibition of protein phosphatase-1 resulting from the dopamine- and cyclic AMP-stimulated phosphorylation of DARPP-32 may lead to the decreased dephosphorylation of a protein phosphorylated in response to a glutamate-induced elevation of calcium ion (Z in Fig. 3); this phosphoprotein would then exert an inhibitory effect (negative feedback) on glutamate excitability (Nestler et al., 1984). Further biochemical and electrophysiological studies may help to further elucidate the molecular mechanisms involved in mediating the physiological responses to dopamine as well as the interactions between dopamine and other neurotransmitters.

The interaction of dopamine and cyclic AMP with other first and second messenger systems at the level of protein phosphorylation is also possible by another mechanism. DARPP-32 and protein phosphatase-2B are both highly concentrated within medium-sized spiny neurons of the basal ganglia (see above), and are likely to be present in the same cells. Given the cellular colocalization of DARPP-32 and protein phosphatase-2B and the observation that DARPP-32 is a particularly effective substrate for this protein phosphatase in vitro, a physiological role for protein phosphatase-2B in catalyzing the dephosphorylation of DARPP-32 in vivo is likely. The calcium-induced dephosphorylation of DARPP-32 by protein phosphatase-2B provides a possible mechanism by which calcium ion, acting as a second messenger, may antagonize some of the effects of the dopamine-induced cyclic AMP signal in dopaminoceptive neurons.

The discussion above describes two potential

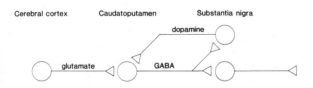

Fig. 4. Simplified schematic diagram of the synaptic organization of some of the major afferent and efferent connections of the caudatoputamen. The GABAergic medium-sized spiny neurons of the caudatoputamen, which contain DARPP-32, receive major afferent projections from the cerebral cortex (glutamatergic) and the substantia nigra pars compacta (dopaminergic). The major efferent projections of the caudatoputamen are to the globus pallidus and entopeduncular nucleus (not shown) and to the substantia nigra pars reticulata. GABA, GABAergic medium-sized spiny neuron.

interactions between the cyclic AMP and calcium second messenger systems which may be mediated through the regulation of the state of phosphorylation of DARPP-32 and the concomitant control of protein phosphatase-1 activity. These interactions provide molecular mechanisms by which a protein phosphatase inhibitor is able to mediate either synergistic or antagonistic effects between two first messengers through the second messengers cyclic AMP and calcium ion. A synergistic effect of cyclic AMP on the effects of calcium could occur by the cyclic AMP-dependent phosphorylation of DARPP-32, leading to the inhibition of the dephosphorylation by protein phosphatase-1 of specific substrate proteins for calcium-dependent protein kinases. Alternatively, calcium may antagonize the effects of cyclic AMP by activating protein phosphatase-2B, and thereby lead to the dephosphorylation of DARPP-32 and possibly other substrate proteins for cyclic AMP-dependent protein kinase. It is clear that a variety of types of interactions between neurotransmitters are possible at the level of the regulation of protein phosphatase inhibitor activity. It is likely that these interactions occur in many different types of neurons and between various pairs of neurotransmitters.

Conclusions

The regulation of protein phosphatase activity by the reversible phosphorylation of specific protein phosphatase inhibitors appears to be a particularly important mechanism of cellular regulation in the brain. In addition to inhibitor-1, which is present in several tissues including brain (see Hemmings et al., 1984a and unpublished observations), two cell type-specific protein phosphatase inhibitors have been identified in brain. One of these, DARPP-32, is present in dopaminoceptive neurons possessing D-1 dopamine receptors and may function as a protein phosphatase inhibitor specific for the dopamine system. The other, G-substrate, which is specifically localized to the Purkinje cells of the cerebellum (Schlichter et al., 1980; Detre et al., 1984), is a specific substrate for cyclic GMP-dependent protein kinase (Aswad and Greengard, 1981b). G-substrate resembles DARPP-32 and inhibitor-1 in many of its biochemical properties (Aswad and Greengard, 1981a; Hemmings et al., 1984b), and has been found to inhibit a protein phosphatase isolated from cerebellum (P.F. Simonelli, H.-C. Li. A.C. Nairn, and P. Greengard unpublished observations). The study of these two neuronal phosphoproteins indicates that the regulation of protein phosphatase activity by the phosphorylation and activation of specific inhibitor proteins is a prominent regulatory mechanism in brain, and suggests that this mechanism may be common to the actions of several neurotransmitters which act through cyclic nucleotides. Studies on the role of

TABLE III

DARPP-32 research applications

Physiology	Role of DARPP-32 in mediating physiological responses to dopamine
	Role of DARPP-32 in mediating interactions between dopamine and other neurotransmitters
Neuroanatomy	Marker for D-1 dopaminoceptive cells
	Analysis of dopaminoceptive neuron projections
	Phylogeny of dopaminoceptive neurons
Neuropharmacology	Measure of postreceptor response to D-1 dopamine receptor activation
Developmental neurobiology	Differentiation of dopaminoceptive cells in vivo and in tissue culture
Clinical studies	Characterization of autopsy tissue in diseases of the basal ganglia (e.g. Huntington's disease and Parkinson's disease)
	Determination in biological fluids as an index of pathology of D-1 dopaminoceptive neurons

DARPP-32 in the control of the phosphorylation of specific endogenous proteins in dopaminoceptive neurons should provide additional insights into the molecular mechanisms of dopamine action, in particular its interactions with other neurotransmitters.

In conclusion, DARPP-32 is a phosphoprotein specifically enriched in dopaminoceptive neurons possessing D-1 dopamine receptors. Table III summarizes some of the types of studies in which DARPP-32 has provided useful information or holds promise for future studies. Biochemical studies have shown that DARPP-32 functions as a potent inhibitor of protein phosphatase-1 in vitro, and that it may be involved in mediating some of the physiological effects of dopamine by inhibiting this enzyme in vivo. Regulation of the state of phosphorylation of DARPP-32 may also mediate specific interactions between the dopamine acting through cyclic AMP and other first messengers acting through calcium ion. Future studies of phosphoproteins of the basal ganglia, and of DARPP-32 in particular, should lead to further elucidation of the molecular mechanisms underlying dopamine regulation of neuronal function. Inhibition of protein phosphatase-1 activity by the dopamine- and cyclic AMP-stimulated phosphorylation of DARPP-32 may be an important component of the biochemical mechanisms involved in producing the neurophysiological effects of dopamine acting at D-1 dopamine receptors on dopaminoceptive cells.

References

Aitken, A. and Cohen, P. (1982) Isolation and characterisation of active fragments of protein phosphatase inhibitor-1 from rabbit skeletal muscle. *FEBS Lett.*, 147:54–58.

Aitken, A., Bilham, T. and Cohen, P. (1982) Complete primary structure of protein phosphatase inhibitor-1 from rabbit skeletal muscle. *Eur. J. Biochem.*, 126:235–246.

Aswad, D.W. and Greengard, P. (1981a) A specific substrate from rabbit cerebellum for guanosine 3':5'-monophosphate-dependent protein kinase. I. Purification and characterization. *J. Biol. Chem.*, 256:3487–3493.

Aswad, D.W. and Greengard, P. (1981b) A specific substrate from rabbit cerebellum for guanosine 3':5'-monophosphate-dependent protein kinase. II. Kinetic studies on its phosphorylation by guanosine 3':5'-monophosphate-dependent and adenosine 3':5'-monophosphate-dependent protein kinases. *J. Biol. Chem.*, 256:3494–3500.

Bouyer, J.J., Park, D.H., Joh, T.H. and Pickel, V.M. (1984) Chemical and structural analysis of the relation between cortical inputs and tyrosine hydroxylase-containing terminals in the rat neostriatum. *Brain Res.*, 302:267–275.

Bunney, B.S. and Aghajanian, G.K. (1973) Electrophysiological effects of amphetamine on dopaminergic neurons. In E. Usdin and S.H. Snyder (Eds.), *Frontiers in Catecholamine Research*, Pergamon Press, New York, pp. 957–962.

Burd, G.D., Paton, J.A., Hemmings, H.C. Jr., Heintz, J. and Nottebohm, F. (1986) Dopamine innervation of newly-generated neurons in the forebrain of adult canaries, *J. Histochem. Cytochem.* 34:109.

Clement-Cormier, Y.C., Kebabian, J.W., Petzold, G.L. and Greengard, P. (1974) Dopamine-sensitive adenylate cyclase in mammalian brain: A possible site of action of antipsychotic drugs. *Proc. Natl. Acad. Sci. U.S.A.*, 71:1113–1117.

Clement-Cormier, Y.C., Parrish, R.G., Petzold, G.L., Kebabian, J.W. and Greengard, P. (1975) Characterization of a dopamine-sensitive adenylate cyclase in rat caudate nucleus. *J. Neurochem.*, 25:143–149.

Cohen, P. (1982) The role of protein phosphorylation in the neural and hormonal control of cellular activity. *Nature*, 296:613–620.

Detre, J.A., Nairn, A.C., Aswad, D.W. and Greengard, P. (1984) Localization in mammalian brain of G-substrate, a specific substrate for guanosine 3':5'-monophosphate-dependent protein kinase. *J. Neurosci.*, 4:2843–2849.

DiFiglia, M., Pasik, P. and Pasik, T. (1976) A Golgi study of neuronal types in the neostriatum of monkeys. *Brain Res.*, 114:245–256.

Dimova, R., Vuillet, J. and Seite, R. (1980) Study of the rat neostriatum using a combined Golgi-electron microscope technique and serial sections. *Neuroscience*, 5:1581–1596.

Divac, I., Fonnum, F. and Storm-Mathisen, J. (1977) High affinity uptake of glutamate in terminals of corticostriatal axons. *Nature*, 266:377–378.

Foster, G.A., Schultzberg, M., Hökfelt, T., Goldstein, M., Hemmings, H.C. Jr., Ouimet, C.C., Walaas, S.I. and Greengard, P. (1986) Development of DARPP-32, a dopamine- and adenosine 3':5'-monophosphate-regulated phosphoprotein, in the prenatal rat central nervous sytem, and its relationship to the arrival of presumed dopaminergic innervation. *J. Neurosci.* (in press).

Freund, T.F., Powell, J.F. and Smith, A.D. (1984) Tyrosine hydroxylase-immunoreactive boutons in synaptic contact with identified striatonigral neurons, with particular references to dendritic spines. *Neuroscience*, 13:1189–1215.

Greengard, P. (1978) Phosphorylated proteins as physiological effectors. *Science*, 199:146–152.

Groves, P.M. (1983) A theory of the functional organization of the neostriatum and the neostriatal control of voluntary movement. *Brain Res. Rev.*, 5:109–132.

Hemmings, H.C. Jr. and Greengard, P. (1986) DARPP-32, a dopamine- and cyclic AMP-regulated phosphoprotein: Regional, tissue and phylogenetic distribution. *J. Neurosci.* 6:1469–1481.

Hemmings, H.C. Jr., Greengard, P., Tung, H.Y.L. and Cohen, P. (1984a) DARPP-32, a dopamine-regulated neuronal phosphoprotein, is a potent inhibitor of protein phosphatase-1. *Nature*, 310:503–505.

Hemmings, H.C. Jr., Nairn, A.C., Aswad, D.W. and Greengard, P. (1984b) DARPP-32, a dopamine- and adenosine 3':5'-monophosphate-regulated phosphoprotein enriched in dopamine-innervated brain regions. II. Purification and characterization of the phosphoprotein from bovine caudate nucleus. *J. Neurosci.*, 4:99–110.

Hemmings, H.C. Jr., Nairn, A.C. and Greengard, P. (1984c) DARPP-32, a dopamine- and adenosine 3':5'-monophosphate-regulated neuronal phosphoprotein. II. Comparison of the kinetics of phosphorylation of DARPP-32 and phosphatase inhibitor-1. *J. Biol. Chem.*, 259:14491–14497.

Hemmings, H.C. Jr., Williams, K.R., Konigsberg, W.H. and Greengard, P. (1984d) DARPP-32, a dopamine- and adenosine 3':5'-monophosphate-regulated neuronal phosphoprotein. I. Amino acid sequence around the phosphorylated threonine. *J. Biol. Chem.*, 259:14486–14490.

Hemmings, H.C. Jr., Nairn, A.C. and Greengard, P. (1986a) Protein kinases and phosphoproteins in the nervous system. In J.B. Martin and J.D. Barchas (Eds.), *Neuropeptides in Neurologic and Psychiatric Disease, Research Publications: Association for Research in Nervous and Mental Disorders, Vol. 64*, Raven Press, New York, pp. 47–69.

Hemmings, H.C. Jr., Nestler, E.J., Walaas, S.I., Ouimet, C.C. and Greengard, P. (1986b) Protein phosphorylation and neuronal function: DARPP-32, an illustrative example. In G.M. Edelman, W.E. Gall, and W.M. Cowan (Eds.), *New Insights Into Synaptic Function*, John Wiley and Sons, New York.

Hemmings, H.C. Jr., Walaas, S.I., Ouimet, C.C. and Greengard, P. (1986c) Dopamine receptors: Regulation of protein phosphorylation. In I. Creese and C.M. Fraser (Eds.), *Receptor Biochemistry and Methodology, Vol. 9: Structure and Function of Dopamine Receptors*, Alan R. Liss, New York.

Huang, F.L. and Glinsmann, W.H. (1976) Separation and characterization of two phosphorylase phosphatase inhibitors from rabbit skeletal muscle. *Eur. J. Biochem.*, 70:419–426.

Ingebritsen, T.S. and Cohen, P. (1983a) Protein phosphatases: Properties and role in cellular regulation. *Science*, 221:331–338.

Ingebritsen, T.S. and Cohen, P. (1983b) The protein phosphatases involved in cellular regulation. I. Classification and substrate specificities. *Eur. J. Biochem.*, 132:255–261.

Kebabian, J.W. and Calne, D.B. (1979) Multiple receptors for dopamine. *Nature*, 277:93–96.

Kebabian, J.W., Petzold, G.L. and Greengard, P. (1972) Dopamine-sensitive adenylate cyclase in the caudate nucleus of rat brain and its similarity to the 'dopamine receptor.' *Proc. Natl. Acad. Sci. U.S.A.*, 69:2145–2149.

King, M.M., Huang, C.Y., Chock, P.B., Nairn, A.C., Hemmings, H.C. Jr., Chan, K.-F.J. and Greengard, P. (1984) Mammalian brain phosphoproteins as substrates for calcineurin. *J. Biol. Chem.*, 259:8080–8083.

Krebs, E.G. and Beavo, J.A. (1979) Phosphorylation-dephosphorylation of enzymes. *Annu. Rev. Biochem.*, 48:923–959.

Kuo, J.F. and Greengard, P. (1969) Cyclic nucleotide-dependent protein kinases. IV. Widespread occurrence of adenosine 3':5'-monophosphate-dependent protein kinase in various tissues and phyla of the animal kingdom. *Proc. Natl. Acad. Sci. U.S.A.*, 64:1349–1355.

Lindvall, O. and Björklund, A. (1978) Organization of catecholamine neurons in the rat central nervous system. In L.L. Iversen, S.D. Iversen and S.H. Snyder (Eds.), *Handbook of Psychopharmacology, Vol. 9*, Plenum Press, New York, pp. 139–231.

MacDermott, A.B., Mayer, M.L., Westbrock, G.L., Smith, S.J. and Barker, J.L. (1986) NMDA-receptor activation increases cytoplasmic concentration in cultured spinal cord neurones. *Nature*, 321:519–522.

McGeer, P. L., McGeer, E. G., Scherer, U. and Singh, K. (1977) A glutamatergic corticostriatal path? *Brain Res.*, 128:369–373.

Miller, R.J. and McDermed, J. (1979) Dopamine-sensitive adenylate cyclase. In A.S. Horn, J. Korf and B.H.C. Westerink (Eds.), *The Neurobiology of Dopamine*, Academic Press, London, pp. 159–177.

Molloy, A.G. and Waddington, J.L. (1984) Dopaminergic behaviour stereospecifically promoted by the D_1 agonist *R*-SK + F 38393 and selectively blocked by the D_1 antagonist SCH 23390. *Psychopharmacology*, 82:409–410.

Moore, R.Y. and Bloom, F.E. (1978) Central catecholamine neuron systems: Anatomy and physiology of the dopamine systems. *Annu. Rev. Neurosci.*, 1:129–169.

Nairn, A.C., Hemmings, H.C. Jr. and Greengard, P. (1985) Protein kinases in the brain. *Annu. Rev. Biochem.*, 54:931–976.

Nestler, E.J. and Greengard, P. (1980) Dopamine and depolarizing agents regulate the state of phosphorylation of Protein I in the mammalian superior cervical sympathetic ganglion. *Proc. Natl. Acad. Sci. U.S.A.*, 77:7479–7483.

Nestler, E.J. and Greengard, P. (1982) Distribution of Protein I and regulation of its state of phosphorylation in the rabbit superior cervical ganglion. *J. Neurosci.*, 2:1011–1023.

Nestler, E.J. and Greengard, P. (1983) Protein phosphorylation in the brain. *Nature*, 305:583–588.

Nestler, E.J. and Greengard, P. (1984) *Protein Phosphorylation in the Nervous System*, Wiley-Interscience, New York.

Nestler, E.J., Walaas, S.I. and Greengard, P. (1984) Neuronal phosphoproteins: Physiological and clinical implications. *Science*, 225:1357–1364.

Nimmo, G.A. and Cohen, P. (1978) The regulation of glycogen metabolism: Purification and characterization of protein phosphatase inhibitor-1 from rabbit skeletal muscle. *Eur. J. Biochem.*, 87:341–351.

Ouimet, C.C., Hemmings, H.C. Jr. and Greengard, P. (1983) Light and electron microscopic immunocytochemistry of a dopamine- and cyclic AMP-regulated phosphoprotein (DARPP-32) in rat brain. *Soc. Neurosci. Abstr.*, 9:82.

Ouimet, C.C., Miller, P.E., Hemmings, H.C. Jr., Walaas, S.I.

and Greengard, P. (1984) DARPP-32, a dopamine- and adenosine 3':5'-monophosphate-regulated phosphoprotein enriched in dopamine-innervated brain regions. III. Immunocytochemical localization. *J. Neurosci.*, 4:111–124.

Pasik, P., Pasik, T. and DiFiglia, M. (1979) The internal organization of the neostriatum in mammals. In I. Divac and G.E. Öberg (Eds.), *The Neostriatum*, Pergamon Press, New York, pp. 5–36.

Pickel, V.M., Beckley, S.C., Joh, T.H. and Reis, D.J. (1981). Ultrastructural immunocytochemical localisation of tyrosine hydroxylase in the neostriatum. *Brain Res.*, 225:373–385.

Reiner, A., Brauth, S.E. and Karten, H.J. (1984) Evolution of the amniote basal ganglia. *Trends Neurosci.*, 7:320–325.

Rosengarten, H., Schweitzer, J.W. and Friedhoff, A.J. (1983) Induction of oral dyskinesis in naive rats by D_1 stimulation. *Life Sci.*, 33:2479–2482.

Schlichter, D.J., Detre, J.A., Aswad, D.W., Chehrazi, B. and Greengard, P. (1980) Localization of cyclic GMP-dependent protein kinase and substrate in mammalian cerebellum. *Proc. Natl. Acad. Sci. U.S.A.*, 77:5537–5541.

Siggins, G.R., Hoffer, B.J. and Ungerstedt. U. (1974) Electrophysiological evidence for involvement of cyclic adenosine monophosphate in dopamine responses of caudate neurons. *Life Sci.*, 16:779–792.

Siggins, G.R., Hoffer, B.J., Bloom, F.E. and Ungerstedt, U. (1976) Cytochemical and electrophysiological studies of dopamine in the caudate nucleus. In M.D. Yahr (Ed.), *The Basal Ganglia*, Raven Press, New York, pp. 227–248.

Sonnhof, U. and Bührle, C. (1981) An analysis of glutamate-induced ion fluxes across the membrane of spinal motoneurons of the frog. *Adv. Biochem. Psychopharmacol.*, 27:195–204.

Stewart, A.A., Ingebritsen, T.S., Manalan, A., Klee, C.B. and Cohen, P. (1982) Discovery of Ca^{2+}- and calmodulin-dependent protein phosphatase. *FEBS Lett.*, 137:80–84.

Stoof, J.C. and Kebabian, J.W. (1981) Opposing roles for D-1 and D-2 dopamine receptors in efflux of cyclic AMP from rat neostriatum. *Nature*, 294:366–368.

Stoof, J.C. and Kebabian, J.W. (1984) Two dopamine receptors: biochemistry, physiology and pharmacology. *Life Sci.*, 35:2281–2296.

Treiman, M. and Greengard, P. (1985) D-1 and D-2 dopamin-

ergic receptors regulate protein phosphorylation in the rat neurohypophysis. *Neuroscience*, 15:713–722.

Tsou, K. and Greengard, P. (1982) Regulation of phosphorylation of proteins I, IIIa, and IIIb in rat neurohypophysis in vitro by electrical stimulation and by neuroactive agents. *Proc. Natl. Acad. Sci. U.S.A.*, 79:6075–6079.

Walaas, S.I., Aswad, D.W. and Greengard, P. (1983a) A dopamine- and cyclic AMP-regulated phosphoprotein enriched in dopamine-innervated brain regions. *Nature*, 301:69–71.

Walaas, S.I., Nairn, A.C. and Greengard, P. (1983b) Regional distribution of calcium- and cyclic AMP-regulated protein phosphorylation systems in mammalian brain. I. Particulate systems. *J. Neurosci.*, 3:291–301.

Walaas, S.I., Nairn, A.C. and Greengard, P. (1983c) Regional distribution of calcium- and cyclic AMP-regulated protein phosphorylation systems in mammalian brain. II. Soluble systems *J. Neurosci.*, 3:302–311.

Walaas, S.I. and Greengard, P. (1984) DARPP-32, a dopamine- and adenosine 3':5'-monophosphate-regulated phosphoprotein enriched in dopamine innervated brain regions. I. Regional and cellular distribution in rat brain. *J. Neurosci.*, 4:84–98.

Walaas, S.I., Ouimet, C.C., Hemmings, H.C. Jr. and Greengard, P. (1986) DARPP-32, a dopamine-regulated neuronal phosphoprotein in the basal ganglia. In G.N. Woodruff (Ed.), *Dopamine Systems and Their Regulation*, Macmillan Press, London.

Wallace, R.W., Tallant, E.A. and Cheung, W.Y. (1980) High levels of a heat-labile calmodulin-binding protein (CaM-BP_{80}) in bovine neostriatum. *Biochemistry*, 19:1831–1837.

Williams, K.R., Hemmings, H.C. Jr., LoPresti, M.B., Konigsberg, W.H. and Greengard, P. (1986) DARPP-32, a dopamine- and cyclic AMP-regulated neuronal phosphoprotein: Primary structure and homology with protein phosphatase inhibitor-1. *J. Biol. Chem.*, 261:1890–1903.

Wood, J.G., Wallace, R.W., Whitaker, J.N. and Cheung, W.Y. (1980) Immunocytochemical localization of calmodulin and a heat-labile calmodulin-binding protein (CaM-BP_{80}) in basal ganglia of mouse brain. *J. Cell Biol.*, 84:66–76.

Woodruff, G.N., McCarthy, P.S. and Walker, R.J. (1976) Studies on the pharmacology of neurones in the nucleus accumbens of the rat. *Brain Res.*, 115:233–242.

W.H. Gispen and A. Routtenberg (Eds.)
Progress in Brain Research, Vol. 69
© 1986 Elsevier Science Publishers B.V. (Biomedical Division)

CHAPTER 14

Molecular mechanisms involved in the desensitization of dopamine receptors in slices of corpus striatum

Ingeborg Hanbauer and Enrico Sanna

Hypertension-Endocrine Branch, National Heart, Lung, and Blood Institute, Bethesda, MD 20792, U.S.A.

In the nervous system, communication between neurons occurs at structurally specialized junctions termed synapses. In the past, synaptic transmission was considered to depend on the action of a single chemical signal. In such a simple system the working model for studying the mechanisms operative in synaptic communication included: release of specific transmitter, recognition of the transmitter by specialized postsynaptic membrane sites, transmembrane signaling mediated by a second messenger, transmission of a signal to a transducer system, and physiological response. Recently the documentation of the coexistence of more than one neuromodulator in the same axon has raised the possibility that multiple signals may participate. Although for dopaminergic transmission the consequences of this new vista have not been completely assessed, several lines of evidence have indicated the coexistence of dopamine and cholecystekinin octapeptide in dopaminergic neurons present in mesolimbic structures (Hokfelt et al., 1980).

The multiple of chemical signals at a synaptic connection has to be conceptualized on the basis of the complexity of the receptorial system. Hence a receptor system modulated by multiple signals has multiple recognition sites and additional coupling mechanisms for allosteric modulation of the action of the primary neurotransmitter. For example, allosteric regulatory sites modulate the efficiency of the interaction of γ-aminobutyric acid (GABA) at its specific recognition sites during GABAergic transmission. This modulation was shown to be expressed by a change in the duration of the opening bursts of the Cl^- channel, which functions as the transducer at GABAergic synapses (Guidotti et al., 1983; Borman and Clapham, 1985). Instead, in the dopaminergic system the modulatory functions which have been described up to this point of time are limited to the coupling of dopamine recognition sites to the transducer, adenylate cyclase, mediated by the N_s and N_i subunits of the GTP-binding protein. On the basis of differences in ligand affinity of dopamine recognition sites (Seeman, 1980; Stoof et al., 1981), different manifestations of physiological responses (Attie et al., 1980; Cote et al., 1982) and because of the existence of distinct coupling proteins (Cassell and Selinger, 1977), the existence of two subtypes of physiological functional dopamine receptors has been proposed. The D-1 receptor is directly coupled with adenylate cyclase through the N_s-GTP binding protein, and promotes the increased formation of cAMP. The D-2 receptor is coupled to adenylate cyclase through the N_i-GTP binding protein, and inhibits the activation of adenylate cyclase (Kebabian and Calne, 1979). The experimental outcome of studies on S49 cells and platelet membranes suggests that the inhibitory activity of the N_i subunit is not exerted on the catalytic subunit of adenylate cyclase, but rather on the level of the stimulatory coupling protein (Gilman, 1984).

In addition to a short-term interaction between a transmitter and its postsynaptic receptor sites, there is another dimension of transmitter–receptor

TABLE I

Modulation of synaptic transmission

Fast events	Transmembrane signaling (second, messenger formation)	Enzymes (cyclase, phospholipase), ion channels
	Feedback traces of fast event	Membrane protein phosphorylation
Slow events	Supersensitivity	Lack of feedback traces
	Subsensitivity	Temporal summation of feedback traces

function, which can be viewed as long-term modulation of a receptor. Such long-term changes of a receptor are triggered by an oscillation in the efficiency of chemical signal transduction. This functional change involves an alteration of the supramolecular structure of the receptor. The scheme shown in Table I suggests that changes in the supramolecular structure of the ·dopamine receptor are not elicited by a rapid receptor response to a chemical signal; rather they are determined by the continuous summation of changes brought about by each fast event.

The present chapter summarizes work from our laboratory which was carried out to elucidate the biochemical changes that occur during desensitiz-ation of the dopamine receptor. Our data indicate that prolonged occupancy of dopamine recog-nition sites confers subsensitivity to various dopa-mine-mediated mechanisms, which include radio-ligand recognition sites and the regulatory subunit of adenylate cyclase. In addition, our data demon-strate that desensitization of dopamine receptors is associated with ·an increased phosphorylation mediated by a cAMP-dependent protein kinase of proteins located at postsynaptic membranes.

Desensitization of D-1 dopamine receptor-coupled adenylate cyclase

The regulatory process termed 'desensitization' has been extensively studied in β-adrenergic recep-tors, which are present in a wide variety of cells (Shear et al., 1976; Chuang and Costa, 1979; Su et

al., 1980; Iyengar et al., 1981). These studies indicate that the down-regulation of β-adrenergic receptor-linked adenylate cyclase involves alter-ation of several mechanisms that are associated with the function of β-adrenergic receptors.

Prolonged incubation of striatal slices with dopamine attenuates the responsiveness of adeny-late cyclase to subsequent stimulation by dopa-mine (Memo et al., 1982).

Studies carried out with specific ligands for D-1, D-2 and β-adrenergic recognition sites (Table II) corroborate the findings on the desensitization of dopamine receptor elicited by dopamine by showing that only prolonged incubation with the D-1 receptor ligand SKF38393 (2,3,4,5-tetra-hydro-7, 8-dihydroxy-1-phenyl-1 H-3-benzozepine) reduced the responsiveness of adenylate cyclase to subsequent stimulation by dopamine. In contrast, prolonged exposure of striatal slices to LY141865 (*trans:*4, 4a, 5, 6, 7, 8, 8a, 9-octahydro-5-propyl-2H-pyrazolol), a D-2 receptor agonist (Tsuruta et al., 1981) and isoproterenol, a β-adrenergic receptor agonist, did not alter the responsiveness of adeny-late cyclase to dopamine. Additional support for a specific involvement of D-1 recognition sites in the down-regulation of adenylate cyclase is given by experiments carried out in the presence of dopa-mine receptor antagonists. The data in Table II show that preincubation with 10^{-6} M haloperidol, an antagonist for D-1 and D-2 receptors, could partially prevent the desensitization. In contrast,

TABLE II

Desensitization of dopamine-stimulated adenylate cyclase in striatal slices

Addition to medium		Dopamine-stimulated increase in cAMP (pmol/mg prot/min)[a]
Preincubation	Incubation	
None	None	208 ± 24
None	SKF 38393	105 ± 8*
None	LY 141865	188 ± 12
None	Isoproterenol	168 ± 11
Haloperidol	Dopamine	158 ± 12
Sulpiride	Dopamine	104 ± 8*

[a]The numbers represent mean $\pm$ SEM of three separate experiments done in triplicate.
*$p < 0.01$ for difference for control.

preincubation with 10^{-6} M sulpiride, a specific D-2 receptor antagonist (Trabucchi et al., 1975) failed to block the desensitization of the cyclase system. In addition, several lines of investigation indicate that the phenomenon of dopamine receptor subsensitivity is closely associated with a decrease of the affinity of dopamine recognition sites and a decrease of the coupling efficiency of the GTP-binding protein. When striatal slices are incubated for 30 min or longer in the presence of 10^{-4} M dopamine, the K_D value for the specific binding of $[^3H]N$-propyl-norapomorphine to crude synaptic membranes is increased (Memo et al., 1982). A similar extent of increase in K_D is obtained when the specific binding of $[^3H]N$-propyl-norapomorphine to control striatal membrane preparations is measured in the presence of 0.1 mM GTP. These findings are in agreement with reports in the literature showing that in striatal membranes GTP decreases the affinity of specific recognition sites for dopamine receptor agonists (Creese et al., 1979). Moreover, measurements of the IC_{50} of $[^3H]$spiroperidol binding with dopamine as a displacer indicate that the affinity for dopamine is greatly reduced in slices incubated with 10^{-4} M dopamine for 30 min (Table III). Taking these data into consideration, it can be proposed that prolonged incubation of striatal slices with dopamine, or incubation of crude synaptic membranes in the presence of high concentrations of GTP promote an interconversion from a high to a low affinity state of the receptor (Memo et al., 1981; Sibley et al., 1982).

Since the coupling of dopamine recognition

TABLE III

Inhibition of $[^3H]$spiroperidol binding by dopamine in membranes prepared from striatal slices after incubation with 10^{-4} M dopamine

Treatment	IC_{50} (μM)[a]
Control	0.56 ± 0.12
Desensitized	3.8 ± 0.21*

[a] The data are expressed as mean $\pm$ SEM of three experiments in triplicate.
*$p < 0.05$.

TABLE IV

Effect of cholera toxin on cAMP formation in striatal slices incubated in the absence and presence of 10^{-4} M Dopamine

Addition to incubation medium	cAMP (pmol/mg prot)[a]	
	Control	Desensitized
None	1.8 ± 0.2	2.1 ± 0.2
Cholera toxin	3.8 ± 0.2*	2.8 ± 0.2

Slices were incubated for 30 min in the presence or absence of 10^{-4} M dopamine. Cholera toxin (100 $\mu g/ml$) was added and the incubation continued for 40 min. The cyclic AMP content was measured by radioimmunoassay.
[a] Values are the mean $\pm$ SEM of three separate experiments done in triplicate.
*$p < 0.001$ for difference from control.

sites to the catalytic subunit of adenylate cyclase is mediated through the N_s subunit of the GTP-binding protein (Ross et al., 1977; Lad et al., 1980; Londos et al., 1981) we studied the stimulation of adenylate cyclase in control and desensitized slices by directly activating the regulatory subunit. Cholera toxin was shown to catalyze the ADP-ribosylation of the N_s subunit of the GTP binding protein and thereby mediated the activation of adenylate cyclase (Gill and Meren, 1978; Gilman, 1984). As shown in Table IV, the increase in cAMP formation elicited by cholera toxin (100 $\mu g/ml$) in control slices is greatly reduced in desensitized slices. Since cholera toxin acts on the adenylate cyclase system by promoting the formation of the N_s-GTP complex (Gilman, 1984), it is possible to speculate that the reduced functional efficiency of N_s may be related to alteration of its affinity for GTP or to a change in the number of GTP binding sites.

In summary, the present data suggest that in caudate nucleus the dopamine-sensitive adenylate cyclase is a part of a multimolecular receptor complex consisting of various proteins with highly specific functions. The activity of adenylate cyclase is regulated by a tissue-specific distribution of D-1 or D-2 recognition sites coupled to the catalytic subunit of the enzyme by N_s or N_i subunits, respectively.

Increased phosphorylation of membrane proteins

In neuronal membranes phosphorylation and dephosphorylation elicit changes in the fluidity of membranes by altering the conformation of the proteins. This appears to be an important mechanism in the regulation of the functional state of membranes (Gazitt et al., 1976; Greengard, 1978). In the past various laboratories demonstrated that the physiological function of first messengers at the target cell can be expressed through regulating the state of phosphorylation of specific proteins. Phosphorylation can occur on one or numerous protein substrates depending on the protein kinase involved (Adelstein et al., 1982; Freedman and Jamieson, 1982), and may result in the generation of specific biological responses. It has been shown that first messengers can activate protein kinase either directly (Zwiers et al., 1980; Cohen et al., 1982; Roth and Cassell, 1983), or

indirectly through a second messenger (Krueger et al., 1977; Greengard, 1978; Rodnight, 1982). The transduction of a chemical signal through neuronal membranes appears to involve a complex membrane-bound phosphorylating system, which is responsive to a second messenger and increased Ca^{2+} flux. This inference is supported by findings showing that the phosphorylation of synapsin I can be catalyzed by a protein kinase stimulated via neuro-transmitters or membrane-depolarizing agents (Forn and Greengard, 1978; Nestler and Greengard, 1980, 1984; Dolphin and Greengard, 1981).

Increasing evidence in the literature suggests that phosphorylation of membrane proteins may play a role in the desensitization of neurotransmitter-stimulated adenylate cyclase (Anderson and Jaworski, 1979; Ehrlich et al., 1977, 1982; Stadel et al., 1983; and, Memo and Hanbauer, 1984). In this chapter evidence is provided that the desensit-

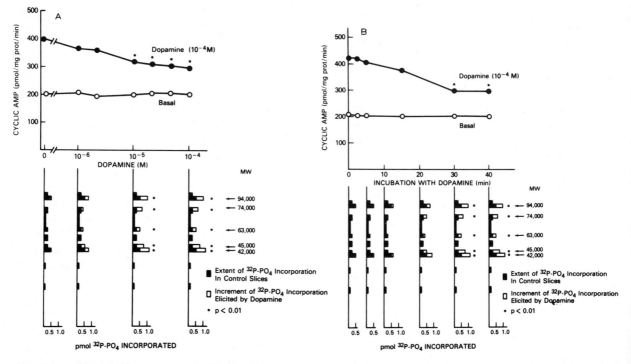

Fig. 1. Comparison of time course (A) and dose–response relationship (B) of dopamine-elicited alterations in the responsiveness of adenylate cyclase to dopamine stimulation and phosphorylation of membrane proteins. Striatal slices were incubated in the presence of [^{32}P]NaH$_2$PO$_4$ with various concentrations of dopamine as indicated. Crude synaptosomal fractions were extracted with 50 mM Tris buffer, pH 7.4, containing 1% n-octylglucoside. The solubilized protein fractions were resolved on 10% acrylamid slab gels.

ization of striatal dopamine receptors is associated with phosphorylation of various membrane proteins. The data in Figs. 1A and 1B show that the length of incubation and the concentration of dopamine required to elicit desensitization of dopamine-sensitive adenylate cyclase are comparable to those required to increase membrane protein phosphorylation. The dopamine-promoted modification of the phosphorylation pattern of membrane proteins occurs when dopamine receptors in striatal slices are exposed to dopamine (10^{-5} to 10^{-4} M) for at least 30 min. Increased incorporation of $^{32}PO_4$ occurred predominantly in protein bands with the apparent molecular weights of 42 000, 45 000, 63 000, 74 000 and 94 000.

To obtain information as to whether the enhanced phosphorylation of these protein bands occurs as the result of a specific interaction of dopamine with the D-1 dopamine receptor, we studied the effects of specific D-1 and D-2 dopamine receptor agonists. The data in Table V indicate that incubation in the presence of SKF38393 elicited a similar phosphorylation pattern as was obtained with dopamine. In contrast when striatal slices are incubated in the presence of LY141865 an enhanced $^{32}PO_4$ incorporation occurs only in one band with the molecular weight of 42 000. This difference in phosphorylation pattern suggests that the prolonged stimulation of D-1 or D-2 dopamine receptors results in the manifestation of specific feedback traces. In the case of D-1 receptor-promoted membrane phosphorylation, the protein bands with the molecular weights of 45 000, 63 000 and 74 000 may be specifically associated with the subsensitive state of the dopamine receptor. In addition, the relationship between D-1 dopamine receptor and the phosphorylation of these specific protein bands is supported by findings showing that sulpiride failed to prevent the dopamine-mediated increase (Fig. 2). In contrast, haloperidol, a blocker of D-1 and D-2 receptors, curtailed the increase of membrane protein phosphorylation. Since the transmembrane signaling of D-1 receptor agonists is mediated by cyclic AMP, which subsequently leads to the activation of cAMP-dependent protein kinase, we studied the effect of cholera toxin on the incorporation of $^{32}PO_4$ in striatal membrane proteins. The data in Table V demonstrate that the phosphorylation pattern obtained is similar to that with D-1 dopamine receptor agonists. In the past, various laboratories have described the occurrence of phosphoproteins in specific areas of the nervous system (Routtenberg, 1979; Bar et al., 1980) as well as in specific subcellular locations (for review see Nestler and Greengard, 1984).

Although it is generally accepted that in caudate nucleus the D-1 dopamine receptor is most likely located on cholinergic interneurons

TABLE V

Increased phosphorylation of membrane protein bands from striatal slices incubated in presence of various drugs

Drugs added to incubation medium	Phosphorylation (pmol $^{32}PO_4^{3-}$) of band: (MW × 10^{-3})				
	42	45	63	74	94
None	0.45	0.33	0.33	0.33	0.62
SKF38393 (10^{-5} M)	1.4	0.80	0.65	0.75	1.1
Cholera toxin (100 g/ml)	1.7	0.79	0.50	0.77	1.7
LY141865 (10^{-5} M)	1.0	0.49	0.30	0.40	0.55

The numbers represent the mean of three similar experiments. Striatal slices were preincubated for 20 min. Thereafter, the various drugs and [^{32}P]NaH$_2$PO$_4$ (250 µCi/ml) were added and the incubation was continued for 40 min.

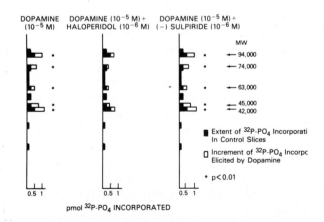

Fig. 2. Effect of preincubation of striatal slices with haloperidol (10^{-6} M) or (−)sulpiride (10^{-6} M) on the increased phosphorylation of several membrane protein bands elicited by prolonged incubation with dopamine (10^{-5} M).

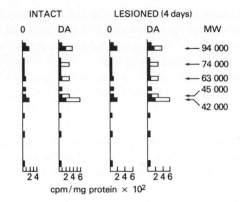

Fig. 3. Effect of transection of the nigra-striatal fiber tract on the increased phosphorylation of several membrane protein bands elicited by prolonged incubation with (10^{-5} M) dopamine (DA).

(Lehmann and Langer, 1983), it was important in our studies to verify the location of the phosphoproteins, which appear to be altered during desensitization of the dopamine receptor. In a group of rats the nigrastriatal fibers were transected unilaterally four days prior to the experiment. At this time period after transection the presynaptic dopaminergic terminals are degenerated, while supersensitivity of the postsynaptic dopamine receptor has not yet been developed. The results in Fig. 3 show that the electrophoretic pattern and the extent of $^{32}PO_4$ incorporation in various membrane protein bands are similar in intact and lesioned rats. These data support our present view which suggests that the enhanced phosphorylation of specific membrane protein bands is one of the molecular events brought about by prolonged occupancy of D-1 dopamine recognition sites. Recently, evidence for the presence of the phosphoprotein DARPP-32 in dopaminoceptive postsynaptic neurons was presented by Walaas and Greengard (1984). However, our studies covered only changes occurring at the level of membrane proteins, while DARPP-32, which is a specific marker for dopaminoceptive cells, is a cytosolic protein.

Conclusion

This chapter summarizes our present concepts on the molecular mechanism associated with the desensitization of striatal dopamine receptors. Prolonged occupancy of D-1 dopamine recognition sites decreases their affinity for agonists and reduces the coupling efficiency of the G/F protein. Our data further indicate that, during desensitization of dopamine-sensitive adenylate cyclase, intracellular signals are amplified leading to an increase in the phosphorylation of specific proteins located in striatal membranes. Although we have not yet characterized the chemical and functional properties of these phosphoproteins, we can assume on the basis of pharmacological studies that the phosphorylation of the proteins with the apparent molecular weights of 45 000, 63 000 and 74 000 is one of the snyaptic events that are associated with the regulation of the functional state of the D-1 dopamine receptor. It is possible to speculate that a subunit of the dopamine recognition sites, the regulatory subunit of adenylate cyclase or a subunit of the voltage-dependent Ca^{2+} channel could be protein substrates for a cAMP-dependent protein kinase that is activated through the increase of second messenger content. In fact, it has been shown that the responsiveness of the GABA receptor to modulator proteins was altered by phosphorylation catalyzed by specific protein kinases (Guidotti et al., 1983). Moreover, it has been suggested that in cardiac muscle a cAMP-dependent protein kinase is operative in the phosphorylation of a protein closely associated to the Ca^{2+} channel and may trigger an increase in membrane conductance (Reuter, 1983). The scheme in Table VI depicts our present working model, which proposes that two types of synaptic events may be involved in establishing dopamine receptor subsensitivity. Firstly, a D-1 dopamine receptor, cAMP protein kinase-mediated phosphorylation of ion channel proteins that modulates membrane conductance. Secondly a Ca^{2+} mobilizing receptor-linked signaling system may be involved in the phospholipase C-mediated formation of diacylglycerol and subsequent activation of protein kinase C. Since the signal transduction of the Ca^{2+} mobilizing system appears to be facilitated by the N_i-GTP binding protein subunit, it is tempting to speculate whether the D-2

TABLE VI

Transfer of fast synaptic events to membrane proteins

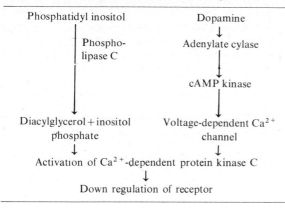

dopamine receptor may play a role in this Ca^{2+}-requiring modulation of synaptic membranes.

Acknowledgment

Dr. Enrico Sanna was supported in part by a grant from the Scottish Rite Research Program, N.M.J., U.S.A. The authors thank Mr. A.G. Wright, Jr., for his excellent technical assistance.

References

Adelstein, R.S., Sellers, J.R., Conti, M.A., Pato, M.D. and de Lanerolle, P. (1982) Regulation of smooth muscle contractile proteins by calmodulin and cyclic AMP. *Fed. Proc.*, 41:2873–2878.

Anderson, W.B. and Jaworski, C.J. (1979) Isoproterenol-induced desensitization of adenylate cyclase responsiveness in cell-free system. *J. Biol. Chem.*, 254:4596–4601.

Attie, M.F., Brown, E.M., Gardner, D.G., Spiegel, A.M. and Aurbach, G.D. (1980) Characterization of the dopamine-responsive adenylate cyclase of bovine parathyroid cells and its relationship to parathyroid hormone secretion. *Endocrinology*, 107:1776–1781.

Bar, P.R., Schotman, P., Gispen, W.H., Tielen, A.M. and Lopes da Silva, F.H. (1980) Changes in synaptic membrane phosphorylation after tetanic stimulation in the dentate area of rate hippocampal slices. *Brain Res.*, 198:478–484.

Bormann, J. and Clapham, D.E. (1985) γ-Aminobutyric acid receptor channels in adrenal chromaffin cells: A patch-clamp study. *Proc. Natl. Acad. Sci. U.S.A.*, 82:2168–2172.

Cassel, D. and Selinger, Z. (1977) Mechanism of adenylate cyclase activation by cholera toxin: Inhibition of GTP hydrolysis at the regulatory site. *Proc. Natl. Acad. Sci. U.S.A.*, 74:3307–3311.

Chuang, D.-M. and Costa, E. (1979) Evidence for internalization of the recognition site of β-adrenergic receptors during receptor subsensitivity induced by (−)-isoproterenol. *Proc. Natl. Acad. Sci. U.S.A.*, 76:3024–3028.

Cohen, S., Carpenter, G. and King, L., Jr. (1982) Epidermal growth factor–receptor–protein kinase interactions. Co-purification of receptor and epidermal growth factor-enhanced phosphorylation activity. *J. Biol. Chem.*, 255:4834–4842.

Cote, T.E., Eskay, R.L., Frey, E.A., Grewe, C.W., Munemura, M., Stoof, J.C. and Tsuruta, K. (1982) Biochemical and physiological studies of the beta-adrenoceptor and the D-2 dopamine receptor in the intermediate lobe of the rat pituitary gland: A review. *Neuroendocrinology*, 35:217–224.

Creese, I., Usdin, T.B. and Snyder, S.H. (1979) Dopamine receptor binding regulated by guanine nucleotides. *Mol. Pharmacol.*, 16:69–76.

Dolphin, A.C. and Greengard, P. (1981) Neurotransmitter- and neuromodulator-dependent alterations in phosphorylation of protein I in slices of rat facial nucleus. *J. Neurosci.*, 1:192–203.

Ehrlich, Y.H., Rabjohns, R.R. and Routtenberg, A. (1977) Experimental input alters the phosphorylation of specific proteins in brain membranes. *Pharmacol. Biochem. Behav.*, 6:169–177.

Ehrlich, Y.H., Whittemore, S.R., Garfield, M.K., Graber, S.G. and Lenox, R.H. (1982) Protein phosphorylation in the regulation and adaptation of receptor function. *Prog. Brain Res.*, 56:375–396.

Forn, J. and Greengard, P. (1978) Depolarizing agents and cyclic nucleotides regulate the phosphorylation of specific neuronal proteins in rat cerebral cortex slices. *Proc. Natl. Acad. Sci. U.S.A.*, 75:5195–5199.

Freedman, S.D. and Jamieson, J.D. (1982) Hormone-induced protein phosphorylation. III. Regulation of the phosphorylation of the secretagogue-responsive 29 000-dalton protein by both Ca^{2+} and cAMP in vitro. *J. Cell Biol.*, 195:918–923.

Gazitt, Y., Ohad, I. and Loyter, A. (1972) Phosphorylation and dephosphorylation of membrane proteins as a possible mechanism of structural rearrangement of membrane components. *Biochim. Biophys. Acta*, 436:1–14.

Gill, D.M. and Meren, R. (1978) ADP-ribosylation of membrane proteins catalyzed by cholera toxin: Basis of the activation of adynylate cyclase. *Proc. Natl. Acad. Sci. U.S.A.*, 75:3050–3054.

Gilman, A.G. (1984) Guanine nucleotide-binding regulatory proteins and dual control of adenylate cyclase. *J. Clin. Invest.*, 73:1–4.

Greengard, P. (1978) Phosphorylated proteins as physiological effectors. *Science*, 199:146–152.

Guidotti, A., Corda, M.G., Wise, B.C., Vaccarino, F. and Costa, E. (1983) GABAergic synapses: Supramolecular organization and biochemical regulation. *Neuropharmacology*, 22:1471–1479.

Hokfelt, T., Rehfeld, J.F., Skirboll, L., Ivemark, B., Goldstein, M. and Marley, K. (1980) Evidence for the coexistence of dopamine and cholecystekinin in mesolimbic neurons, *Nature*, 285:476–478.

Iyengar, R., Bhat, M.K., Riser, M.E. and Birnbaumer, L. (1981) Receptor-specific desensitization of the S49 lymphoma cell adenylyl cyclase. *J. Biol. Chem.*, 256:4810–4815.

Kebabian, J.W. and Calne, D.B. (1979) Multiple receptors for dopamine. *Nature*, 277:93–96.

Krueger, B.K., Forn, J. and Greengard, P. (1977) Depolarization-induced phosphorylation of specific proteins mediated by calcium ion flux in rat brain synaptosomes. *J. Biol. Chem.*, 252:2764–2773.

Lad, P.M., Nielsen, T.B., Preston, M.S. and Rodbell, M. (1980) The role of the guanine nucleotide exchange reaction in the regulation of the β-adrenergic receptor and in the actions of catecholamines and cholera toxin on adenylate cyclase in turkey erythrocyte membranes. *J. Biol. Chem.*, 255:988–995.

Lehmann, J. and Langer, S.Z. (1983) The striatal cholinergic interneuron: Synaptic target of dopaminergic terminals? *Neuroscience*, 10:1105–1120.

Londos, C., Cooper, D.M.F. and Rodbell, M. (1981) Receptor-mediated stimulation and inhibition of adenylate cyclases: The fat cell as a model system. *Adv. Cycl. Nucleotide Res.*, 14:163–171.

Memo, M. and Hanbauer, I. (1984) Phosphorylation of membrane proteins in response to persistent stimulation of adenylate cyclase-linked dopamine receptors in slices of striatum. *Neuropharmacology*, 23:449–455.

Memo, M., Lovenberg, W. and Hanbauer, I. (1982) Agonist-induced subsensitivity of adenylate cyclase coupled with a dopamine receptor in slices from rat corpus striatum. *Proc. Natl. Acad. Sci. U.S.A.*, 79:4456–4460.

Nestler, E.J. and Greengard, P. (1980) Dopamine and depolarizing agents regulate the state of phosphorylation of protein I in the mammalian superior cervical sympathetic ganglion. *Proc. Natl. Acad. Sci. U.S.A.*, 77:7479–7483.

Nestler, E.J. and Greengard, P. (1984) *Protein Phosphorylation in the Nervous System.* John Wiley and Sons, New York.

Reuter, H. (1983) Calcium channel modulation by neurotransmitters, enzymes and drugs. *Nature*, 301:569–574.

Rodnight, R. (1982) Aspects of protein phosphorylation in the nervous system with particular reference to synaptic transmission. *Prog. Brain Res.*, 56:1–25.

Ross, E.M., Maguire, M.E., Sturgill, T.W., Biltonen, R.L. and Gilman, A.G. (1977) Relationship between the β-adrenergic receptor and adenylate cyclase. *J. Biol. Chem.*, 252:5761–5775.

Roth, R.A. and Cassell, D.J. (1983) Insulin receptor: Evidence that it is a protein kinase. *Science*, 219:299–301.

Routtenberg, A. (1979) Anatomical localization of phosphoprotein and glycoprotein substrates of memory. *Prog. Neurobiol.* 12:85–113.

Seeman, P. (1980) Brain dopamine receptors. *Pharmacol. Rev.* 32:229–313.

Sibley, D.R., De Lean, A. and Creese, I. (1982) Anterior pituitary dopamine receptors. *J. Biol. Chem.*, 257:6351–6361.

Shear, M., Insel, P.A., Melmon, K.L. and Coffino, P. (1976) Agonist-specific refractoriness induced by isoproterenol. *J. Biol. Chem.*, 251:7572–7576.

Stadel, J.M., Nambi, P., Shorr, R.G.L., Sawyer, D.F., Caron, M.G. and Lefkowitz, R.J. (1983) Catecholamine-induced desensitization of turkey erythrocyte adenylate cyclase is associated with phosphorylation of the β-adrenergic receptor. *Proc. Natl. Acad. Sci. U.S.A.*, 80:3173–3177.

Stoof, J.C. and Kebabian, J.W. (1981) Opposing roles of D-1 and D-2 dopamine receptors in efflux of cyclic AMP from rat neostriatum. *Nature*, 294:366–368.

Su, Y.-F., Harden, T.K. and Perkins, J.P. (1980) Catecholamine-specific desensitization of adenylate cyclase. *J. Biol. Chem.*, 255:7410–7419.

Trabucchi, M., Longoni, R., Fresia, P. and Spano, P.F. (1975) Sulpiride: A study of the effects on dopamine receptors in rat neostriatum and limbic forebrain. *Life Sci.*, 17:1551–1556.

Tsuruta, K., Frey, E.A., Grewe, C.W., Cote, T.E., Eskay, R.L. and Kebabian, J.W. (1981) Evidence that LY 141865 specifically stimulates the D-2 dopamine receptor. *Nature*, 292:463–465.

Walaas, S.I. and Greengard, P. (1984) DARPP-32, a dopamine and adenosine 3′,5′-monophosphate-regulated phosphoprotein enriched in dopamine-innervated brain regions. I. Regional and cellular distribution in the rat brain. *J. Neurosci.*, 4:84–98.

Zwiers, H., Schotman, P. and Gispen, W.H. (1980) Purification and some characteristics of an ACTH-sensitive protein kinase and its substrate protein in rat brain membranes. *J. Neurochem.*, 34:1689–1699.

W.H. Gispen and A. Routtenberg (Eds.)
Progress in Brain Research, Vol. 69
© 1986 Elsevier Science Publishers B.V. (Biomedical Division)

CHAPTER 15

Structural and functional aspects of epidermal growth factor (EGF) and its receptor

L.H.K. Defize and S.W. de Laat

Hubrecht Laboratory, International Embryological Institute, Uppsalalaan 8, 3584 CT Utrecht, The Netherlands

Introduction

Polypeptide growth factors play an essential role in the regulation of cell proliferation and differentiation. They exert their mitogenic or differentiating activity at nanomolar concentrations by binding to specific high-affinity receptor molecules localized in the plasma membrane. The ultimate biological action of a polypeptide growth factor is dependent on the nature of the target cell. The number of identified growth factors is still rapidly growing. Several of these factors have been purified to homogeneity and their primary amino acid sequence has been determined completely or in part, including epidermal growth factor (EGF) (Savage et al., 1972) and platelet-derived growth factor (PDGF) (Waterfield et al., 1983; Westermark et al., 1983).

The study of growth factors and their receptors has been intensified in recent years by the discovery that at least some of these molecules show a striking homology with certain oncogene products: this *sis* oncogene encodes for a product homologous to PDGF (Doolittle et al., 1983; Waterfield et al., 1983), the *erb-B* oncogene product is homologous to the intracellular domain of the EGF receptor (Downward et al., 1984; Ullrich et al., 1984), and very recently a significant homology has been found between the *fms* oncogene and the colony stimulating factor (CSF-1) receptor of mononuclear phagocytes (Sherr et al., 1985). Furthermore, there is evidence that other oncogene products and also tumor promotors interfere with

certain growth factor receptor-mediated cellular responses (Berridge and Irvine, 1984) in exerting their transforming or promoting activity. Thus, knowledge of the mode of action of growth factors seems indispensable for understanding the mechanisms of carcinogenesis.

Growth factors may serve as diffusible signal molecules in the interaction between cells and tissues, in which the interaction will depend on the production and secretion of the growth factor as well as on the expression of functional receptor molecules in the target cells. Such interactions could play a role in the regulation of differential growth of embryonic and somatic tissues, but also in the outgrowth of tumors (for a review see De Laat et al., 1983). In particular in the latter situation these interactions could differ from the classical endocrine type. A number of polypeptide growth factors have been isolated from tumor cells, but also from cells equivalent to early embryonic cells (Heath and Isacke, 1984; Stern and Heath, 1983), which are capable, in themselves or in combination, to induce mitogenic stimulation as well as a transformed phenotype in normal cells (for a review see Sporn and Roberts, 1985). These so-called transforming growth factors (TGFs) could control the growth behavior of neighboring cells (paracrine stimulation) but also of the producing cell itself (autocrine stimulation), provided that the appropriate receptor molecules are expressed at the cell surface.

TGFα binds to and activates the EGF receptor and has only mitogenic and no transforming activity: to call it a TGF is thus misleading. TGFβ binds to specific receptor sites, has no mitogenic activity, but modulates the action of EGF or TGFα such that the target cell acquires a transformed phenotype. TGFs which utilize the PDGF receptor have also have been identified (Van Zoelen et al., 1984) but their complete characterization is still awaiting. It might be expected that more information on the nature of TGFs, their mode of action, and their role in embryonic and tumor growth, will emerge rapidly.

How the growth factor–receptor interaction leads to the stimulation of cell proliferation and/or to new patterns of gene expression is still largely obscure, despite the great attention given to this important question. Among the various growth factors, EGF and its receptor have probably been studied in most detail. For that reason we will focus this chapter mainly on the nature of these molecules and the intracellular signal pathways activated by their interaction. Furthermore, we will describe some of our recent work on the control of EGF receptor expression during neuronal differentiation and its possible relevance for the establishment, and the maintenance of the neuronal phenotype.

Epidermal growth factor (EGF); structural and functional aspects

EGF was first discovered in extracts of mouse submaxillary glands, by Stanley Cohen (1959). It was given its name because, when injected into newborn mice, it induced precocious eye-lid opening and incisor eruption, due to growth stimulation of epidermal cells and enhancement of keratinization (Cohen, 1962, 1965). Later it turned out that urogastrone, a polypeptide that is acid stable, like EGF, and has gastric anti-secretory properties, and which is found in human urine, was almost identical to mouse EGF. Comparison of the primary amino acid sequence of mouse EGF and human EGF urogastrone, reveals that the polypeptides have 37 amino acids in common, whereas they differ in 16 amino acids (Fig. 1B) (Gregory, 1975). Of specific importance is the alignment of the cysteine residues, which are an important feature in the determination of the tern-

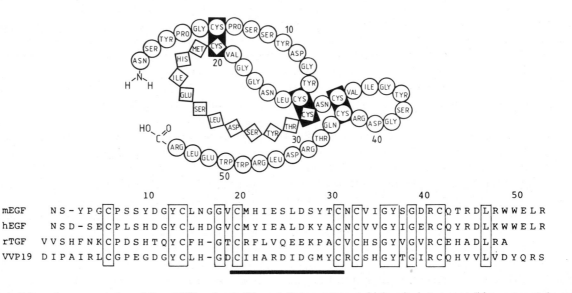

Fig. 1. A: Schematic representation of the mEGF molecule. The putative receptor-combining site is represented by squares (adapted from Savage et al., 1973). B: Amino acid sequences of mouse EGF (mEGF), human EGF (hEGF), rat TGFα (rTGF) and the vaccinia virus early protein P19 (VVP19). Amino acids common in all four sequences are boxed. Deletions of amino acids to obtain optimal alignment are represented by a hyphen. The putative combining region is underlined. Single-letter amino acid abbreviations are used: A = Ala; C = Cys; D = Asp; E = Glu; F = Phe; G = Gly; H = His; I = Ile; K = Lys; L = Leu; M = Met; N = Asn; P = Pro; Q = Gln; R = Arg; S = Ser; T = Thr; V = Val; W = Trp; Y = Tyr.

ary structure of the EGFs through formation of disulfide bridges (Savage et al., 1973). Holladay et al. (1976) have constructed a space-filling model of the mouse EGF molecule. This model, based on the study of the unfolding thermodynamics and thermal stability of EGF, predicts a compact globular structure that is thermodynamically very stable.

The physiological role and the tissue distribution of EGF are still rather elusive. Rich sources for the factor are excretion products like urine, saliva, sweat and milk. The richest source found so far is human urine, which contains microgram quantities of EGF (Dailey et al., 1978). EGF has been found in a variety of tissues, but only in very low concentrations. A recent study by Kasselberg et al. (1985) has confirmed and extended the work of others. Using the immunostaining PAP method, EGF-like material was found in tissues such as placenta, kidney, stomach, bone marrow, submandibular gland and duodenum. In two other studies, EGF was found in human cerebrospinal fluid (Hirata et al., 1982) and in fore- and midbrain structures of the rat (Fallon et al., 1984). The variety of tissues in which EGF is found leads to the proposition that it has no single tissue source (Kasselberg et al., 1985) and that it exerts multiple functions, depending on the nature of the target tissue. EGF can thus function as growth stimulating and/or differentiation inducing agent in fetal development (Thornburn et al., 1985) and wound healing (EGF is tightly associated with blood platelets; Oka and Orth, 1983), and as neurotransmitter/neuromodulator substance in the central nervous system (Fallon et al., 1984).

Biosynthesis of EGF

Recent investigations into the biosynthesis of EGF have yielded some unexpected and exciting results. EGF can be isolated from mouse submaxillary glands as part of a high molecular weight complex, in which two EGF molecules are bound to a trypsin-like, arginine esteropeptidase-active binding protein (EGF-BP) (Taylor et al., 1970). It was proposed that EGF is synthesized as a large pro-EGF molecule which is turned into the biologically active form through cleavage by its binding protein. Such a pro-EGF molecule was isolated from mouse submaxillar glands by Frey et al. (1979). It was isolated using an anti-EGF antiserum, and has a molecular mass of 9 kDa. Even larger pro-EGF molecules have been found in human urine (Hirata and Orth, 1979). Recent investigations using molecular cloning techniques have shown that EGF is synthesized as part of a large precursor with a molecular mass of 128–133 kDa. In addition to EGF this so-called prepro-EGF molecule (Scott et al., 1983) contains eight EGF-related sequences, which upon degradation of prepro-EGF could yield other biologically active polypeptides. Pro-EGF is possibly an intermediate cleavage product from prepro-EGF (Gray et al., 1983; Scott et al., 1983). Interestingly, the precursor has all the properties of a plasma membrane-spanning protein. Moreover, there is a significant amino acid sequence homology between prepro-EGF and the low density lipoprotein (LDL) receptor (Russell et al., 1984; Yamamoto et al., 1984), while a structural homology between prepro-EGF, the LDL receptor and the human EGF receptor is reflected in repetitive cysteine-rich sequences, a feature which is thought to give membrane receptors a rigid three-dimensional structure (Ullrich et al., 1984). It could thus well be that prepro-EGF not only functions as EGF precursor but also as a transmembrane receptor molecule (Pfeffer and Ullrich, 1985). Another implication from the fact that EGF is contained within a membrane-anchored protein, is that it could exert its signaling function in situ, by direct interaction with receptors in neighboring cells. There is, however, no evidence yet for such an interaction. The distribution of prepro-EGF has been investigated (Rall et al., 1985) in various adult mouse tissues. The authors report a high abundance in the submaxillar gland, but also in the kidney. In fact, the amount in the latter tissues is only 2 times lower than in the former. The abundance of EGF, however, is 2000 times less in the kidney than in the submaxillar gland. It thus seems that prepro-EGF is not processed to EGF in the kidney. The reason for this is unclear. The relative abundance of prepro-EGF in other tissues is rather low, but the number of tissues where the molecule is found is extensive, again indicating that EGF has no single source, and probably acts only locally.

EGF–EGF receptor binding

Not much is known about the way in which EGF interacts with its specific membrane receptor. Komoriya et al. (1984), using synthetic peptides, have identified the putative receptor combining site of EGF (see Fig. 1A), which is claimed to be cysteine residue number 20 to cysteine residue number 31. αTGF (see above) competes with EGF for binding to the receptor (De Larco, 1978). Comparison of the primary amino acid sequence of αTGF (Marquardt et al., 1983) with that of EGF reveals a significant homology between both factors. Surprisingly, however, the homology in the putative binding region is restricted to the two terminal cysteine residues only in case of mEGF and to an additional 2 residues in case of hEGF (Fig. 1B). So, either αTGFs bind in a different manner to the receptor and compete with EGF due to steric hindrance, or they do bind to the receptor in a way analogous to EGF. In the latter case, it is conceivable that the three-dimensional structure of the ligands, which due to the 100% alignment of the cysteine residues is probably almost identical, determines the specificity of the binding to the receptor.

Using computer analysis of protein sequence data, three groups independently reported the existence of EGF-homologous sequences in several proteins (Blomquist et al., 1984; Brown et al., 1985, Reisner, 1985). One of these proteins, the vaccinia virus 19-kDa protein (VVP19), which is transcribed from the virus genome early after infection, is included in Fig. 1B. Again there is 100% homology with respect to the localization of the cysteine residues. Twardzik et al. (1985) have found that vaccinia virus-infected cells release an acid-stable 25-kDa polypeptide, which competes with EGF for binding to the EGF receptor and is mitogenic for receptor-bearing cells. It is not clear yet whether the VVP19 polypeptide and the 25-kDa polypeptide are identical, but several experimental data support this contention. This could thus be another example of a polypeptide capable of interacting with the EGF receptor, which has

only its three-dimensional structure in common with the 'natural' ligand EGF.

EGF receptor; structural aspects

The first evidence that EGF binds in a specific saturable manner to a cellular receptor came from EGF binding studies on human fibroblasts (Hollenberg and Cuatracasas, 1973). The finding of Fabricant et al. (1977) that the human epidermoid carcinoma line A431 possesses an extraordinary amount of EGF veceptors (2×10^6/cell) and thus provide an excellent source to study receptor structure and function, resulted in numerous attempts to characterize the receptor molecule. ^{125}I-EGF cross-linking experiments and sodium dodecyl sulfate gel electrophoresis analysis showed the molecular mass of the receptor to be between 145 and 190 kDa (Das et al., 1977; Sayhoun et al., 1978; Baker et al., 1979; Hock et al., 1979; Linsley et al., 1979; Wrann and Fox, 1979). Cohen et al. (1980) purified the receptor from A431 plasma membrane preparations using an EGF affinity column. They found a major band of 150 kDa in their gels, and a minor band of 170 kDa. It turned out later (Cassel and Glaser, 1982; Gates and King, 1982) that the native receptor is represented by the latter band and that the conversion of the 170 kDa to the 150 kDa form is due to the proteolytic action of a Ca^{2+}-sensitive protease present in the membrane preparation. Metabolic labeling of newly synthesized receptor in the presence of tunicamycin, an inhibitor of N-linked glycosylation, showed that the receptor is heavily glycosylated (Mangelsdorf-Soderquist and Carpenter, 1984) and that the protein core of the receptor has a molecular mass of 130 kDa.

A very important finding concerning the function of the EGF receptor came from Carpenter et al. (1979). They found that membrane preparations of A431 cells, upon treatment with EGF, incorporated three times more $^{32}P_i$ into endogenous membrane proteins when $[\gamma\text{-}^{32}P]ATP$ was used as phosphate donor. It was shown by King et al. (1980) that the receptor itself is a major substrate for this EGF-stimulated kinase activity (autophosphorylation). Purification of the EGF receptor on an EGF affinity column did not lead to separation of the tyrosine kinase from the EGF binding activity, suggesting that these two features reside in the same molecule. Hunter and Cooper (1981) reported that the kinase phosphorylates proteins on tyrosine residues. This was a very intriguing finding, since it was already known that tyrosine phosphorylation is also linked to the mitogenic action of pp60[src], the transforming protein of the Rous sarcoma virus (RSV) (Hunter and Sefton, 1980). It is now clear that tyrosine kinase activity is linked to transformation by a number of acutely oncogenic retroviruses as well as to the mitogenic action of a number of other growth factor receptor systems. (For a review covering both topics see Hunter and Cooper, 1985.) The latter include the PDGF receptor (Ek et al., 1982), the insulin receptor (Kasuga et al., 1981) and the insulin like growth factor-1 (IGF-1) receptor (Rubin et al., 1983).

The first step in unraveling the receptor's primary structure was taken by Downward et al. (1984), who sequenced a set of six tryptic peptides derived from affinity purified human EGF receptor. The sources of receptors were human placenta and A431 plasma membranes. Based on these sequences, Ullrich et al. (1984) prepared synthetic oligonucleotides to screen a human cDNA library. From several overlapping cDNA clones the entire nucleotide sequence of the cDNA coding for the receptor could be deduced. Parts of these sequences were confirmed independently by two other groups (Xu et al., 1984; Lin et al., 1984) using different procedures.

From the sequence data, the following picture of the receptor emerges (Fig. 2). The receptor consists of a single chain of 1186 amino acids, which crosses the plasma membrane only once. A short stretch of 23 predominantly hydrophobic amino acids traverses the membrane. The NH_2-terminus of the receptor contains the extracellular binding domain for EGF and is heavily glycosylated. Furthermore, it contains two cysteine-rich regions, which can be aligned and which probably give the external part of the receptor a rigid, two-lobal structure (Hunter, 1984). The internal, COOH-terminal part of the receptor contains the tyrosine kinase activity. It displays extensive homology with the v-erb B oncogene of avian

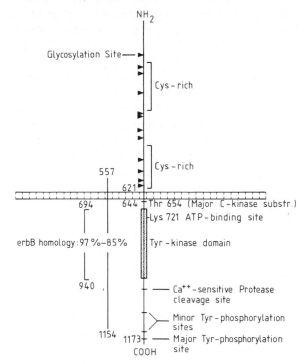

Fig. 2. Highly schematic linear representation of the EGF receptor structure. The horizontal hatched bar represents the plasma membrane. The numbers indicate individual amino acids according to the numbering system proposed by Ullrich et al. (1984). For further details see text.

erythroblastosis virus (AEV). In the kinase domain, this homology is as high as 97%. This has led to the hypothesis that the transforming activity of the v-erb B product is due to the expression of a truncated EGF receptor-like molecule in the plasma membrane. In this view, the extracellular EGF binding domain is thought to act as a regulator for the intracellular tyrosine kinase activity. Because the erb B product lacks this control, it is constantly activated, and therefore transforms the cell in which it is expressed (Downward et al., 1984). It has recently been shown that the v-erb B product indeed has a tyrosine kinase activity (Gilmore et al., 1985) and that it is present at the cell surface of AEV-infected rat-1 cells (Hayman and Beug, 1984). Several other features of the intracellular part of the receptor are depicted in Fig. 2. Lysine residue 721 lies within the ATP binding site of the receptor (Russo et al., 1985). The indicated threonine residue on position 654 is a substrate for protein kinase C (see below). Phosphorylation of this residue (Hunter et al., 1984; Davis and Czech, 1985) decreases the EGF affinity and lowers the tyrosine kinase activity (Cochet et al., 1984; Fearn and King, 1985), which could function as a regulatory feedback mechanism in the growth factor-signaling pathway. The most extensively autophosphorylated tyrosine residue (number 1173) on the receptor is found in the Ca^{2+}-sensitive protein cleavable (terminal part of the receptor). Whether autophosphorylation of the receptor is necessary for its function is not clear yet. Receptor preparations of which the COOH-terminus lacks due to proteolytic cleavage are still active as a protein kinase (Chinkers and Brugge, 1984). Hunter and Cooper (1985) favor a model in which the C-terminal 20 kDa part acts as a tyrosine kinase regulating moiety, which upon phosphorylation due to EGF binding leaves the kinase accessible to other substrates. That autophosphorylation of the receptor in an intramolecular reaction was reported by two groups (Biswas et al., 1985; Weber et al., 1984). Based on in vitro studies, using solubilized and purified receptor preparations, the first group conclude that the regulation of receptor kinase activity occurs via an equilibrium shift due to EGF, from a dimeric, inactive form to a monomeric, active form of the receptor kinase. However, how this model fits within the widely accepted view that EGF causes receptor clustering (see below) in unclear.

Signal transduction

The biological action of EGF is initiated by its binding to the EGF receptor. Typically, EGF shows saturation binding within 1 h at 37°C, after which the binding capacity of the cells gradually decreases (down regulation). Carpenter and Cohen (1976) were the first to postulate that, subsequent to the initial binding of EGF, the EGF receptor complex is internalized, after which the ligand is being degraded in the lysosomes. This process of receptor-mediated ligand endocytosis is a common property of polypeptide hormones (for reviews see

Pastan and Willingham, 1981a,b). Several methods have been applied to monitor the fate of the EGF receptor complex. In each case EGF was shown to bind to dispersed mobile receptors on the cell surface followed by aggregation of the EGF–receptor complexes into regions coated with a specific protein, clathrin (Gordon et al., 1978; Schlessinger et al., 1978; Haigler et al., 1979). This process of patching or macroclustering is temperature-dependent and energy-independent and occurs within 10–15 min at 37°C. It is followed by temperature- and energy-dependent endocytosis in clathrin-coated vesicles. Evidence exists that rapid microclustering of a limited number of EGF–receptor complexes precedes the above microclustering (Zidovetzki et al., 1981), and it has been suggested that the microclustering of receptors is required and sufficient for the induction of DNA synthesis (Schechter et al., 1979; Schreiber et al., 1981). This latter notion has been questioned recently (Defize et al., submitted).

Early responses

How EGF–receptor interaction leads to mitogenic stimulation is still poorly understood. In attempting to unravel the signal transduction machinery, most attention has been given to the analysis of the earliest receptor-mediated responses. Interestingly, these early responses are very similar for the various growth factors, which suggests that common molecular pathways are utilized in reaching the ultimate biological effect.

The EGF receptor, like many other growth factor receptors, shows tyrosine-specific protein kinase activity (Ushiro and Cohen, 1980; for a recent review see Hunter and Cooper, 1985). EGF binding induces a rapid stimulation of receptor kinase activity, which results in autophosphorylation of the receptor itself at several tyrosine residues, as well as in the phosphorylation of exogenous substrates (see above). So far, no function has yet been established for any of the phosphorylated substrate molecules, nor for the autophosphorylation reaction. It is also unclear whether the enhanced tyrosine phosphorylation is required for mitogenic stimulation, but recent studies from our laboratory indicate that it is certainly not a sufficient trigger for the induction of DNA synthesis (see below).

A common feature of many agonists of membrane receptors is their ability to induce the breakdown of phospoinositides in the plasma membrane (for recent reviews see Berridge and Irvine, 1984; Nishizuka, 1984; Hokin, 1985). In animal cells, inositol-containing phosphatides comprise less than 10% of the total phospholipid. Two phosphorylated forms of phosphatidyl inositol (PI) can be found in the plasma membrane, i.e. phosphatidyl inositol 4-phosphate (PIP) and phosphatidyl inositol 4,5-biphosphate (PIP$_2$). It is generally accepted that agonist activation of membrane receptors stimulates the hydrolysis of these phosphoinositides, which results in the production of second messengers. In this general scheme, binding of the agonist to its receptors stimulates PIP$_2$ cleavage by phospholipase C through some unknown mechanisms. As a result inositol 4,4,5-triphosphate (IP$_3$) and 1,2-diacylglycerol (DG) are produced, which both serve as second messengers. IP$_3$ is an effective mobilizer of cytoplasmic Ca^{2+} (Ca_i^{2+}), probably from stores such as the endoplasmic reticulum (Berridge and Irvine, 1984). DG is a potent activator of the Ca^{2+}- and phospholipid-dependent protein kinase C which phosphorylates proteins at serine and threonine residues. Importantly, phorbol ester tumor promotors such as 12-O-tetradecanoyl-phorbol-13-acetate (TPA) bear a structural similarity to DG and mimic DG in stimulating protein kinase C (Nishizuka, 1984). This feature can be used experimentally to bypass certain receptor-mediated responses.

The evidence implicating phosphoinositides in the action of growth factors is limited and rather circumstantial, but so far the data are consistent with the above scheme. Sawyer and Cohen (1981) have shown that EGF stimulates PI turnover and the production of DG, and the same holds for PDGF (Habenicht et al., 1981). Consequently, it might be expected that protein kinase C activity will be enhanced by EGF. Evidence hereto has been obtained by comparing the effects of EGF and TPA on receptor phosphorylation as well as on other secondary responses. In vitro, purified protein kinase C preparations will phosphorylate the EGF receptor at a threonine residue (Thr654) which is located nine amino acids from the membrane on the cytoplasmic domain of the receptor (see above). The same threonine becomes phosphorylated when cells are exposed to tumor promotors or to EGF (Cochet et al., 1984; Decker, 1984; Iwashita and Fox, 1984). Thus, it seems likely that the interaction between EGF and its receptor leads to phosphoinositide breakdown, DG production and protein kinase C activation, which in turn causes phosphorylation of the EGF receptor. This feedback mechanism may have a role in the modulation of receptor activity since the phosphorylation of the receptor at Thr654 is associated with a reduction in its tyrosine kinase activity (Cochet et al., 1984; Friedman et al., 1984) and tumor promotors reduce the EGF binding capacity of cells (Lee and Weinstein, 1978; Shoyab et al., 1979). Together, there studies indicate that phosphorylation of the EGF receptor by protein kinase C is an important modulator of the conformation of the receptor molecule, as it affects both the extracellular domain (binding capacity) as well as the cytoplasmic catalytic domain.

An alternative line of evidence for the involvement of phosphoinositide breakdown comes from studies on the generation of ionic signals by growth factors (see De Laat et al., 1984, 1985; Moolenaar et al., 1986). Such signals are among the earliest detectable mitogen-induced responses in quiescent cells. Generally, growth factors, including EGF, activate a plasma membrane-bound, electroneutral Na^+/H^+ exchanger. The extrusion of protons leads to a rapid alkalinization of the cytoplasm, while the concomitant influx of Na^+ stimulates the Na^+,K^+-ATPase activity as a secondary response (Moolenaar et al., 1981, 1983, 1984a; Schuldiner and Rozengurt, 1982; Cassel et al., 1983; l'Allemain et al., 1984). Evidence has been given that growth factors raise cytoplasmic pH (pH_i) by increasing the sensitivity of the Na^+/H^+ exchanger to intracellular H^+, possibly by inducing a conformational change at the intracellular H^+-binding modifier site (Moolenaar et al., 1983). More recent experiments have implicated protein kinase C in this action (Moolenaar et al., 1984a): TPA as well as the DG derivative 1-oleoyl-2-acetyl-glycerol (OAG) can mimic growth factors in activating Na^+/H^+ exchange and raising pH_i. The simplest model to explain these observations is that upon EGF receptor interaction, the Na^+/H^+ exchanger becomes phosphorylated by protein kinase C, as a result of phosphoinositide breakdown and DG production, and that thereby its apparent affinity for intracellular H^+ is increased (Moolenaar et al., 1984a). Further studies will be needed to verify this hypothesis.

Besides pH_i, intracellular Ca^{2+} (Ca_i^{2+}) appears to be involved in the signal transduction by growth factors. Using the intracellularly trapped fluorescent Ca^{2+} indicator quin-2, it was found that EGF and PDGF induce a rapid but transient increase in Ca_i^{2+} (Moolenaar et al., 1984a,b). This two- to three-fold increase in Ca_i^{2+} represents one of the fastest cellular responses to mitogenic stimulation; it is detectable within 1 s and reaches its maximum within 30–60 s after growth factor addition. While TPA mimicks growth factors in activating Na^+/H^+ exchange, it has no effect on Ca_i^{2+}. This demonstrates that these ionic signal pathways are dissociable (Moolenaar et al., 1984a,b). These observations are consistent with the concept that Ca_i^{2+} mobilization is caused by IP_3 production, while the activation of Na^+/H^+ exchange is connected to the other branch of phosphoinositide breakdown, i.e. DG production and protein kinase C stimulation. Clearly, this concept needs further verification, in particular by detailed analysis of the phosphoinositide metabolism in growth factor-stimulated cells.

As described above, the partial activation of growth factor receptor-mediated responses by tumor promotors has been a fruitful approach in establishing interrelationships among these events. An alternative tool for the dissociation of molecular events in the mitogenic signaling cascade is given by the availability of monoclonal antibodies against the EGF receptor. Recently, we have raised such antibodies (IgGs) against different epitopes of the extracellular domain of the human EGF receptor (Defize et al., submitted), and we have tested three of these, denoted 2E9, 2D11 and

TABLE I

Comparison of the effects of EGF and anti-EGF receptor monoclonal antibodies 2E9, 2D11 and 2G5

	EGF	2E9	2D11	2G5
Precipitation of EGF receptor		+	+	+
EGF binding competition	+	+	–	–
Stimulation of tyrosine kinase	+	+	+	–
Activation of Na^+/H^+ exchange	+	–	–	–
Rise in Ca_i^{2+}	+	–	–	–
Stimulation of DNA synthesis	+	–	–	–

2G5, for their capacity to mimic or to modulate some charactistic EGF-dependent cellular responses including mitogenicity, stimulation of tyrosine kinase activity, cytoplasmic alkalinization and Ca_i^{2+} mobilization (Defize et al., 1986). All three antibodies were able to immunoprecipitate a functional EGF receptor showing EGF-dependent tyrosine kinase activity. 2E9 is so far unique in that it is directed against a peptide determinant at or very close to the EGF binding domain of the receptor. Consequently, 2E9 competitively inhibits ^{125}I-EGF binding to human cells. In contrast, 2D11 and 2G5 recognize bloodgroup A-related carbohydrate structures on the EGF receptor and fail to affect EGF binding.

As summarized in Table I, these antibodies could be used as partial agonists of the EGF receptor. Whereas 2E9 and 2D11 were able to mimic EGF in stimulating tyrosine kinase activity of the EGF receptor in a variety of human cells, both in vivo and in vitro. 2G5 had no such effects. Although minor differences were observed in the rate of substrate phosphorylation induced by EGF, 2E9 and 2D11, respectively, this finding demonstrates that phosphorylation of tyrosine residues at the receptor itself, as well as at other proteins, can be induced by ligands other than EGF, and that the stimulation of the receptor tyrosine kinase does not necessarily involve the EGF binding domain. Very interestingly, none of the antibodies was able to mimic EGF in its ability to raise pH_i or to mobilize Ca_i^{2+}, but 2E9 could inhibit the effect of EGF on Ca_i^{2+}, as expected for a competitive ligand. This implies (by inference) that phosphoinositide breakdown can be dissociated from the stimulation of receptor tyrosine kinase activation. The antibodies were also unable to induce DNA synthesis in quiescent human fibroblasts. Stimulation of tyrosine kinase activity is apparently insufficient to elicit a mitogenic response (for further details see Defize et al., submitted). Whether or not the same holds for phosphoinositide-mediated cellular responses remains to be shown.

Control of growth factor action during neuronal differentiation

Polypeptide growth factors show cell type specificity in their action. This implies that during development different cell lineages acquire specific susceptibilities for the action of different growth factors. In addition it is recognized that during terminal differentiation, such as neuronal differentiation, cells lose their capacity for division, and thus their susceptibility for growth factor action (De Laat et al., 1983). Neuroblastoma cells have been used extensively for studying the regulation of neuronal differentiation in vitro and the emergence of the differentiated phenotype is characteristically associated with an arrest of the cells in the G1 phase of the cell cycle.

Recent studies from our laboratory have used the N1E-115 murine neuroblastoma cell line to study the control of growth factor action during neuronal differentiation. Under conventional culture conditions, serum deprivation is a sufficient stimulus to induce neurite outgrowth in N1E-115 cells. The cells respond to serum removal with a gradual decrease in the rate of DNA synthesis and cessation of cell division within 24–48 h, accompanied by a flattening of the cell body and the formation of thin neurites. Re-addition of serum to such cultures during the initial period of differentiation results in retraction of the neurites, rounding up of the cells, and a synchronous reinitiation of DNA synthesis after 8–10 h (Moolenaar et al., 1981). However, as cells proceed further along the differentiation pathway, their ability to re-enter the growth cycle is gradually abolished (Mummery et al., 1983). N1E-115 cells can also be maintained in a chemically defined serum-free medium supplemented with insulin and EGF. Under these conditions differentiation can be induced by the deletion of these polypeptides from the medium, indicating that growth factors act merely as suppressors of differentiation for these committed cells (Van der Saag et al., submitted). A similar mechanism has been proposed for primary neural crest cells (Ziller et al., 1983).

^{125}I-EGF binding studies have revealed that the loss of mitogenic ability in differentiating N1E-115 cells is correlated with a decrease in EGF binding capacity (Mummery et al., 1983). Depending on the culture condition, the number of EGF receptors per cell is reduced by a factor of 2 to 4 within 48 h of differentiation. As an example: cells growing exponentially in defined serum-free medium have 17 000 EGF receptors at their cell surface. This number is reduced to 8 500 within 48 h of deletion of insulin and EGF. Similar observations have been reported on EGF receptor expression during neuronal differentiation of rat pheochromocytoma cells (Huff et al., 1983). This provides a simple mechanism for the observed loss of susceptibility to growth factor action during neuronal differentiation.

How is the level of EGF receptor expression controlled during differentiation? A possible clue to this problem came from the observation that the decrease in EGF binding capacity coincides with profound alterations in plasma membrane lipid organization, in particular an increase in cholesterol content due to enhanced sterol biosynthesis. Subsequently, the rate of sterol biosynthesis was modulated experimentally, by the addition of 25-OH-cholesterol, a specific inhibitor of HMG-CoA reductase, the rate limiting enzyme of sterol biosynthesis. When applied to differentiating N1E-115 cells, 25-OH-cholesterol suppressed sterol biosynthesis and decreased plasma membrane cholesterol content. As a consequence, neurite outgrowth as well as the loss of EGF receptors were completely blocked, these effects being counteracted by the simultaneous addition of mevalonate, the product of the 25-OH-cholesterol–inhibited HMG-CoA reductase (Van der Saag et al., submitted). These results provide evidence for an essential role of sterol biosynthesis and plasma membrane cholesterol content in the acquisition of the neuronal phenotype, and the loss of proliferative ability in differentiating N1E-115 cells. They also suggest that sterol biosynthesis is under the control of growth factor receptor-mediated signals, possibly through dephosphorylation/phosphorylation of HMG-CoA reductase.

Conclusion

In recent years great advances have been made in the characterization of the molecules involved in the control of cell growth, transformation and differentiation. Nevertheless, we are still far from understanding the mechanisms by which these molecules, such as growth factors, exert their action. As knowledge increases, the complicated nature of the cellular signals generated by the activation of membrane receptors becomes more evident. The apparent intimate relationship between growth factor action and the action of oncogene products and tumor promotors will certainly stimulate further multidisciplinary studies in this field. Even less is known about the developmental regulation of growth-controling mechanism, but the extension of studies like the ones described on neuroblastoma cells might be a first step in gaining further insight. It will be a challenge for future research to characterize in detail the intermediate events between growth factor receptor activation and the control of DNA replication and cell division, and to understand how growth factor production and regulation of receptor expression are involved in the control of cell differentiation and transformation.

Acknowledgements

We thank our colleagues Drs. W.H. Moolenaar, C.L. Mummery, P.T. van der Saag and E.J.J. van Zoelen for their contributions, and Ms. E.J.G.M. Hak for preparing the manuscripts. This work was supported in part by the Koningin Wilhelmina Fonds (Netherlands Cancer Foundation).

References

Baker, J.B., Simmer, R.L., Glenn, K.C. and Cunningham. D.D. (1979) Thrombin and epidermal growth factor become linked to cell surface receptors during mitogenic stimulation. *Nature*, 278:743–745.

Berridge, M.J. and Irvine, R.F. (1984) Inositol triphosphate, a novel second messenger in cellular signal transduction. *Nature*, 312:315–321.

Biswas, R., Basu, M., Sen-Majumdar, A. and Das, M. (1985) Intrapeptide autophosphorylation of the epidermal growth factor receptor: regulation of kinase catalytic function by receptor dimerization. *Biochemistry*, 24:3795–3802.

Blomquist, M.C., Hunt, L.T. and Barker, W.C. (1984) Vaccinia virus 19 kilodalton protein: Relationship to several mammalian proteins, including two growth factors. *Proc. Natl. Acad. Sci. U.S.A.*, 81:7363–7367.

Brown, J.P., Twardzik, D.R., Marquardt, H. and Todaro, G.J. (1985) Vaccina virus encodes a polypeptide homologous to epidermal growth factor and transforming growth factor. *Nature*, 313:491–492.

Carpenter, G. and Cohen, S. (1976) ^{125}I-labeled human epidermal growth factor (EGF(: binding, internalization and degradation in human fibroblasts. *J. Cell Biol.*, 71:159–171.

Carpenter, G., King, L. and Cohen, S. (1979) Rapid enhancement of protein phosphorylation in A431 cell membrane preparations by epidermal growth factor. *J. Biol. Chem.*, 254:4884–4891.

Cassel, D. and Glaser, L. (1982) Proteolytic cleavage of epidermal growth factor receptor. A Ca^{++} dependent, sulfhydryl-sensitive proteolytic system in A431 cells. *J. Biol. Chem.*, 257:9845–9848.

Cassel, D., Rothenberg, P., Zhuang, Y.-X., Deuel, T.F. and Glaser, L. (1983) Platelet-derived growth factor stimulates Na^+/H^+ exchange and induces cytoplasmic alkalinization in NR6 cells. *Proc. Natl. Acad. Sci. U.S.A.* 80:6224–6228.

Chinkers, M. and Brugge, J.S. (1984) Characterization of structural domains of the human epidermal growth factor receptor obtained by partial proteolysis. *J. Biol. Chem.*, 259:11534–11542.

Cochet, C., Gill, G.N., Meisenhelder, J., Cooper, J.A. and Hunter, T. (1984) C-kinase phosphorylates the epidermal growth factor receptor and reduces its epidermal growth factor stimulated tyrosine protein kinase activity. *J. Biol. Chem.*, 259:2553–2558.

Cohen, S. (1959) Purification and metabolic effects of a nerve growth promoting protein from snake venom. *J. Biol. Chem.*, 234:1129–1137.

Cohen, S. (1962) Isolation of a mouse submaxillary gland protein accelerating incisor eruption and eyelid opening in the newborn animal. *J. Biol. Chem.*, 237:1555–1562.

Cohen, S. (1965) The stimulation of epidermal proliferation by a specific protein (EGF). *Dev. Biol.*, 12:394–407.

Cohen, S., Carpenter, G. and King, L. Jr. (1980) Epidermal Growth Factor receptor protein kinase interactions. Copurification of receptor and epidermal growth factor-enhanced phosphorylation activity. *J. Biol. Chem.*, 255:4834–4842.

Dailey, G.E., Kraus, J.W. and Orth, D.N. (1978) Homologous radioimmunoassay for human epidermal growth factor (urogastrone). *J. Clin. Endocrinol. Metab.*, 46:929–935.

Das, M., Miyakawa, T., Fox, C.F., Pruss, R.M., Aharonov, A. and Herschmann, H.R. (1977) Specific radiolabeling of a cell surface receptor for epidermal growth factor. *Proc. Natl. Acad. Sci. U.S.A.*, 74:2790–2794.

Davis, R.J. and Czech, M.P. (1985) Tumor-promoting phorbol esters cause the phosphorylation of epidermal growth factor receptors in normal human fibroblasts at throenine-654. *Proc. Natl. Acad. Sci. U.S.A.*, 82:1974–1978.

Decker, S.J. (1984) Effects of epidermal growth factor and 12-O-tetradecanoylphorbol-13-acetate on metabolism of the epidermal growth factor receptor in normal human fibroblasts. *Mol. Cell Biol.*, 4:1718–1724.

De Laat, S.W., Boonstra, J., Moolenaar, W.H., Mummery, C.L., van der Saag. P.T. and Van Zoelen, E.J.J. (1983) The plasma membrane as the primary target for the action of growth factors and tumour promoters in development. In M.H. Johnson (Ed.), *Development in Mammals, Vol. 5*, Elsevier, Amsterdam, pp. 33–106.

Defize, L.H.K., Moolenaar, W.N., Van der Saag, P.T. and De Laat, S.W. (1986) Dissociation of cellular responses to epidermal growth factor using anti-receptor monoclonal antibodies. *EMBO J.*, 5:1187–1192.

De Laat, S.W., Boonstra, J., Moolenaar, W.H. and Mummery, C.L. (1984) Growth factor action and ionic signal transduction: Characterization and relation to receptor expression. In G. Guroff (Ed.), *Growth and Maturation Factors, Vol. 3*, John Wiley & Sons, New York, pp. 219–250.

De Laat, S.W., Moolenaar, W.H., Defize, L.H.K., Boonstra, J. and Van der Saag, P.T. (1985) Ionic signal transduction in growth factor action. *Biochem. Soc. Symp.* 50:205–220.

De Larco, J.E. and Todaro, G.J. (1978) Growth factors from murine sarcoma virus-transformed cells. *Proc. Natl. Acad. Sci. U.S.A.*, 75:4001–4005.

Doolittle, R.F., Hunkapiller, H.W., Hood, L.E., Devare, S.G., Robbins, K.C., Aaronson, S.A. and Antoniades, H.N. (1983) Simian sarcoma virus onc gene, v-sis, is derived from the gene (or genes) encoding a platelet-derived growth factor. *Science*, 221:275–277.

Downward, J., Yarden, Y., Mayes, E., Scrace, G., Totty, N., Stockwell, P., Ullrich, A., Schlessinger, J. and Waterfield, M.D. (1984) Close similarity of epidermal growth factor receptor and v-erb-B oncogene protein sequences. *Nature*, 307:521–527.

Ek, B., Westermark, B., Wasteson, A. and Heldin, C.-H. (1982) Stimulation of tyrosine-specific phosphorylation by platelet-derived growth factor. *Nature*, 295:419–420.

Fabricant, R.N., De Larco, J.E. and Todaro, G.J. (1977) Nerve growth factor receptors on human melanoma cells in culture. *Proc. Natl. Acad. Sci. U.S.A.*, 74:565–569.

Fallon, J.H., Scroogy, K.B., Loughlin, S.W., Morrison, R.S., Bradshaw, R.A., Knauer, D.J. and Cunningham, D.D. (1984) Epidermal Growth Factor immunoreactive material in the central nervous system: location and development. *Science*, 224:1107–1109.

Fearn, J.C. and King, A.C. (1985) EGF receptor affinity is regulated by intracellular calcium and protein kinase C. *Cell*, 40:991–1000.

Frey, P., Forand, R., Maciag, T. and Shooter, E.M. (1979) The biosynthetic precursor of epidermal growth factor and the mechanism of tis processing. *Proc. Natl. Acad. Sci. U.S.A.*, 76:6294–6298.

Friedman, B., Frackelton, A.R., Ross, A.H., Connors, J.M., Fujiki, H., Sugimura, T. and Rosner, M.R. (1984) Tumor promoters block tyrosine-specific phosphorylation of the epidermal growth factor receptor. *Proc. Natl. Acad. Sci. U.S.A.*, 81:3034–3038.

Gates, R.E. and King, L.E. Jr., (1982) Calcium facilitates endogenous protyeolysis of the EGF receptor-kinase. *Mol. Cell. Endocrinol.*, 27:263–276.

Gilmore, T., DE Clue, J.E. and Martin, G.S. (1985) Protein phosphorylation at tyrosine is induced by the v-erb B gene product in vivo and in vitro. *Cell*, 40:609–618.

Gordon, P., Carpentier, J.L., Cohen, S. and Orci, L. (1978) Epidermal growth factor: morphological demonstration of binding, internalization, and lysosomal association in human fibroblasts. *Proc. Natl. Acad. Sci. U.S.A.*, 75:5025–5029.

Gray, A., Dull, T.J. and Ullrich, A. (1983) Nucleotide sequence of epidermal growth factor cDNA predicts a 128,000 molecular weight protein precursor. *Nature*, 303:722–725.

Gregory, H. (1975) Isolation and structure of urogastrone and its relationship to epidermal growth factor. *Nature*, 257:325–327.

Habenicht, A.J.R., Glomset, J.A., King, W.C., Nist, C., Mitchell, C.D. and Ross, R. (1981) Early changes in phosphatidyl inositol and arachidonic acid metabolism in quiescent Swiss 3T3 cells stimulated to divide by platelet-derived growth factor. *J. Biol. Chem.*, 256:12329–12335.

Haigler, H.T., McKanna, J.A. and Cohen, S. (1979) Direct visualization of the binding and internalization of a ferritin conjugate of epidermal growth factor in human carcinoma cells A431. *J. Cell Biol.* 81:382–395.

Hayman, M.J. and Beug, H. (1984) Identification of a form of the avian erythrosblastosis virus erb B gene product at the cell surface. *Nature*, 309:460–462.

Heath, J.K. and Isacke, C.M. (1984) PC13 embryonal carcinoma-derived growth factor. *EMBO Journal*, 3:2957–2962.

Hirata, Y. and Orth, D.N. (1979) Epidermal growth factor (Urogastrone) in human fluids: Size Heterogeneity. *J. Clinic. Endocrinol. Metab.*, 48:673–679.

Hirata, Y., Uchihashi, M., Nakayima, H., Fujita, T. and Matsuhurn, S. (1982) Presence of human epidermal growth factor in human cerebrospinal fluid. *J. Clin. Endocrinol. Metab.*, 55:1174–1179.

Hock, R.A., Nexö, E. and Hollenberg, M.D. (1979 Isolation of the human placenta receptor for epidermal growth factor-urogastrone. *Nature*, 277:403–405.

Holladay, L.A., Savage, C.R. Jr., Cohen, S. and Puett, D. (1976) Conformation and unfolding thermodynamics of Epidermal Growth Factor and derivatives. *Biochemistry*, 15:2624–2633.

Hollenberg, M.D. and Cuatracasas, P. (1973) Epidermal growth factor: receptors in human fibroblasts and modulation of action by cholera toxin. *Proc. Natl. Acad. Sci. U.S.A.*, 70:2964–2968.

Hokin, L.E. (1985) Receptors and phosphoinositide-generated second messengers. *Annu. Rev. Biochem.*, 54:205–235.

Huff, K., End, D. and Guroff, G. (1981) Nerve growth factor-induced alterations in the response of PC12 pheochromocytoma cells to epidermal growth factor. *J. Cell Biol.*, 88:189–198.

Hunter, T. (1984) The epidermal growth factor receptor gene and its product. *Nature, News and Views*, 311:414–415.

Hunter, T. and Cooper, J.A. (1981) Epidermal growth factor induces rapid tyrosine phosphorylation of proteins in A431 human tumor cells. *Cell*, 24: 741–752.

Hunter, T. and Cooper, J.A. (1985) Protein-tyrosine kinases. *Annu. Rev. Biochem.*, 54:897–930.

Hunter, T. and Sefton, B.M. (1980) Transforming gene product of Rous sarcoma virus phosphorylates tyrosine. *Proc. Natl. Acad. Sci. U.S.A.*, 77:1311–1315.

Hunter, T., Ling, N. and Cooper, J.A. (1984) Protein kinase C phosphorylation of the EGF receptor at a threonine residue close to the cytoplasmic face of the plasma membrane. *Nature*, 311:480–483.

Iwashita, S. and Fox, C.F. (1984) Epidermal growth factor and potent phorbol tumor promoters induce epidermal growth factor receptor phosphorylation in a similar but distinctively different manner in human epidermoid carcinoma A431 cells. *J. Biol. Chem.*, 259:2559–2567.

Kasselberg, A.G., Orth, D.N., Gray, M.E. and Stahlman, M.T. (1985) Immunocytochemical localization of human epidermal growth factor/urogastrone in several human tissues. *J. Histochem. Cytochem.*, 33:315–322.

Kasuga, M., Karlsson, F.A. and Kahn, R. (1981) Insulin stimulates the phosphorylation of the 95,000 dalton subunit of its own receptor. *Science*, 215:185–187.

King, L.E., Carpenter, G. and Cohen, S. (1980) Characterization by electrophoresis of Epidermal Growth Factor-stimulated phosphorylation using A431 membranes. *Biochemistry*, 19:1524–1528.

Komoriya, A., Hortsch, M., Meyers, C., Smith, M., Kanety, H. and Schlessinger, J. (1984) Biologically active synthetic fragments of epidermal growth factor. Localization of a major receptor binding region. *Proc. Natl. Acad. Sci. U.S.A.*, 81:1351–1355.

L'Allemain, G., Franvi, A., Cragoe, E. and Pouysségur, J. (1984) Blockade of the Na^+/H^+ antiport abolishes growth factor-induced DNA synthesis in fibroblasts. *J. Biol. Chem.*, 259:4313–4319.

Lee, L.S. and Weinstein, I.B. (1978) Tumor-promoting phorbol esters inhibit behind of epidermal growth factor to cellular receptors. *Science*, 202:313–315.

Lin, C.R., Chen, W.S., Kruijer, W., Stolarsky, L.S., Weber, W., Evans, R.M., Verma, I.M., Gill, G.N. and Rosenfeld, M.G. (1984) Expression cloning of human EGF receptor complementary DNA: Gene amplification and three related messenger RNA products in A413 cells. *Science*, 224:843-848.

Linsley, P.S., Blifold, C., Wrann, M. and Fox, C.F. (1979) Direct linkage of EGF to its receptor. *Nature*, 278:745–748.

Mangelsdorf-Soderquist, A. and Carpenter, G. (1984) Glycosylation of the Epidermal Growth Factor receptor in A431 cells: The contribution of carbohydrate to receptor function. *J. Biol. Chem.*, 259:12586–12594.

Marquardt, H., Hunkapiller, M.W., Hoperskaya, O.A., Twarazik, D.R., De Larco, J.E., Stephenson, J.R. and Todaro, G.J. (1983) Transforming growth factors produced by retrovirus transformed rodent fibroblasts and human melanoma cells. Amino acid sequence homology with epidermal growth factor. *Proc. Natl. Acad. Sci. U.S.A.*, 80: 4684–4688.

Moolenaar, W.H., Mummery, C.L., Van der Saag, P.T. and De Laat, S.W. (1981) Rapid ionic events and the initiation of growth in serum-stimulated neuroblastoma cells. *Cell*, 23:789–798.

Moolenaar, W.H., Tsien, R.Y., Van der Saag, P.T. and De Laat, S.W. (1983) Na^+/N^+ exchange and cytoplasmic pH in the action of growth factors in human fibroblasts. *Nature*, 304:645–648.

Moolenaar, W.H., Tertoolen, L.G.J. and De Laat, S.W. (1984a) Growth factors immediately raise cytoplasmic free $Ca2^+$ in humay fibroblasts. *J. Biol. Chem.*, 259:8066–8069.

Moolenaar, W.H., Tertoolen, L.G.J. and De Laat, S.W. (1984b) Phorbol ester and diacylglycerol mimic growth factors in raising cytoplasmic pH. *Nature*, 312:371–374.

Moolenaar, W.H. Defize, L.H.K., Van Der Saag, P.T. and De Laat, S.W. (1986) The generation of ionic signals by growth factors. In W. Boron and P. Aronson (Eds.), *Current Topics in Membranes and Transport*, Academic Press, New York, pp. 137–154.

Mummery, C.L., Van der Saag, P.T. and De Laat, S.W. (1983) Loss of EGF binding and cation transport response during differentiation of mouse neuroblastoma cells. *J. Cell. Biochem.*, 21:63–75.

Nishizuka, Y. (1984) The role of protein kinase C in cell surface signal transduction and tumour promotion. *Nature*, 308:693–698.

Oka, Y. and Orth, D.N. (1983) Human plasma epidermal growth factor/β urogastrone is associated with blood platelets. *J. Clin. Invest.*, 72:249–259.

Pastan, I.H. and Willingham, M.C. (1981a) Receptor-mediated endocytosis of hormones in cultured cells. *Annu. Rev. Physiol.*, 43:239:250.

Pastan, I.H. and Willingham, M.C. (1981b) Journey to the center of the cell: role of receptosome. *Science*, 214:504–509.

Pfeffer, S. and Ullrich, A. (1984) Is the precursor a receptor? *Nature, News and Views*, 313:184.

Rall, L.B., Scott, J., Bell, G.I., Crawford, R.J., Penschow, J.D., Niall, H.D. and Coghlan, J.P. (1985) Mouse prepro-epidermal growth factor synthesis by the kidney and other tissues. *Nature*, 313:228–231.

Reisner, A.H. (1985) Similarity between the vaccinin virus 19 K early protein and epidermal growth factor. *Nature*, 313:801–802.

Rubin, J.B., Shia, M.A. and Pilch, P.F. (1983) Stimulation of tyrosine-specific phosphorylation in vitro by insulin-like growth factor I. *Nature*, 305:438–440.

Russell, D.W., Schneider, W.J., Yamamoto, T., Luskey, K.L., Brown, M.S. and Goldstein, J.L. (1984) Domain map of the LDL receptor: Sequence homology with the Epidermal Growth Factor precursor. *Cell*, 37:577–585.

Russo, M.W., Lukas, T.J., Cohen, S. and Staros, J.V. (1985) Identification of residues in the nucleotide binding site of the epidermal growth factor receptor/kinase. *J. Biol. Chem.*, 260:5205–5208.

Savage, C.R. Jr., Inagami, T. and Cohen, S. (1972) The primary structure of Epidermal Growth Factor. *J. Biol. Chem.*, 247:7612–7621.

Savage, C.R. Jr., Hash, J.H. and Cohen, S. (1973) Epidermal Growth Factor: location of disulfide bonds. *J. Biol. Chem.*, 248:7669–7672.

Sawyer, S.T. and Cohen, S. (1981) Enhancement of calcium uptake and phosphatidyl turnover by epidermal growth factor in A431 cells. *Biochemistry*, 20:6280–6286.

Sayhoun, N., Hock, R. and Hollenberg, M.D. (1978) Insulin and epidermal growth factor-urogastrone: Affinity cross-linking to specific binding sites in rat liver membranes. *Proc. Natl. Acad. Sci. U.S.A.*, 75:1675–1679.

Schlessinger, J., Shechter, Y., Willingham, M.C. and Pastan, I.H. (1978) Direct visualization of binding aggregation, and internalization of insulin and epidermal growth factor on living fibroblastic cells. *Proc. Natl. Acad. Sci. U.S.A.*, 75:2659–2663.

Schreiber, A.B., Lax, I., Yarden, Y., Eshhar, Z. and Schlessinger, J. (1981) Monoclonal antibodies against receptor for epidermal growth factor induce early and delayed effects of epidermal growth factor. *Proc. Natl. Acad. Sci. U.S.A.*, 75:7535–7539.

Schuldiner, S. and Rozengurt, E. (1982) Na^+/H^+ antiport in Swiss 3T3 cells: mitogenic stimulation leads to cytoplasmic alkalinization. *Proc. Natl. Acad. Sci. U.S.A.*, 79:7778–7782.

Scott, J., Urdea, M., Quiroga, M., Sanchez-Pescador, R., Fong, N., Selby, M., Rutter, W.J. and Bell, G.I. (1983) Structure of a mouse submaxillary messenger RNA encoding epidermal growth factor and seven related proteins. *Science*, 221:236–240.

Shechter, Y., Hernaez, L., Schlessinger, J. and Cuatracasas, P. (1979) Local aggregation of hormone–receptor complexes is required for activation by epidermal growth factor. *Nature*, 278:835–838.

Sherr, C.J., Rettenmier, C.W., Sacca, R., Roussel, M.F., Look, A.T. and Stanley, E.R. (1985) The *c-fms* proto-oncogene product is related to the receptor for the mononuclear phagocyte growth factor, CSF-1. *Cell*, 41:665–676.

Shoyab, M., De Larco, J.E. and Todaro, G.J. (1979) Biologically active phorbol esters specifically alter affinity of epidermal growth factor receptors. *Nature*, 279:387–391.

Sporn, M.B. and Roberts, A.B. (1985) Autocrine growth factors and cancer. *Nature*, 313:745–747.

Stern, R.L. and Heath, J.K. (1983) In M.H. Johnson (Ed.), *Development in Mammals*, Vol. 5, Elsevier, Amsterdam, pp. 107–134.

Taylor, J.M., Cohen, S. and Mitchell, W.M. (1970) Epidermal Growth Factor: High and low molecular weight forms. *Proc. Natl. Acad. Sci. U.S.A.*, 67:164–171.

Thorburn, G.D., Ross-Young, I., Dolling, M., Walker, D.W., Browne, C.A. and Carmichael, G.C. (1985) Growth factors in fetal development. In G. Guroff (Ed.), *Growth and Maturation Factors*, Vol. 3, John Wiley & Sons, New York, pp. 175–195.

Twardzik, D.R., Brown, J.P., Ranchalis, J.E., Todaro, G.J. and Moss, B. (1985) Vaccinia virus-infected cells release a novel polypeptide functionally related to transforming and epidermal growth factors. *Proc. Natl. Acad. Sci. U.S.A.*, 82:5300–5304.

Ullrich, A., Caussens, L., Hayflick, J.S., Dull, T.J., Gray, A., Tam, A.L.S., Lee, J., Yarden, Y., Libermann, T.A., Schlessinger, J., Downward, J., Mayes, E.L.V., Whittle, N., Waterfield, M.D. and Seebing, P.H. (1984) Human epidermal growth factor receptor cDNA sequence and aberrant expression of the amplified gene in A431 epidermoid carcinoma cells. *Nature*, 309:418–425.

Ushiro, H. and Cohen, S. (1980) Identification and phosphotyrosine as a product of epidermal growth factor-activated protein kianse in A431 cell membranes. *J. Biol. Chem.*, 255:8363–8365.

Van Zoelen, E.J.J., Twardzik, D.R., Van Oostwaard, Th.M.J., Van der Saag, P.T., De Laat, S.W. and Todaro, G.J. (1984) Neuroblastoma cells produce transforming growth factors during exponential growth in a defined hormone-free medium. *Proc. Natl. Acad. Sci. U.S.A.*, 81:4085–4089.

Waterfield, M.D., Scrace, G.T., Whittle, N., Stroobant, P., Johnsson, A., Wasteson, A., Westermark, B., Heldin, C.H., Huang, J.S. and Deuel, T.F. (1983) Platelet-derived growth factor is structurally related to the putative transforming protein p28^sis of simian sarcoma virus. *Nature*, 304:35–39.

Weber, W., Bastus, P.J. and Gill, G.N. (1984) Immunoaffinity purification of the epidermal growth factor receptor: Stoichiometry of binding and kinetics of self-phosphorylation. *J. Biol. Chem.*, 259:14631–14636.

Westermark, B., Heldin, C.-H., Ek. B., Johnsson, A., Mellström, K., Nistér, M. and Wasteson, A. (1983) Biochemistry and biology of platelet-derived growth factor. In G. Guroff (Ed.), *Growth and Maturation Factors*, Vol. 1, John Wiley & Sons, New York, pp. 75–115.

Wrann, M. and Fox, C.F. (1979) Identification of Epidermal Growth Factor receptors in a hyperproducing human epidermoid carcinoma cell line. *J. Biol. Chem.*, 254:8083–8086.

Xu, Y., Ishii, S., Clark, A.J.L., Sullivan, M., Wilson, R.K., Ma, D.P., Roe, B.A., Mertino, G.T. and Pastan, I. (1984) Human epidermal growth factor receptor cDNA is homologous to a variety of RNA's overproduced in A431 carcinoma cells. *Nature*, 309:806–809.

Yamamoto, T., Davis, C.G., Brown, M.S., Schneider, W.J., Casey, M.L., Goldstein, J.L. and Russell, D.W. (1984). The human LDL-receptor: A cysteine rich protein with multiple Alu sequences in its mRNA. *Cell*, 39:27–38.

Zidovetzki, R., Yarden, Y., Schlessinger, J. and Jovin, T.M.

182

(1981) Rotational diffusion of epidermal growth factor complexed to cell surface receptors reflects rapid microaggregation and endocytosis of occupied receptors. *Proc. Natl. Acad. Sci. U.S.A.*, 78:6981–6985.

Ziller, C., Dupin, E., Brazeau, P., Paulér, D. and Le Douarin, N.M. (1983) Early segregation of a neuronal precursor cell line in the neural crest as revealed by culture in a chemically defined medium. *Cell*, 32:627–638.

W.H. Gispen and A. Routtenberg (Eds.)
Progress in Brain Research, Vol. 69
© 1986 Elsevier Science Publishers B.V. (Biomedical Division)

CHAPTER 16

Growth factor activation of protein kinase C-dependent and -independent pathways of protein phosphorylation in fibroblasts: relevance to activation of protein kinase C in neuronal tissues

Perry J. Blackshear,[1] Lisa Wen,[1] Raphael A. Nemenoff,[2] J. Ryan Gunsalus,[3] and Lee A. Witters[4]

[1]*Howard Hughes Medical Institute Laboratories, and Section of Diabetes and Metabolism, Division of Endocrinology, Metabolism and Genetics, Department of Medicine, Duke University Medical Center, P.O. Box 3897, Durham, NC 27710,* [2]*Howard Hughes Medical Institute Laboratories,* [3]*Diabetes Unit, Medical Services, Massachusetts General Hospital, Harvard Medical School, Boston, MA 02114, and* [4]*The Endocrine-Metabolism Division, Departments of Medicine and Biochemistry, Dartmouth Medical School, Hanover, NH 03756, U.S.A.*

Despite recent advances in our knowledge of certain of the actions of insulin and the polypeptide growth factors, we still do not understand at the molecular level how these hormones transduce their signals from their specific membrane receptors to the cell interior. The ignorance applies not only to the classical short-term actions of insulin, such as enhanced glucose transport or inhibition of lipolysis, but also to the longer term effects of insulin and the growth factors, which include induction or repression of certain specific enzymes, increases in protein and mRNA synthesis and even DNA synthesis. Recently, our laboratory has focussed on intracellular changes in protein phosphorylation states as markers for enzymic activities activated or inhibited by insulin and the growth factors, in the hope that these phosphorylation changes might lead to elucidation of kinase and phosphatase activities specific for the action of the agonists. Initial hopes that the discovery of the insulin, epidermal growth factor (EGF) and platelet-derived growth factor (PDGF) receptors as tyrosine-specific protein kinases might lead rapidly to the elucidation of sequential protein phosphorylation events have not been realized. In fact, a large number of experiments designed to search for phosphotyrosine-containing, insulin-stimulated intracellular phosphoproteins in insulin's target cells led to the discovery of no single intracellular protein whose phosphorylation state on a tyrosine residue was changed in response to insulin. We have, therefore, continued to study the changes in serine and threonine phosphorylation states provoked by insulin and the growth factors in a variety of target cells, in the hopes that such phosphorylation state changes will lead backwards to the original mechanism of activation at the cell surface.

In the succeeding pages, we will describe some of our recent studies evaluating insulin and growth factor promoted phosphorylation pathways in fibroblasts and related cell lines, especially as these relate to the activation of protein kinase C and other protein kinase activities by these agents. We will also describe recent data which suggest that the growth factor activated pathways of protein phosphorylation in cells such as fibroblasts apppear to be similar in many ways to the responses elicited by muscarinic cholinergic agonists in certain neuronal tissues.

Studies in fibroblasts and related cells

Insulin- and growth factor-stimulated protein phosphorylation

It has been known for many years that insulin can stimulate the phosphorylation of a number of intracellular proteins in several of its target tissues, including the lipogenic enzymes acetyl CoA carboxylase and ATP citrate lyase, the ribosomal protein S6, and unidentified proteins of molecular weight 46 000, 22 000, 17 000 and others (for review see Avruch et al., 1982, 1985; Denton et al., 1981). In none of these cases studied to date has the insulin-stimulated phosphorylation resulted in a change in enzymic activity, with the possible exception of acetyl CoA carboxylase (Witters, 1985). However, in the same cell types, insulin has also been shown to inhibit the phosphorylation of certain well-known enzymes, and in these cases, the decrease in phosphorylation is usually associated with a change in enzymic activity: these include pyruvate kinase, glycogen synthase, glycogen phosphorylase, HMG CoA reductase, and protein phosphatase inhibitor 1. A central difficulty underlying research into insulin's mechanism of action is how to reconcile these stimulatory and inhibitory phosphorylation responses which occur in the same cell types.

Several years, ago, we noted that several of the polypeptide growth factors also stimulated the phosphorylation of these insulin-stimulated proteins in various target cells on which appropriate receptors were present. For example, in isolated hepatocytes, EGF stimulates the phosphorylation of acetyl CoA carboxylase, ATP citrate lyase, and unidentified 46-kDa protein (Avruch et al., 1985); similarly, in murine fibroblasts and adipocytes of the 3T3-L1 line, insulin, EGF, PDGF, multiplication-stimulating activity and fetal calf serum all stimulated the phosphorylation of the 31-kDa ribosomal protein S6 as well as an unidentified heat-stable, acidic 22 kDa protein which was first discovered as an insulin-stimulated phosphoprotein in rat adipose tissue (Belsham et al., 1980; Blackshear et al., 1982, 1983). The 22-kDa protein was of particular interest to us in this context, for two main reasons: first, because its phosphorylation was not stimulated in response to agents which act by elevating intracellular levels of cAMP, in contrast to the other insulin-stimulated phosphoproteins listed above; and second, because phosphorylation of this protein in response to insulin or the growth factors appeared to be due to a stoichiometric increase in phosphorylation, as evidenced by a shift of the protein toward the anode after insulin-stimulated phosphorylation. This shift was documented by labeling of the protein with [^{35}S]methionine followed by stimulation of the cells with insulin. In the cases in which it was studied, insulin, EGF and PDGF, for example, stimulated the phosphorylation of the 22-kDa protein on similar phosphoamino acid residues, with lack of additivity; these findings suggested that identical site(s) might be phosphorylated by the various agents (Blackshear et al., 1983).

At about that time it became clear that the cell surface receptors for insulin, EGF and PDGF were ligand-activated, tyrosine-specific protein kinases. These observations, coupled with the similarities in the intracellular protein phosphorylations promoted by these agents, suggested the possibility of one or more common mechanisms of action of insulin and the various growth factors. However, despite intensive study, we were unable to directly link the tyrosine-specific protein kinase activity of the insulin receptor to the intracellular phosphorylation state changes induced by insulin. We therefore undertook a series of experiments in which we began comparing the insulin- and growth factor-stimulated protein phosphorylations with those induced by the tumor-promoting phorbol esters and similar compounds. These studies were initially designed to determine if there were any interactions between the insulin- and growth factor-stimulated protein phosphorylation pathways and those mediated by protein kinase C, the receptor for the phorbol esters; unexpectedly, they yielded new information on multiple pathways of growth factor-stimulated serine and threonine protein phosphorylation in intact cells.

Similarities between insulin- and growth factor-promoted protein phosphorylation and phorbol ester-promoted phosphorylation

In several cell types, we found that insulin and

active phorbol esters such as phorbol 12-myristate 13-acetate (PMA) stimulated the phosphorylation of a number of proteins in common (Blackshear, 1986; Blackshear et al., 1985). This was studied in greatest detail in 3T3-L1 fibroblasts and adipocytes, the latter being an extremely insulin-responsive cell type. In these two types of cells, insulin and the growth factors as well as the phorbol esters stimulated the phosphorylation of at least two proteins in common, the 31-kDa ribosomal protein, S6, and the 22-kDa protein alluded to above. In both cases, stimulated phosphorylation of the protein was not additive when maximal concentrations of insulin and PMA were used. The phosphoamino acid specificity of the two stimulations was identical, i.e. the S6 was phosphorylated on serine by both agents, and the 22-kDa protein was phosphorylated on both serine and threonine in response to insulin or PMA. Finally, preliminary peptide mapping studies of the 22-kDa protein suggested that insulin- and PMA-stimulated phosphorylation resulted in nearly identical tryptic peptide patterns on two-dimensional mapping. In other words, several types of circumstantial evidence suggested that insulin and the growth factors on one hand and phorbol esters on the other might be promoting phosphorylation of these proteins on identical sites. There were several possible explanations for these findings. First, one had to consider the possibility that insulin was activating protein kinase C, a suggestion which has been raised by a number of investigators (e.g. Farese et al., 1985; Graves and McDonald, 1985). Second, the unlikely possibility existed that insulin might be activating a protein phosphorylation pathway (which could be activation of a protein kinase or inhibition of a phosphatase), which had identical site and substrate specificity to protein kinase C. Third, insulin and the growth factors could activate a protein phosphorylation pathway, again by activating a kinase or inhibiting a phosphatase, which could be secondarily activated by the primary activation of protein kinase C by the phorbol esters. We embarked on a number of experiments to test these three hypotheses, which are not necessarily exclusive for all cells and tissues. The data described below suggest that the third possibility in the correct one: that phorbol esters activate protein kinase C leading to the secondary activation of a protein phosphorylation pathway activated through an alternative route by insulin. In addition, our studies indicated that both pathways could be activated by certain growth factors.

Use of the 80-kDa protein as an indicator of protein kinase C activity in fibroblasts and other cell types

To distinguish among the three possibilities listed above, we studied the phosphorylation of a cytosolic, acidic, 80-kDa protein (80K), whose phosphorylation state was dramatically increased upon exposure of quiescent, serum-deprived fibroblasts to activate phorbol esters such as PMA. Our studies were conducted primarily in 3T3-L1 fibroblasts and adipocytes (Blackshear et al., 1985); however, phorbol ester-induced phosphorylation of this or a similar protein had been described independently by Rozengurt et al. (1983, 1984) in related mouse fibroblasts, and has now been shown in a wide variety of cell types (Blackshear et al., 1986). The functional identity of this protein remains unknown, as does its true molecular weight; it migrates anomalously on polyacrylamide gels, yielding very high apparent molecular weights on high percentage acrylamide gels and low apparent molecular weights on low percentage acrylamide gels, yielding very abnormal Ferguson plots (P.J. Blackshear, unpublished data). We have accumulated evidence which suggests that the phosphorylation state of this protein in fibroblasts and possibly other cell types may be an accurate reflection of protein kinase C activation in those cells.

This evidence is of several types (described in detail in Blackshear et al., 1985; 1986; Blackshear, 1986). First, phosphorylation of the 80K protein is increased dramatically within a couple of minutes by exposure of quiescent fibroblasts to active phorbol esters but not inactive analogs such as 4α-phorbol-12, 13-didecanoate (4α -PDD). The phosphorylation state of the protein can be quantitated readily because the magnitude of the increase is generally on the order of 20- to 50-fold after the addition of phorbol esters to the cell monolayer. Second, the activated phosphorylation of the 80K protein can be mimicked by a variety of synthetic diacylglycerols, especially those with chain lengths of 6–8 carbons (diC6–diC8). Phosphorylation is not increased by diacylglycerols of shorter chain length, or of much longer chain length. The shorter chain length compounds are also ineffective at activating protein kinase C in vitro, under conditions where the phospholipid added to the reaction mixture is suboptimal; the longer chain lengths are capable of activating the kinase in vitro, but may not promote 80K protein phosphorylation in the intact cells because of difficulty penetrating the cell membrane. However, the three analogues which are maximally effective at promoting 80K protein phosphorylation in the intact cell are also those which are most effective at activating protein kinase C in vitro. In addition, the phorbol esters and active synthetic diacyglycerols promote phosphorylation of the 80K protein in intact cells with identical phosphoamino acid specificity, and produce identical partial proteolytic peptide maps when the protein is digested by staphylococcal V8 protease using the Cleveland technique. The 80K protein is not phosphorylated in response to either dibutyryl cyclic AMP or agents which cause an elevation in intracellular cyclic AMP, at least in the cells we have studied. It is an excellent substrate for protein kinase C in a cell-free system (Blackshear et al., 1986), although the precise stoichiometry of this reaction has not yet been calculated; in addition, again using the partial proteolytic peptide mapping technique, the phosphoamino acid residues and peptide sites on the protein phosphorylated in vitro by protein kinase C and those phosphorylated in intact cells in response to phorbol esters appear to be identical (Blackshear et al., 1986). Finally, as described in more detail below, phosphorylation of the protein is not stimulated by phorbol esters or synthetic diacylglycerols under conditions where the cells have been made temporarily protein kinase C deficient by preincubation with high concentrations of phorbol ester (Blackshear et al., 1985). Thus, for a number of reasons, it seems likely that the 80K protein represents a substrate for protein kinase C in the intact cell, and that its phosphorylation state is a reasonably good marker for protein kinase C activation in these cells.

We were able to determine that several of the polypeptide growth factors which we had studied could activate protein kinase C in these same cells, using the phosphorylation of the 80K protein as an index of protein kinase C activation (Blackshear et al., 1985). PDGF as well as bovine pituitary fibroblast growth factor (FGF) and fetal calf serum all promoted phosphorylation of the 80K protein to a great extent in the quiescent 3T3-L1 fibroblasts. EGF, on the other hand, stimulated phosphorylation of the 80K protein only to a very limited extent; in a large series of studies, the phosphorylation increase averaged only about 50%, as opposed to 20- to 50-fold in studies involving phorbol esters, PDGF or FGF. In contrast to the other growth factors, insulin was completely *ineffective* at stimulating the phosphorylation of the 80K protein over a wide dosage range and over a broad range of exposure times. In addition, PMA but not insulin stimulated phosphorylation of the 80K protein in fully differentiated 3T3-L1 adipocytes, which contain many more insulin receptors than the 3T3-L1 fibroblasts from which they are derived (Rubin et al., 1978). Although insulin and the other growth factors stimulated the phosphorylation of a large number of proteins in common, all of which were also phosphorylated in response to phorbol esters, they could finally be distinguished by the response of the 80K protein phosphorylation. Based on this type of analysis, it seemed clear that PDGF, FGF, and serum could activate protein kinase C in intact fibroblasts, whereas EGF was much less effective and insulin was completely ineffective. Circumstantial data arguing the PDGF could activate protein kinase C included the fact that PDGF is known to increase intracellular concentrations of diacylglycerols in quiescent 3T3 cells (Habenicht et al., 1981), and also our findings that the phosphoamino acid specificity and partial proteolytic peptide maps of the 80K protein after phosphorylation in response to PDGF were identical to those found after exposure of the cells to PMA or synthetic diacylglycerols. Finally, phosphorylation of the 80K protein in response to PDGF or FGF was not seen in the cells made temporarily protein kinase C deficient (see below).

Based on this analysis, we concluded that the first of our three possibilities would not prove to be the case: that is, that insulin might be activating protein kinase C in these cells. We were left then with the other two possibilities: that insulin might be activating a pathway similar to protein kinase C; or that protein kinase C might be activating a secondary pathway, activated by insulin through a different mechanism.

Studies in 'down-regulated' cells

To investigate these remaining possibilities, we utilized a technique first described by Rozengurt and his colleagues in related 3T3 cell lines, which they have termed 'down-regulation' of protein kinase C in response to phorbol esters (Collins and Rozengurt, 1982; Rodriguez-Pena and Rozengurt, 1984). They first found that exposure of cells to fairly high concentrations of phorbol esters for long periods of time resulted in desensitization of subsequent cellular responses to these mitogens; and further evaluation led to the discovery that not only was specific phorbol binding eliminated in these cells, but protein kinase C activity was no longer detectable after such down-regulation. We performed similar studies in the 3T3-L1 fibroblasts and adipocytes (Blackshear et al., 1985); after a 16-h exposure to 16 μM PMA, the confluent fibroblasts contained no detectable protein kinase C, which we assessed by three independent criteria:

(*a*) they had no detectable specific phorbol dibutyrate (PDBu) binding (also seen after 16 h of exposure to 20 μM PDBu, followed by 'washout' of the PDBu;
(*b*) they had no detectable protein kinase C activity either in a soluble cellular fraction or in a detergent-extracted particulate fraction; and
(*c*) protein kinase C immunoreactivity was completely absent in a total cellular homogenate when compared to an identical homogenate prepared from cells exposed to the vehicle alone, dimethyl sulfoxide (DMSO).

In other words, using techniques available to us at the time, we could find no evidence that there were significant amounts of protein kinase C in the cells down-regulated in response to PMA. A further discussion of this phenomenon is beyond the

scope of this chapter; however, both Collins and Rozengurt (1982) and we (P.J. Blackshear, unpublished data) have determined that the down-regulation process is a completely reversible phenomenon. Although no studies of these points have been conducted, to our knowledge, it seems possible that the phorbol esters are inhibiting either translation of protein kinase C mRNA or transcription of the protein kinase C gene, and that normal proteolytic processes degrade the kinase until it is virtually gone from the cell interior. Removal of the inhibitory stimulus could then lead to resynthesis of the protein kinase C, once again in balance with the proteolytic removal mechanisms.

Using this down-regulated model of 3T3-L1 fibroblasts, we then explored the phosphorylation responses to the phorbol esters and various growth factors which we were studying. In the down-regulated cells, PMA, active diacylglycerols such as diC7, PDGF and FGF were no longer effective at stimulating phosphorylation of the 80K protein (Blackshear et al., 1985). This suggested what we had inferred from other studies, that stimulated phosphorylation of the 80K protein was impossible in the absence of protein kinase C. However, somewhat to our surprise, insulin and PDGF stimulated phosphorylation of the 22-kDa protein in a completely normal fashion in the protein kinase C-deficient cells. This was particularly reassuring since it has been known for some time that phorbol esters can compromise the function of certain growth factor receptors, such as the EGF receptor; however, in the down-regulated cells, the insulin and the PDGF receptors were still able to transduce the signal of these ligands in what appeared to be a normal manner. Similarly, insulin, FGF and PDGF were all able to promote phosphorylation of the ribosomal protein S6 in the down-regulated cells (Fig. 1). As expected, neither PMA nor active synthetic diacylglycerols were able to stimulate phosphorylation of either the 22-kDa or 31-kDa protein in the down-regulated cells, indicating that intact protein kinase C was necessary for this component of the phosphorylation response to phorbol esters or diacylglycerols.

These findings led to the following working

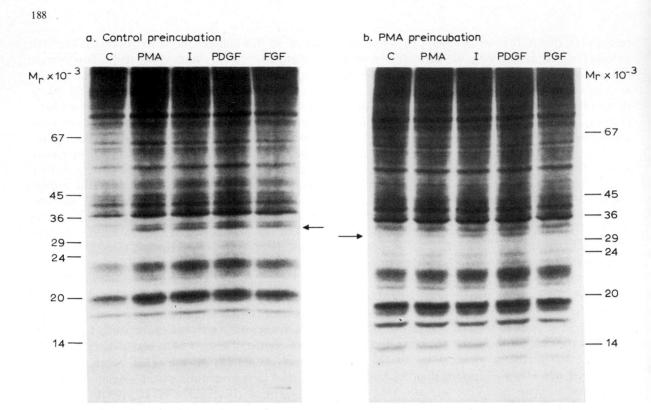

Fig. 1. Effects of preincubation of PMA on ribosomal protein S6 phosphorylation. Confluent 3T3-L1 fibroblasts were washed three times in serum-free Dulbecco's modified Eagle medium (DMEM), then incubated for 18 h in the same serum-free medium containing 1% (w/v) bovine serum albumin (crystallized and lyophilized; Sigma, St. Louis, MO). After 2 h of this incubation, to the cells was added (final concentration) either 0.1% (v/v) dimethyl sulfoxide (DMSO) (a) or 16 μM PMA in 0.1% DMSO (b) for the remaining 16 h. The cells were then washed three times with 4 ml Krebs Ringer bicarbonate buffer, then incubated for 2 h in Krebs Ringer bicarbonate buffer containing 1% (w/v) bovine serum albumin and 0.1 mCi/ml $^{32}P_i$, exposed to control conditions (C), PMA (1.6 μM), insulin (1 mU/ml; I), PDGF (approximately 10^{-9} M) or FGF (125 ng/ml) for 15 min, washed, homogenized and extracted as described (Blackshear et al., 1983) except that 1% (v/v) Triton X100, 1% (v/v) NP40 and 0.5% (w/v) sodium deoxycholate were used in place of Zwittergent. Equal amounts of trichloroacetic acid-precipitable radioactivity were loaded into each gel lane. Autoradiographs of the resulting gels are shown here; the positions of molecular weight markers run in adjacent lanes are shown. The arrows indicate the position of the 31-kDa ribosomal protein S6. Other details of experimental procedure are contained in Blackshear et al. (1983, 1985).

hypothesis (Blackshear et al., 1985): in normal cells, PMA, diacylglycerols, PDGF, FGF and serum all led to the activation of protein kinase C which led in turn to phosphorylation of the 80-kDa protein and also to the phosphorylation of the 22-kDa and 31-kDa proteins. Insulin, on the other hand, led to the phosphorylation of the 22-kDa and 31-kDa proteins in either normal cells or protein kinase C deficient cells, but did not stimulate phosphorylation of the 80-kDa protein under any circumstances, indicating its lack of direct activation of protein kinase C. PDGF and FGF, as well as EGF

to a much lesser extent, under conditions of complete apparent protein kinase C deficiency, could also lead to the phosphorylation of the 22-kDa or 31-kDa proteins through a completely protein kinase C-independent pathway, that is, they could activate the insulin-like or 'I' pathway which would lead to phosphorylation of the 22-kDa and 31-kDa proteins in the complete absence of protein kinase C. However, under these conditions, neither PMA nor diacylglycerols were effective at promoting the phosphorylation of these latter two proteins. In other words, an intact protein kinase C pathway appeared

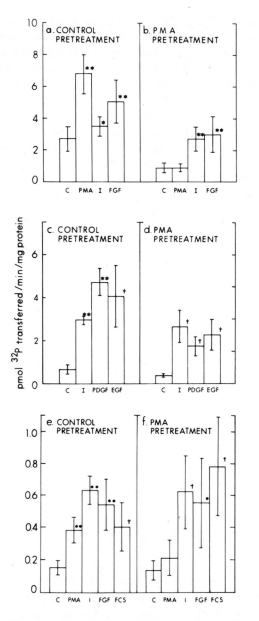

Fig. 2. Effects of preincubation with PMA on ribosomal protein S6 kinase activity. Recently confluent (within 24 h) 3T3-L1 fibroblasts (a–d), or cells which had been confluent for 48–72 h (e,f) were incubated in serum-free medium in 0.1% DMSO (a,c,e) or 16 µM PMA in 0.1% DMSO (b,d,f) and exposed to hormones or other agents, including 10% (v/v) fetal calf serum (FCS) for 15 min as described in the legend to Fig. 1, except that no $^{32}P_i$ was included in the incubation medium. PDGF (HPLC purified; 2 units/ml), EGF (1 µg/ml) and FGF (125 ng/ml) were from Collaborative Research (Lexington, MA). The cells were then washed, homogenized and centrifuged, and the resulting supernatants were snap-frozen in dry ice/acetone and stored at −90°C, exactly as described (Novak-Hofer and Thomas, 1984). The samples were then thawed, and ribosomal protein S6 kinase activity in the supernatant fraction from each plate of cells was assayed as described (Novak-Hofer and Thomas, 1984). Each bar represents the mean ± S.D. of duplicate determinations from 3–6 plates of cells, *, $p < 0.05$; **, $p < 0.001$; †, $p < 0.01$ when compared to control, using Student's t-test.

to be necessary for the phosphorylation of the 80K, as well as the 22-kDa and 31-kDa proteins in response to PMA or synthetic diacylglycerols.

This working hypothesis still left open the question of whether PMA and the synthetic diacylglycerols might be stimulating the phosphorylation of the 22-kDa and 31-kDa proteins as substrates for protein kinase C, or whether they might be activating the insulin-stimulated or I pathway, which would in turn lead to the phosphorylation of these proteins. To investigate these possibilities, we studied the activation state of a possible linking protein kinase, a ribosomal protein S6 kinase first described by Novak-Hofer and Thomas (1984). They found that EGF as well as serum could activate this ribosomal protein S6 kinase in intact quiescent fibroblasts. More recent studies by Tabarini et al. (1985) also established that this kinase could be activated by insulin and tumor-promoting phorbol esters in 3T3-L1 fibroblasts and adipocytes. We investigated the activation state of this kinase in quiescent 3T3-L1 fibroblasts which had been exposed either to serum-free, control conditions, or high concentrations of phorbol esters in order to down-regulate the protein kinase C. In the normal cells, we found that the ribosomal protein S6 kinase was activated by insulin, EGF, PDGF, FGF, serum, and PMA (Fig. 2a,c,e). However, in the cells made temporarily protein kinase C deficient by down-regulating with PMA, insulin and the growth factors maintained their stimulatory effect on the kinase, whereas PMA was no longer effective at activating the S6 kinase (Fig. 2b,d,f). In other words, the presence of protein kinase C was mandatory for the PMA-mediated activation of the ribosomal protein S6 kinase, whereas this was not the case for its activation by insulin and the other growth factors. These findings strongly support

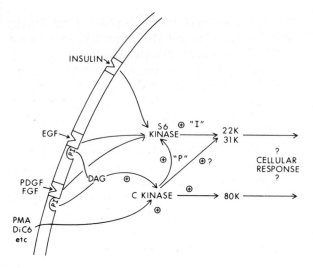

Fig. 3. Proposed scheme for the interactions of phorbol esters and diacylglycerols, growth factors and insulin in intact fibroblasts. The pathways diagrammed here represent possible interactions of the various agents discussed in the text on intact 3T3-L1 fibroblasts; this scheme represents a minor modification of the one proposed in Blackshear et al. (1985). PI, polyphosphoinositides; DAG, endogenous diacylglycerols liberated by 'turnover' of membrane phospholipids; C kinase, protein kinase C; 'P', the pathway leading from activated protein kinase C to activation of the S6 kinase; 'I', the S6 kinase pathway activated by insulin. + denotes activation of the pathway. See the text for further details.

the third possibility raised at the beginning of this section: that is, that phorbol esters and synthetic diacylglycerols activate protein kinase C, which in turn activates the ribosomal protein S6 kinase, leading to some of the intracellular phosphorylation events which are held in common between the growth factors and PMA, notably the phosphorylation of the ribosomal protein S6. This current working hypothesis is represented schematically in Fig. 3. There probably will be other protein kinase C-activated secondary kinases. For example, we have not been able to detect phosphorylation of the 22-kDa protein by the ribosomal protein S6 kinase, nor has the PMA-stimulated tyrosine phosphorylation of a 42-kDa protein (Gilmore and Martin, 1983) been adequately explained; this will probably be due to activation of a secondary protein tyrosine kinase by protein kinase C itself.

These findings have several interesting corol-

laries. Obviously, one cannot assume that proteins whose phosphorylation state is increased upon exposure of the cells to PMA are substrates for protein kinase C, since they could well be substrates for one of these secondarily activated protein kinases. In addition, it seems obvious that PDGF, for example, activates at least three distinct protein kinase moieties upon binding to its cell surface receptors: the tyrosine-specific receptor kinase, protein kinase C, and the ribosomal S6 kinase. Finally, it is also clear that activation of two of these kinases by growth factors leads to the same intracellular event, i.e. activation of ribosomal protein S6 phosphorylation. Why PDGF and FGF require these apparently redundant phosphorylation pathways to achieve exactly the same end is not clear.

In summary, we determined in intact fibroblasts and cultured adipocytes that growth factors such as PDGF and FGF were able to activate at least two distinct phosphorylation pathways in these cells: one involving the activation of protein kinase C, presumably through increases in intracellular diacylglycerols mediated by enhanced polyphosphoinositide turnover; and the other involving the activation of a separate, insulin-stimulated phosphorylation pathway which does not appear to interact with protein kinase C. However, the two pathways clearly interact at a more distal point with activated protein kinase C able to activate the insulin-stimulated phosphorylation pathway(s), one of which is represented by the ribosomal protein S6 kinase. These results suggest that the great similarity among the substrates and (presumably) sites phosphorylated by insulin and PMA are a result of protein kinase C activation of the insulin-stimulated pathway. Major questions which remain unresolved about this pathway include the mechanism of the insulin-stimulated activation of the S6 kinase, as well as the molecular nature of this kinase and its method of activation by protein kinase C.

Relevance of the fibroblast findings to neuronal protein phosphorylation

In comparing the phosphorylation of the 80K

protein in living fibroblast cells and related cells to the phosphorylation of the same protein in vitro by protein kinase C, we inadvertently discovered that the 80K protein from rat adipose tissue belonged to a small group of mainly acidic proteins which remain in solution after boiling, i.e. are heat-stable (Blackshear et al., 1986). In an attempt to find out more about this potentially interesting substrate protein, we performed a tissue survey in which heat-stable proteins from various rat tissues were subjected to phosphorylation by protein kinase C. The 80K substrate protein appeared to be fairly ubiquitous in rat tissues but, somewhat surprisingly, appeared to be most prominent in brain (Blackshear et al., 1986), as is the case with protein kinase C itself. This finding suggested the possibility that the 80K protein kinase C substrate might be of some relevance to neuronal function, perhaps in response to agents which promote polyphosphoinositide turnover in nervous tissue, including muscarinic cholinergic agonists in some systems (Masters et al., 1985), and light in the retina (Schmidt, 1983a,b).

In order to facilitate studies of the molecular characterization of the 80K protein, we purified this protein using preparative two-dimensional electrophoresis and raised polyclonal antibodies to it in rabbits. We were then able to use these antibodies to compare the 80K protein to protein kinase C itself, as well as to characterise the related protein in various tissues and species. Details of these studies have been described in detail in Blackshear et al. (1986), and are summarized in the suceeding pages.

Comparison of the 80K protein with protein kinase C

Although at first we, as well as Rozengurt et al. (1983), suspected that the 80K protein might be protein kinase C itself, since its phosphorylation was stimulated by the same agonists which activated protein kinase C, it rapidly became clear that this was not the case. To summarise a large series of studies aimed at clarifying this issue, we were able to distinguish between protein kinase C and the 80K protein by at least eight physical criteria. To do this, we partially purified protein

kinase C from 3T3-L1 fibroblasts, subjected it to autophosphorylation, and then compared it to the ^{32}P-labeled 80K protein from intact fibroblasts of the same type. In these comparisons, the 80K protein could be differentiated from protein kinase C in the following ways:

(*a*) It migrated anomalously on polyacrylamide gel electrophoresis, compared to the more orthodox migration characteristics of protein kinase C.

(*b*) Its had an acidic isoelectric point of approximately 4.4, compared to the isoelectric point of the kinase of about 5.8. The two phosphoproteins could be clearly separated by more than 1.5 pH units by co-electrophoresis in two dimensions.

(*c*) The two phosphoproteins eluted at different salt concentrations on anion-exchange chromatography.

(*d*) Differences in heat-stability: while the 80K protein was heat-stable, protein kinase C from the same source was not.

(*e*) Partial proteolytic peptide maps, using staphylococcal V8 protease, clearly distinguished between the two on the basis of their anomalous migration characteristics, as well as their characteristic peptide maps.

(*f*) The fibroblast studies described above indicated that in the cells which were effectively protein kinase C deficient, the 80K was just as prominent a phosphoprotein as in the cells with the normal complement of protein kinase C.

(*g*) The anti-80K protein antiserum cross-reacted with the 80K protein from bovine brain and porcine brain, but did not cross-react with protein kinase C from porcine brain (kindly provided by Drs. Peggy R. Girard and J.F. Kuo of Emory University).

(*h*) A polyclonal antiserum directed against pig brain protein kinase C (another generous gift from Drs. Girard and Kuo) did not cross-react with any component of the heat-stable proteins from either pig or cow brain.

Therefore, based on at least these physical criteria, we believe that the 80K protein is distinct from protein kinase C in the various tissues in which we have examined it.

Based on a number of physical characteristics

of this protein, we suspected that the 80K protein might be similar or identical to a protein described by Greengard and his associates in rat brain synaptosomes and labeled as the 87K protein (Wu et al., 1982; for review, see Nairn et al., 1985). Indeed, based on the ability of our antiserum to the heat-stable 80K protein from bovine brain to recognize purified 87K protein (Albert et al., 1984) (generously provided by Katherine A. Albert and Dr. Paul Greengard) and the exact co-migration of the two phosphoproteins on two-dimensional electrophoresis, we can conclude at the present time that the two proteins, at least from bovine brain, are identical. However, this left open the question of whether there were tissue or species differences in the 80K protein; this appeared to be likely since we had already noted that the bovine brain phosphoprotein migrated with a somewhat higher molecular weight than the analogous protein from mouse fibroblasts, and that the analogous protein from chicken fibroblasts had an apparent molecular weight of 60 000 on sodium dodecylsulfate (SDS) gels, although all of these molecular weight estimations are suspect because of the anomalous migration characteristics of the protein. In any event, using the anti-80K antibody from bovine brain and our ability to label the protein both in vivo and in vitro with protein kinase C, we performed a comparison of the protein from various tissues and species. These studies are described in detail in Blackshear et al. (1986), and are summarized below.

First, we prepared heat-stable proteins from a variety of mammalian brains, subjected them to one-dimensional electrophoresis and identified the 80K protein using the Western blotting procedure. By this means, we found antibody cross-reactivity to the 80K protein from all of the species examined, including cow, pig, mouse, rat, rabbit and human, but there was no antibody cross-reactivity to a heat-stable preparation of proteins from human placenta. However, there were some differences in the antibody cross-reactivity pattern. For example, comparing cow, pig and human, the antibody directed to the bovine brain protein appeared to cross-react strongly with proteins of identical molecular weight from all three species. The rabbit protein, however,

although comprising a reasonable fraction of the heat-stable brain proteins (as determined by Coomassie blue staining) and migrating with an identical apparent molecular weight to the bovine protein, appeared to have lower affinity for the antibody. The mouse and rat 80K proteins, however, which again represented reasonable amounts of protein in the heat-stable fraction, seemed to migrate at an apparent molecular weight of approximately 3 000 lower on whatever type of SDS gel electrophoresis they were subjected to. In other words, while all of the proteins were recognized by the antibody to the bovine brain protein, cow, pig and human protein appeared to have the highest affinity for the antibody, whereas the rat, rabbit and mouse had lower affinity and the rat and mouse proteins appeared to have a lower molecular weight as well. These relationships were confirmed independently by co-migrating the proteins on two-dimensional electrophoresis, and recognizing them by their characteristic staining pattern on the gels. Once again, the cow, rabbit and human 80K proteins co-migrated exactly on two-dimensional electrophoresis, whereas the rat and mouse both migrated at a somewhat lower apparent molecular weight and with a slightly more acidic isoelectric point than the cow protein. These species differences do not appear to be artifacts of the heat-stable preparation itself since the mouse and cow ^{32}P-labeled 80K proteins from the respective fibroblasts also failed to co-migrate in the same relationship as the brain heat-stable proteins. The most pronounced species difference we have noted is the apparent 20 000 molecular weight difference between the mouse fibroblast and chicken embryo fibroblast proteins (Blackshear, 1986), which behave similarly in terms of acidic isoelectric point, multiple phosphorylated spots, and 20- to 50-fold stimulated phosphorylation with PMA.

A remaining major question was whether the proteins from different tissues in the same species were identical or isomeric forms. We addressed this question by subjecting to co-migration on two-dimensional electrophoresis ^{32}P-labeled 80K proteins from fibroblasts of various species exposed to PMA, or rat epididymal fat pads exposed to PMA, with the relevant proteins from

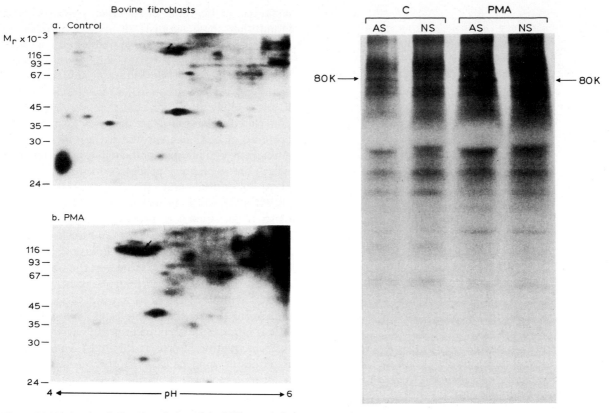

Fig. 4. PMA-stimulated phosphorylation of the 80K protein in bovine skin fibroblasts. Serum-deprived primary bovine skin fibroblasts were labeled with $^{32}P_i$ and exposed to control conditions (a; 0.01% DMSO) or PMA (b; 1.6 µM in 0.01% DMSO) for 15 min exactly as described for mouse fibroblasts in Blackshear et al. (1985). The ^{32}P-proteins were then separated by two-dimensional electrophoresis and autoradiographs of the two gels are shown here. The positions of molecular weight markers are shown on the left; the approximate pH gradient is shown at the bottom. The arrow points to the 80K protein whose phosphorylation is markedly stimulated by PMA in these cells. See the text for further details.

Fig. 5. Immunoprecipitation of the 80K protein from bovine skin fibroblasts. The ^{32}P-proteins from the bovine fibroblast samples described in the legend for Fig. 4 (both control and PMA-stimulated) were diluted 1:10 with immunoprecipitation buffer (10 mM Tris HCl (pH 7.5), 140 mM NaCl, 2.5 mM EDTA, 0.5% Triton X-100, 0.5% sodium deoxycholate, 0.05% SDS), then incubated overnight at 4°C with a 1:100 dilution of either preimmune rabbit serum (NS) or antiserum directed against the bovine brain 80K protein (AS). Immune complexes were then precipitated with *Staphylococcus aureus* cells, the pellets were washed vigorously, and proteins eluted with boiling SDS were separated by electrophoresis on the 15% acrylamide gel. An autoradiograph of this gel is shown here. C, cells exposed to control conditions; PMA, cells exposed to PMA. The arrows indicate the position of the ^{32}P-labeled 80-kDa protein (80K).

heat-stable preparations of brain. In all three cases examined, the mouse, rat and cow, the ^{32}P-labeled fibroblast (or fat pad) 80K protein co-migrated exactly with the analogous 80K Coomassie blue-stained protein from the brain of the same animal species. Similarly, the antibody raised against the bovine brain protein was effective at specifically immunoprecipitating the ^{32}P-labeled 80K protein from PMA-stimulated bovine fibroblasts (Figs. 4 and 5). Therefore, we believe that the proteins from brain and fibroblasts (or fat pads) from individual species are very similar or identical, at least based on the determinants of co-electrophoresis in both dimensions and co-immunoreactivity.

In other tissue comparisons, we compared crude cellular supernatants from bovine pituitary, retina and brain; as shown in Fig. 6, the retina

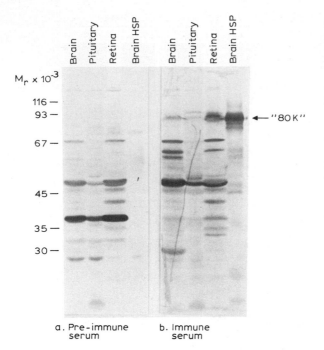

Fig. 6. Western blotting of crude cytosolic supernatants of various bovine neuronal tissues. A crude cytosolic fraction was prepared from frozen bovine pituitary, retina and brain, and equal amounts of protein were subjected to electrophoresis with a smaller amount of bovine brain heat-stable proteins (HSP). The proteins were then transferred to nitrocellulose, and allowed to react with either preimmune serum or an antiserum directed against the bovine brain 80K protein, as described in Blackshear et al. (1986). The retina appeared to contain more immunoreactive 80K protein (indicated by the arrow) than the brain, which contained more than the pituitary. See the text for further details.

contained more immunoreactive material per unit supernatant protein than did the brain, which contained more than the pituitary. Thus. the retina appears to possess the highest concentration of the protein of any tissue tested to date. Clearly, detailed analysis of various brain and nerve fractions, as well as immunocytochemistry, will help in the elucidation of the relative prevalence of the protein in various anatomical areas.

A major remaining question is: What relevance does the protein kinase C-mediated stimulation of growth in fibroblasts have to a neuronal process mediated by the same kinase? In preliminary experiments, we have exposed a variety of cultured neuronal cell types to phorbol esters and in some

instances muscarinic cholinergic agonists, and found that these agonists promoted phosphorylation of the 80K protein in these cells as well, where it appeared to be an equally or perhaps more prominent protein kinase C substrate than in the murine fibroblasts (Blackshear et al., 1986). It seems likely, therefore, that this protein is phosphorylated in response to agents which activate protein kinase C in neuronal tissues, for example muscarinic cholinergic agonists in appropriate cell types. The metabolic processes mediated by this phosphorylation, and the relationship of the growth-promoting properties of PMA in fibroblasts to an equivalent process in neuronal tissue, await elucidation of the functional identity of the 80K protein and other protein kinase C-activated pathways in both tissues. However, the ubiquity of the 80K protein, and its phosphorylation in response to phorbol esters in a wide variety of cell and tissue types (Blackshear et al., 1986), suggest that it might be a fairly widespread early response to the activation of protein kinase C. An attractive hypothesis would be that the 80K protein is itself a protein kinase of some type, activated or inhibited by protein kinase C-dependent phosphorylation. Whatever the functional identity of the protein, however, it seems likely that elucidation of the molecular characteristics, phosphorylation site determinants and phosphorylation stoichiometry of this and other protein kinase C substrate proteins will eventually help in our understanding of how this important mediator of cell membrane signals functions in a variety of tissues.

Acknowledgments

We are very grateful to several of our colleagues who collaborated in some of the studies described here, especially Drs. Peggy R. Girard and J.F. Kuo, who supplied us with pig brain protein kinase C and antiserum to the kinase; Katherine A. Albert and Paul Greengard, who provided us with purified 87K protein and with whom we had many stimulating discussions; Robert M. Bell and Berry R. Ganong, who provided the synthetic diacylglycerols; James E. Niedell for an early gift of protein kinase C and many helpful discussions; and R.R. Minor for supplying us with bovine skin fibroblasts. We are also very grateful to Dr. Joseph Avruch, in whose laboratory the S6 kinase assays were performed. We also thank Elizabeth Kennington, Jane Tuttle, Jenni Lessin and Stephanie Quamo for technical assistance, and Lessie Detwiler for typing the manuscript. LW is an Associate, RAN is an Assistant Investigator, and PJB is an Investigator of the Howard Hughes Medical Institute.

Supported in part by grants AM 35712 and 17776 from the National Institutes of Health.

References

Albert, K.A., Wu, W.C.-S., Nairn, A.C. and Greengard, P. (1984) *Proc. Natl. Acad. Sci. U.S.A.*, 81:3622–3625.

Avruch, J., Alexander, M.C., Palmer, J.L., Pierce, M.W., Nemenoff, R.A., Blackshear, P.J., Tipper, J.P. and Witters, L.A. (1982) *Fed. Proc.*, 41:2629–2633.

Avruch, J., Nemenoff, R.A., Pierce, M.W., Kwok, Y.C. and Blackshear, P.J. (1985) Protein phosphorylation as a mode of insulin action. In Czech, M.P. (Ed.), *Molecular Basis of Insulin Action*, Plenum Press, New York, pp. 263–296.

Belsham, G.J., Bownsey, R.W., Hughes, W.A. and Denton, R.M. (1980) *Diabetologia*, 18:307–312.

Blackshear, P.J. (1986) Protein Phosphorylation in Cultured Cells: Interactions Among Insulin, Growth Factors and Phorbol Esters. In P. Stalfors, J. Donner and P. Belfrage (Eds.), *Mechanisms of Insulin Action*, Elsevier, Amsterdam. pp. 211–227.

Blackshear, P.J., Nemenoff, R.A. and Avruch, J. (1982) *Biochem. J.*, 204:817–824.

Blackshear, P.J., Nemenoff, R.A. and Avruch, J. (1983) *Biochem. J.*, 214:11–19.

Blackshear, P.J., Witters, L.A., Girard, P.R., Kuo, J.F. and Quamo, S.N. (1985) *J. Biol. Chem.*, 260:13304–13315.

Blackshear, P.J., Wen, L., Glynn, B.P. and Witters, L.A. (1986) *J. Biol. Chem.*, 261:1459–1469.

Collins, M.K.L. and Rozengurt, E. (1982) *J. Cell. Physiol.*, 112:42–50.

Denton, E.M., Brownsey, R.W. and Belsham, G.L. (1981) *Diabetologia*, 21:347–362.

Farese, R.V., Standaert, M.L., Barnes, D.E., Davis, J.S. and Pollet, R.J. (1985) *Endocrinology*, 116:2650–2655.

Gilmore, T. and Martin, G.S. (1983) *Nature*, 306:487–490.

Graves, C.B. and McDonald, J.M. (1985) *J. Biol. Chem.*, 260:11286–11292.

Habenicht, A.J.R., Glomset, J.A., King, W.C., Nist, C., Mitchell, C.D. and Ross, R. (1981) *J. Biol. Chem.* 256:12329–12335.

Masters, S.B., Harden, T.K. and Brown, J.H. (1984) *Mol. Pharmacol.* 25:149–155.

Nairn, A.C., Hemmings, H.C. Jr, and Greengard, P. (1985) *Annu. Rev. Biochem.*, 54:931–976.

Novak-Hofer, I., and Thomas, G. (1984) *J. Biol. Chem.*, 259:5995–6000.

Rodriguez-Pena, A. and Rozengurt, E. (1984) *Biochem. Biophys. Res. Commun.*, 120:1053–1059.

Rozengurt, E., Rodriguez-Pena, M. and Smith, K.A. (1983) *Proc. Natl. Acad. Sci. U.S.A.*, 80:7244–7248.

Rozengurt, E., Rodriguez-Pena, A., Coombs, M.D. and Sinnett-Smith, J. (1984) *Proc. Natl. Acad. Sci. U.S.A.*, 81:5748–5752.

Rubin, C.S., Hirsch, A., Fung, C. and Rosen, O.M. (1978) *J. Biol. Chem.*, 253:7570–7578.

Schmidt, S.Y. (1983) *J. Biol. Chem.*, 258:6863–6768.

Schmidt, S.Y. (1983) *J. Neurochem.*, 40:1630–1638.

Tabarini, D., Heinrich, J. and Rosen, O.M. (1985) *Proc. Natl. Acad. Sci. U.S.A.*, 82, 4369–4373.

Witters, L.A. (1985) Regulation of acetyl CoA carboxylase by insulin and other hormones. In Czech, M.P. (Ed.) *Molecular Basis of Insulin Action*, Plenum Press, New York, pp. 315–326.

Wu, W.C.-S. Walaas, S.I., Nairn, A.C. and Greengard, P. (1982) *Proc. Natl. Acad. Sci. U.S.A.*, 79:5249–5253.

W.H. Gispen and A. Routtenberg (Eds.)
Progress in Brain Research, Vol. 69
© 1986 Elsevier Science Publisher B.V. (Biomedical Division)

CHAPTER 17

Extracellular protein phosphorylation systems in the regulation of neuronal function

Y.H. Ehrlich[1,2], M.G. Garfield[1,3], T.B. Davis[1,2], E. Kornecki[1], J.E. Chaffee[1,4] and R.H. Lenox[1]

[1]*Neuroscience Research Unit, Department of Psychiatry and the Departments of* [2]*Biochemistry,* [3]*Pharmacology and* [4]*Physiology–Biophysics, University of Vermont College of Medicine, Burlington, VT 05405, U.S.A.*

Introduction

Several lines of investigation have provided evidence that extracellular adenosine triphosphate (ATP) exerts potent effects on the activity of excitable cells, neurons and muscle (for a recent review see Burnstock, 1985). Holton and Holton (1954) first suggested that ATP is released from nerve endings and plays a role in chemical transmission. Since then, it has been shown that ATP is present in synaptic vesicles of cholinergic and adrenergic neurons (Silinsky, 1975; Winkler, 1976; Zimmerman, 1982; Castel et al., 1984), and that ATP is secreted in association with classical neurotransmitters at certain synapses and neuromuscular junctions (Silinsky and Hubbard, 1973; Silinsky, 1975; Winkler, 1976; Phillis and Wu, 1981). Burnstock (1972, 1975) has reported findings suggesting that, in addition to the release of ATP as a co-transmitter, there also may exist specific purinergic neurons which secrete ATP as the principal neurotransmitter.

The question as to whether ATP molecules that are secreted by stimulated neurons have a direct physiological function had been a matter of debate. Released ATP can be rapidly hydrolyzed by extracellular enzymes to adenosine, which is a potent neuroregulator (Silinsky, 1975, 1984; Phillis and Wu, 1981). However, numerous studies have demonstrated transmission systems in which ATP itself is more effective than adenosine (Burnstock, 1985), and thus clarified the initial controversy.

Based on evidence obtained primarily from electophysiological studies, Burnstock (1981) has classified two types of purinergic receptors. The type named P_1 is most sensitive to adenosine and responds to ATP only after it has been hydrolyzed. Receptors of the P_2 type are stimulated much more potently by ATP than by adenosine (Burnstock, 1981; 1985). This classification has been generally accepted. Within the context of this chapter it should be mentioned that many of the responses mediated by P_2-purinoreceptors can be elicited by non-hydrolyzable analogs of ATP. Such responses can be mediated by ATP-binding proteins, and may not necessarily involve an ATP-utilizing enzyme. On the other hand, some neuronal responses, discussed below, were shown to require native, hydrolyzable ATP (Silinsky and Ginsborg, 1983). Such responses may be mediated by extracellular protein phosphorylation systems.

In addition to its role as a neurotransmitter, extracellular ATP can also serve as a modulator, regulating the activity of other neurohormones (for several reviews, see Daly et al., 1983). One well-documented modulatory effect of extracellular ATP is the inhibition of evoked quantal acetylcholine secretion (Riberio and Walker, 1975; Silinsky, 1975; Burnstock, 1985). Recent studies have demonstrated that when ATP is applied extracellularly to preganglionic nerves, it inhibits acetylcholine release. However, application of adenosine or a slowly degradable derivative of

ATP to the same nerves were without effect (Silinsky and Ginsborg, 1983). The authors have concluded that this modulation of synaptic function by ATP does not appear to be mediated by either adenosine receptors (P_1), nor by P_2-purinergic receptors. The mechanisms underlying this modulatory action of extracellular ATP may be mediated by an ATP-utilizing enzyme. In this chapter we present evidence consistent with the suggestion (Ehrlich et al., 1982; Ehrlich, 1984) that the modulation of certain neuronal functions by extracellular ATP involves the activity of extra-cellular protein kinases which phosphorylate pro-teins localized at the outer surface of the plasma membrane of neural cells.

Clonal cell lines: a model for investigating the function of neuronal phosphoproteins

The complexity and heterogeneity of cell pop-ulations in the nervous system may account, in a large part, for the fact that the information available to date on the specific functions of neuronal phosphoproteins is rather limited. In comparison, considerable progress in elucidating the function of specific protein phosphorylation systems in non-neural tissues has been achieved in studies utilizing *homogeneous* populations of cloned cells grown in culture. Studies of different clones of neuroblastoma cells have provided a model for investigating, in culture, various molecular events associated with neuronal differ-entiation (Prasad, 1980), including protein phosphorylation (Ehrlich et al., 1977a, 1978). Nonetheless, many attempts to induce complete neuronal maturation in clones of neuroblastoma cells have failed. It has been suggested, therefore, that neuroblastoma cells do not express all the genes for proteins that might be required for synaptic communication (Nirenberg et al., 1983). Clonal cell lines with the ultimate property of mature neurons, namely, the competence for synaptogenesis, have been obtained by somatic hybridization of neuroblastoma with glioma cells (for a most recent review, see Hamprecht et al., 1985). These hybrid cells express numerous neuronal-specific enzymes, ion-channels and receptors characteristic of mature neurons (ibid).

When neuroblastoma × glioma hybrid cells (NG cells) are treated in culture for several days with agents that increase the intracellular levels of cyclic AMP, they are shifted from a dividing state to a well-differentiated, synapse-competent state (Nirenberg et al., 1983; Hamprecht et al., 1985). NG cell lines provide, therefore, a homogeneous cell population most suitable for investigating molecular events which regulate certain functions of mature neurons. Our recent studies demon-strate the advantage of utilizing such a population of NG cells in investigations aiming to elucidate the role of specific phosphoproteins in neuronal function.

Neuroblastoma × glioma cells of the clone NG108-15 (obtained from Dr. M. Nirenberg; NIH, Bethesda, MD) are grown in our laboratory as described previously (see, e.g., McGee et al., 1978), except that the final concentration of fetal calf serum added to the growth medium is 5% instead of 10%. The morphological appearance of these cells is shown in Fig. 1A. Treatment for 4 days with 1 mM dibutyryl cyclic AMP (dBcAMP) induces in these cells growth arrest and morpho-logical differentiation (Fig. 1B). When dBcAMP-treated cells are further exposed to treatment with 5 µM cytosine arabinoside for 3 days, the remaining cells can be maintained in culture for an additional period of at least 4 weeks. During this period, some of the cells develop very large cell bodies and extend long and thick neurites with structures resembling nerve endings (Fig. 1C). Although under the conditions developed to date we cannot obtain sufficient amounts of cells as shown in Fig. 1C for detailed biochemical investi-gation, these cells are most suitable for electro-physiological studies. On the other hand, detailed analysis of protein phosphorylation activity could be carried out during the transition of NG108-15 cells from the multiplying state (Fig. 1A) to the differentiated (Fig. 1B), synapse-competent state Results of such studies are summarized below.

Phosphorylative modifications induced during differntiation of NG108–15 cells in culture

The potential of various protein kinases to phosphorylate different intrinsic protein substrates

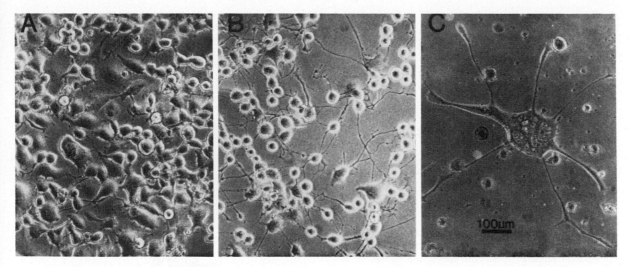

Fig. 1. Morphology of neuroblastoma × glioma cells grown and differentiated in culture. A: Photograph of NG108-15 cells grown under conditions promoting cell division (medium supplemented with 5% fetal bovine serum). B: NG108-15 cells differentiated in culture by treatment for 4 days with 1 mM dibutyryl cyclic AMP. C: Cells were differentiated as in B, then treated for 3 days with 5 μM of cytosine arabinoside, and the photograph taken 18 days later. All three panels were photographed with the same magnification (see bar in panel C).

may alter during the differentiation of NG cells. To determine these alterations we have carried out endogenous protein phosphorylation assays (Ehrlich, 1984), using the reaction conditions employed in our previous studies of rat brain protein phosphorylation systems (Ehrlich et al., 1974–1982). Fig. 2 shows a densitometric scan of an autoradiogram of endogenously phosphorylated proteins in isotonic homogenates which were prepared from non-differentiated or differentiated NG108-15 cells, and then incubated in vitro with $[\gamma^{-32}P]ATP$. It can be clearly seen that treatment for 6 days with 1 mM dBcAMP induced bidirectional changes in the endogenous phosphorylation of specific protein components. The most prominent alterations detected under these reaction conditions were a decrease in the phosphorylation of a protein with apparent M_r of 100–kDa, and the emergence of phosphorylation of a protein with M_r of approximately 80-kDa (Fig. 2). The finding that the phosphorylation of a 80-kDa protein is greatly increased in NG cells during a period of massive neurite outgrowth (see Fig. 1B) is consistent with the reports that such a phosphorylation system is enriched in nerve growth-cone particles (see Chapter 19), and associated with growth regulation (Chapter 16).

Analysis of endogenous protein phosphorylation activity in well-defined subcellular fractions prepared from a homogeneous population of NG108-15 cells has proven to be most revealing with respect to the role of protein phosphorylation in neuronal function. In a highly purified fraction of plasma membranes isolated from non-differentiated NG cells, the endogenous phosphorylation of proteins was found to be very low compared to the activity observed in the cytosol from such cells (see N in Fig. 3). After dBcAMP-induced differentiation there was a marked increase of endogenous protein phosphorylation activity in the plasma membranes (see D in Fig. 3). It should be emphasized that a high ratio of protein phosphorylation activity in the plasma membranes, as compared to the cytosol, is a feature characteristic of excitable cells, and rarely found non-neural tissues (Rodnight, 1983; Ehrlich, 1984). These results support the evidence for the neuronal nature of differentiated NG cells, and serve to identify which specific phosphoproteins have the potential for involvement in neuronal functions

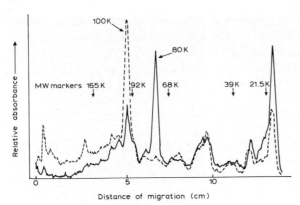

Fig. 2. Endogenously phosphorylated proteins in non-differentiated (dashed line) and differentiated (full line) NG108-15 cells. Aliquots containing 40 µg protein of an isotonic homogenate prepared from cells grown and treated as described in the legend to Fig. 1 were incubated for 2 min at 30°C with 1 µM [γ-^{32}P]ATP (10 µCi/reaction) in the presence of 20 mM HEPES buffer (pH 7.4) and 10 mM MgCl$_2$. Sodium dodecylsulfate-solubilized proteins were resolved by slab gel electrophoresis, then autoradiographed and scanned as described by Whittemore et al. (1984).

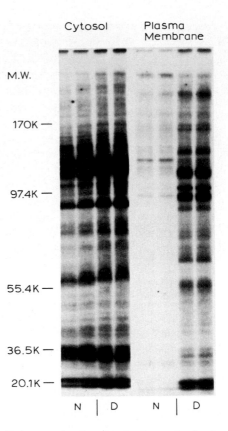

Fig. 3. Endogenously phosphorylated proteins in the cytosol and purified plasma membrane fractions of non-differentiated (N) and dibutyrl cyclic AMP-differentiated (D) NG108-15 cells. Shown above are autoradiographs of duplicate reactions with each sample, carried out as described in the legend to Fig. 2, but with the purified subcellular fractions.

which emerge in NG cells during cyclic AMP-induced differentiation. Fig. 3 also demonstrates that the phosphorylative modifications induced in the plasma membranes of differentiating NG cells are highly specific. While total phosphorylation activity increased, the endogenous phosphorylation of several endogenous protein substrates decreased (see, e.g., the phosphoproteins with apparent M_r of > 200 kDa and 131 kDa, marked with arrowheads in Fig. 3). The multiplicity of endogenous protein phosphorylation systems present in a homogenous population of neural cells, as shown here, provides further experimental support to the notion that specificity in the regulation of various neuronal functions by phosphorylative activity is determined by the nature of the protein substrate (Ehrlich, 1979). Furthermore, these results provide the data basis needed to carry out experiments designed to determine the role of specific phosphoproteins in: (a) the regulation of presynaptic functions expressed by differentiated NG108-15 cells (McGee et al., 1978; Nirenberg et al., 1983), and (b) the adaptation of receptor activity induced in neural cells by treat-

ment with psychotropic drugs (Ehrlich, 1984; Kornecki et al., 1984a; Hamprecht et al., 1985).

The measurement of endogenous protein phosphorylation in cell-free assays has been a method of choice for biochemical characterization of the activity of protein kinases which utilize ATP (Ueda et al., 1973) or GTP (Ehrlich et al., 1982a) as co-substrates in the phosphorylation of specific protein components in brain membranes. In addition, these in vitro reactions have proven useful for implicating certain specific phosphoproteins in alterations induced in brain tissue in vivo in response to training experience (Ehrlich et al., 1977; Morgan and Routtenberg, 1981), various psychotropic drugs (reviewed by Ehrlich, 1979,

1984), electroconvulsive shock (Ehrlich et al., 1980) and long term potentiation (see Chapter 18). As demonstrated above, in studies of cells grown in culture these in vitro reactions provide the means to detect changes in the *potential* of protein kinase(s) to phosphorylate certain specific proteins. Such potential changes in activity which are induced during the differentiation of NG cells may remain latent until an additional stimulus (e.g. active synaptogenesis, cell depolarization, receptor stimulation) elicits their expression. With cells grown in culture, such hypotheses can be conveniently tested by labeling the phosphoproteins of intact cells with inorganic $^{32}P_i$. In conducting studies with this conventional procedure, we follow the guidelines and precautions detailed by Garrison (1983). The results of these experiments, however, cannot be discussed in detail within the context of this chapter. The remainder of this report focusses on studies in which we utilize a novel approach: the phosphorylation of surface proteins by extracellular ATP.

The interaction of extracellular ATP with intact neural cells

Phosphorylation of Surface Proteins

The preceding sections of this chapter have cited studies which utilized NG108-15 cells to provide new insights into molecular mechanisms underlying neuronal maturation, and demonstrated that these cells can be particularly suitable for investigating the role of membrane-bound protein phosphorylation systems in the regulation of presynaptic activity. We have proposed previously that protein phosphorylation systems may be involved in mechanisms underlying the modulatory effects of *extracellular* ATP on certain presynaptic functions (Ehrlich, 1984). However, protein kinase activity which utilizes extracellular ATP to phosphorylate proteins localized at the outer surface of the plasma membrane (an ecto-protein kinase) has never been demonstrated conclusively in neurons. The first step in investigating the role of extracellular protein phosphorylation systems in neuronal

function must be to prove that ecto-protein kinase activity indeed phosphorylates specific protein substrates at the surface of neural cells. We have utilized intact, viable NG108-15 cells to provide evidence for the existence of such activity and begun to explore its role in neuronal function.

In the initial phase of this investigation, NG108-15 cells were grown in the presence of 5% fetal calf serum until they reached 80–90% confluency, and then harvested by gently shaking the culture flasks. The cells were then washed extensively in a medium without serum, and assayed for endogenous protein phosphorylation by extracellular ATP. These assays were carried out in a medium mimicking the extracellular environment of cells in the nervous system (see legend to Fig. 4). When intact NG108-15 cells were incubated with $[\gamma\text{-}^{32}P]ATP$, there was incorporation of ^{32}P into trichloroacetic acid (TCA)-precipitable proteins. This incorporation was linearly proportional to cell number (Fig. 4)

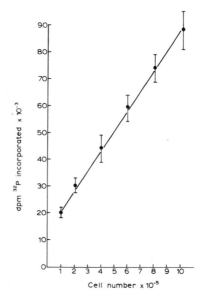

Fig. 4. Extracellular ATP as a co-substrate in endogenous phosphorylation activity. Intact NG108-15 cells were washed twice and gently resuspended in a Krebs–Ringer medium containing 145 mM NaCl, 5 mM KCl, 0.8 mM MgCl$_2$, 1.8 mM CaCl$_2$, 20 mM glucose and 25 mM HEPES buffer, adjusted to pH 7.4 with NaOH. The reaction was then initiated by adding $[\gamma\text{-}^{32}P]$-ATP (initial concentration 2 μM) and stopped after 10 min incubation at 37°C. ^{32}P incorporation into proteins was measured in TCA precipitates of the reaction products.

202

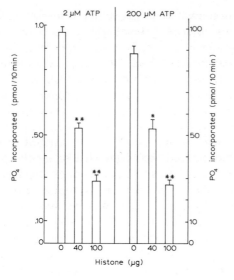

Fig. 5. Histones inhibit endogenous ecto-protein kinase activity in NG108-15 cells. Assays were carried out as described in the Legend to Fig. 4, with 10^5 cells/reaction and either 2 µM (left panel) or 200 µM (right panel) extracellular [γ-^{32}P]ATP. Type I histone (Sigma) was added (40 or 100 µg/ml) 1 min prior to the ATP. *$p < 0.05$; **$p < 0.001$.

and increased linearly with reaction time up to at least 10 min. Over 80% of the ^{32}P incorporated under these conditions was found to be bound to protein in phosphomonoester linkages, as expected from products of protein kinase activity.

When the concentration of ATP added to the extracellular medium was 2 µM, we measured incorporation of 0.96 ± 0.025 pmol PO_4/2 × 10^5 cells/10 min, and with 200 µM ATP the incorporation was 88 ± 3 pmol PO_4. This value was increased by $45 \pm 6\%$ when the exogenous protein α-casein (40 µg) was added to the extracellular medium of cells incubated with [γ-^{32}P]ATP. The phosphorylation of an exogenous protein substrate by intact cells utilizing extracellular ATP provides evidence that the protein kinase involved is an ecto-enzyme. In contrast to the phosphorylation of casein by intact cells, addition of histones *inhibited* the endogenous phosphorylation activity measured when intact NG108-15 cells were incubated with extracellular ATP (Fig. 5). This finding suggests that ecto-

protein kinase may be one of the targets for the cytotoxic effects of histones on intact cells, reported by Kubler et al. (1982). Furthermore, since we have found that histones are readily phosphorylated by lysed cells, we conclude that the phosphorylating activity measured with intact cells (Figs. 4 and 5) is not likely to be carried out by protein kinases of intracellular origin. Using the same reaction conditions, we have measured the ecto-protein kinase activity of NG108-15 cells as a function of extracellular ATP concentration between 100 and 1000 µM. Lineweaver–Burke analysis of the data ($R = 0.98$) indicated that the apparent K_m of this activity for ATP is 525 µM.

Effects of extracellular ATP on intracellular adenylate cyclase activity

Based on previous studies in our laboratory, we have suggested that membrane-bound protein phosphorylation systems may play a role in the desensitization of receptor-coupled adenylate cyclase activity in neuronal cells (Whittemore et al., 1981, 1984). To examine the potential of ecto-protein kinase activity for involvement in such a regulatory process, we have measured the effects of extracellular ATP on intracellular generation of cyclic AMP in intact NG108-15 cells. In these experiments we labeled the intracellular ATP pools of the intact cells by preincubation with tritiated adenine, as previously described (Ehrlich et al., 1982; Lenox et al., 1985). Washed cells were then reincubated with increasing concentrations of extracellular ATP, and analyzed for de novo formation of tritiated cyclic AMP. Fig. 6A demonstrates that basal cyclic AMP generation in intact NG108-15 cells was stimulated by 100 µM extracellular ATP, and that this stimulation was reversed at higher ATP concentrations. Prostaglandin E_1 (PGE$_1$) receptors in NG108-15 cells mediate stimulation of adenylate cyclase. As can be seen in Fig. 6B, PGE$_1$-stimulated generation of intracellular cyclic AMP in intact NG108-15 cells is potently inhibited by extracellular ATP. The $K_{0.5}$ for this inhibitory effect was found to be 510 µM extracellular ATP.

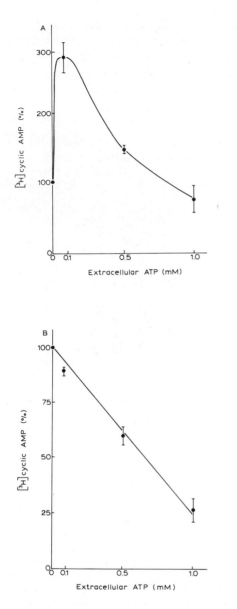

Fig. 6. Effects of extracellular ATP on intracellular cyclic AMP generation in intact NG108-15 cells. A: Basal activity of non-stimulated cells. B: Activity in cells stimulated with 0.5 µM PGE$_1$. Assays were carried out essentially as described by Lenox et al. (1985), using intact NG cells prelabeled with [^{3}H]adenine (Ehrlich et al., 1982b). The reaction time was 10 min and 1 mM R020-1724 (Ehrlich et al., 1977a) was used as phosphodiesterase inhibitor. Results are presented as percent of control (100%), measured without adding extracellular ATP. Stimulation with PGE$_1$ (B) caused a 22-fold increase in cyclic [^{3}H]AMP formation, compared to basal conditions (A). Values represent mean ± S.E.M. from 3 experiments.

Extracellular ATP Stimulates the uptake of calcium ions by neural cells

Studies in the laboratory of B. Hamprecht (see his review, 1985) have demonstrated that the treatment with a calcium-ionophore, A23187, inhibits the PGE$_1$-stimulated formation of cyclic AMP in intact NG108-15 cells. To examine whether a similar mechanism underlies the effects of extracellular ATP on this activity, we have measured the uptake of ^{45}Ca^{2+} in intact NG108-15 cells incubated under conditions identical to those used in the assays of cyclic AMP generation (see Fig. 6). Table I demonstrates that extracellular ATP caused a dose-dependent increase in the uptake of ^{45}Ca^{2+} into NG108-15 cells resuspended in a physiological buffer. Half maximal increase of ^{45}Ca^{2+} uptake was induced by 520 µM ATP. The ATP-induced increase in the uptake of Ca^{2+} ions was additive with the uptake induced by 50 mM KCl. This finding suggests that the mechanism activated by extracellular ATP is different from that operating in depolarization-induced calcium uptake. Studies of non-neural cells have provided evidence that extracellular ATP (0.1–1.0 mM) causes increase in passive membrane permeability (Dicker et al., 1980). It is possible that a similar mechanism operates in NG108-15 cells, and that ecto-protein kinase activity with a relatively high K_m (0.5 mM) for extracellular ATP mediates an increase in

TABLE 1
Effects of extracellular ATP on ^{45}Ca^{2+} uptake by NG108-15 cells

Extracellular ATP (mM)	^{45}Ca^{2+} uptake (dpm ^{45}CaCl$_2$/5 × 10^5 cells/12 min)[a]
0	8 828 ± 349
0.1	12 217 ± 1 408
1.0	59 919 ± 1 590

[a]Values are means ± S.D. of triplicate determination from a representative assay. Uptake was measured with cells resuspended in the buffer used for measuring ecto-kinase activity (see legend to Fig. 4), with 1 µCi of ^{45}CaCl$_2$ added per reaction tube.

204

passive influx of Ca^{2+} ions. This influx could be the cause of a decrease in the sensitivity of intracellular adenylate cyclase to stimulation by PGE_1. Based on electrophysiological considerations, Silinsky (1975) has calculated that after repetitive stimulation, the concentration of extracellular ATP in the cleft of cholinergic synapses would be at least 100 µM. Any consideration of a potential physiological role for neuronal ecto-protein kinase with high K_m for ATP must be reserved for feedback mechanisms, or for adaptive processes induced by repetitive stimulation (see Chapter 18).

Identification of the endogenous substrates for ecto-protein kinase in neural cells

The ectokinase activity measured in our initial studies (Figs. 4 and 5) may have arisen from a contaminating serum protein kinase, or reside on membrane fragments formed from some cells which break during harvest. To exclude these possibilities, we have grown NG108-15 cells in a chemically defined, serum-free medium (Bottenstein, 1981). The assays of endogenous protein phosphorylation activity utilizing extracellular ATP were then carried out with these cells while still attached to the bottom of individual wells in 96-well plates. Under these assay conditions, we have successfully reproduced results such as we have presented previously with cells that were harvested after growth in serum-containing medium, and then assayed in suspension (Ehrlich et al., 1982b). Accordingly, the pattern of phosphorylated proteins in intact NG108-15 cells incubated with extracellular [γ-^{32}P]-ATP was found to be qualitatively different from that observed in cells incubated under identical conditions with equivalent amounts of radioactive inorganic $^{32}P_i$. Moreover, kinetic studies (Ehrlich et al., 1986) have provided evidence that the phosphorylation of specific protein components seen in intact NG108-15 cells incubated with extracellular [γ-^{32}P]ATP for up to 20 min cannot be attributed to $^{32}P_i$ liberated by ecto-ATPases, which may then label intracellular ATP pools and, in turn, intracellular proteins.

The protein substrates phosphorylated by

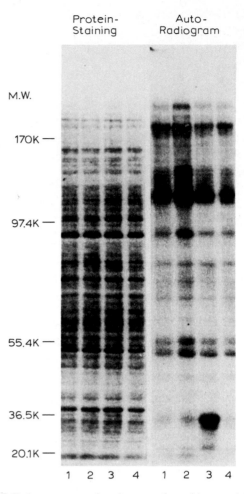

Fig. 7. Endogenous protein substrates of ecto-kinase activity in intact NG108-15 cells grown in a chemically defined, serum-free medium. Assays were carried out with cells attached to the bottom of the plate (96 wells), with each well containing 100 µl of the medium specified in Fig. 4 and supplemented with 1 µM Verapamil (lane 1), no additions (lane 2), α-casein (lane 3) or 1 µM veratridine (lane 4). Sodium dodecylsulfate gel electrophoresis was conducted as described in Figs. 2 and 3. Reaction time was 10 min and the concentration of added [γ-^{32}P]ATP was 1 µM (10 µCi per well).

extracellular [γ-^{32}P]ATP in intact NG108-15 cells are demonstrated in Fig. 7. An autoradiogram which was obtained from an assay carried out in our standard reaction buffer (see Legend to Fig. 4) is depicted in lane 2. Lane 3 demonstrates that intact NG108-15 cells can utilize extracellular ATP to phosphorylate the exogenous protein, casein, when added to the extracellular medium. Mild pretreatment of the surface of intact cells with 0.01% trypsin (10 min/37°C) eliminated this activity (Ehrlich et al., 1986). Based on these results, and other findings reported elsewhere, we have concluded that NG108-15 cells have an ecto-protein kinase which phophorylates endogenous protein substrates localized at the cell surface.

The potential role of ecto-protein kinase in neuronal function

When NG108-15 cells are treated for 4–10 days with 1 mM dBcAMP their growth is arrested, they become non-tumorigenic and develop many physiological and biochemical · properties characteristic of mature neurons, including the competence to form functional synapses (Nirenberg et al., 1983; Hamprecht et al., 1985). On the basis of over 100 reports cited in the two reviews quoted above (ibid), it would be expected that, if ecto-protein kinase is associated with the neuronal functions of NG108-15 cells, its activity should increase after cyclic AMP-induced differentiation of these cells. Fig. 8 demonstrates that such is indeed the case (compare lanes marked with D and N in left panel). Quantitation of these results revealed that after differentiation there was a greater than two-fold increase in the phosphorylation of surface proteins by extra-cellular ATP in NG108-15 cells. Labeling of the surface proteins of intact NG108-15 cells with ^{125}I by the Iodogen method (Tuszynski et al., 1983) or by Iodobeads (Kornecki et al., 1984b) did not reveal major differences between differentiated and non-treated cells (Fig. 8 in right panel). Several of the surface-iodinated protein bands co-migrated with proteins phosphorylated by extracellular ATP. The changes in phosphorylation seen in Fig. 8 may thus be due to increase in ectokinase activity rather than in the amount of its protein substrates. Additional support for the suggestion that ecto-protein kinase activity is associated with neuronal functions was obtained from our finding that another clonal cell line which has been studied extensively for its neuronal properties, the PC12 cells (Greene and Tishler, 1976), also demonstrates ecto-protein kinase activity (Chaffee

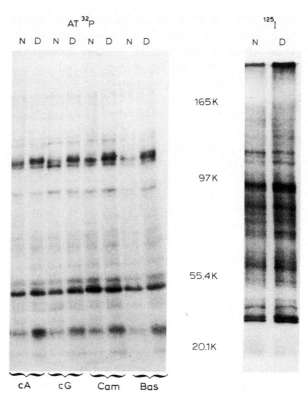

Fig. 8. Left: Ectokinase activity in differentiated (D) and non-differentiated (N) NG108-15 cells. Assays were carried out under basal (Bas) conditions (no additions), as detailed in the legend to Fig. 7, or by adding the [γ-^{32}P]ATP 30 s after the addition of 1 unit calmodulin (Cam), 1 µM cyclic AMP (cA) or 1 µM cyclic GMP (cG), which had no detectable effects on the measured activity. Right: The two lanes on the right show the pattern of surface-iodinated proteins (^{125}I) of 'N' and 'D' cells, separated in a 7–14% exponential gel gradient, as the phosphorylated surface proteins shown on the left panel (AT^{32}P).

et al., in preparation). In contrast, in clonal cells of non-neural origin (e.g. A431 cells), this activity was found to be about 10 to 100 times lower than in NG108-15 cells.

Certain specific neuronal functions, such as depolarization-induced acetylcholine release (McGee et al., 1978) and voltage-sensitive calcium channel activity (Nirenberg et al., 1983) were shown to operate in NG108-15 only after the cells had been induced to differentiate by agents that increase cyclic AMP levels, but not in untreated cells. We have found recently that when NG108-15 cells that had been differentiated by treatment with 1 mM dBcAMP are depolarized with 50 mM KCl. there is a selective increase in the phosphorylation of one specific protein component (126 kDa) by ecto-kinase activity. In non-treated NG108-15 cells, phosphorylation of this protein component was not seen, neither under resting nor under depolarizing conditions. These findings have demonstrated that ecto-protein kinase activity is evoked by depolarization in differentiated NG108-15 cells. Detailed studies of the surface phosphoprotein of 126 kDa should enable us to determine the role of ecto-protein kinase in the regulation of neuronal functions evoked by depolarization.

Conclusions and future directions

In the studies described above, cells of the neuroblastoma × glioma hybrid line NG108-15, grown and differentiated in a chemically defined (serumfree) medium, were used to demonstrate the presence of an ecto-protein kinase and specific substrates for its activity at the surface of neural cells. Intact cells incubated in a physiological buffer catalyzed the transfer of the γ-^{32}P from extracellular ATP to specific membrane proteins. The evidence for the ecto-enzymatic nature of this activity includes the following:

(a) Intact, attached cells phosphorylated exogenous protein (casein) added to the extracellular medium.

(b) Mild treatment of intact cells with 0.01% trypsin removed the phosphate incorporated from extracellular ATP and eliminated the ectokinase activity.

(c) A different time-course of protein phosphorylation was observed in intact cells incubated with equivalent amounts of either [γ-^{32}P]ATP or inorganic ^{32}P$_i$.

(d) The spectrum of cell proteins phosphorylated by extracellular ATP was different from that obtained by labeling intracellular ATP pools. Only differentiated, but not dividing NG108-15 cells, responded to depolarization by 50 mM KC1 with increased phosphorylation of one specific protein by ecto-kinase activity.

The results reported here suggest several directions for future investigations on the role of extracellular protein phosphorylation activity in regulating specific neuronal functions. An ecto-protein kinase with a relatively high K_m for ATP (0.5 mM) may be involved in the changes in passive membrane permeability (Dicker et al., 1980) that can be induced in neurons by repetitive stimulation (Silinsky et al., 1975; Chapter 18), and in its effects on receptor sensitivity (Ehrlich et al., 1982). Ecto-protein kinase may also function as a key enzyme in the phosphorylation of neural cell adhesion molecules (N-CAM's; Edelman, 1983; Lyles et al., 1984). The specific protein substrate of ecto-kinase activity whose phosphorylation is selectively stimulated by depolarization could play a regulatory role in the function of voltage-sensitive Ca^{2+} channels (Nirenberg et al., 1983) or in other events associated with evoked acetylcholine release (McGee et al., 1978). These two processes operate in differentiated NG cells, and either one may be involved in the modulation of quantal neurotransmitter release by extracellular ATP (Silinsky and Ginsborg, 1983). The role of ecto-protein kinase in the regulation of these pre-

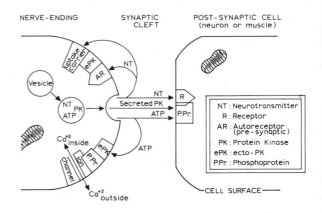

Fig. 9. Schematic presentation of the *hypothetical* involvement of extracellular protein phosphorylation systems in synaptic function. ATP released from stimulated neurons can be utilized by two types of extracellular protein kinases. A membrane-bound ecto-kinase, and a secreted, soluble protein kinase. Phosphorylation of proteins at the outer surface of the nerve terminal by ecto-kinase activity may regulate presynaptic functions, such as Ca^{2+} channels, neurotransmitter release and/or re-uptake. The secreted, soluble protein kinase may phosphorylate surface proteins of the postsynaptic cell and regulate, for example, receptor function.

synaptic activities can now be conveniently investigated in a homogeneous population of NG cells. Similar studies with primary cultures of embryonic brain neurons could reveal a role for extracellular protein phosphorylation systems in neuronal development and maturation.

In the process described above, an ecto-protein kinase could function as a *receptor* for extracellular ATP when the latter modulates presynaptic activity (see Fig. 9). Recently, we have found that depolarization of differentiated NG108-15 cells can cause the secretion of soluble protein kinase activity to the extracellular medium (Ehrlich and Kornecki, 1986). This soluble protein kinase may utilize extracellular ATP to phosphorylate target proteins on the outer surface of *post*synaptic cells. A protein kinase secreted from stimulated nerve endings may thus play the role of a *neurohormone*, an enzyme functioning as first messenger in intercellular communications. Experimental testing of the working hypothesis illustrated in Fig. 9 may prove that extracellular protein phosphorylation plays a significant role in regulating the function of cells in the peripheral and central nervous system.

Acknowledgements

We are grateful to Drs. M. Hacker, E. Hendley and S. Weiss for many helpful discussions, to W. Ohlsson, I. Galbraith and J. Wesson for expert technical assistance, to P. Smith for typing the manuscript and to D. Hardwick for preparing the figures. The studies reported here were supported by USAFOSR grant 84-0331, NIH grant MH-35735, NSF grant BNS82-09265 and an ACS Institutional Research Grant.

References

Bottenstein, J. (1981) Differentiated properties of neuronal cell lines. In G. Sato (Ed.), *Functionally Differentiated Cell Lines*, Alan R. Liss, New York, pp. 155–184.

Burnstock, G. (1972) Purinergic nerves. *Pharmacol Rev.*, 24:509–581.

Burnstock, G. (1975) Purinergic transmission. In L.L. Iverson, S.D. Iversen and S.H. Snyder (Eds.), *Handbook of Psychopharmacology, Vol. 5*, Plenum Press, New York, pp. 131–194.

Burnstock, G. (1981) Neurotransmitters and trophic factors in the autonomic nervous system. *J. Physiol.*, 313:1–35.

Burnstock, G. (1985) Purinergic mechanisms broaden their sphere of influence, *Trends Neurosci. Res.*, 5:6.

Caster, M., Gainer, H. and Pellman, H.D. (1984) Neuronal secretory systems. *Int. Rev. Cytol.*, 88:303–459.

Daley, J.W., Kuroda, Y., Phillis, J.W., Shimizu, H. and Ui, M. (Eds.) (1983) Roles of adenosine and adenine nucleotides in the central nervous system. *Physiology and Pharmacology of Adenosine Derivatives*, Raven Press, New York.

Dicker, P., Heppel, L.A. and Rozengurt, E. (1980) Control of membrane permeability by external and internal ATP in 3T6 cells grown in serum-free medium. *Proc. Natl. Acad. Sci. U.S.A.*, 77:2103–2107.

Edelman, G.M. (1983) Cell adhesion molecules. *Science*, 219:450–457.

Ehrlich, Y.H. (1979) Phosphoproteins as specifiers for mediators and modulators in neuronal function. *Adv. Exp. Med. Biol.*, 116:75–102.

Ehrlich, Y.H. (1981) Protein phosphorylation neuronal receptors and seizures in the CNS. In C. Waterlain, A.V. Delegado-Escueta and R. Porter (Eds.), *Advances in Neurology, Vol. 34*, Raven Press, New York, pp. 345–352.

Ehrlich, Y.H. (1984) Protein phosphorylation: role in the function, regulation and adaptation of neural receptors. In A. Lajtha (Ed.),; *Handbook of Neurochemistry, Vol. 6*, Plenum, New York, pp. 541–574.

Ehrlich, Y.H. and Kornecki, E. (1986). Secretion of protein kinase from stimulated neural cells and activated platelets. *Trans. Am. Soc. Neurochem.* 17:1 (abstract).

Ehrlich, Y.H. and Routtenberg, A. (1974) Cyclic AMP regulates the phosphorylation of three proteins of rat cerebal cortex membranes for thirty minutes. *FEBS Lett.*, 45:237–243.

Ehrlich, Y.H., Brunngraber, E.G., Sinah, P.K. and Prasad, K.N. (1977a) Specific alterations in phosphorylation of cytosol proteins from differentiating neuroblastoma cells grown in culture. *Nature*, 265:238–240.

Ehrlich, Y.H., Rabjohns, R. and Routtenberg, A. (1977b) Experiential-input alters the phosphorylation of specific proteins in brain membranes. *Pharmacol. Biochem. Behav.*, 6:169–174.

Ehrlich, Y.H., Prasad, K.N., Davis, L.G., Sinah, P.K. and Brunngraber, E. (1978) Endogenous phosphorylation of specific proteins in subcellular fractions from malignant and cAMP-induced differentiated neuroblastoma cells in-culture. *Neurochem. Res.*, 3:803–813.

Ehrlich, Y.H., Volovka, J., Davis, L.G. and Brunngraber, E.G. (Eds.) (1979) *Modulators, Mediators and Specifiers in Brain Function*, Plenum Press, New York.

Ehrlich, Y.H., Reddy, M.N., Keen, P. and Davis, L.G. (1980) Transient changes in the phosphorylation of cortical membrane proteins after electroconvulsive shock. *J. Neurochem.*, 34:1327–1330.

Ehrlich, Y.H., Wittemore, S.R., Lambert R., Ellis, J., Graber, S.G. and Lenox, R.H. (1982a) GTP-preferring protein phosphorylating systems in brain membranes: Possible role in adenylate cyclase regulation. *Biochem. Biophys. Res. Commun.*, 107:669–706.

Ehrlich, Y.H., Whittemore, S.R., Garfield, M.K., Graber, S.G. and Lenox, R.H. (1982b) Protein phosphorylation in the regulation and adaptation of receptor function. In W.H. Gispen and A. Routtenberg (Eds.), *Progress in Brain Research, Vol. 56*, Elsevier/North Holland, Amsterdam, pp. 375–396.

Ehrlich, Y.H., Davis, T.B., Bock, E., Kornecki, E., and Lenox, R.H. (1986) Ecto-protein kinase activity on the external surface of neural cells. *Nature*, 320:67–70.

Garrison, J.C. (1983) Measurement of hormone-stimulated protein phosphorylation in intact cells. *Meth. Enzymol.*, 99:20–36.

Greene, L.A. and Tischler, A. (1976) Establishment of a noradrenergic clonal line of rat adrenal pheochromocytoma cells which respond to nerve growth factor. *Proc. Natl. Acad. Sci. U.S.A.*, 73:2424–2428.

Hamprecht, B., Glaser, T., Reiser, G., Bayer, E. and Propst, F. (1985) Culture and characteristics of hormone-responsive neuroblastoma × glioma hybrid cells. *Meth. Enzymol.*, 109:316–341.

Holton, F.A. and Holton, P. (1954) The capillary dilator substances in dry powders of spinal roots: a possible role of ATP in chemical transmission from nerve endings. *J. Physiol. (London)*, 126:124–140.

Kornecki, E., Ehrlich, Y.H. and Lenox, R.H. (1984a). Platelet-activating factor-induced aggregation of human platelets specifically inhibited by triazolobenzodiazepines. *Science*, 226:1454–1456.

Kornecki, E., Davis, T.B. and Ehrlich, Y.H. (1984b) Iodination of membrane surface proteins of neuroblastoma × glioma cells. *Trans. Am. Soc. Neurochem.*, 15:164.

Kubler, D., Pyerin, W. and Kinzel, V. (1982) Protein kinase activity and substrates at the surface of intact Hela cells. *J. Biol. Chem.*, 257:322–329.

Lenox, R.H., Ellis, J., Van Riper, D. and Ehrlich, Y.H. (1985) α_2-Adrenergic receptor-mediated regulation of adenylate cyclase in the intact human platelet: Evidence for a receptor reserve. *Mol. Pharmacol.*, 27:1–7.

Lyles, J.M., Linnemann, D. and Bock, E. (1984) Biosynthesis of the D2-cell adhesion molecule: Post-translational modifications intracellular transport and developmental changes. *J. Cell Biol.*, 99:2082–2091.

McGee, R., Simpson, P., Christian, C., Mata, M., Nelson, P. and Nirenberg, M. (1978) Regulation of acetylcholine release from neuroblastoma × glioma hybrid cells. *Proc. Natl. Acad. Sci. U.S.A.*, 75:1314–1318.

Morgan, D.G. and Routtenberg, A. (1981) Brain pyruvate dehydrogenase: phosphorylation and enzyme activity altered by a training experience. *Science*, 214:470–471.

Nirenberg, M., Wilson, S., Higashida, H., Rotter, A., Krueger, K., Busis, N., Ray, R., Kenimer, J.G. and Adler, M. (1983) Modulation of synapse formation by cyclic adenosine monophosphate. *Science*, 222:793–799.

Phillis, J.W. and Wu, P.H. (1981) Roles of adenosine and adenine nucleotides in the central nervous system. In J.W. Daly, Y. Kuroda, J.W. Phillis, H. Shimizu and M. Ui (Eds.), *Physiology and Pharmacology of Adenosine Derivatives*, Raven Press, New York, pp. 219–236.

Prasad, K.N. (1980) *Regulation of Differentiation in Mammalian Nerve Cells*, Plenum, New York.

Ribeiro, J.A. and Walker, J. (1975). The effects of adenosine triphosphate and adenosine disphosphate on transmission at the rat and frog neuromuscular junctions. *Br. J. Pharmacol.*, 54:213–218.

Rodnight R. (1983) Protein kinases and phosphatases. In A. Lajtha (Ed.), *Handbook of Neurochemistry*, Plenum, New York, pp. 195–217.

Silinsky, E.M. (1975) On the association between transmitter secretion and the release of adenine nucleotides from mammalian motor nerve terminals. *J. Physiol.*, 247:145–162.

Silinsky, E.M. (1984) On the mechanism by which adenosine receptor activation inhibits the release of acetycholine from motor nerve endings. *J. Physiol.*, 346:243–256.

Silinsky, E.M. and Ginsborg, B.L. (1983) Inhibition of acetylcholine release from preganglionic frog nerves by ATP but not adenosine. *Nature*, 305:327–328.

Silinsky, E.M. and Hubbard, J.I. (1973) Release of ATP from rat motor nerve terminals. *Nature*, 243:404–405.

Tuszynski, G.P., Knight, L.C., Kornecki, E. and Srivastava, S. (1983) Labeling of platelet surface proteins with ^{125}I by the iodogen method. *Anal. Biochem.*, 130:166–170.

Ueda, T., Maeno, H. and Greengard P. (1973) Regulation of endogenous phosphorylation of specific proteins in synaptic membrane fractions from rat brain by adenosine 3′:5′-monophosphate, *J. Biol. Chem.*, 248:8295–8305.

Whittemore, S.R., Lenox, R.H., Hendley, E.D., and Ehrlich, Y.H. (1981) Protein phosphorylation mediates effects of isoproterenol on adenylate cyclase activity in rat cortical membranes. *Neurochem. Res.*, 6:777–787.

Whittemore, S.R., Graber, S.G., Lenox, R.H., Hendley, E.D. and Ehrlich, Y.H. (1984) Activation of adenylate cyclase by preincubation of rat cerebral-cortical membranes under phosphorylating conditions: Role of ATP, GTP and divalent cations. *J. Neurochem.*, 42:1685–1696.

Winkler, H. (1976) The composition of adrenal chromaffin granules: an assessment of controversial results. *Neuroscience*, 1:65–80.

Zimmerman, H. (1982) Biochemistry of the isolated cholinergic vesicles. In R.L. Klein, H.Lagercrantz and H. Zimmerman (Eds.), *Neurotransmitter Vesicles*, Academic Press, New York, pp. 271–304.

SECTION IV

Plasticity

W.H. Gispen and A. Routtenberg (Eds.)
Progress in Brain Research, Vol. 69
© 1986 Elsevier Science Publishers B.V. (Biomedical Division)

CHAPTER 18

Synaptic plasticity and protein kinase C

Aryeh Routtenberg

Northwestern University, Evanston, IL 60201, U.S.A.

With the assistance of: R. Akers, S. Chan, P. Colley, D. Linden, D. Lovinger, K. Murakami, R. Nelson and F-S. Sheu

Introduction

The present chapter focusses on the role of protein kinase C in the expression of synaptic plasticity. One theme to emerge from our studies is that protein kinase C specifically regulates the durability or persistence of the enhanced synaptic response, possibly by preventing decay of the response. It does not appear to play a role in the response initiation stages.

Another theme is that protein kinase C, as a multifunctional enzyme, may be capable of organizing the major cellular events underlying the persistence of synaptic plasticity by regulating the phosphorylation state of different substrate proteins. It will be suggested that these substrates could then regulate synaptic growth, neurotransmitter release, receptor number and ionic conductance. In the first section of this chapter the evidence that the durability of synaptic plasticity is regulated by protein kinase C and its substrates is considered. In the second section evidence is reviewed that implicates protein kinase C as participating in the regulation of several different cellular processes.

This chapter is dedicated to Donald Olding Hebb (1904–1985) whose insights more than thirty years ago provided the theoretical foundation for much of the current work on synaptic plasticity and information storage, including the empirical results presented herein.

Synaptic plasticity: models (long-term potentiation) and memory

The long-range goal in this laboratory is to understand how information is stored in the nervous system. One hypothesis, for which no suitable alternative has yet been proposed, is that there is a "growth process or metabolic change" that occurs in a network of synapses that is, in fact, the physical substrate of information storage (Hebb, 1949; p. 51).

We have challenged the nervous system of intact animals with training situations which would generate information storage processes. This would leave a biochemical residual which would then allow us to observe and describe the metabolic consequences of training situation challenge. Based on the hypothesis that information storage is associated with post-translational modification of proteins already present within the synaptic junction (Routtenberg, 1982b), we focussed our study on the metabolism of brain phosphoproteins. The intent was to cast a wide net at both behavioral and biochemical levels and establish whether a training situation would provide a set of candidate phosphoprotein molecules for subsequent detailed analysis.

Our first report in 1975 provided such a candidate. This was a 47-kDa protein, termed band F then and protein F1 now, which was altered in its phosphorylation as a consequence of training (Routtenberg et al., 1975; Ehrlich et al., 1977). If this alteration in protein phosphorylation observed following training were specifically re-

212

lated to alterations in synaptic strength, then it should be possible to observe alterations in protein F1 in relation to electrophysiological measures of synaptic strength. To study this problem we chose the long-term potentiation (LTP) paradigm developed by Bliss and Lomo (1973). By stimulating a particular pathway leading into the hippocampus at high frequency, these authors altered the synaptic strength of the monosynaptic perforant path dentate gyrus granule cell connection (see, e.g., Ruth et al., 1982). The alteration in synaptic strength was specific to these particular synapses located on the outer 2/3 of the granule cell dendritic tree. Other synapses on the inner 1/3 of the dendrite of granule cells showed no increase in synaptic strength. Of special interest to the use of this system as a model of information storage is the fact that the physiological enhancement of the response can persist for days or months (Bliss and Gardner-Medwin, 1973; Douglas and Goddard, 1975; Barnes and McNaughton, 1980). The intact hippocampal system was therefore used so that we could study both short-term plasticity in acute preparations and long-term plasticity in chronic studies (see also Abraham et al., 1985).

Prior to the initiation of the LTP paradigm, stimulating electrodes were placed in the bottleneck of Lomo (1971) to maximize the number of perforant path fibers activated (Fig. 1). Using recording micropipettes in the dentate gyrus we established that the activation was local, and not a broadcast field potential, by performing a laminar profile along the dendritic tree of the granule cell. As shown in Fig. 2, a reversal of potential is observed. In the dendrites, an initial negative wave, the extracellular excitatory postsynaptic potential (EPSP) (Andersen et al., 1966; Lomo, 1971), represents the sink or current inflow and the site of maximum synaptic activation. At the cell body current flows out at the source and is detected as a positive wave. This sink–source relation is also observed, but in reverse, when the consequent extracellular population spike is studied under laminar profile. Here the wave is negative (sink) in the cell body region and positive (source) in the dendritic zone. One can establish the extent of this local synaptic invasion along the dorsal–ventral

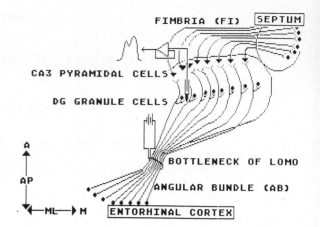

Fig. 1. Highly schematic diagram to show that perforant path/angular bundle stimulation at Lomo's bottleneck leads to widespread activation of dentate gyrus (DG) granule cells. A: Micropipette is marched along the DG to determine the extent of invasion and guide subsequent dissection for biochemical analysis.

(or septo–temporal) axis of the hippocampus by marching the pipette along this axis and performing successive laminar profiles (see Fig. 1. in Routtenberg (1984) for an example). This electrophysiological map guides subsequent dissection of tissue for phosphorylation analysis, enabling a maximization of the biochemical signal to noise ratio.

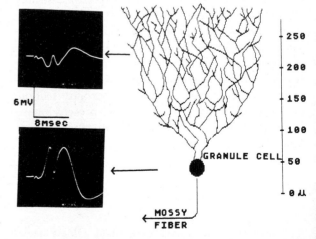

Fig. 2. Local monosynaptic input to granule cell dendrites demonstrated by potential reversal in the dipole layer as a recording micropipette is advanced from the dendritic zone to the granule cell body. See text for detailed discussion.

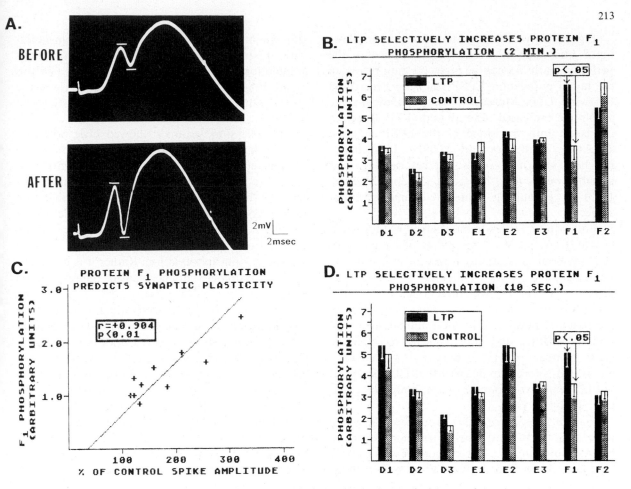

Fig. 3. Long-term potentiation (LTP) and protein phosphorylation in the intact hippocampal formation. A: Field potentials recorded from the granule cell layer of the dentate gyrus. Single 0.1-ms stimuli were delivered to the angular bundle perforant path either before (baseline) or 9 min after LTP initiation. Spike amplitude was measured as the potential between the two horizontal white bars. B: A selective increase in the in vitro phosphorylation (2 min reaction) of protein F1 was observed in animals sacrificed 9 min after LTP initiation relative to animals given low-frequency, non-potentiating stimulation. No other protein studied exhibited altered phosphorylation following LTP ($n = 10$ in LTP group, $n = 8$ in low-frequency group). The hippocampus was rapidly cooled by application of liquid nitrogen to a retaining cup overlying the exposed cortical surface. The portion of the dorsal hippocampus containing the granule cells locally activated by angular bundle stimulation was dissected in the cold room ($4°C$), and homogenized in a 30 mM potassium phosphate buffer. Aliquots of this homogenate were then preincubated for 30 s and incubated with 5 μM [^{32}P]ATP at a temperature of $30°C$. The reaction was terminated after 2 min by the addition of a sodium dodecylsulfate stop solution. Final concentrations of reaction constituents were: 2 mM Mg^{2+} 1 mM ethylenediaminetetraacetic acid (EDTA), 30 mM potassium phosphate, 1 mg/ml hippocampal homogenate protein, and 2 mM dithiothreitol. Protein concentration was determined by the Lowry method with bovine serum albumin as standard (29). Aliquots containing 50 μg protein were layered on 10% polyacrylamide gels. The electrophoretically separated proteins were stained, dried, and exposed to Kodak x-omat film. Autoradiographs were quantified densitometrically, and phosphorylation was expressed as the percentage of the total densitometric area under the peak, using a computer-based integration program. Protein bands D1, D2, and E3 density values can be multiplied by 2, 5, and 10 respectively to obtain the absolute densitometric values for the area under the curve. Phosphorylation of individual bands for LTP and control animals was compared using t for uncorrelated means. C: Phosphorylation of protein F1 predicts the increase in the population spike amplitude observed following LTP ($n = 10$). Probability levels for the regression coefficient were determined using a t-test. D: Protein F1 phosphorylation was selectively increased 5 min after LTP when a 10-s in vitro phosphorylation assay was employed. The identical tissue samples as in Fig. 1B were used. Procedures for in vitro phosphorylation, separation of individual protein bands, and their densitometric analysis were as in Fig. 1B with the exception that aliquots were incubated with [^{32}P]ATP for 10 s rather than 2 min (Lovinger et al., 1986).

Fig. 3A shows the potentiated response following 8 brief high-frequency trains applied to the perforant path. As can be seen, the rate of rise of the initial population EPSP (the slope) increased following LTP. Moreover, the population spike amplitude increased several fold. LTP therefore increased both the slope of the EPSP and the amplitude of the population spike. This change has been shown to persist for several days and possibly weeks (e.g., Bliss and Gardner-Medwin, 1973) in chronically implanted unanesthetized subjects.

Following LTP procedures which last for 4 min (8 400 Hz trains of 0.4-ms pulses delivered every 30 s) the brain was rapidly frozen in situ, stopping brain electrical activity in less than 5 s. Subsequent dissection of the hippocampal tissue in the cold room was followed by in vitro phosphorylation of the tissue of both experimental animals receiving LTP procedures and controls who received the same number of pulses but at low frequency (0.2 Hz). It is to be emphasized that LTP is carried out in the in vivo hippocampus, followed by phosphorylation in vitro.

Fig. 3B shows that LTP produced a selective increase in the in vitro phosphorylation of protein F1. As shown in Fig. 3C this increase was directly related to the increase in population spike amplit-

ude ($r = +0.904$, $p < 0.01$) as well as the translation ratio ($r = +0.845$, $p < 0.01$) which is the ratio of the population spike to the population EPSP (Wilson et al., 1984). Thus, protein F1 phosphorylation is directly linked to the change in the plasticity of LTP.

Because some animals showed little potentiation of the response, there exists a built-in control for the effects of high-frequency stimulation, i.e. failure to show potentiation. As seen in Fig. 1C, animals that showed a potentiated response barely above control levels, showed control levels of protein F1 phosphorylation. Thus, high-frequency stimulation alone is not sufficient to elevate protein F1 phosphorylation. Rather it is necessary that a physiologic enhancement of the response is observed.

One theme in this chapter which is noted here for the first time is that the alteration in protein F1 phosphorylation observed does not appear to be of rapid onset. Thus, in the experiment just reviewed the increase in F1 phosphorylation was not observed 1 min after the termination of the LTP procedure (the 1 min group), but was first seen 5 min after LTP (the 5 min group; Routtenberg et al., 1983, 1985). Related observations to be reviewed have subsequently been made under different circumstances and using different end-points

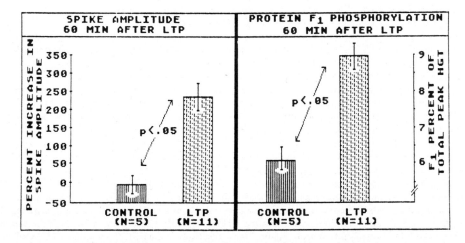

Fig. 4. Protein F1 phosphorylation is increased 1 h after LTP. Using the same procedures as described in Fig. 3, LTP was monitored for 60 min after the initiation of high-frequency stimulation and prior to study of in vitro phosphorylation. Control animals received low-frequency (0.2 Hz) stimulation only. See text for further details.

suggesting that the protein kinase C/F1 mechanism is not associated with the initiation of the plastic response but rather its persistence.

Given this perspective, one would predict that at time points beyond 5 min one should still observe an increase in protein F1 phosphorylation. Consistent with this expectation, an enhanced population spike response was observed 1 h after LTP initiation, as shown in Fig. 4 (left panel). Under these conditions a significant increase was observed in protein F1 phosphorylation (Fig. 4, right panel) that was directly related to the persistence of the response ($r = +0.606$, $p < 0.02$; Routtenberg et al., 1985). To determine whether this persistence extended beyond 1 h and over days, we have studied protein phosphorylation patterns 3 days after potentiating stimulation using the high-frequency stimulation parameters in our acute studies. The animals were chronically implanted with electrodes in the perforant path and dentate gyrus. A similar increase in synaptic strength is observed in these chronically prepared subjects. Because of its long-term nature, this change in synaptic efficacy has been referred to as long-term enhancement (LTE) by McNaughton (1982).

As shown in Fig. 5A, we observed an increase in the in vitro phosphorylation of protein F1 3 days after high-frequency stimulation was applied (Lovinger et al., 1985). This increase was selective for protein F1 (Fig. 5B). This selective increase in F1 phosphorylation was directly related to growth of the population spike amplitude (Fig. 5C) and the population EPSP or synaptic response (Fig. 5D). That is, those animals that showed growth had greater F1 phosphorylation than those that showed decay of the response.

Using the hippocampal slice preparation, Bar et al. (1980) reported that there was no significant effect of LTP on protein B-50, now considered to be identical to protein F1 (see, e.g., Nelson and Routtenberg, 1985). This failure to find an effect on LTP may be considered at odds with our results on protein F1 (Routtenberg et al., 1983). Recently, however, Schrama et al. (Chapter 20) have repeated their study and now do find a significant effect of LTP on their B-50 protein, confirming our initial observation. The effect is less striking, however, possibly because it is not

possible to stimulate the bottleneck of Lomo (vide supra) in the slice and protein kinase C activity may be diminished in the slice relative to the in vivo situation. Nonetheless, there now exists inter-laboratory confirmation of our observation of an LTP-induced alteration in protein F1 phosphorylation.

In summary, data from acutely anesthetized and chronic preparations indicated that alterations in protein F1 phosphorylation was not an immediate response to high-frequency stimulation, but had a relatively slow onset and persisted for several days. Moreover, these effects were selective for protein F1. Alterations were not observed, for example, in cyclic AMP-dependent substrates such as synapsin, nor were alterations observed in the alpha subunit of pyruvate dehydrogenase, a 41-kDa phosphoprotein (Morgan and Routtenberg, 1980, 1981).*

These results enabled us to reach our first goal, namely to establish that post-translational modification by phosphorylation of particular brain proteins could be related to alterations in synaptic strength. With this affirmative answer pointing to protein F1 we then set out to characterize the substrate and its kinase.

Purification of protein kinase C and protein F1

The selective increase in protein F1 phosphory-

---

*Earlier studies indicated that a 41-kDa protein, protein F2, was also altered by training (Routtenberg and Benson, 1980). This latter result has since been confirmed by another laboratory (Hoch et al., 1984). Following the identification of F2 as the alpha subunit of pyruvate dehydrogenase (α-PDH; Morgan and Routtenberg, 1980), considerable interest was focussed on the potential role of this molecule in regulating synaptic strength (Browning et al., 1982) and information storage (Routtenberg, 1982). While this molecule is no doubt of importance in such processes, understanding its precise role has been delayed. Without a probe that can specifically and selectively alter the consequences of α-PDH activity, one is likely to influence the whole range of cellular functions as a consequence of alterations of intermediary metabolism. Potential approaches might focus on the functional differences between presynaptic and postsynaptic (dendritic α-PDH is regulating synaptic strength (Akers et al., 1982).

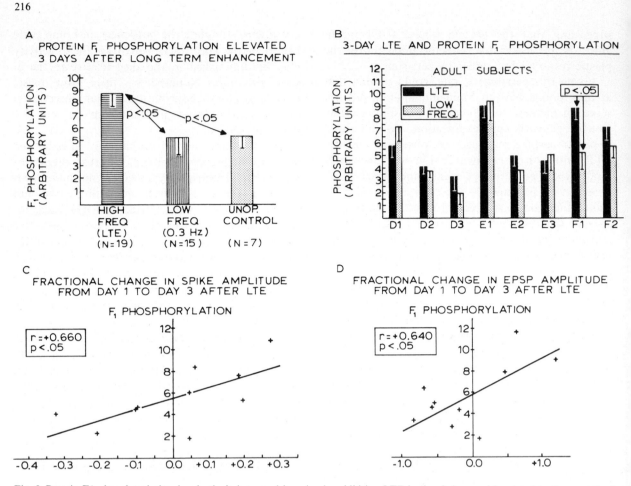

Fig. 5. Protein F1 phosphorylation is selectively increased in animals exhibiting LTE lasting 3 days and is related to the growth of LTE. A: Animals given high-frequency stimulation and sacrificed 3 days later show increased protein F1 phosphorylation in vitro relative to animals sacrificed 3 days after low-frequency stimulation or unoperated animals (LTE, $n = 19$; low frequency, $n = 15$; unoperated control, $n = 7$). Phosphorylation values for F1 were compared using an ANOVA test for groups of unequal size. B: Selectivity of the LTE–F1 relationship is demonstrated by the fact that no other protein assayed exhibits altered phosphorylation in enhanced animals relative to low-frequency animals. Values are mean $\pm$ SEM phosphate incorporation quantified as described in the text, and compared using a t-test for uncorrelated means. To obtain actual phosphorylation values, multiply bands D2 and E3 by 3. C: Dorsal hippocampal protein F1 phosphorylation varies in direct proportion to the growth or decay of the change in spike amplitude (EA) over the 3 days following induction of LTE in perforant path synapses. The fractional change in SA from day 1 to day 3 after LTE was calculated by dividing the difference between the percent change on days 1 and 3 by the percent change on day 1. D: Dorsal hippocampal Protein F1 phosphorylation varies in direct proportion to the growth or decay of the change in EPSP amplitude (EA) over the 3 days following induction of LTE in perforant path synapses. The fractional change in EA was calculated as in part C. The observation that protein F1 phosphorylation state is greater in animals that exhibited growth of LTE than in animals that showed decay of LTE provides the first evidence of a functional role for a specific brain phosphoprotein in the long-term maintainence of synaptic plasticity. (Lovinger et al., 1985).

lation after LTP could be related to an increase in substrate or an increase in kinase activity. By isolating the components we could assess their relative contributions to the increase in protein F1

phosphorylation. One goal of these purification studies was to assess the contribution of component processes of the endogenous phosphorylation system to the synaptic plasticity of LTP. Moreover, by identifying the substrate and kinase the effects on LTP of their selective manipulation becomes feasible.

In order to identify and establish the kinase for protein F1 it is necessary to purify both substrate and kinase and determine whether the purified substrate can be phosphorylated by the purified kinase in the presence of the appropriate effectors. With such information it should be possible to understand the mechanism for alteration in protein F1 phosphorylation and to relate such modifications to underlying cellular processes.

Recent evidence has shown that protein F1 is a substrate for protein kinase C (Akers and Routtenberg, 1985; Nelson and Routtenberg, 1985; Chan et al., 1986). This confirms the initial observation of Aloyo et al. (1983) based on the assumption that protein F1 is the same as protein B-50 (Zwiers et al., 1982; see Chapter 4 and Addendum) Discussion of issues and background surrounding the identification of substrate and kinase have been presented elsewhere (Routtenberg, 1984, 1985a, 1985b, 1985c) and will not be reviewed further here.

Purification of protein kinase C was carried out by Dr. Kentaro Murakami who modified currently available methods, to obtain a protein kinase of high purity and high yield (Murakami et al., 1985). This kinase has the properties of protein kinase C described by Nishizuka and co-workers (Takai et al., 1977; Kikkawa et al., 1982; Nishizuka, 1984a, 1984b; Chapter 3): dependence on phosphatidylserine; calcium requirement reduced by diolein and by tumor-promoting phorbol esters. In addition, as recently reported by Murakami et al. (1985), we have discovered that protein kinase C can be fully activated by oleic acid. The physiological significance of this important new observation awaits empirical clarification.

Purification of protein F1 was carried out by Dr. Shew Chan using a series of liquid column chromatographic steps as outlined in Fig. 6. As shown in Fig. 7, protein F1 was phosphorylated by a phosphatidylserine-dependent process (Chan et al., 1986). This phosphorylation reaction was not stimulated by cyclic AMP. We have also been unable to phosphorylate protein F1 with calmodulin kinase II (gift of Dr. Mary Kennedy) with either a crude preparation of calmodulin kinase I or the calmodulin kinase, phosphorylase B kinase. While we do not rule out a role for another calmodulin kinase in phosphorylating protein F1, at this time the evidence, using both exogenous effectors and exogenous kinases in a purified system, is that protein kinase C is the major kinase for the F1 substrate.

These results indicated that protein kinase C can directly phosphorylate the protein F1 substrate in an isolated, purified system. It is also important to establish that these components normally form an endogenous system. For this purpose we have studied the effects of phosphatidylserine and phorbol ester on the endogenous phosphorylation of protein F1 in osmotically shocked crude synaptic plasma membranes. We found that protein F1 was stimulated in its phosphorylation by both substances (Akers and Routtenberg, 1985), which are known to activate protein kinase C (Chapter 3). In addition, exogenous protein kinase C stimulated its phosphorylation.

We have recently studied this system using two-dimensional gel electrophoresis (Nelson and Routtenberg, 1985). Protein F1 in our system is a 47-kDa, $pI = 4.5$ phosphoprotein. It is not stimulated by cyclic AMP, but it is stimulated by calcium, phosphatidylserine and phorbol ester. Protein F1 in rat has no co-migrating phosphoproteins using two-dimensional gels in which the entire pH range is surveyed (NEPHGE gels). The quantitative analysis of one-dimensional gels in the LTP experiments therefore represents a quantification of this single F1 protein. The same may not be true for the analysis of synapsin (proteins D_1 and D_2) which did not change with functional treatment. In this case, there is an acidic (4.0) protein kinase C-dependent protein substrate that can co-migrate with synapsin, a highly basic molecule (10.4). Thus, two-dimensional analysis of functional manipulations will be necessary to determine the role of synapsin and, parri passu, the acidic co-migrator.

218

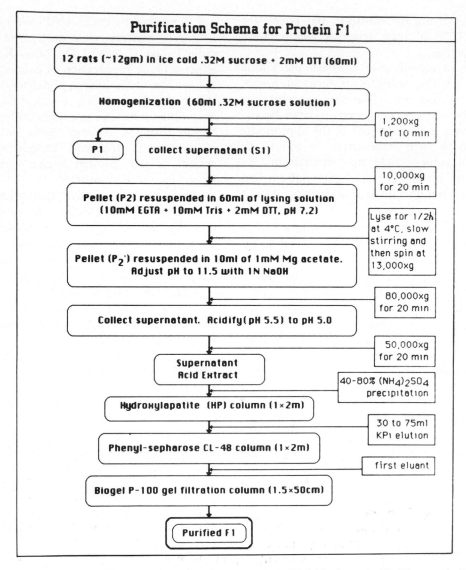

Purification Schema for Protein F1

12 rats (~12gm) in ice cold .32M sucrose + 2mM DTT (60ml)

Homogenization (60ml .32M sucrose solution)

1,200×g for 10 min

P1   **collect supernatant (S1)**

10,000×g for 20 min

Pellet (P2) resuspended in 60ml of lysing solution (10mM EGTA + 10mM Tris + 2mM DTT, pH 7.2)

Lyse for 1/2h at 4°C, slow stirring and then spin at 13,000×g

Pellet (P₂') resuspended in 10ml of 1mM Mg acetate. Adjust pH to 11.5 with 1N NaOH

80,000×g for 20 min

Collect supernatant. Acidify(pH 5.5) to pH 5.0

50,000×g for 20 min

Supernatant Acid Extract

40-80% (NH₄)₂SO₄ precipitation

Hydroxylapatite (HP) column (1×2m)

30 to 75ml KPᵢ elution

Phenyl-sepharose CL-4B column (1×2m)

first eluant

Biogel P-100 gel filtration column (1.5×50cm)

Purified F1

Fig. 6. Steps used in the purification (estimated to be greater than 500-fold) of protein F1 (Chan et al., 1986).

What mechanisms are responsible for the LTP-induced increase in protein F1 phosphorylation?

As pointed out in the first volume of this series (Routtenberg, 1982b) alterations in the in vitro phosphorylation of a substrate following a functional manipulation only indicates that an alteration has been preserved and detected. It does not indicate what the alteration might be. The selective increase in protein F1 phosphorylation after LTP may be the result of an alteration in its kinase, the amount of substrate or its phosphatase, i.e. any one of the components of the endogenous F1 phosphorylation system. In the present case it is possible that alterations of protein kinase C occur minutes or hours following LTP, whereas at longer time intervals (days) alterations in the amount of the F1 substrate occur. Thus, an in-

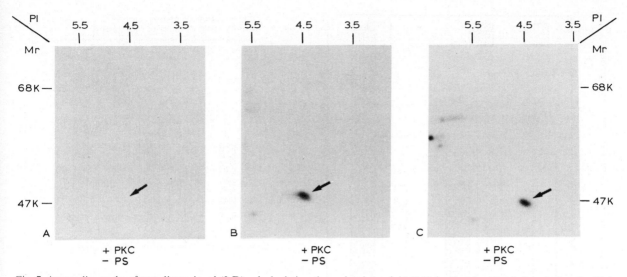

Fig. 7. Autoradiographs of two-dimensional (2-D) gels depicting the molecular weight (M_r), isoelectric point (pI) and phosphatidyl-serine (PS) dependency of F1 in the P-100 gel filtration column purified fraction. A: 2-D autoradiograph of the P-100 purified fraction when PS was not added for phosphorylation reaction. In the absence of PS, no F1 phosphorylation by purified exogenous kinase C (PKC) was found. B: Autoradiograph when 50 µg/ml PS was added. Protein F1, the only phosphoprotein in this fraction, was found at the position of $M_r = 47$ kDa and p$I = 4.5$, which matched the phosphorylated protein F1 in a HP fraction (c) under the same phosphorylation conditions. The microheterogeneity of the two phosphorylated bands also appeared to be similar. (From Chan et al., 1985.)

crease in F1 phosphorylation detected at different points in time may be the result of different mechanisms.

In considering the particular mechanism within the endogenous phosphorylation system for the increase in protein F1 phosphorylation following LTP we were led to consider the possibility that activation of protein kinase C would be most important. This was first suggested by our finding of a significant and selective increase in F1 phosphorylation using a brief, 10-s in vitro reaction (Fig. 3D). We estimate (see Morgan, 1981) that less than 1% of sites are phosphorylated using 7.5 µM ATP and a 10-s reaction. This short reaction emphasizes the role of kinase-substrate affinity, and de-emphasizes the contribution of vacant phosphorylatable sites, amount of substrate or in vitro phosphatase activity to the increase in F1 phosphorylation.

This led our laboratory to evaluate the hypothesis that LTP increased protein kinase C activity. We were especially interested in the sug-

gestion that protein kinase C activation occurs as a consequence of translocation of the kinase from the cytosol to the membrane (Kikkawa et al., 1983). To study this issue in individual animals after LTP, Ray Akers in our laboratory developed a method for partially purifying the kinase from separate membrane and cytosol fractions of the unilateral dorsal hippocampus of individual rat subjects. After kinase extraction each sample was partially purified using DEAE minicolumns which also removed substances that interfere with the kinase assay (Kraft and Anderson, 1983). Protein kinase C assays were performed using exogenous histone H_1 as substrate (see Fig. 8 caption for description of methods).

As shown in Fig. 8 we found that LTP increased *membrane* protein kinase C activity 1 h but not 1 min after high-frequency stimulation (Akers et al., 1986). Moreover, at 1 h there was a significant decrease in the activity of cytosolic protein kinase C while total kinase C activity remained unchanged (Fig. 9). These results sug-

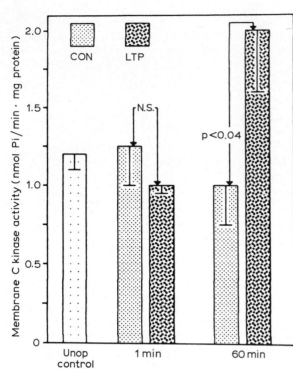

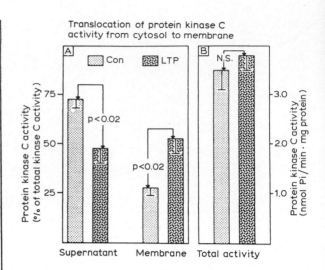

Translocation of protein kinase C
activity from cytosol to membrane

Fig. 9. LTP stimulation shifts the subcellular distribution of PKC activity. Methods as described in the legend to Fig. 1. All animals were sacrificed 1 h after the delivery of LTP stimulation. All values mean $\pm$ S.E.M.; all $n = 6$.

Fig. 8. Protein kinase C activity is increased in membranes 1 h after LTP stimulation. The extent of perforant path activation of the dentate gyrus of male albino rats was first determined. High-frequency repetitive stimulation (LTP) (8 trains of 8 pulses of 100 Hz), or low-frequency control stimulation (LFC) (64 pulses at 0.1 Hz) was then delivered. 1 min or 1 h later, the animals were sacrificed by rapid freezing in liquid nitrogen. The innervated regions of the dorsal hippocampus were dissected on a block of dry ice, and homogenized in 50 mM Tris (pH 7.2), 0.1 mM EDTA, and 10 mg/ml leupeptin. To obtain particulate and soluble fractions for each dorsal hippocampus, homogenates were spun at $100\,000 \times g$ for 1 h, and the resulting supernatants were collected. The pellets were washed, and the supernatants were combined. The supernatants, containing PKC activity from the soluble or cytosolic fraction, were then applied to a 0.4×1.0 cm DEAE–cellulose minicolumn, equilibrated with 50 mM Tris (pH 7.2), 2 mM EGTA, and 2 mM EDTA. The column was washed, and PKC activity was eluted with 0.3 M NaCl. To obtain particulate PKC activity, the $100\,000 \times g$ pellet was resuspended in 50 mM Tris (pH 7.2), 0.1% Triton X-100, 2 mM EDTA, 2 mM EGTA, and 10 mg/ml leupeptin, and stirred for 1 h at 4°C. Following centrifugation at $100\,000 \times g$ for 1 h to remove debris, the supernatants, containing PKC activity extracted from membranes, were applied to DEAE–cellulose minicolumns, and PKC activity was eluted as before. PKC activity was determined in the following assay mix: 50 mM Tris (pH 7.2), 1.5 mM $CaCl_2$, 0.5 mM EGTA, 0.5 mM EDTA, 100 mg histone H_1, 3–5 mg enzyme preparation, and 0.5 mm [γ-^{32}P]ATP (specific activity

gest that high-frequency stimulation translocated kinase C from the cytosol to the membrane. However, this translocation did not occur immediately as there was no detectable change 1 min after the termination of LTP procedures. This latter result is consistent with the theme noted earlier that protein kinase C plays a role in the persistence of the response but not in its initiation.

If this translocation were central to the plasticity of LTP one would expect that the level of kinase activity in the membrane should be directly related to the extent of change of the potentiated response. We have found that there is a direct relation, in fact, with the persistence of the response 1 h after the initiation of LTP ($r = +0.875$, $p < 0.05$). There was no relation of protein kinase C activity to the amplitude of the enhanced res-

50 cpm/pmol), ± 100 mg/ml phosphatidylserine. The reaction was run for 10 min at 30°, quenched with the addition of a saturated EDTA solution, and spotted onto phosphocellulose paper. The papers were washed and counted by liquid scintillation spectrometry. PKC activity was taken as the difference between activity seen in the presence or absence of phosphatidylserine. All enzyme assays were linear with respect to time and enzyme concentration. All values are mean $\pm$ S.E.M; $n = 6$ for all groups except naive controls, where $n = 7$.

ponse following LTP. This again suggests that protein kinase C translocation to the membrane plays a specific role in the maintenance of the response, possibly in preventing its decay to baseline, rather than participating in the extent of initial enhancement. This is coherent with our earlier findings (Lovinger et al., 1985) that protein F1 phosphorylation was not related to the amplitude of the response 3 days after LTP procedures but was directly related to the persistence of the enhanced response.

The results to this point are consistent with the following sequence of events schematically depicted in Fig. 10. High frequency activity in the perforant path, either generated by LTP or endogenous high-frequency activity (Ranck, 1975), induces the translocation of protein kinase C from the cytoplasm to the membrane. At the membrane, the kinase interaction with protein F1 is increased, giving rise to an increase in protein F1 phosphorylation. Thus, in our earlier in vitro phosphorylation studies the increase in F1 phosphorylation could be the result of an increased enzyme–substrate association.

If this scenario were correct and a stable enzyme/substrate complex at the membrane were formed, then one might expect that the increase in protein F1 phosphorylation induced by LTP would be preserved in a membrane pellet prepared from a high-speed $150\,000 \times g$ spin. As shown in Fig. 11, we have indeed observed in the 5 min

post-LTP experiment that the extent of protein F1 phosphorylation was directly related to the amplitude of the enhanced response ($r = +0.74$, $p < 0.05$). Analysis of each phosphoprotein band revealed that no other band showed such a direct relationship. Interestingly, animals that showed a potentiated response barely above control levels, showed control levels of protein F1 phosphorylation. Thus, the critical factor in leading to the elevation in F1 phosphorylation was not the tetanizing high-frequency stimulation but rather the consequence of the tetanus, the enhanced physiological response.

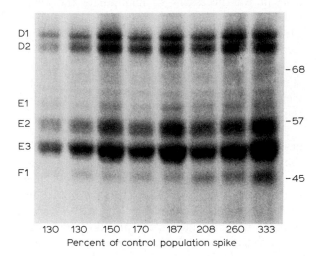

Fig. 11. Phosphorylation of membrane-bound protein F1 is directly related to long-term potentiation. Autoradiogram showing in vitro phosphorylation of hippocampal membrane proteins from animals exhibiting varying degrees of population spike amplitude (SA) potentiation (indicated by the percentages beneath each sample) following LTP. Note the close correspondance between the increase in SA and the increase in protein F1 phosphorylation ($r = +0.85$, $p < 0.05$). No other phosphoprotein analyzed exhibits a significant relationship between phosphorylation and LTP (DI: $r = 0.06$; D2: $r = +0.20$; E1: $r = +0.09$; E2: $r = +0.032$; E3: $r = -0.27$; $p > 0.20$ for all bands. Dissection and tissue preparation were as described in Fig. 3B with the exception that hippocampal samples were homogenized in 50 mM sucrose and subjected to centrifugation at $150\,000 \times g$ for 10 min. The resultant pellet was then resuspended in the potassium phosphate buffer as described in Fig. 3B. Procedures for protein phosphorylation, separation and analysis of phosphorylation of individual protein bands were performed as in Fig. 1B. Labels for the major phosphoproteins D1–F1 are to the left. Molecular weight (in kDa) is indicated to the right of the autoradiogram (Lovinger et al., 1986).

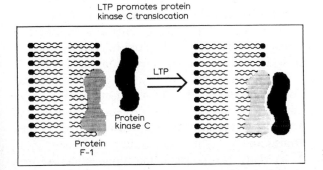

Fig. 10. Schematic depiction of the hypothesized translocation of protein kinase C to the membrane based on the results in Figs. 8 and 9. Note that physical translocation or stronger attachment of kinase to the membrane would lead to an increase in protein F1 phosphorylation.

222

Can translocation of protein kinase C by phorbol esters regulate synaptic plasticity?

The experiments reviewed to this point have demonstrated convergent lines of evidence directly associating the synaptic plasticity of LTP with alterations in the protein F1/protein kinase C system. It is clear, however, that demonstration of such an association, no matter how persuasive, leaves unanswered the issue of the centrality of this mechanism to the expression of that plasticity. Moreover, if kinase C/F1 were central, what would be the precise role of this endogenous phosphorylation system? To answer such questions it was necessary to manipulate the kinase C/F1 system and observe its effects on synaptic plasticity. If such manipulations produced no effects on LTP then the association would be only that. On the other hand, if LTP were affected in a significant fashion, then this would strengthen the view that the kinase C/F1 system was central to the synaptic plasticity mechanism.

Biochemical evidence gathered previously suggested that LTP-induced translocation of the kinase might be a critical step in regulating synaptic plasticity. If we could translocate kinase C from the cytosol to the membrane then the role of this translocation in LTP could be assessed. A class of tumor-promoting agents, the phorbol esters, activate protein kinase C (Castagna et al., 1983) and, indeed, translocate this kinase to the membrane (Kraft and Anderson, 1983). By using 5-barreled pipettes for both recording and ionotophoretic ejection of drugs into the hippocampus, we determined the effect of the phorbol ester 12-O-tetradecanoyl phorbol-13-acetate (TPA) on the LTP response.

As shown in Fig. 12, TPA had a significant effect on the persistence of the enhanced response (Lovinger et al., 1985; Routtenberg et al., 1986) It is important to note that this persistence occurred in the population EPSP, the synaptic wave, as well as the population spike. Interestingly, TPA had little effect on the initial magnitude of the response. Nor did TPA have any significant effect by itself on the population EPSP or population spike prior to LTP. The effect of TPA, rather, was to enhance the persistence of the potentiated res-

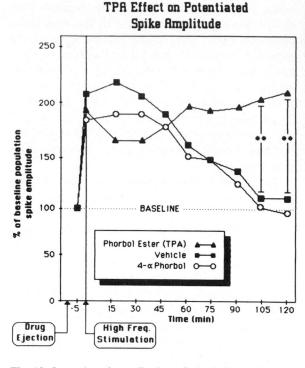

Fig. 12. Iontophoretic application of phorbol ester into the hilar dentate gyrus prevents decay and induces growth of potentiated response. Animals ejected with TPA prior to high-frequency stimulation show a growth in potentiation beyond the initial increase in response beginning at 45 min until 2 h. The percentage of initial potentiation seen in the TPA-ejected animals was significantly different (df = 1,10) with $p < 0.025$ (*), $p < 0.005$ (**) or $p < 0.001$ (***) from 4-α-phorbol and vehicle (dimethylsulfoxide/Tris) controls at the last five time points.

ponse, perhaps by preventing its decay. Note that neither the inactive phorbol ester, 4-α phorbol, nor the Tris/dimethyl sulfoxide vehicle had any substantial effect. These decay curves were not different from the decay observed in control subjects in which no iontophoretic ejection was used.

We are currently evaluating the biochemical consequences of the TPA injection. We have shown that TPA increases protein F1 phosphorylation in a synaptosomal preparation (Akers and Routtenberg, 1985) and initial evidence indicates that iontophoretic injections of TPA produce their effect by increasing protein F1 phosphorylation (Routtenberg et al., 1986). It is worthwhile considering in a provisional fashion, given the implication of protein kinase C involvement, what these findings might signify with respect to the role that protein kinase C might play in the regulation of synaptic plasticity.

The fact that TPA alone had no effect on the size of the initial enhanced response, nor induced an increase in the amplitude by itself, suggests that protein kinase activation may play no role in initiation. Rather, protein kinase C, as noted earlier, regulates the persistence of plasticity.

An additional factor other than TPA would therefore appear to be necessary to initiate the enhanced response. What might this factor be? Since low-frequency stimulation of the perforant path by itself did not produce potentiation, it is clear that this factor was derived from the consequences of high-frequency stimulation. One such consequence of high-frequency activity in the hippocampus is an elevation of intracellular calcium (Morris et al., 1983). There is precedent (Michell, 1983; Nishizuka et al., 1984) for considering the possibility that the elevation of intracellular calcium on the one hand and the TPA-induced translocation and activation of protein kinase C on the other hand work synergistically to produce the persistent response.

An important feature of our iontophoretic experiments was that two high-frequency trains were used since preliminary studies indicated that when eight high-frequency trains (the number of trains applied in our biochemical studies) were used the persistent response was not altered by TPA. The failure of TPA to alter LTP generated by 8 trains may itself be suggestive evidence that LTP sets into motion a process engendered by TPA when 2 trains are used.

Neither TPA alone nor the tetanus of two high-frequency stimulus trains was capable of producing an enduring plastic change of large magnitude. However, when the two were active concurrently, a significant large and enduring plastic change occurred. This result is schematically shown in Fig. 13, which suggests that a synergism exists between the effects of the high-frequency stimulation tetanus and the activation of protein kinase C.

Because there are some rather obvious parallels with the proposal by Nishizuka that a synergism exists between calcium and the activation of kinase C by diacylglycerol, our results provide the first suggestive evidence in the central nervous system for this proposed synergism (Fig. 13). A similar view, based on evidence from non-neural systems, has also been proposed (Rasmussen and Barrett, 1984). It is to be emphasized that the synergism we have described operates in two time domains: response initiation and response persistence. Thus, protein kinase C may regulate or modulate the duration of the change in synaptic strength, while calcium-related events, which appear not to involve this kinase, initiate synaptic change.

In the last section of the paper the executable synaptic mechanisms by which the increase in synaptic strength is maintained are considered.

Protein kinase C orchestrates cellular mechanisms necessary for the maintenance of synaptic plasticity

Studies on synaptic plasticity have suggested several different candidate mechanisms for the alteration in synaptic strength. Earlier hypotheses suggested the physical growth of synaptic boutons (Hebb, 1949) as a model for information storage. It was later suggested that another bulbous protuberance, the dendritic spine, might grow and increase overall synaptic strength (e.g., Ruiz-Marcos and Valverde, 1969). Evidence that growth of presynaptic and postsynaptic structures may occur following the synaptic plasticity of LTP has been reported by several different laboratories (Fifkova and van Harreveld, 1973; Lee et al., 1980; Desmond and Levy, 1983; Greenough, 1984).

A second mechanism that alters synaptic strength involves an alteration in the release of transmitter substance. This proposal has its origins in the demonstration of post-tetanic potentiation (Lloyd, 1949) and the view that high-frequency stimulation increases transmitter mobilization by swelling presynaptic terminals (Eccles, 1953). This potentiation lasted for typically less than a minute and was thus not considered an especially accurate candidate model for long-term memory. A far superior model of information storage that paralleled the time domains of learning and forgetting was the demonstration of long-term potentiation (LTP) in the hippocampus by

224

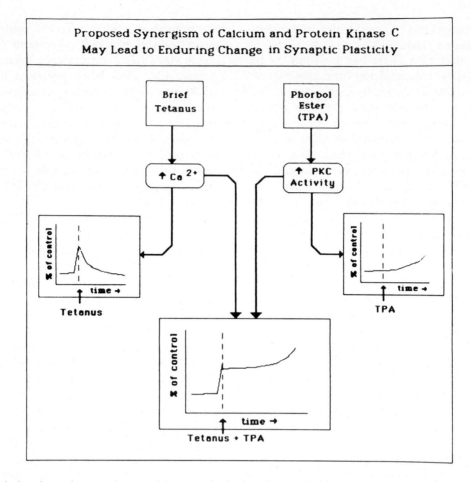

Fig. 13. An enduring change in synaptic strength may require both an increase in intracellular calcium (Ca^{2+}) and an increase in protein kinase C (PKC) activity. In the experiment shown in Fig. 12, neither the brief tetanus nor the phorbol ester alone was able to produce a prolonged change. However, when the two were combined, a change greater than the sum of the two occurred. As discussed in the text, the calcium elevation limb is suggested to be responsible primarily for response initiation while the PKC limb is responsible primarily for response persistence.

Bliss and Lomo (1973a). One proposal to account for the potentiated response is an increase in efficacy due to enhanced release of transmitter (Bliss and Dolphin, 1984).

A third candidate mechanism for enduring synaptic change involves an increase in the number of effective receptors for the released neurotransmitters. It is now well known that receptor number can be up- or down-regulated by transmitter agonists or antagonists (Snyder, 1984). Using the LTP model a specific proposal has been made that an increase in glutamate receptors is important for the enduring plastic change (Lynch and Baudry, 1984).

A fourth candidate mechanism has been proposed to regulate synaptic strength via an alteration in ion channel properties (Kandel and Schwartz, 1982; Alkon, 1984). In one case, the alteration is of a calcium-dependent potassium channel in the postsynaptic cell body (Alkon, 1984). In another model it is of a special calcium channel presumed to be present on the presynaptic terminal (Kandel and Schwartz, 1982) In both cases, it is posited that a change in channel protein

Multi-Functional Protein Kinase C
Coordinates Regulation of Synaptic Plasticity

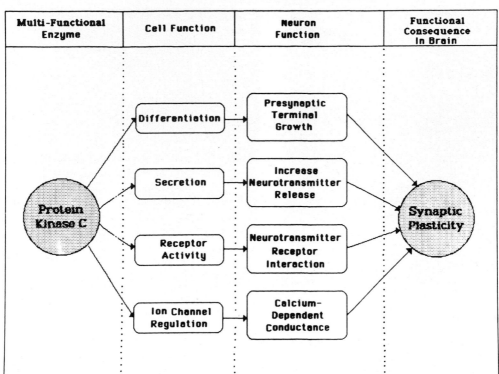

Fig. 14. Summarizing scheme of cell and neuron functions underlying protein kinase C activation leading to an enduring plastic change. Focus of the change may be on the presynaptic terminal, based on the evidence from Girard et al. (1985) localizing the enzyme to this site. Prior formulations on the mechanisms of synaptic plasticity have focussed on only one neuron function. In this scheme, it is proposed that protein kinase C, by virtue of its multifunctional character, can recruit these functions for the purpose of promoting a plastic change that endures.

conformation mediated by protein phosphorylation is responsible for the endurance of the plastic change.

These four candidate mechanisms, while often considered as mutually exclusive alternatives, may form a consortium of devices that are necessary for the final product, a plastic synaptic change which endures. In the next few paragraphs the evidence is briefly reviewed that such mechanisms are regulated by protein kinase C. The possibility is then raised that this kinase plays a crucial role in orchestrating the sequence of events necessary to the expression of synaptic plasticity.

This view is schematically depicted in Fig. 14.

In this diagram the cell biologic functions now ascribed to protein kinase C are suggested to occur in brain, and such brain functions are suggested to converge on the consequence, synaptic plasticity.

Growth

The type of growth referred to here is one of differentiation of axonal processes, rather than cell proliferation. Evidence for a role of protein kinase C comes from cell culture studies using TPA. In particular, it has been shown that phorbol ester, at

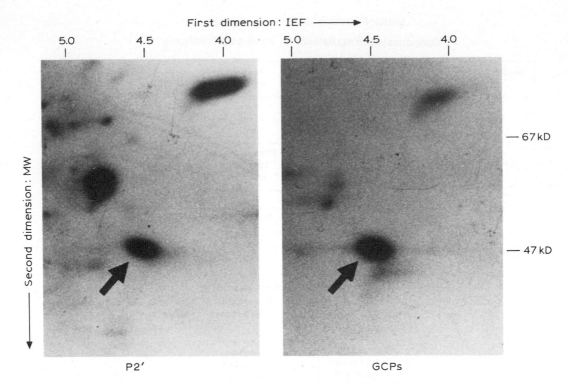

First dimension: IEF ⟶

Second dimension: MW

—67kD

—47kD

P2′   GCPs

Fig. 15. Comigration and similar microheterogeneity on two-dimensional autoradiograms of phosphorylated pp46 (right panel) and protein F1 (left panel). Phosphoproteins from p2′ fractions of adult rat hippocampal formation and GCPs were separated by IEF-SDS. Molecular mass markers are indicated in the figure (bovine serum albumin, 68 kDa; catalase, 60 kDa; fumarase, 48 kDa). F1 in p2′ and pp46 in GCPs are indicated by arrows. The specific activity of $[\gamma\text{-}^{32}P]$ATP used in p2′ fraction was 20 times higher than that used in GCPs so that radioactive phosphate incorporation between the two samples would be roughly equal.

low dosages (1.6 nM TPA) is a potent stimulator to neurite outgrowth (Hsu et al., 1984). Presuming that protein kinase C activation occurs under this circumstance some association is likely to exist between kinase activation and neurite outgrowth. Consistent with this expectation is the finding that TPA binding sites are especially abundant in areas of neuronal growth and synaptogenesis (Dunphy et al., 1980; Murphy et al., 1983). Given the evidence that protein kinase C may be the receptor for phorbol ester (Ashendel et al., 1983; Kikkawa et al., 1983; Kraft and Anderson, 1983; Niedel et al., 1983) and that protein kinase C is localized to the presynaptic terminal (Girard et al., 1985) it is tempting to believe that growth of the presynaptic terminal is strongly associated with the presence of protein kinase C. Such growth could provide

for the enduring nature of the plastic response without involvement in the initial change of the response itself.

The view that protein kinase C is associated with growth of presynaptic terminals is also supported by studies of purified growth cone particles (GCP) demonstrating the presence of protein substrates for protein kinase C (Katz et al., 1985). One of these substrates, pp46, appeared to be similar in physical properties to protein F1 as reviewed elsewhere (Chapter 19). In collaboration with this group, we have studied the two-dimensional profiles of GCP in relation to lyzed synaptosomes from adult rats (p2′) to determine whether the kinase C substrate, protein F1, might be present within GCP (Nelson et al., 1985). We have found, indeed, that protein F1 is present in

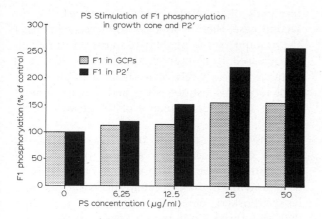

Fig. 16. Stimulation of protein F1 and pp46 phosphorylation by PS. Graph compares the sensitivity of protein F1 from P_2 and pp46 from GCPs to increasing concentrations of PS. Samples were incubated on ice in the presence of 0.15% Triton X-100 for 1 min. Final reaction conditions were the same as in Fig. 1 except that only one specific activity of $[\gamma\text{-}^{32}P]ATP$ was used and samples contained a final concentration of 0.075% Triton X-100.

abundance in this preparation (Fig. 15), that it is indeed similar to pp46 and that it is readily stimulated by the addition of TPA, phosphatidyl-serine and purified protein kinase C. Comparison of phosphopeptide maps of protein F1 in adult brain and the growth cone protein pp46 of Katz et al. (1985) further supported the claim that these substrates are likely to be equivalent. One may wish to be cautious about their identity, however, since certain differences did emerge between the proteins even though their molecular weight (47 kDa) and their isoelectric point (4.5) were identical. To our surprise we have found that the level of phosphorylation in GCP was 20 times greater than that present in the adult p2′. In addition, the extent of stimulation of pp46 in 17-day embryos by phosphatidylserine was less than the stimulation of protein F1 in adult p2′ (see Fig. 16). These two results indicated that the regulation of pp46 and protein F1 phosphorylation by protein kinase C may change during the development of the nervous system.

Because the growth cone is in some respects a primitive precursor of the presynaptic terminal, our results suggest that the kinase C/F1 system is likely to be present within the presynaptic portion of the synapse. This view is supported by the work of Girard et al. (1985) and Gispen et al. (1985) who claimed, respectively, that kinase C and F1 (as B-50) are localized to the presynaptic terminal and that both proteins are absent from postsynaptic structures. It is possible that protein F1 and protein kinase C system are restricted to the pre-synaptic terminal. Such an exclusive presynaptic localization, if true, would be of functional importance, suggesting that synaptic plasticity may emanate from presynaptic events. In addition, a presynaptic localization of protein kinase C raises an issue with regard to understanding the role of the phosphoinositide response purported to occur in postsynaptic structures in the hippocampus (Chapter 1). It should be noted that Nishizuka and co-workers (Chapter 3) have recent immuno-cytochemical evidence that, in contrast to the assertion of Girard et al. (1985), protein kinase C is in fact located in dendrites.

Several lines of evidence have been reviewed which converge on the attractive hypothesis that protein F1 and its kinase, C, play an important role in presynaptic terminal growth leading to an alteration in synaptic strength (Routtenberg, 1985). This hypothesis, now dressed in modern clothes, differs surprisingly little from the prescient view espoused by Hebb nearly 40 years ago. He noted that "When one cell repeatedly assists in firing another, the axon of the first cell develops synaptic knobs (or enlarges them if they already exist). ... This seems to me the most likely mechanism of a lasting effect ..." (Hebb, 1949, p. 63). Hebb went on to propose that the joint firing of an axon of passage and a nearby dendrite could produce "a thickening of the fiber – a synaptic knob – or add to a thickening already present" (ibid., p. 65).

Hebb's hypothesis fits well with subsequent evidence from several laboratories indicating that presynaptic terminal growth, related to either sprouting or insertion of membrane vesicles into the plasma membrane, occurs following activation (e.g. Pysh and Wiley, 1973) and that increases in synaptic number occur following LTP (Lee et al., 1981; Desmond and Levy, 1983; Greenough, 1984). Moreover, it has recently been observed (Nelson and Routtenberg, 1985) that protein F1 may also be similar to the growth-associated protein, GAP-43, observed in greater abundance during axonal regeneration (Skene and Willard, 1981a, 1981b; Heacock and Agranoff, 1982; Benowitz and Lewis, 1983). Taken together with the association of protein F1 with the growing tips of axons during development (Nelson et al., 1985), it becomes attractive to imagine that synaptic plasticity in the adult involves a growth of the axon terminal similar to that occurring in development or regeneration but in muted form.

It is yet to be established whether the alterations in synaptic structure so far observed after induction of LTP are exclusively a presynaptic phenomena or, as seems more likely, involves a coordinated morphologic alteration in the postsynaptic structure. Carlin and Siekevitz (1983) have suggested, in fact, that the synaptic spinule described by Tarrant and Routtenberg (1977) may represent a dendritic spine that is splitting into two spines. In their model, the focus is on an increase in the number of spines with a coordinated enlargement of the presynaptic terminal so that it synapses on these splitting spines. An alternative view is that sprouting of the presynaptic terminal occurs with a coordinated increase in size or number of dendritic spines, so that there is an increase in the number of individual synaptic junctions.

One final point with respect to the role of protein kinase C and growth concerns the likely participation of the cytoskeleton in the transmogrification of the synapse consequent to high-frequency activity. The role of protein kinase C in the regulation of cytoskeletal processes has been described (e.g. Burn et al., 1985). Moreover, it has been proposed that certain cytoskeletal elements may participate in the process of synaptic plasticity (Lynch and Baudry, 1984). It would be surprising indeed if the alterations in shape and the growth of synaptic elements during the process of plasticity did not involve the regulation of cytoskeletal proteins by protein kinase C.

Secretion and transmitter release

There are two ways in which an increase in transmitter release are likely to be affected. In one case, there would be an increase in the number of terminals that release neurotransmitter. In the second case, there would be an increase in either the amount or the qualitative nature of transmitter released from individual terminals. The first instance is clearly related to the growth of presynaptic terminals just described, and may be thought of as a specific consequence of the growth mechanism.

Although by no means mutually exclusive, the second case, increase in amount or nature of transmitter release, may be mediated by activation of a protein kinase C mechanism. Nishizuka and his co-workers demonstrated several years ago that the thrombin-induced release of serotonin from platelets is mediated by kinase C phosphorylation of a 40-kDa substrate (Nishizuka et al., 1983; see also, Rank et al., 1983). Although the function of this substrate is not known, it has been shown using limited proteolysis that sites of phosphorylation of this peptide precisely match those phosphorylated by purified protein kinase C. Thus, a protein kinase C mechanism is directly implicated in stimulus–secretion coupling.

These results have prompted the question as to the role of this kinase in neurotransmitter release. Using TPA, the kinase C-activating phorbol ester, an increased release of acetylcholine from nerve terminals has been demonstrated (Publicover, 1985). It is still necessary to establish what specific role protein kinase C plays in this release process.

The activation of protein kinase C following LTP could conceivably increase transmitter release. Such a view is supported by a recent series of experiments from Bliss and co-workers, who have suggested that LTP is, in fact, derived from an increase in release of transmitter. Using the push–pull cannula, this laboratory has demonstrated that following LTP there is an increase in the amount of transmitter released (Feasey et al., 1985; Lynch and Bliss, 1985; Lynch et al., 1985).

These experiments do not differentiate between the increased release of transmitter from a given terminal and the increased release of transmitter caused by an increase in the number of terminals that would occur following growth. One conception that m y favor the latter interpretation comes from quantal analysis studies of transmission of Ia fibers in spinal cord in which it has been claimed that the release of one quanta from a terminal saturates the available receptors (Jack et al., 1981a, 1981b). In such a case it would seem of little use to increase the amount of transmitter released, as saturating levels would have already been reached.

One possibility mentioned briefly just above is that the nature of the transmitter changes when plasticity is engendered, i.e. a transmitter-like agent is released post-synaptically (sic) only at times of high-frequency stimulation. Such a compound might have a special action on the protein kinase C system. An example of this might be the action of an insulin-like growth factor (Koontz and Iwahashi, 1981; Puro and Agardh, 1984). This is suggested by the finding that insulin has been shown to stimulate the phosphorylation of protein F1 (Akers and Routtenberg, 1984) possibly by activating protein kinase C (see Chapter 16).

Receptor regulation

If the release of transmitter saturates the receptors, then a possible mechanism for overcoming this limitation would be to increase the number of receptors beyond the level of transmitter saturation. There is now good evidence to indicate that protein kinase C plays a central role in receptor activity. (For a general discussion of the role of protein phosphorylation in receptor regulation see Chapter 12), Cochet et al. (1985) have shown that epidermal growth factor (EGF) receptor activation is regulated by protein kinase C phosphorylation. Hunter et al. (1985) have shown that this occurs at threonine residue 654 near the cytoplasmic face of the plasma membrane. This kinase C regulation reduces the EGF-induced increase in tyrosine protein kinase activity, possibly by blocking via an allosteric change the affinity of EGF for the receptor. Another possible mechanism for receptor regulation has been raised by Beguinot et al. (1985), who suggested that phosphorylation of these threonine residues on the EGF receptor causes internalization of the receptor. It is clear that if this type of regulation holds for different receptor types activation of protein kinase C could regulate receptor number during the expression of synaptic plasticity.

Receptor regulation may therefore be important for synaptic plasticity. Baudry and Lynch (1980) proposed that LTP increases the number of glutamate binding sites. They suggested the hypothesis that this increase in related to an uncovering of cryptic receptors mediated by a protease, Calpain I. Thus, blockade of this protease by leupeptin decreases the number of glutamate binding sites. Issues surrounding certain difficulties with this model have been discussed elsewhere (Foster and Fagg, 1984; Routtenberg, 1984). Moreover, the failure of leupeptin to alter LTP-induced plasticity represents a serious difficulty for the proposed model.

Since protein kinase C is a substrate for Calpain I the effects of leupeptin on the glutamate receptor may be mediated through protein kinase C. One apparent difficulty with this hypothesis is that it is claimed that the glutamate receptor altered by LTP is postsynaptic, yet a presynaptic localization for protein kinase C has been suggested (Girard et al., 1985). There is, however, a recent suggestion that the blockade of LTP by the glutamate blocker aminophosphonovaleric acid may be a presynaptic effect (Lynch et al., 1985). It is conceivable therefore that glutamate blockade may occur at presynaptic loci and thus influence the protein kinase C localized there.

There is little doubt that protein kinase C can regulate receptor activity and that receptor activity may be related to alterations in synaptic strength. This would not preclude alterations in postsynaptic receptors mediated by a mechanism other than that involving protein kinase C. It is conceivable, based on the presynaptic localization of the kinase, that protein kinase C activation following LTP alters receptors ('autoreceptors') in the presynaptic membrane. It is to be re-emphasized that this receptor change could be related to the persistence of the plastic response and also to its initiation.

Ion conductance and channel properties

There is evidence that protein kinase C is capable of regulating ion channels. Two recent reports, one in the *Aplysia* and one in the hippocampal slice, suggest that TPA is capable of altering calcium conductance (DeRiemer et al., 1985; see Chapters 7 and 8) and calcium-dependent potassium conductance (Baraban, 1985). It may be noted that in both studies TPA was reported not to affect many of the parameters of the cell's physiology, suggesting that its effects may be selective. It may however be premature to discuss the implications of these results until detailed reports are available. Yet it may be noted that DeRiemer et al. were able to duplicate the effect of TPA with intracellular injection of partially purified protein kinase C. This suggests the possibility that activation of protein kinase C alters ion channel proteins in the membrane. Such ionic current alterations could be responsible, in part, for the plasticity of LTP, in particular, and for synaptic plasticity in general. Two recent proposals demonstrating alterations in ion conductance in relation to synaptic plasticity (Kandel and Schwartz, 1982; Alkon, 1984) have suggested a role for cyclic AMP-dependent or calcium/calmodulin-dependent kinases (Acosta-Uriquidi et al., 1984; see also Chapter 9 for the role of these kinases on ion channel function). The role of calcium/phospholipid-dependent kinases in regulating ionic conductance during the expression of synaptic plasticity has recently been studied (see Chapters 7 and 8; Farley and Auerbach, 1986).

In summary of this section, the participation of protein kinase C is the regulation of cellular processes of growth, secretion, receptor activity and ion conductance has been reviewed. As illustrated in Fig. 14, these different mechanisms may all participate in a coordinated fashion in the expression of plasticity. In each case, a role for such mechanisms in the expression of synaptic plasticity has been proposed by different laboratories. However, it is not necessary to consider that the different mechanisms for plasticity that have been proposed are mutually exclusive. Rather, there is a coordinated participation that is suggested to be orchestrated by the multifunctional nature of the protein kinase C mechanism. As has been suggested as a theme throughout this chapter, the role of the kinase would be in the persistence of the change: no recrudescence of terminal growth, a persistent change in the capacity for increase in transmitter release, increase in receptor number and probability of ion channel opening.

The protein kinase C–protein F1 connection

Our studies over the past ten years began with the substrate of protein kinase C, protein F1. It is appropriate, then, to conclude this chapter with a consideration of the possible function of protein F1. Two alternative categories of function may be considered. In one category, protein F1 may be directly associated with only one of the cellular functions just reviewed and would thus be growth-related, secretion-associated or perhaps a receptor or an ion channel protein. In the second category, there is the possibility that protein F1 plays a role in all of these processes, regulating these functions. An example of this latter type of regulatory role would be that proposed by Zwiers et al. (1982) in which protein B-50, which is thought to be identical to protein F1, regulates diphosphoinositide (DPI) kinase, which catalyzes the phosphorylation of DPI to triphosphoinositide (TPI). TPI is likely to be the substrate for the receptor-mediated activation of phospholipase C (Berridge, 1983) which hydrolyzes TPI and provides two signals to the cell: diacylglycerol (DG), leading to activation of protein kinase C, and inositol trisphosphate (IP_3), which leads to the release of calcium from intracellular stores. Intracellular injection of IP_3 can mimic the extracellular muscarinic action of acetylcholine and may, in general, be capable of mimicking the cell's particular function (e.g. Oron et al., 1985). It is attractive to think that the IP_3 limb of receptor-mediated phospholipase C action may be related to response initiation, while the protein kinase C limb may be related to response durability or persistence. These two responses would each then contribute to the enhanced plasticity following LTP.

The phosphorylation state of protein F1 would be increased in direct relation to the synergistic activation of protein kinase C by DG and IP_3-released calcium. If protein F1 phosphorylation inhibits DPI kinase then a negative feedback exists since protein kinase C activation would lead to F1 phosphorylation which would decrease DPI kinase activity (by inhibition). This would decrease available TPI and thereby reduce the receptor-activated phospholipase C elevation of DG and IP_3, de-activating protein kinase C and decreasing the phosphorylation state of protein F1. The regulatory or fine-tuning of such a system is apparent since the decrease in protein F1 phosphorylation would then remove the negative feedback influence.

The translocation of protein kinase C to the membrane (Fig. 9), possibly mediated by calcium (Walsh et al., 1984), increases the association of substrate and kinase, thereby providing an additional negative feedback loop. The need for regulatory control of the protein kinase C system is clearly evident in its putative role in tumor promotion (Castagna et al., 1982; Ashendel and Boutwell, 1983). It is not so obvious in brain, where the regulation of synaptic terminal growth, of both a negative and positive nature, is likely to be under considerable control, to permit, for example, both the rigid lamination of the hippocampus *and* its synaptic plasticity.

References

Abraham, W.C., Bliss, T.V.P. and Goddard, G.V. (1985) Heterosynaptic changes accompany long-term but not short-term potentiation of the perforant path in the anaesthetized rat. *J. Physiol.*, 363:335–349.

Acosta-Uriquidi, J., Alkon, D.L. and Neary, J.T. (1984) Ca^{++}-dependent protein kinase injection in a photoreceptor mimics biophysical effects of associative learning. *Science*, 224:1254–1257.

Akers, R. and Routtenberg, A. (1984) Brain protein phosphorylation: Selective action of insulin. *Life Sci.*, 35:809–813.

Akers, R. and Routtenberg, A. (1985) Protein kinase C phosphorylates a 47kd protein directly related to synaptic plasticity. *Brain Res.*, 334:147–151.

Akers, R.F., Cain, S.T. and Routtenberg, A. (1982) Brain pyruvate dehydrogenase: subcellular compartmentalization of functional regulation. *Neurosci. Abstr.*, 8:795.

Akers, R., Lovinger, D., Colley, P., Linden, D. and Routtenberg, A. (1986) Translocation of protein kinase C activity after long-term potentiation may mediate synaptic plasticity. *Science*, 231:587–589.

Alkon, D. (1984) Calcium-mediated reduction of ionic currents: a biophysical memory trace. *Science*, 226:1037–1045.

Aloyo, V.J., Zwiers, H. and Gispen, W.H. (1983) Phosphorylation of B-50 protein by calcium-activated,

phospholipid-dependent protein kinase and B-50 protein kinase. *J. Neurochem.*, 41:649–653.

Andersen, P., Blackstad, T.W. and Lomo, T. (1966) Location and identification of excitatory synapses on hippocampal pyramidal cells. *Exp. Brain Res.*, 1:236–248.

Ashendel, C.L., Staller, J.M. and Boutwell, R.K. (1983) Protein kinase activity associated with a phorbol ester receptor purified from mouse brain. *Cancer Res.*, 43:4333–4337.

Bar, P.R., Schotman, P., Gispen, W.H., Lopes da Silva, F.H. and Tielen, A.M. (1980) Changes in synaptic membrane phosphorylation after tetanic stimulation in the dentate area of the rat hippocampal slice. *Brain Res.*, 198:478–484.

Baraban, J.M., Snyder, S.H. and Alger, B.E. (1985) Protein kinase C regulates ionic conductance in hippocampal pyramidal neurons: electrophysiological effects of phorbol esters. *Proc. Natl. Acad. Sci. U.S.A.*, 82:2538–2542.

Barnes, C.A. and McNaughton, B.L. (1980) Spatial memory and hippocampal synaptic plasticity in senescent and middle-aged rats. In D.G. Stein (Ed.), *The Psychobiology of Aging: Problems and Perspectives*, Elsevier/Holland, Amsterdam, pp. 253–272.

Baudry, M. and Lynch, G. (1980) Regulation of hippocampal glutamate receptors: Evidence for the involvement of a calcium-activated protease. *Proc. Natl. Acad. Sci. U.S.A.*, 77:2298–2302.

Beguinot, L., Hanover, J.A., Ito, S., Richert, N.D., Willingham, M.C. and Pastan, I. (1985) Phorbol esters induce transient internalization without degradation of unoccupied epidermal growth factor receptors. *Proc. Natl. Acad. Sci. U.S.A.*, 82:2774–2778.

Benowitz, L.I. and Lewis, E.R. (1983) Increased transport of 44 000- to 49 000-dalton acidic proteins during regeneration of the goldfish optic nerve: a two-dimensional gel analysis. *J. Neurosci.*, 3:2153–2163.

Berridge, M.J. (1983) Rapid accumulation of inositol triphosphate reveals that agonists hydrolyse polyphosphoinositides instead of phosphatidylinositol. *Biochem. J.*, 212:849–858.

Bliss, T.V.P. and Dolphin, A.C. (1984) Where is the locus of long term potentiation? In G. Lynch, J.L. McGaugh and N.M. Weinberger (Eds.), *Neurobiology of Learning and Memory*, The Guilford Press, New York, pp. 451–458.

Bliss, T.V.P. and Gardner-Medwin, A.R. (1973) Long-lasting potentiation of synaptic transmission in the dentate area of the unanesthetized rabbit following stimulation of the perforant path. *J. Physiol.*, 232:357–374.

Bliss, T.V.P. and Lomo, T. (1973) Long-lasting potentiation of synaptic transmission in the dentate area of the anaesthetized rabbit following stimulation of the perforant path. *J. Physiol.*, 232:334–356.

Bliss, T.V.P., Dolphin, A.C. and Feasey, K.J. (1984) Elevated calcium induces a long-lasting potentiation of commissural responses in hippocampal CA3 cells of the rat in vivo. *J. Physiol.*, 350:13–14.

Browning, M., Baudry, M. and Lynch, G. (1982) Evidence that high frequency stimulation influences the phosphorylation of

232

pyruvate dehydrogenase and that the activity of this enzyme is linked to mitochondrial calcium sequestration. In W. Gispen and A. Routtenberg (Eds.), *Brain Phosphoproteins: Characterization and Function. Progress In Brain Research*, *Vol. 56*, Elsevier/Holland, Amsterdam, pp. 317–338.

Burn, P., Rotman, A., Meyer, R.K. and Burger, M.M. (1985) Diacylglycerol in large alpha-actinin/actin complexes and in the cytoskeleton of activated platelets. *Nature*, 314:469–492.

Carlin, R.K. and Siekevitz, P. (1983) Plasticity in the central nervous system: do synapses divide? *Proc. Natl. Acad. Sci. U.S.A.*, 80:3517–3521.

Castagna, M., Takay, Y., Kambuchi, K., Samo, K., Kikkawa, U. and Nishizuka, Y. (1982) Direct activation of calcium-activated, phospholipid-dependent protein kinase by tumor-promoting phorbol esters. *J. Biol. Chem.*, 257:7847–7851.

Chan, S.Y., Murakami, K. and Routtenberg, A. (1985) Purification of a kinase C substrate: brain phosphoprotein F1 and the discovery of an endogenous kinase C inhibitory factor. *Soc. Neurosci.*, 11:927.

Chan, S.Y., Murakami, K. and Routtenberg, A. (1986) Phosphoprotein F1: Purification and characterization of a brain kinase C substrate related to plasticity. *J. Neurosci.* (in press).

Cochet, C., Gill, G.N., Meisenhelder, J., Cooper, J.A. and Hunter, T. (1984) C-kinase phosphorylates the epidermal growth factor receptor and reduces its epidermal growth factor-stimulated tyrosine protein kinase activity. *J. Biol. Chem.*, 259:2553–2558.

DeRiemer, S.A., Strong, J.A., Albert, K.A., Greengard, P. and Kaczmarek, L.K. (1985) Phorbol ester and protein kinase C enhance calcium current in *Aplysia* neurones. *Nature*, 313:313–315.

Desmond, N.L. and Levy, W.B. (1983) Synaptic correlates of associative potentiation/depression: An ultrastructural study in the hippocampus. *Brain Res.*, 265:21–30.

Douglas, R.M. and Goddard, G.V. (1975) Long-term potentiation of the perforant path-granule cell synapse in the rat hippocampus. *Brain Res.*, 86:205–215.

Dunphy, W.G., Delclos, K.B. and Blumberg, P.M. (1980) Characterization of specific binding of [3H]phorbol 12,13-dibutyrate and [3H]phorbol 12-myristate 13-acetate to mouse brain. *Cancer Res.*, 40:3635–3641.

Eccles, J.C. (1953) *The Neurophysiological Basis of Mind*, Clarendon Press, Oxford, p. 314.

Ehrlich, Y.H., Rabjohns, R.R. and Routtenberg, A. (1977) Experiential-input alters the phosphorylation of specific proteins in brain membranes. *Pharmacol. Biochem. Behav.*, 6:354–360.

Ellis, L., Katz, F. and Pfenninger, K.H. (1985) Nerve growth cones isolated from fetal rat brain. II. Cyclic adenosine 3′:5′-monophosphate (cAMP)-binding proteins and cAMP-dependent phosphorylation. *J. Neurosci.*, 5:1399–1401.

Farley, J. and Auerbach, S. (1986) Protein kinase C activation induces conductance changes in *Hermissenda* photoreceptors like those seen in associative learning. *Nature*, 319:220–223.

Feasey, K., Lynch, M.A., Errington, M.L.G. and Bliss, T.V.P. (1985) Long-term potentiation in two different hippocampal pathways is associated with increased release but not in-

creased uptake of ^{14}C-glutamate. *Neurosci. Lett.*, 21:544.

Fifkova, E. and Von Harreveld, A. (1977) Long-lasting morphological changes in dendritic spines of dentate granular cells following stimulation of the entorhinal area. *J. Neurocytol.*, 6:211–230.

Foster, A.C. and Fagg, G.E. (1984) Acidic amino acid binding sites in mammalian neuronal membranes: their characteristics and relationship to synaptic receptors. *Brain Res. Rev.*, 7:103–164.

Girard, P.R., Mazzei, G.J., Wood, J.G. and Kuo, J.F. (1985) Polyclonal antibodies to phospholipid/Ca^{2+}-dependent protein kinase and immunochemical localization of the enzyme in rat brain. *Proc. Natl. Acad. Sci. U.S.A.*, 82:3030–3034.

Gispen, W.H., Leunissen, J.L.M., Oestreicher, A.B., Verkleij, A.J. and Zwiers, H. (1985) Presynaptic localization of B-50 phosphoprotein: the (ACTH)-sensitive protein kinase substrate involved in rat brain polyphophoinositide metabolism. *Brain Res.*, 328:381–385.

Hebb, D.O. (1949) *The Organization of Behavior*, Wiley, New York, p. 335.

Hoch, D.B., Dingledine, R.J. and Wilson, J.E. (1984) Long-term potentiation in the hippocampal slice: Possible involvement of pyruvate dehydrogenase. *Brain Res.*, 28:1–10.

Hsu, L., Natyzak, D. and Laskin, J.D. (1984) Effects of tumor promoter 12-O-tetradecanoylphorbol-13-acetate on neurite outgrowth from chick embryo sensory ganglia. *Cancer Res.*, 44:4607–4614.

Hunter, T., Ling, N. and Cooper, J.A. (1984) Protein kinase C phosphorylation of the EGF receptor at a threonine residue close to the cytoplasmic face of the plasma membrane. *Nature*, 311:480–483.

Jack, J.J.B., Redman, S.J. and Wong, K. (1981a) Modification to synaptic transmission at group Ia on cat spinal motoneurones by 4-aminopyridine. *J. Physiol.*, 321:111–126.

Jack, J.J.B., Redman, S.J. and Wong, K. (1981b) The components of synaptic potentials evoked in cat spinal motoneurones by impulses in single group Ia afferents. *J. Physiol.*, 321:65–94.

Kandel, E.R. and Schwartz, J.H. (1982) Molecular biology of learning: Modulation of transmitter release. *Science*, 218:433–443.

Katz, F., Ellis, L. and Pfenninger, K.H. (1985) Nerve growth cones isolated from fetal rat brain. III. Calcium-dependent protein phosphorylation. *J. Neurosci.*, 5:1402–1411.

Kikkawa, U., Takai, Y., Minakuchi, R., Inohara, S. and Nishizuka, Y. (1982) Calcium-activated, phospholipid-dependent protein kinase from rat brain. *J. Biol. Chem.*, 257:13341–13348.

Kikkawa, U., Takai, Y., Tanaka, Y., Miyake, R. and Nishizuka, Y. (1983) Protein kinase C as a possible receptor protein of tumor-promoting phorbol esters. *J. Biol. Chem.*, 258:11442–11445.

Koontz, J.W. and Iwahashi, M. (1981) Insulin as a potent, specific growth factor in a rat hepatoma cell line. *Science*, 211:947–949.

Kraft, A.S. and Anderson, W.B. (1983) Phorbol esters increase the amount of Ca^{2+}, phospholipid-dependent protein kinase associated with plasma membrane. *Nature*, 301:621–623.

Lee, K.S., Schottler, F., Oliver, M. and Lynch, G. (1980) Brief bursts of high frequency stimulation produce two types of structural change in rat hippocampus. *J. Neurophysiol.*, 44:247–258.

Lloyd, D.P.C. (1949) Post-synaptic potentiation of response in monosynaptic reflex pathways of the spinal cord. *J. Gen. Physiol.*, 33:147–170.

Lomo, T. (1971) Patterns of activation in a monosynaptic cortical pathway: The perforant path input to the dentate area of the hippocampal formation. *Exp. Brain Res.*, 12:18–45.

Lovinger, D.M., Akers, R.F., Nelson, R.B., Barnes, C.A., McNaughton, B.L. and Routtenberg, A. (1985a) A selective increase in the phosphorylation of protein F1, a protein kinase C substrate, directly related to three-day growth of long-term synaptic enhancement. *Brain Res.*, 343:137–145.

Lovinger, D.M., Colley, P., Linden, D., Mukarami, K. and Routtenberg, A. (1985b) Phorbol ester, which induces protein kinase C (PKC) translocation to the membrane, prevents decay of long term potentiation. *Soc. Neurosci.*, 11:927.

Lovinger, D., Akers, R., Colley, P., Linden, D. and Routtenberg, A. (1986) Direct relation of synaptic plasticity to phosphorylation of membrane protein F1: Potential association with protein kinase C translocation. *Brain Res.*, (in press).

Low, P.S., Waugh, S.M., Zinke, K. and Drenckhahn, D. (1985) The role of hemoglobin denaturation and band 3 clustering in red blood cell aging. *Science*, 227:531–533.

Lynch, G. and Baudry, M. (1984) The biochemistry of memory: A new and specific hypothesis. *Science*, 224:1057–1063.

Lynch, M.A. and Bliss, T.P.V. (1985) Long-term potentiation in commisural input to hippocampal CA3 cells is accompanied by a sustained increase in release of endogenuous aspartate. *Neurosci. Letters Suppl.*, 21:544.

Lynch, G., McGaugh, J.L. and Weinberger, N.M. (1984) *Neurobiology of Learning and Memory*, Guilford Press, New York, p. 528.

Lynch, M.A., Errington, M.L. and Bliss, T.V.P. (1985) Long-term potentiation and the sustained increase in glutamate release which follow tetanic stimulation of the perforant path are both blocked by d(−)-aminophosphovaleric acid. *Soc. Neurosci.* 11:438.

McNaughton, B. (1982) Long-term synaptic enhancement and short-term potentiation in rat fascia dentata act through different mechanisms. *J. Physiol.*, 324:249–262.

Michell, R.H. (1983) Ca^{2+} and protein kinase C: two synergistic cellular signals. *TIBS*, 8:263–265.

Morgan, D.G. (1981) *The Phosphorylation of Brain Pyruvate Dehydrogenase and its Response to Behavioral Experience*. Dissertation, Northwestern University, Evanston, IL.

Morgan, D.G. and Routtenberg, A. (1980) Evidence that a 41 kDa phosphoprotein is pyruvate dehydrogenase. *Biochem. Biophys. Res. Commun.*, 95:509–512.

Morgan, D.G. and Routtenberg, A. (1981) Brain pyruvate dehydrogenase: Phosphorylation and enzyme activity altered by a training experience. *Science*, 214:470–471.

Morris, M.E., Krnjevic, K. and Ropert, N. (1983) Changes in free Ca^{++} recorded inside hippocampal neurons in response to fimbrial stimulation. *Soc. Neurosci.*, 9:395.

Murakami, K., Chan, S.Y. and Routtenberg, A. (1985) Direct stimulation of protein kinase C (PKC): unsaturated fatty acids (oleate, arachidonate) are sufficient. *Soc. Neurosci.*, 11:927.

Murphy, K.M.M., Gould, R.J., Oster-Granite, M.L., Gearheart, J.D. and Snyder, S.H. (1983) Phorbol esters receptors: autoradiographic identification in the developing rat. *Science*, 222:1036–1038.

Nelson, R.B. and Routtenberg, A. (1985) Characterization of the 47kD protein F1 (p*I* 4.5), a kinase C substrate directly related to neural plasticity. *Exp. Neurol.*, 89:213–224.

Nelson, R.B., Routtenberg, A., Hyman, C. and Pfenninger, K. H. (1985) A phosphoprotein, F1, directly related to neuronal plasticity in adult rat brain may be identical to a major growth cone membrane protein *Soc. Neurosci.*, 11:927.

Nishizuka, Y. (1984a) The role of protein kinase C in cell surface signal transduction and tumour promotion. *Nature*, 308:693–697.

Nishizuka, Y. (1984b) Turnover of inositol phospholipids and signal transduction. *Science*, 225:1365–1370.

Nishizuka, Y., Takai, Y., Kishimoto, A., Kikkawa, U. and Kaibuchi, K. (1984) Phospholipid turnover in hormone action. *Rec. Progr. Horm. Res.*, 40:301–345.

Oron, N., Dascal, N., Nadler, E. and Lupu, M. (1985) Inositol 1,4,5,-triphosphate mimics muscarinic response in xenopus oocytes. *Nature*, 313:141–143.

Publicover, S.J. (1985) Stimulation of spontaneous transmitter release by the phorbol ester 12-*O*-tetradecanoylphorbol-13-acetate, an activator of protein kinase C. *Brain Res.*, 333:185–187.

Puro, D.G. and Agardh, E. (1984) Insulin-mediated regulation of neuronal maturation. *Science*, 225:1170–1172.

Ranck, J.B. (1973) Studies on single neurons in dorsal hippocampal formation and septum in unrestrained rats. I. Behavioral correlates and firing repertoires. *Exp. Neurol.*, 41:461–555.

Rasmussen, H. and Barret, P. (1984) Calcium messenger system: an integrated view. *Physiol. Rev.*, 64:938–984.

Rink, T.J., Sanchez, A. and Hallam, T.J. (1983) Diacylglycerol and phorbol ester stimulate secretion without raising cytoplasmic free calcium in human platelets. *Nature*, 305:317–319.

Routtenberg, A. (1982a) Identification and back-titration of brain pyruvate dehydrogenase: functional significance for behavior. In W.H. Gispen and A. Routtenberg (Eds.), *Brain phosphoproteins: Characterisation and Function, Progress in Brain Research, Vol. 56*, Elsevier Biomedical Press, Amsterdam, pp. 349–394.

Routtenberg, A. (1982b) Memory formation as a post-translational modification of brain proteins. In C.A. Marsden and H. Matthies (Eds.), *Mechanisms and Models os Neural Plasticity. Proc. VIth Int. Neurobiol. IBRO Symp. Learning and Memory*, Raven Press, New York, pp. 17–24.

Routtenberg, A. (1984) Brain phosphoproteins, kinase C and protein F1 protagonists of plasticity in particular pathways. In G. Lynch, J. McGaugh and N. Weinberger (Eds.), *Memory Neurobiology*, Guilford Press, New York, pp. 479–490.

234

Routtenberg, A. (1985a) Phosphoprotein regulation of memory formation: enhancement and control of synaptic plasticity by protein kinase C and protein F1. *Ann. N.Y. Acad. Sci.*, 444:203–209.

Routtenberg, A. (1985b) Protein kinase C activation leading to protein F1 phosphorylation regulate synaptic plasticity by presynaptic terminal growth. *Behav. Neurol Biol.*, 44:186–200.

Routtenberg, A. (1985c) Protein kinase C and substrate protein F1 relation to synaptic plasticity and growth. In B. Will and P. Schmidt (Eds.), *Brain Plasticity, Learning and Memory*, Plenum Press, New York.

Routtenberg, A., Ehrlich, Y.H. and Rabjohns, R. (1975) Effect of a training experience on phosphorylation of a specific protein in neocortical and subcortical membrane preparations. *Fed. Proc.*, 34:293.

Routtenberg, A., Lovinger, D., Cain, S., Akers, R. and Steward, O. (1983) Effects of long-term potentiation of perforant path synapses in the intact hippocampus on in vitro phosphorylation of a 47kD protein (F1). *Fed. Proc.*, 42:755.

Routtenberg, A., Nelson, R.B., Akers, R., Murakami, K., Chan, S., Colley, P. and Lovinger, D. (1985) Protein kinase C and its substrate protein F1: Pivotal role in synaptic plasticity. *J. Neurochem.*, 44:135.

Routtenberg, A., Colley, P., Linden, D., Lovinger, D. and Murakami, K. (1986) Phorbol ester promotes growth of synaptic plasticity. *Brain Res.*, 378:374–378.

Ruiz-Marcos, A. and Valverde, F. (1969) The temporal evolution of the distribution of dendritic spines in the visual cortex of normal and dark-raised mice. *Exp. Brain Res.*, 8:284–294.

Ruth, R.E., Collier, T.J. and Routtenberg, A. (1982) Topography between entorhinal cortex and the dentate septo-temporal axis in rats. I. Medial and intermediate entorhinal projecting cells. *J. Comp. Neurol.*, 209:69–78.

Skene, J.H.P. and Willard, M. (1981a) Axonally transported proteins associated with axon growth in rabbit central and peripheral nervous system. *J. Cell Biol.*, 89:96–103.

Skene, J.H.P. and Willard, M. (1981b) Changes in axonally transported proteins during axon regeneration in toad retinal ganglion cells. *J. Cell. Biol.*, 89:86–95.

Snyder, S.H. (1984) Drug and neurotransmitter receptors in the brain. *Science*, 224:22–31.

Takai, Y., Kishimoto, A., Iwasa, Y., Kawahara, Y., Mori, T. and Nishizuka, Y. (1977) Calcium-dependent activation of a multifunctional protein kinase by membrane phospholipids. *J. Biol. Chem.*, 254:3692–3695.

Tarrant, S. and Routtenberg, A. (1977) The synaptic spinule in the dendritic spine: electron microscopic study of the hippocampal dentate gyrus. *Tissue Cell*, 9:461–473.

Walsh, M.P., Valentine, K.A., Ngai, P.K., Carruthers, C.A. and Hollenberg, M.D. (1984) Ca^{++}-dependent hydrophobic-interaction chromatography. *Biochem. J.*, 224:117–127.

Wilson, R.C. and Levy, W.B. (1981) Changes in translation of synaptic excitation to dentate granule cell discharge accompanying long-term potentiation. II. An evaluation of mechanisms utilizing dentate gyrus dually innervated by surviving and sprouted crossed tempo-dentate imputs. *J. Neurophysiol.*, 46:339–335.

Zwiers, H., Jolles, J., Aloyo, V.J., Oestreicher, A.B. and Gispen, W.H. (1982) ACTH and synaptic membrane phosphorylation in rat brain. In W.H. Gispen and A. Routtenberg (Eds.), *Function of brain phosphoproteins, Progress in Brain Research*, Vol. 56, Elsevier/North Holland, Amsterdam, pp. 405–417.

W.H. Gispen and A. Routtenberg (Eds.)
Progress in Brain Research, Vol. 69
© 1986 Elsevier Science Publishers B.V. (Biomedical Division)

CHAPTER 19

Protein phosphorylation in the nerve growth cone

Karl H. Pfenninger, Carolyn Hyman* and Robert S. Garofalo**

Department of Cellular and Structural Biology, University of Colorado Health Sciences Center, 4200 E. Ninth Avenue, Denver, CO 80110, U.S.A.

Introduction

The nerve growth cone is the irregularly shaped terminal enlargement of the growing neurite. It is its leading edge, endowed with the capacity of finding the path to the appropriate target area and forming a synapse with an appropriate target cell. Therefore, the nerve growth cone is a developmentally regulated structure which precedes the axon's mature terminal enlargement, the presynaptic ending.

Not until recently has a detailed biochemical analysis of nerve growth cones been possible. Subcellular fractions enriched in sheared-off fragments from nerve growth cones have recently been prepared by Pfenninger et al. (1983) and by Gordon-Weeks and Lockerbie (1984). These so-called growth cone particles (GCPs) contain a set of organelles that is equivalent to that of nerve growth cones, as well as a number of growth-associated proteins (Simkowitz and Pfenninger, 1983; Ellis et al., 1985b; Wallis et al., 1985; Willard et al., 1985; Meiri et al., 1986; Simkowitz et al., submitted). We believe, therefore, that the major characteristics of the GCP fraction are representative of those of axonal nerve growth cones.

Knowledge of phosphoproteins and kinase activities of the GCP fraction can serve to sort out its components and is of primary interest for

answering the questions: (*a*) are the well-known synaptic phosphoproteins already present prior to synaptogenesis and (*b*) can we identify in GCPs developmentally regulated phosphoproteins that might be involved in growth regulation?

Substrates of cyclic nucleotide-dependent protein kinases

The observations reviewed in this article are the results of phosphorylation studies begun in this laboratory by Flora Katz and Leland Ellis. In those earlier studies, GCPs were pelleted, homogenized and exposed to [^{32}P]ATP in the presence or absence of various cofactors (Ellis et al., 1985a; Katz et al., 1985); the protocols closely followed those developed by Greengard and his colleagues for adult brain and synaptosomes (Lohmann et al., 1978; Kennedy and Greengard, 1981; Wu et al., 1982). A listing of the most prominent GCP phosphoproteins and their possible correlation with phosphoproteins described elsewhere is presented in Table I.

When fetal rat brain homogenates, low-speed pellets or low-speed supernatants are incubated with [^{32}P]ATP in the presence of various cofactors, phosphoproteins are difficult to detect, i.e. protein kinase activity per unit protein is very low (Fig. 1; cf. Lohmann et al., 1978). However, in particulate subfractions of the low-speed supernatant such as the GCP fraction, various phosphoproteins are evident. This basic observation applies to the substrates of cyclic AMP (cAMP)- and calcium-dependent kinases. However, substrates of cGMP-dependent kinase have not been detected in our assays.

---

*Present address: Department of Cell Biology, NYU Medical Center, 550 First Avenue, New York, NY 10016, U.S.A.

**Present address: Memorial Sloan Kettering Cancer Center, 1275 Park Avenue, New York, NY 10021, U.S.A.

TABLE I

Prominent phosphoproteins of growth cone particles

M_r (kDa)	Kinase dependence	Major	Identity (? = tentative)	Synapto-somal	Comments	Ref.
300	cAMP, CaCM		MAP 2 (?)		doublet	1
80	cAMP, CaCM		synapsin I	+	basic, doublet	1
80	cAMP, CaPL	+	presynaptic 87 kDa	+	acidic, cytosol	2
77	cAMP		protein IIIa (?)	+		1
60	CaCM		synapsin I kinase (?)	+		4
56	cAMP		protein IIIb (?)	+		1
53	cAMP		R II	+		3
52	cAMP	+	protein IIb· (?)	+		5
52	CaCM	+	tubulin	+		6
49	CaCM		synapsin I kinase (?)	+		4
46	CaCM, CaPL	+	GAP 43, F1/B-50	+	acidic, membrane	7
40	CaPL	+		+	acidic, cytosol	2

References: 1, for review, see Nestler and Greengard, 1983; 2, Wu, Walaas, Nairn and Greengard, 1982; 3, Rangel-Aldao, Kupiec and Rosen, 1979; 4, Kennedy, McGuiness and Greengard, 1983; 5, Lohmann, Walter and Greengard, 1980; 6, Burke and DeLorenzo, 1981; 7, Willard, Meiri and Glicksman, 1985; Nelson and Routtenberg, 1985; Zwiers, Schotman and Gispen, 1980;

Substrates of cAMP kinase include proteins at 300, 80, 77, 56, 53, and 52 kDa (see Table I). As resolved by two-dimensional gel electrophoresis, the 80-kDa region contains several substrates including: a basic doublet at 80 kDa (according to our calibration), which is also phosphorylated by a calcium/calmodulin-dependent kinase. It co-migrates in two-dimensional gels with synapsin I, shares V8 protease phosphopeptides with it (Ellis et al., 1985a) and cross-reacts with an antibody to it (kindly provided by Dr. Greengard's laboratory). A further, but very acidic (p*I* 4.0) 80-kDa substrate can also be phosphorylated by a calcium/phospholipid-dependent kinase, presumably protein kinase C (see below), and may correspond to a presynaptic substrate described by Wu et al. (1982). While the 53-kDa substrate of cAMP-dependent kinase appears to be one of its regulatory subunits, RII, the substrates of 52, 56 and 77 kDa may correspond to synaptosomal phosphoproteins IIb, IIIb, and IIIa, respectively (Table I; Ellis et al., 1985a). Some substrates, especially those at 52 and 56 kDa appear to be concentrated in GCP membranes, but none are radiolabeled if GCP lysate, i.e. the soluble protein

content of GCPs, is analyzed separately (Fig. 1). Overall, there is a variety of major and minor cAMP-dependent kinase substrates in the GCP fraction but none of them is as prominant as the substrates of calcium-dependent kinases described below.

Substrates of calcium-dependent protein kinases

Many phosphoproteins are detected in GCPs if phosphorylation is carried out in the presence of calcium. Consistent with this observation is the finding that GCPs contain significant amounts of calmodulin and several calmodulin binding proteins (Hyman and Pfenninger, 1985). Minor GCP substrates of calcium/calmodulin kinase include, as already mentioned, synapsin I and the subunits of synapsin I kinase (Fig. 2A; NEPHGE). In addition, there are four major polypeptide species, one of which (52 kDa) is presumably tubulin (Fig. 2; IEF; Katz et al., 1985). The three remaining proteins have molecular masses of 80, 46, and 40 kDa. One of these, the 46-kDa species (pp46), is the only major target of a calcium/calmodulin-dependent kinase in GCPs.

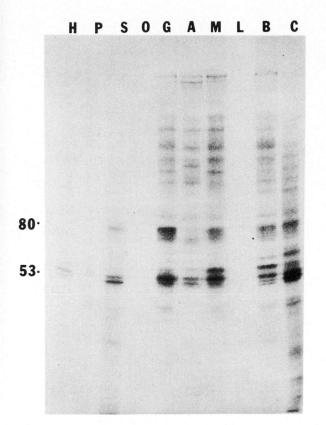

H P S O G A M L B C

80·

53·

Fig. 1. cAMP-dependent protein phosphorylation in subfractions of fetal rat brain (17 days gestation). Autoradiogram of a 5–15% acrylamide gradient gel. Each lane contained 17 µg protein, phosphorylated (15 s at 30°C) in the presence of 5 µM cAMP, approximately 1 µg purified catalytic subunit of the cAMP-dependent kinase, 5 µM [^{32}P]ATP and 0.1% Triton X-100. H, whole brain homogenate; P, low-speed pellet; S, low-speed supernatant (parent fraction of O–C); O, high-speed supernatant; G, pelleted GCPs; A, low-density fraction containing GCPs; M and L, crude membranes and lysate, respectively, of GCPs; B and C, heterogeneous, heavier subfractions of S. B and C contain glial and neuritic fragments as well as disrupted GCPs and various organelles. For detailed description of fractions, see Pfenninger et al. (1983). Molecular masses are indicated on the left, in kDa. Note that phosphoproteins are difficult to detect in H, P, O, and L, but prominent in particulate subfractions of S. (From Ellis et al., 1985b).

This protein is acidic (pI 4.3), exhibits a characteristic microheterogeneity (with the more acidic isoform migrating at a slightly lower apparent molecular weight) and co-migrates with a major, developmentally regulated membrane protein of GCPs (Ellis et al., 1985b; Katz et al., 1985; Simkowitz et al., submitted). Furthermore, pp46 appears to be identical to a growth-associated protein, GAP 43 (see below).

Phosphorylation of the 80- and 40-kDa proteins (pp80 and pp40) can be stimulated with phosphatidylserine and diolein in the presence of a low concentration of the detergent Triton X-100 (0.05%), indicating the action of protein kinase C (Katz et al., 1985). At high concentrations of detergent (0.1% Triton X-100) the phosphorylation of pp46 is also enhanced. The phorbol ester 12-O-tetradecanoylphorbol-13-acetate (TPA) is believed to bind to and activate protein kinase C (for review, see Nishizuka, 1984). Accordingly, TPA increases the radioactivity incorporated into pp80, pp40 and also into pp46 (Nelson et al., 1986; Hyman and Pfenninger, in preparation).

GCPs can be prepared sealed (Hyman and Pfenninger, 1985) and then incubated in the presence of a small amount (0.01%) of the detergent saponin for permeabilization of the plasmalemma, in a high K$^+$, low Na$^+$ medium containing ATP and co-factors. In this system the time course of phosphorylation following the addition of calcium is different for pp46 (phosphorylated immediately) than for pp40 and pp80 (delay of about 10 s).

Overall, pp40, pp46 and pp80 (acidic) are the most prominent kinase substrates in GCPs. pp46 is the only major substrate of a calcium/calmodulin kinase, but all three may be the target of protein kinase C. However, the time courses of phosphorylation and the detergent requirements of phosphorylation by protein kinase C are different for pp46 than for pp40 and pp80. These findings also indicate that protein kinase C activity is high in GCPs and, thus, in growth cones. This conclusion is consistent with the observation that a particularly high density of TPA receptor, believed to be protein kinase C, is associated with nervous system structures rich in growing axons (Murphy et al., 1983).

Phosphorylation and metabolism of phosphatidylinositol

Sodium dodecylsulfate–polyacrylamide gels (SDS-PAGE) used to resolve radiolabeled phospho-

238

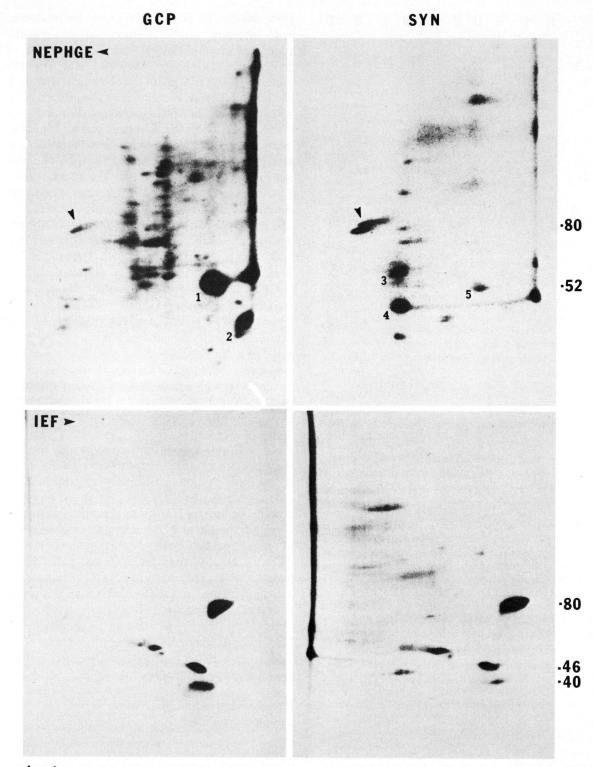

proteins of GCPs contain in the dye front area a number of radioactive bands, including one which becomes progressively more radioactive with time and whose phosphorylation is influenced by calcium concentration; the presence of relatively high calcium levels inhibits the incorporation of ^{32}P (Fig. 3; SDS-PAGE). Material corresponding to that running in this dye-front position can be extracted from GCPs with chloroform–methanol and then analyzed by thin-layer chromatography (Fig. 3; TLC). Radioactive spots can be seen to co-migrate with phosphatidic acid (PA) and/or phosphatidylinositol (PI) (which are often not separated in the chromatographic system used), phosphatidylinositol 4-monophosphate (PIP) and phosphatidylinositol 4,5-bisphosphate (PIP$_2$; Hyman et al., 1985). In other words, GCPs contain the enzymes required for phosphorylation of PI. Preliminary experiments with radiolabeled inositol as precursor suggest the release of inositol 1,4,5-trisphosphate (IP$_3$) in GCPs (Garofalo and Pfenninger, in preparation). Therefore, it appears that GCPs are also capable of cleavage of PIP$_2$ into IP$_3$ and sn-1,2-diacylglycerol. It is likely that the enzyme cascade involved in this process is receptor-activated as in all other systems described (Berridge and Irvine, 1984), and that the release of diacylglycerol, together with calcium, stimulates protein kinase C. As described by a number of investigators (see, e.g., Joseph et al., 1984; Berridge and Irvine, 1984; Nishizuka, 1984), IP$_3$ liberated into the cytosol probably leads to the discharge of calcium from an intracellular compartment, presumably endoplasmic reticulum. Such reticulum is abundant in growth cones (Tennyson, 1970; Yamada et al., 1971; Bunge, 1973) and GCPs (Pfenninger et al., 1983) and has been reported to contain calcium (P.R. Gordon-Weeks and R.O. Lockerbie, personal communication). Interestingly, exogenous IP$_3$ added to intact, permeabilized GCPs stimulates phosphorylation of the protein kinase C substrates pp40 and pp80 (but not of pp46), and this stimulation can be blocked by first depleting intracellular calcium stores (Hyman and Pfenninger, in preparation). This result suggests a role of IP$_3$ in the release of calcium in the growth cone. It should be noted that PI phosphorylation and metabolism are very active processes in GCPs, even in the resting state. This is evident from the density in radioautograms (of SDS–polyacrylamide gels) of the phospholipid band relative to that of the phosphopeptide bands and from the time course of labeling of PIP$_2$ resolved by TLC (Fig. 3).

Comparisons with subfractions of the mature brain

GCP phosphoproteins have been compared with those in synaptosomes and those in a P$_2'$ fraction from hippocampus. As evident in Table I, all major GCP phosphoproteins except for the 300-kDa species appear to have equivalents in the synaptosome fraction. For some of these, such as synapsin I, pp80 (acidic), pp46 and pp40, the identification of GCP and synaptosome species is based on substantial evidence: for others this correlation is tentative at present (Ellis et al., 1985a; Katz et al., 1985). The similarities of

Fig. 2. Autoradiograms of calcium-dependent kinase substrates separated by two-dimensional gel electrophoresis. Top panels, GCP and synaptosomal (SYN) proteins phosphorylated (15 s at 30°C) in the presence of 0.2 mM EGTA and 0.5 mM CaCl$_2$ (GCP) or 0.7 mM CaCl$_2$ and 0.5 µg/50 µl exogenous calmodulin (SYN). Polypeptides were separated by non-equilibrium pH gradient gel electrophoresis (NEPHGE) and SDS-PAGE. Bottom panels, proteins of GCPs (11 µg) and synaptosomes (22 µg) phosphorylated (15 s at 30°C) in the presence of 0.7 mM CaCl$_2$ and then separated by isoelectric focussing (IEF) and SDS-PAGE. Molecular masses are indicated on the right, in kDa. Note that exposures of X-ray film differ for all four samples. NEPHGE gels show that synapsin I (arrowhead) is a minor phosphoprotein in GCPs but a major species in synaptosomes. The numbered proteins are: 1 and 5, tubulin; 2, acidic 40-kDa protein; 3 and 4, putative subunits of synapsin-I kinase; the 46-kDa species is seen as a small spot between 1 and 2. IEF is more suitable to resolve the acidic phosphoproteins. Note the domineering presence of the three GCP phosphoproteins, pp80, pp46, and pp40: tubulin is seen as a more basic group of spots at 52 kDa. When larger protein amounts are used in the assay and after sufficiently long exposure, pp80, and pp46, and pp40 can also be detected in the synaptosome fraction. (From Katz et al., 1985).

240

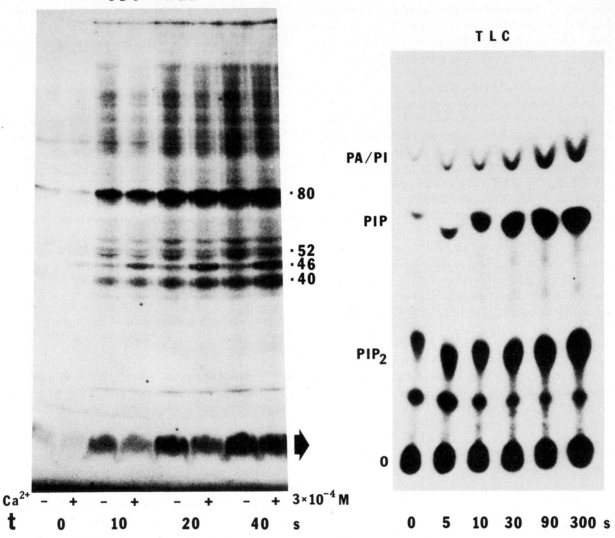

SDS−PAGE

TLC

PA/PI

PIP

PIP₂

· 80

· 52
· 46
· 40

0

Ca²⁺ − + − + − + − + 3×10⁻⁴ M

t   0   10   20   40   s   0   5   10   30   90 300 s

Fig. 3. Autoradiograms of SDS-PAGE and thin-layer chromatogram (TLC) of phosphorylated GCP components. The different lanes show time courses of phosphorylation: from 0–40 s, in the presence or absence of 0.3 mM CaCl₂, for the samples analyzed by SDS-PAGE; and from 0–300 s, in the presence of 0.3 mM CaCl₂, for the chloroform–methanol extracts analyzed by TLC. Molecular mass markers are indicated in kDa. Note the material that is phosphorylated in time- and calcium-dependent manner and runs near the dye front in SDS-PAGE. Phosphoinositides (PI, PIP, PIP₂) radiolabeled by GCPs co-migrate with this material.

phosphoprotein patterns are obvious when auto-radiograms of two-dimensional gels are compared (Fig. 2). However, in samples with similar protein content, there are major differences in the quantities of ³²P incorporated into specific substrates. As already mentioned, synapsin I is clearly present in GCPs, but it is a minor species so that long exposures are required to make it visible. In contrast, pp40, pp46 and pp80 are very prominent phosphoproteins in GCPs; they are present in synaptosomes, but the incorporation of radioactivity on a protein basis is reduced 7 to 20 fold, and they are minor species compared to synapsin I and its kinase.

Of particular interest is pp46, which is a major membrane protein of GCPs. Studies in this laboratory have demonstrated that pp46 is synthesized at a rapid rate and transported into the growing axon by developing retinal ganglion cells, but its synthesis and its presence in synaptic terminals in the adult are greatly reduced (Simkowitz et al., submitted). Therefore, pp46 is a growth-regulated or growth-associated protein. Indeed, collaborative studies with the Willard laboratory have shown that, in terms of its electrophoretic mobility in two dimensions, phosphorylation, V8 protease phosphopeptide fragments, and immunochemical properties, pp46 is identical to the growth-associated protein GAP43 discovered by Willard and his colleagues (Table II; Skene and Willard, 1981; Willard et al., 1985; Meiri et al., 1986).

Of further interest is the comparison of pp46 with hippocampal phosphoproteins. As reviewed elsewhere in this volume, the adult hippocampus contains the phosphoproteins F1 and B-50 (probably identical), which have electrophoretic mobilities similar to that of pp46 (e.g., Zwiers et al., 1980; Nelson and Routtenberg, 1985). Long-term potentiation (LTP) enhances the in vitro phosphorylation of protein F1 in a crude

TABLE II

Comparison of growth cone pp46, GAP 43 and F1

	pp46	GAP 43	F1
M_r: 43–47 kDa	+	+	+
pI: 4.3–4.5	+	+	+
Kinase specificity: CaCM	+	+	+
CaPL, TPA	+[a]	+	+
V8 protease phosphopeptide: 23, 13, 11 kDa	+	+	+
Immunochemical relationship	+	+	nd

[a]Requires high Triton X-100 concentration for CaPL stimulation.
Abbreviations: CM, calmodulin; PL, phospholipid; *TPA*, 12-O-tetradecanoylphorbol-13-acetate, nd, not done.
(From Meiri et al., 1986; Nelson et al., 1985, submitted; cf. Willard et al., 1985; Nelson and Routtenberg, 1985; Simkowitz et al., submitted.)

synaptosome fraction, P_2', from adult hippocampus (Routtenberg et al., 1985). A collaborative effort between the Routtenberg and Pfenninger laboratories has recently demonstrated that F1 and pp46 co-electrophorese in two dimensions, share V8 protease phosphopeptides, and exhibit the same kinase specificity, i.e., can be phosphorylated by both calcium/calmodulin-dependent and C kinases (Table II; Nelson et al., 1985, submitted). It is probable, therefore, that pp46 is identical to F1 (and, probably, B-50).

Conclusions

Our findings indicate that growth cones contain protein kinase activities that resemble those of synaptosomes qualitatively. However, major quantitative differences exist. Particularly striking is the simple pattern of major substrates of calcium-dependent kinases. Three of these substrates, pp40, pp46 and pp80 and/or their phosphorylation are developmentally regulated. Thus they are candidates for molecules involved in growth regulation. This is consistent with a number of observations made by other laboratories suggesting that calcium plays an important role in neurite growth: at least in some types of neurons, the predominant ion channel in the growing axon appears to be that for calcium (Llinas and Sugimori, 1979; Spitzer, 1979; Strichartz et al., 1980; Grinvald and Farber, 1981; Meiri et al., 1981; MacVicar and Llinas, 1985; O'Lague et al., 1985); in the presence of the calcium ionophore A23187, the application of calcium ion mimics the chemotactic effect of NGF on growth cones in culture (Gundersen and Barrett, 1980); furthermore, potassium depolarization leads to calcium-dependent spreading of nerve growth cones (Anglister et al., 1982).

The prominent role of protein kinase C in the phosphorylation of growth cone proteins is of further significance. Protein kinase C has been implicated in a number of growth-regulatory processes as well as leukocyte chemotaxis (Laskin et al., 1981; Snyderman and Goetzl, 1981; Volpi et al., 1983; Dougherty et al., 1984; Berridge and Irvine, 1984; Hsu et al., 1984; Nishizuka, 1984). These functions can be expected to have

242

equivalents in the nerve growth cone because the primary growth factor effects appear to occur at this site, at least in the case of nerve growth factor-sensitive peripheral neurons (Campenot, 1977; Gundersen and Barrett, 1980; Pfenninger and Johnson, 1981). As already mentioned, the activation of protein kinase C appears to be a receptor-mediated phenomenon involving PIP_2 cleavage, the generation of diacylglycerol and the IP_3-triggered release of calcium from an intracellular store. In many of the systems described, the agent activating this enzyme cascade is a peptide hormone. We are currently searching for a factor that activates breakdown of PIP_2 and stimulates protein kinase C in GCPs. Such a factor is likely to be a growth-promoting activity in the CNS.

The comparisons of protein kinase activities in GCPs with those in other systems have led to new insights in a second area of interest: a phosphoprotein associated with LTP in the hippocampus is likely to be identical to a growth-associated membrane protein of the growth cone. A second phosphoprotein characteristic of growth cones, pp80 (acidic) may also be associated with LTP (see Fig. 2 in Nelson and Routtenberg, 1985). LTP may involve the modification of ion channels as described in other paradigms of learning (e.g., Kandel and Schwartz, 1982). However, pp46 is so abundant in growth cone membranes that it is not likely to be an ion channel. On the other hand, long-term modifications of the electrical properties of a neuronal circuit may involve morphological alterations of connectivity. Indeed, morphometric analysis suggest that such changes occur during LTP (Van Harreveld and Fifkova, 1975; Desmond and Levy, 1983; Lee et al., 1980). Interestingly, inhibition of protein synthesis seems to block LTP (Stanton and Sarvey, 1984). Therefore, the discovery that a growth-associated protein may be involved in LTP is particularly exciting and may indicate the persistence of developmental mechanisms in the adult nervous system under physiological conditions. In broader terms, if LTP is indeed a valid paradigm of long-term memory, memory mechanisms may, at least in part, involve limited axonal sprouting and synaptogenesis (Pfenninger, submitted). Thus, research on nerve growth cones may open new avenues towards a molecular understanding of mechanisms of neural plasticity and memory in the adult.

Acknowledgements

This research was supported by NIH Grant NS 21729, NSF Grant BNS 83-10248 and matching funds from the Stifel Paralysis Research Foundation and the Matheson Foundation. Carolyn Hyman and Robert S. Garofalo are fellowship awardees of the Muscular Dystrophy Association of America and the Pharmaceutical Manufacturers Association Foundation, Inc.

References

Anglister, L., Farber, I.C., Shahar, A. and Grinvald, A. (1982) Localization of voltage-sensitive calcium channels along developing neurites: their possible role in regulating neurite elongation. Dev. Biol., 94:351–365.

Berridge, M.J. and Irvine, R.F. (1984) Nature, 312:315–321.

Bunge, M.B. (1973) Fine structure of nerve fibers and growth cones of isolated sympathetic neurons in culture. J. Cell Biol., 56:713–735.

Burke, B.E. and DeLorenzo, R.S. (1981) Ca^{2+}- and calmodulin-stimulated endogenous phosphorylation of neurotubulin. Proc. Natl. Acad. Sci. U.S.A., 78:991–995.

Campenot, R.B. (1977) Local control of neurite development by nerve growth factor. Proc. Natl. Acad. Sci U.S.A., 74:4516–4519.

Desmond N.L. and Levy, W.B. (1983) Synaptic correlates of associative potentiation/depression: an ultrastructural study in the hippocampus. Brain Res., 265:21–30.

Dougherty, R.W., Godfrey, P.P., Hoyle, P.C., Putney, J.W. and Freer, R.J. (1984) Secretagogue-induced phosphoinositide metabolism in human leukocytes. Biochem. J., 222:307–314.

Ellis,L., Katz, F. and Pfenninger, K.H. (1985a) Nerve growth cones isolated from fetal rat brain. II. Cyclic adenosine 3':5'-monophosphate (cAMP)-binding proteins and cAMP-dependent protein phosphorylation. J. Neurosci., 5:1393–1401.

Ellis, L., Wallis, I., Abreu, E. and Pfenninger, K.H. (1985b) Nerve growth cones isolated from fetal rat brain. IV. Preparation of a membrane subfraction and identification of a membrane glycoprotein expressed on sprouting neurons. J. Cell Biol., 101:1977–1989.

Gordon-Weeks, P.R. and Lockerbie, R.O. (1984) Isolation and partial characterisation of neuronal growth cones from neonatal rat forebrain. Neuroscience, 13:119–136.

Grinvald, A. and Farber, I. (1981) Optical recording of Ca^{++} action potentials from growth cones of cultured neurons using a laser microbeam. Science, 212:1164–1169.

Gundersen, R.W. and Barrett, R.A. (1980) Characterization

of the turning response of dorsal root neurites toward nerve growth factor. *J. Cell. Biol.*, 87:546–554.

Hsu, L., Natyzak, D. and Laskin, J.D. (1984) Effects of the tumor promoter 12-*O*-tetradecanoylphorbol-13-acetate on neurite outgrowth from chick embryo sensory ganglia. *Cancer Res.*, 44:4607–4614.

Hyman, C. and Pfenninger, K.H. (1985) Intracellular regulators of neuronal sprouting: Calmodulin binding proteins of nerve growth cones. *J. Cell. Biol.*, 101:1153–1160.

Hyman, C., Garofalo, R.S. and Pfenninger, K.H. (1984) Protein and lipid phosphorylation in nerve growth cones. *J. Cell Biol.*, 101:395a.

Joseph, S.K., Thomas, A.P., Williams, R.J., Irvine, R.F. and Williamson, J.R. (1984) *myo*-Inositol 1,4,5-trisphosphate, a second messenger for the hormonal mobilization of intracellular Ca^{2+} in liver. *J. Biol. Chem.* 259:3077–3081.

Kandel, E.R., and Schwartz, J.H. (1982) Molecular biology of learning: Modulation of transmitter release. *Science*, 218:433–443.

Katz, F., Ellis, L. and Pfenninger, K.H. (1985) Nerve growth cones isolated from fetal rat brain. III. Calcium-dependent protein phosphorylation. *J. Neurosci.*, 5:1402–1411.

Kennedy, M.B. and Greengard, P. (1981) Two calcium/calmodulin-dependent protein kinases, which are highly concentrated in brain, phosphorylate protein I at distinct sites. *Proc. Natl. Acad. Sci. U.S.A.*, 78:1293–1297.

Kennedy, M.B., McGuiness, I. and Greengard, P. (1983) A calcium/calmodulin-dependent protein kinase from mammalian brain that phosphorylates synapsin. I. Partial purification and characterization. *J. Neurosci.*, 3:818–831.

Laskin, D.L., Laskin, J.D., Weinstein, I.B. and Carchman, R.A. (1981) Induction of chemotaxis in mouse peritoneal macrophages by phorbol ester tumor promotors. *Cancer Res.*, 41:1923–1928.

Lee, K.S., Schottler, F., Oliver, M. and Lynch, G. (1980) Brief bursts of high-frequency stimulation produce two types of structural change in rat hippocampus. *J. Neurophysiol.*, 44:247–258.

Llinas, R. and Sugimori, M. (1979) Calcium conductances in Purkinje cell dendrites: their role in development and integration. In M. Cuenod, G.W. Kreutzberg and F.E. Bloom (Eds.), *Development and Chemical Specificity of Neurons, Progress in Brain Research, Vol. 51*. Elsevier/North Holland Biomedical Press, Amsterdam, pp. 323–334.

Lohmann, S.M., Ueda, T. and Greengard, P. (1978) Ontogeny of synaptic phosphoproteins in brain. *Proc. Natl. Acad. Sci. U.S.A.*, 75:4037–4041.

Lohmann, S.M., Walter, U. and Greengard, P. (1980) Identification of endogenous substrate proteins for cAMP-dependent protein kinase in bovine brain. *J. Biol. Chem.*, 255:9985–9992.

MacVicar, B.A. and Llinas, R.R. (1985) Barium action potentials in regenerating axons of the lamprey spinal cord. *J. Neurosci. Res.*, 13:323–335.

Meiri, H., Parnas, I. and Spira, M. (1981) Membrane conductance and action potential of a regenerating axonal tip. *Science*, 211:709–711.

Meiri, K.F., Pfenninger, K.H. and Willard, M.B. (1986) Growth-associated protein, GAP-43, a polypeptide that is induced when neurons extend axons, is a component of growth cones and corresponds to pp46, a major polypeptide of a subcellular fraction enriched in growth cones. *Proc. Natl. Acad. Sci. U.S.A.*, 83:3537–3541.

Murphy, K.M.M., Gould, R.J., Oster-Granite, M.L., Gearhart, J.D. and Snyder, S.H. (1983) Phorbol ester receptors: autoradiographic identification in the developing rat. *Science*, 222:1036–1038.

Nelson, R.B. and Routtenberg, A. (1985) Characterization of protein F1 (47 kDa, 4.5 p*I*): a kinase C substrate directly related to neural plasticity. *Exp. Neurol.*, 89:213–224.

Nelson, R.B., Routtenberg, A., Hyman, C. and Pfenninger, K.H. (1985) A phosphoprotein (F1) directly related to neural plasticity in adult rat brain may be identical to a major growth cone membrane protein (pp46). *Soc. Neurosci. Abstr.*, 11, 927.

Nestler, E.J. and Greengard, P. (1983) Protein phosphorylation in the brain. *Nature*, 305:583–588.

Nishizuka, Y. (1984) The role of protein kinase C in cell-surface signal transduction and tumour promotion. *Nature*, 308:693–698.

O'Lague, P.H., Huttner, S.L., Vandenberg, C.A., Morrison-Graham, K. and Horn, R. (1985) Morphological properties and membrane channels of the growth cones induced in PC12 cells by nerve growth factor. *J. Neurosci. Res.*, 13:301–321.

Pfenninger, K.H. and Johnson, M.P. (1981) Neve growth factor stimulates phospholipid methylation in growing neurites. *Proc. Natl. Acad. Sci. U.S.A.*, 78:7797–7800.

Pfenninger, K.H., Ellis, L., Johnson, M.P., Friedman, L.B. and Somlo, S. (1983) Nerve growth cones isolated from fetal rat brain. I. Subcellular fractionation and characterization. *Cell.* 35:573–584.

Rangel-Aldao, R., Kupiec, J.W. and Rosen, O.M. (1979) Resolution of phosphorylated and dephosphorylated cAMP-binding proteins of cardiac muscle by affinity labeling and two-dimensional electrophoresis. *J. Biol. Chem.*, 254:2499–2508.

Routtenberg, A., Lovinger, D. and Steward, O. (1985) Selective increase in the phosphorylation of a 47-kDa protein (F1) directly related to long-term potentiation. *Behav. Neural Biol.*, 43:3–11.

Simkowitz, P. and Pfenninger, K.H. (1983) Rapidly transported proteins of nerve growth cones and synaptic endings are markedly different. *Neurosci. Abst.*, 98:1422–1433.

Skene, J.H.P. and Willard, M. (1981) Axonally transported proteins associated with axon growth in rabbit central and peripheral nervous systems. *J. Cell Biol.*, 89:96–103.

Snyderman, R. and Goetzl, E.J. (1981) Molecular and cellular mechanisms of leukocyte chemotaxis. *Science*, 213:830–837.

Spitzer, N.C. (1979) Ion channels in development. *Annu. Rev. Neurosci.*, 2:363–397.

Stanton, P.K. and Sarvey, J.M. (1984) Blockade of long-term potentiation in rat hippocampal CA1 region by inhibitors of protein synthesis. *J. Neurosci.*, 4:3080–3088.

Strichartz, G., Small, R., Nicholson, C., Pfenninger, K.H. and

244

Llinas, R.R. (1980) Ionic mechanism for impulse propagation in growing non-myelinated axon: saxitoxin binding and electrophysiology. *Soc. Neurosci. Abstr.*, 6:660.

Tennyson, V.M. (1970) The fine structure of the axon and growth cone of the dorsal root neuroblast of the rabbit embryo. *J. Cell Biol.*, 44:62–79.

Van Harreveld, A. and Fifkova, E. (1975) Swelling of dendritic spines in the fascia dentata after stimulation of the perforant path fibers as a mechanism of post-tetanic potentiation. *Exp. Neurol.*, 49:736–739.

Volpi, M., Yassin, R., Naccache, P.H. and Shaafi, R.I. (1983) Chemotactic factor causes rapid decreases in phosphatidylinositol 4,5-bisphosphate and phosphatidylinositol 4-monophosphate in rabbit neutrophils. *Biochem. Biophys. Res. Commun.*, 112:957–964.

Wallis, I., Ellis, L., Suh, K. and Pfenninger, K.H. (1985) Immunolocalization of a neuronal growth-dependent membrane glycoprotein. *J. Cell Biol.*, 101:1990–1998.

Willard, M.B., Meiri, K. and Glicksman, M. (1985) Changes of state during neuronal development: regulation of axon elongation. In G.M. Edelman, W.E. Gall and W.M. Cowan, eds.), *Molecular Bases of Neural Development*, Neurosciences Research Foundation, New York, pp. 341–361.

Wu, W.C.-S., Walaas, S.I., Nairn, A.O. and Greengard, P. (1982) Calcium/phospholipid regulates phosphorylation of a M_r '87K' substrate protein in brain synaptosomes. *Proc. Natl. Acad. Sci. U.S.A.*, 79:5259–5253.

Yamada, K.M., Spooner, B.S. and Wessels, N.K. (1971) Ultrastructure and function of growth cones and axons of cultured nerve cells. *J. Cell Biol.*, 49:614–635.

Zwiers, H., Schotman, P. and Gispen, W.H. (1980) Purification and some characteristics of an ACTH-sensitive protein kinase and its substrate protein in rat brain membranes. *J. Neurosci.*, 34:1689–1699.

W.H. Gispen and A. Routtenberg (Eds.)
Progress in Brain Research, Vol. 69
© 1986 Elsevier Science Publishers B.V. (Biomedical Division)

CHAPTER 20

Long-term potentiation and 4-aminopyridine-induced changes in protein and lipid phosphorylation in the hippocampal slice

Loes H. Schrama[1], Pierre N.E. De Graan[1], Wytse J. Wadman[2], Fernando H. Lopes da Silva and W.H. Gispen[1]

[1]*Division of Molecular Neurobiology, Rudolf Magnus Institute for Pharmacology and Institute of Molecular Biology, University of Utrecht, Padualaan 8 3584 CH Utrecht and* [2]*Department of Animal Physiology, University of Amsterdam, Kruislaan 320, 1098 SM Amsterdam, The Netherlands*

Introduction

Many parts of the nervous system show the phenomenon of synaptic plasticity. Synaptic plasticity is the ability of the nervous system to adapt its response to previous experiences. One of the most intensively studied models for synaptic plasticity is long-term potentiation (LTP). LTP can be evoked in many parts of the brain by the application of a brief series of high-frequency electrical stimuli (a tetanus) (Bliss, 1979; Eccles, 1983; Lynch and Baudry, 1984). Tetanization of, for instance, the perforant path fibers in the rat hippocampus results in a marked, long-lasting increase in the response of the monosynaptic perforant path–granule cell subsystem to a test stimulus (Tielen et al., 1982). LTP, which can be evoked in vivo as well as in vitro, has been implicated as a physiological substrate for memory and learning (Bliss, 1979; Bliss and Dolphin, 1982; Eccles, 1983; Lynch and Baudry, 1984) and is thought to be a monosynaptic phenomenon. In vivo repetitive tetanization of certain brain areas over a period of several days (kindling) leads to much more generalized electrophysiological responses and epileptiform activity and eventually to generalized convulsions

(Goddard et al., 1969). In vitro such generalized epileptiform activity may be induced by convulsants like 4-aminopyridine (Llinás et al., 1976; Gustafsson et al., 1982; Buckle and Haas, 1982; Hermann and Gorman, 1981; Galvan et al., 1982).

The molecular mechanisms underlying these forms of synaptic plasticity are still largely unknown. Several lines of evidence point to a crucial role of calcium in LTP (Baimbridge and Miller, 1981; Kuhnt et al., 1985; Dolphin, 1985) and in epileptogenesis (Griffiths et al., 1982). The increased calcium influx during LTP is thought to result postsynaptically in the activation of Ca^{2+}-dependent proteases, thereby unmasking postsynaptic glutamate receptors (Lynch and Baudry, 1984). As a presynaptic component of LTP, the increased calcium flux is thought to enhance presynaptic transmitter release (Dolphin et al., 1982). Application of the potassium conductance blocker 4-aminopyridine (4-AP) also increases the intracellular calcium concentration (Agoston et al., 1983; Griffiths et al., 1982), thereby enhancing synaptic transmission (Llinás et al., 1976; Gustafsson et al., 1982; Buckle and Haas, 1982; Hermann and Gorman, 1981; Galvan et al., 1982).

The intracellular Ca^{2+} concentration may regulate the state of phosphorylation of especially membrane- and vesicle-bound proteins. From many observations the general concept has been developed that cyclic phosphorylation and dephosphorylation of proteins may regulate ion permeability of the membrane and synaptic transmission (c.f. Nestler and Greengard, 1984). Although the exact relationship between neurotransmission and protein phosphorylation still has to be clarified, it is clear that the increase in intracellular calcium concentration plays a crucial role in both processes (Miller, 1985).

In both synaptic plasticity models (LTP and 4-AP) we have been studying changes in protein phosphorylation. These two synaptic plasticity models in the in vitro hippocampal slice have been chosen because of their well-defined electrophysiological responses. This permits correlative studies between the degree of changes in electrophysiological parameters and protein phosphorylation. After establishing such correlated effects on phosphorylation of proteins, the affected phosphoproteins and their kinases have to be identified in order to verify the causal relationship between the observed changes in protein phosphorylation and the changes in synaptic plasticity.

LTP and protein phosphorylation

In our first series of studies we found highly reproducible changes in the phosphorylation of a 52-kDa protein and less reproducible but significant changes in B-50 phosphorylation (Bär et al., 1980, Lopes da Silva et al., 1982a, 1982b), when a short tetanus (15 pulses/s, 15 s) was applied to the perforant path–granule cell subsystem of the hippocampus. The degree of LTP was calculated from the changes in the excitatory postsynaptic potential (EPSP) or the population spike (PoPSP). The effects on the degree of phosphorylation of the two protein bands were not observed when the frequency of stimulation was reduced and the duration of the tetanus was increased, conditions not leading to LTP (Bär et al., 1980). Omission of extracellular calcium from the bathing medium, a condition which inhibits LTP and neurotransmission (Dunwiddie and

Lynch, 1979) also failed to produce changes in either 52-kDa protein or B-50 phosphorylation, indicating a relationship between the observed changes in protein phosphorylation and synaptic transmission. Most of our initial studies were devoted to the 52-kDa protein, since this protein showed most consistent changes in protein phosphorylation after tetanization. More recently, however, we have studied B-50 phosphorylation in relation to LTP in more detail.

LTP and B-50 phosphorylation

The initial experiments on the effects of tetanization on B-50 phosphorylation showed a 19% stimulation ($2p < 0.1$), but the results were rather variable (Bär et al., 1980). Recent data from Routtenberg's group point to an important role for protein F1 in LTP induced in the hippocampus in vivo (Routtenberg and Lovinger, 1985; Lovinger et al., 1985; see also Chapter 18). Since B-50 and protein F1 appear to be identical (see Addendum), these results prompted us to reinvestigate the effects of tetanization on B-50 phosphorylation. Therefore after application of two tetani of 50 pulses/s for 2 s, given 5 min apart, a time-course of B-50 phosphorylation and LTP was made. The tetanized slices were processed to give a crude synaptosomal plasma membrane fraction at 10, 20, 35 and 65 min after application of the first tetanus. The correlation between the percentage stimulation of B-50 phosphorylation and the degree of potentiation of each individual slice was calculated at each time-point. The correlation between the degree of potentiation of an individual slice and the degree of B-50 phosphorylation only reached significance 10 min after application of the first tetanus (Fig. 1).

B-50 is a nervous tissue-specific protein (Kristjansson et al., 1982), first isolated by Zwiers et al. (1980) in our laboratory and predominantly found in the presynaptic terminals (Gispen et al., 1985a). The phosphorylation state of B-50 has been implicated to modulate the activity of phosphatidylinositol 4-phosphate (PIP) kinase. Many studies have shown an inverse relationship between the degree of B-50

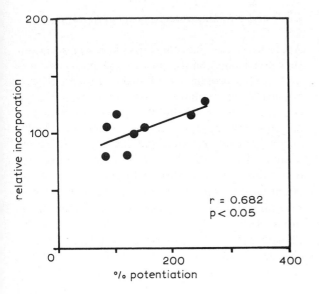

Fig. 1. Correlation between the phosphorylation of B-50 and the degree of potentiation of a hippocampal slice. Hippocampal slices were stimulated twice in the perforant path (100 pulses/s, 2 s) with a time-interval of 5 min. Recordings were made from the granular cell layer of the fascia dentata (cf. Bär et al., 1980; Tielen et al., 1982). 10 min after application of the first tetanus, the slices were individually processed and the crude synaptosomal plasma membrane fraction was phosphorylated with $[\gamma\text{-}^{32}P]ATP$ (cf. Bär et al., 1980; Tielen et al., 1982). The incorporation of phosphate into B-50 was measured by scanning of the autoradiogram after SDS-PAGE, expressed as % stimulation over B-50 phosphorylation in control slices (set to 100%). A significant linear relationship between the degree of phosphorylation of B-50 and the change in amplitude of the PSP was found with a correlation coefficient of 0.682 ($p < 0.05$).

phosphorylation and the amount of phosphatidylinositol 4,5-bisphosphate (PIP_2) formed (Gispen et al., 1985b; Chapter 4). Moreover, it was shown that in a semi-purified system phospho-B-50 inhibited PIP-kinase activity, whereas dephospho-B-50 did not (Van Dongen et al., 1985). This implies that phosphorylation of B-50 protein reduces the amount of substrate available for receptor-mediated degradation of PIP_2 (Gispen et al., 1985b; see also Chapter 4). If B-50 protein is indeed involved in the modulation of polyphosphoinositide (PPI) metabolism in hippocampal tissue, it is not surprising that Bär et al. (1984) reported changes in the turnover of these phospholipids in response to tetanic stimulation of hippocampal slices.

LTP and polyphosphoinositide metabolism

Hokin and Hokin (1954) were the first to demonstrate that cholinergic receptor activation in the pancreas led to stimulation of amylase secretion and an enhanced labeling of phospholipids. The turnover of two minor phospholipids, phosphatidylinositol (PI) and phosphatidic acid (PA), appeared to be responsible for this 'phospholipid labeling effect' (Hokin and Hokin, 1959). Michell (1975, 1979) has initiated a renewed interest in PPI metabolism, by proposing a PI response in relation to the mobilization of the second messenger Ca^{2+} after receptor activation. The current view on the role of PPI metabolism in relation to receptor-mediated elevation of the intracellular calcium concentration is that PIP_2 is degraded by phospholipase C to yield two products, inositol trisphosphate (IP_3) and diacylglycerol (DG). IP_3 serves as a signal to mobilize Ca^{2+} from intracellular stores (Berridge and Irvine, 1984). DG stimulates the Ca^{2+}/phospholipid-dependent protein kinase C (Nishizuka, 1984a, 1984b), which phosphorylates B-50 (Aloyo et al., 1982, 1983).

In a recent study we examined the effects of tetanic stimulation of the perforant pathway in rat hippocampal slices on the metabolism of PPIs and PA (Bär et al., 1984). The changes in PPI metabolism in relation to LTP were studied employing two different methods, both of which involved labeling of the slice with inorganic phosphate. Firstly, slices were prelabelled for 10 min, after they were subjected to high-frequency stimulation and immediately processed. Secondly, the slices were first tetanized, after which the label was added 2 min to 4 h after tetanization for a total time period of 10 min. After 10 min incubation almost all label was recovered in PIP_2, PIP, PI and PA, whereas the other phospholipids had only incorporated 4% of the total radioactivity in the phospholipid fraction. The results obtained with both methods were essentially similar and only the results obtained with the second method are discussed. Control incubations involved the application of a low-frequency stimulus (1 pulse/4s for 15 min), a stimulation frequency inducing neither LTP nor significant changes in any of the phospholipids studied (open symbols,

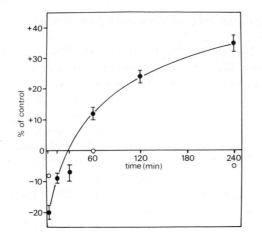

Fig. 2. Labeling of PIP$_2$ after tetanization of the hippocampal slice. Hippocampal slices were subjected to a high-frequency stimulation of 15 pulses/s for 15 s (HI-STIM) or a low-frequency stimulation of 1 pulse/4 s for 15 min (LOW-STIM) in the perforant path. At various time-points after stimulation, the slices were incubated with labeled inorganic phosphate for 10 min, after which the slices were processed, and phospholipids separated by thin-layer chromatography (Bär et al., 1984). The incorporation of phosphate into PIP$_2$ was determined by liquid scintillation counting and expressed as % of control incorporation into non-stimulated slices. Open symbols represent LOW-STIM, closed symbols represent HI-STIM.

Fig. 2). The time-course for the formation of PIP$_2$ is shown in Fig. 2. At short intervals after tetanization a decrease of 20% was observed, whereas after longer time intervals there was a time-dependent increase in labeling of PIP$_2$ (Bär et al., 1984). The results obtained for PA labeling were the same as for PIP$_2$ both with respect to magnitude and time-dependency of the effect (data not shown, see Bär et al., 1984).

These results indicate that at the onset of LTP there is a decrease in the amount of label incorporated into PIP$_2$, suggesting a decreased PIP$_2$-kinase activity, concomitant with an increased B-50 labeling (see page 246). These data are in line with the hypothesis that the degree of B-50 phosphorylation plays a regulatory role in PPI metabolism. They probably reflect an increase in active, membrane-bound protein kinase C (Nishizuka, 1984a, 1984b), resulting in an increase in the degree of B-50 phosphorylation and a concomitant inhibition of PIP-kinase activity leading to a decrease of label into PIP$_2$.

LTP and 52 kDa-protein phosphorylation

Apart from the changes in B-50 phosphorylation, very consistent changes in the phosphorylation of a 52-kDa protein band were observed after application of a tetanus to the perforant path (Bär et al., 1980). To establish a possible correlation between the changes in the degree of 52-kDa protein phosphorylation and the degree of potentiation, Tielen et al. (1983) have studied the quantitative relationship between the degree of potentiation and the degree of 52-kDa protein phosphorylation in synaptosomal plasma membranes (SPM). The percentual change in 52-KDa phosphorylation was therefore correlated with the change in amplitude of the EPSP per individual slice. A semi-logarithmic plot of these data fits a straight line with a correlation coefficient of 0.71 ($p < 0.005$) (Tielen et al., 1983). These results suggest that there may be a quantitative correlation between electrophysiological synaptic changes and synaptic membrane protein phosphorylation for at least two phosphoprpteins, e.g. B-50 and a 52-kDa phosphoprotein.

The next step in our studies on the relation between the phosphorylation of membrane-bound phosphoproteins and synaptic plasticity was the identification of the 52-kDa phosphoprotein. The in vitro phosphorylation of the 52-kDa protein was not dependent on calcium/calmodulin nor on cyclic nucleotides (Bär et al., 1982; De Graan, unpublished observations). Both the relative molecular weight and the phosphorylation characteristics of the 52-kDa protein resemble those of a phosphoprotein called pp50, which has been characterized in coated vesicles (Pauloin et al., 1982; Pauloin and Jollès, 1984; Pauloin et al., 1984; Kadota et al., 1982; Campell et al., 1984). We have carried out a series of experiments to compare the 52-kDa phosphoprotein in SPM and pp50 in coated vesicles isolated from rat brain according to the method of Pearse and Robinson (1984; Schrama et al., 1986). In order to compare the two phosphoproteins accurately, both phosphoproteins were purified by separation from other proteins using sodium dodecylsulfate polyacrylamide gel electrophoresis (SDS-PAGE). The proteins were cut from the gel after identification by autoradiography and subsequently eluted electro-phoretically.

The tentative identification of the 52-kDa phosphoprotein as pp50 from coated vesicles involved several biochemical techniques, such as molecular weight determination by SDS-PAGE, determination of isoelectric point (IEP), phos-phoamino acid analysis and peptide mapping. The results obtained with this study are summarized in Table I and show that the 52-kDa phosphoprotein and pp50 are identical on basis of the following criteria:

(a) relative molecular weight on 11% SDS-PAGE;
(b) insensitivity of phosphorylation to cyclic AMP, calcium and calmodulin;
(c) the phosphate accepting amino acids, serine and threonine in both phosphoproteins;
(d) isoelectrical point range, 9.0–6.5 for both proteins;
(e) peptide mapping, both the products formed and the time-course for digestion by two different proteases were identical for both phosphoproteins.

With respect to phospho-amino acid analysis and isoelectric focussing our results agree very well with those presented by Campbell et al. (1984). We believe that the 52-kDa phosphoprotein present in

SPM and the pp50 protein from coated vesicles are similar if not identical.

Coated vesicles are a special class of intra-cellular organelles which have been recognized in several tissues including the nervous system. They have been implicated in a number of intracellular processes such as receptor-mediated endocytosis (Goldstein et al., 1979, 1982, Steinman et al., 1983), secretory pathways (Palade, 1975; Rothman and Fine, 1980, Rothman et al., 1980), intracellular protein traffic (Rothman et al., 1980) and presy-naptic membrane recycling after neurotransmitter release (Heuser and Reese, 1973; Fried and Blau-stein, 1976, 1978; Kadota and Kadota, 1982, Miller and Heuser, 1984, see also Chapter 21). The exact role of pp50 phosphorylation in the function of coated vesicles, both with respect to the coating/decoating process and to the coated vesicle transport mechanism are still unclear. Pre-liminary data from Pauloin and Jollès (Chapter 21) suggest that the introduction of negatively charged phosphate groups into pp50 could des-tabilize the interaction between certain coat proteins and the vesicle (see Fig. 7). This notion is substantiated by the fact that the activation of the pp50 kinase by clathrin light chains promotes the phosphorylation of pp50 (Pauloin and Jollès, 1984) and allows the dissociation of clathrin from the vesicles (Schmid et al., 1984).

4-Aminopyridine and protein phosphorylation

In the LTP model for synaptic plasticity we have found consistent changes in the phosphorylation of the 52-kDa protein and B-50 correlated with altered synaptic plasticity. Apart from the LTP model, we also employed another model to study the role of protein phosphorylation in synaptic plasticity. In this model, we used the convulsant drug 4-aminopyridine (4-AP) in the hippocampal slice system. This convulsant probably blocks transient potassium channels associated with an influx of calcium (Griffiths et al., 1982; Thesleff, 1980; Nicholson et al., 1976; Pant et al., 1983; Agoston et al., 1983). The result of application of 4-AP to nervous tissue is an enhancement of synaptic transmission, probably as a result of the influx of calcium (Buckle and Haas, 1982; Gustaf-

TABLE 1

Comparison between the 52-kDa phosphoprotein in SPM and pp50 in coated vesicles

	52 kDa	pp50
Relative molecular weight on 11% SDS–PAGE	52 kDa	52 kDa
Sensitivity of phospho-rylation to:		
cAMP	0[a]	0
calcium	0	0
calmodulin	0	0
Phosphate acceptor amino acids	serine, threonine	serine, threonine
Isoelectric point range	9.0–6.5	9.0–6.5
Peptides formed after mapping with S. aureus protease V8	43,33,20 kDa	43,33,20 kDa

[a] Phosphorylation not sensitive to modulator

sson et al., 1982; Llinás et al., 1976; Hermann and Gorman, 1981; Galvan et al., 1982).

4-AP-induced changes in protein phosphorylation

Incubation of rat hippocampal slices for 30 min with 10^{-5} M 4-AP resulted in changes in the post-hoc phosphorylation of 3 phosphoprotein bands (Fig. 3). The most prominent change after 4-AP incubation is an enhancement of 50-kDa protein phosphorylation. Furthermore, a stimulation was found of the phosphorylation of a 80-kDa protein band and an inhibition of a 48-kDa protein band. The effect of 4-AP on stimulation of 50-kDa protein phosphorylation was strongly dose-dependent (Fig. 4), with a maximal stimulation of 108% at 10^{-4} M 4-AP. The half maximal effective concentration was calculated to be 5×10^{-7} M. The stimulation of 80-kDa protein phosphorylation was only observed at 10^{-5} M (Fig. 4). The dose-dependency of the inhibition of 48-kDa protein phosphorylation was not as pronounced as that observed for the stimulation of 50-kDa protein phosphorylation. The 48-kDa protein was identified as B-50 and the 80-kDa phosphoprotein is most probably synapsin I (Nestler and Greengard, 1984).

Incubation of crude synaptosomal membranes with 4-AP in vitro did not affect the degree of phosphorylation of any of the protein bands studied at a concentration of 10^{-7}–10^{-4} M 4-AP. At 10^{-3} M 4-AP only the 50-kDa protein phosphorylation was inhibited by 40% (data not shown). Since the direct 4-AP effects on membrane phosphorylation in vitro were only found at very high concentrations it is not likely that the changes observed after incubation of the hippocampal slice are the result of a direct effect of the convulsant on protein kinases, protein phosphatases or substrate proteins.

Tentative identification of the 50-kDa phosphoprotein affected by 4-AP

In SPM the phosphorylation of the 50-kDa protein is highly sensitive to calmodulin (Fig. 5; see also Bär et al., 1982). In the presence of 0.5 mM EGTA and 0.6 mM calcium a dose-

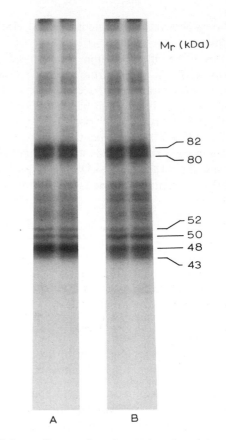

Fig. 3. Autoradiogram of membrane phosphoproteins after 4-AP treatment. Hippocampal slices were incubated for 30 min with 10^{-5} M of the convulsant 4-AP and processed as described in the legend of Fig. 1. The crude synaptosomal membrane fraction was phosphorylated with radioactive ATP in the presence of 7.5 µM ATP, 10 mM Na-acetate, 10 mM Mg-acetate, 0.1 mM Ca-acetate (pH 6.5) for 15 s. Tracks A show the autoradiogram after control incubation, tracks B after 4-AP incubation. The numbers to the right of the figure indicate the relative molecular weight of the most prominent phosphoprotein bands present in the crude membrane fraction, as calculated from the migration of marker proteins run alongside the gel.

dependent stimulation of 50-kDa protein phosphorylation by calmodulin (EC_{50} 2.3 U/25 µl) was found (Fig. 5, closed symbols). Interestingly, a second phosphoprotein doublet (58/60 kDa) was also found to be highly calmodulin sensitive (Fig. 5, open symbols). In fact, the EC_{50} was strikingly similar (3.0 U/25 µl).

The subcellular distribution of the 50- and

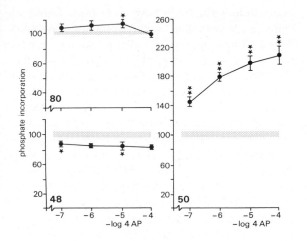

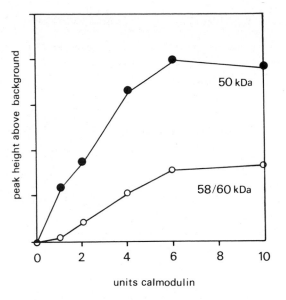

Fig. 4. Dose-dependency of the modulation of protein phosphorylation after 4-AP treatment. After incubation of the hippocampal slices with various concentrations of 4-AP, the incorporation of phosphate into 3 phosphobands was measured by scanning of the autoradiogram. The numbers in the lower left corner refer to the relative molecular weight of the respective phosphobands. The hatched bars indicate the mean $\pm$ S.E.M. of the control incubations, vertical bars indicate the mean $\pm$ S.E.M. of the incorporation in the 4-AP-treated group. The significance between controls and 4-AP treatment was calculated by Student's t-test (*, $2p < 0.05$; **, $2p < 0.01$).

Fig. 5. Concentration-dependency for calmodulin stimulation of 50- and 58/60-kDa phosphoproteins. SPM (10 µg) was freshly prepared and phosphorylated with radioactive ATP in 25 µl, in the presence of various concentrations of calmodulin. 0.6 mM Ca-acetate, 10 mM Na-acetate, 10 mM Mg-acetate and 0.5 mM EGTA (pH 6.5). The incorporation into the 50- and 58/60-kDa phosphoproteins was calculated as described in the legend of Fig. 1.

58/60-kDa phosphoproteins was studied in several subcellular fractions of rat hippocampus using three different in vitro phosphorylation conditions, viz. (1) 0.5 mM EGTA, (2) 0.5 mM EGTA and 0.6 mM Ca^{2+} and (3) 0.5 mM EGTA, 0.6 mM Ca^{2+} and 5 U calmodulin. These 3 phosphorylation conditions allow the identification of calmodulin-sensitive phosphorylation, since they discriminate between calcium- and calcium/calmodulin-sensitive protein phosphorylation, by comparing the relative incorporation of label of the EGTA (1) versus the EGTA–calcium condition (2) and the EGTA–calcium (2) versus the EGTA–calcium–calmodulin condition (3). The result of the post-hoc phosphorylation of the various subcellular fractions is shown in Fig. 6. In the presence of EGTA (1) the 50-kDa phosphoprotein is only present in the mitochondria, whereas residual phosphorylation of the 58/60-kDa protein is observed in the vesicles and light (l)SPM. In the presence of calcium (2), 50-kDa protein

phosphorylation is observed in all fractions except 1-SPM, and 58/60-kDa protein phosphorylation is not found in the mitochondria and to a small extent in 1-SPM. In the presence of both calcium and calmodulin (3) the 50- and 58/60-kDa phosphoproteins are present in all fractions studied. Marked stimulation of 50- and 58/60-kDa protein phosphorylation is only observed in the vesicles, 1-SPM and mitochondria. The fact that calmodulin stimulation of phosphorylation is only observed in these 3 fractions can probably be explained by the fact that these three fractions have all been 'washed' by sucrose density centrifugation and, in the case of the vesicles and l-SPM, by a succeeding centrifugation step to collect the membranes (Kristjansson et al., 1982). These wash steps will remove loosely bound calmodulin from the membranes, resulting in an enhanced calmodulin sensitivity of in vitro phosphorylation of these fractions.

Changes in phosphorylation of proteins after

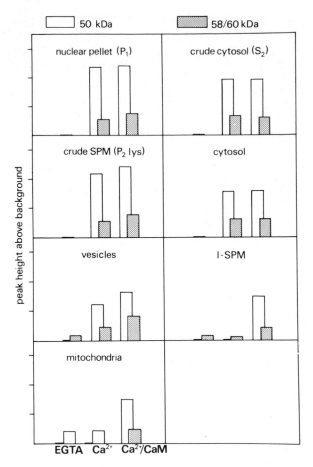

Fig. 6. Subcellular distribution of the 50- and 58/60-kDa phosphoproteins. Endogenous phosphorylation in the subcellular fractions was studied under three different conditions: 0.5 mM EGTA (EGTA), 0.5 mM EGTA and 0.6 mM Ca^{2+} (Ca^{2+}), and 0.5 mM EGTA, 0.6 mM Ca^{2+} and 5U calmodulin (Ca^{2+}/CaM). The various fractions studied were: the first $1000 \times g$ pellet from the homogenate (P_1), the $10\,000 \times g$ supernatant (S_2) and the resulting pellet (P_2), which was lyzed in water before phosphorylation. Furthermore, four fractions of the gradient to prepare SPM as described by Kristjansson et al. (1982), viz. the synaptosomal cytosol (cytosol), the vesicle-enriched 0.4 M sucrose fraction (vesicles), the light synaptosomal plasma membranes (1-SPM) and the mitochondria-enriched pellet (mitochondria). The incorporation of phosphate in the two phosphoprotein bands studied was expressed as peak height above background. Open bars indicate the incorporation into the 50-kDa band, stippled bars indicate the incorporation into the 58/60-kDa band.

incubation with 4-AP have also been found by Pant et al. (1983) in squid optic lobe synaptosomes. They incubated synaptosomes in the presence of 4-AP and $[\gamma\text{-}^{32}P]$ATP in the presence of external calcium. The observed effects of 4-AP were on high-molecular weight proteins, but the major phosphoprotein of 50 kDa was unaffected. Whether the observed changes were on calmodulin-dependent protein kinases has not been investigated.

In the kindling model for epilepsy (see page 245), the major changes in SPM phosphorylation were observed in a 50-kDa protein (Wasterlain and Farber, 1982, 1984; Goldenring et al., 1986). The phosphorylation of this phosphoprotein was also found to be sensitive to calcium and calmodulin. This protein was identified as the α or ρ subunit of calmodulin kinase II (CaM K II) (Goldenring et al., 1986).

Our data strongly suggest that the 50-kDa and 58/60-kDa phosphoproteins are identical to the α/ρ and β/σ subunits of CaM K II and indicate that this kinase is involved in the molecular mechanism underlying epileptogenesis and hence synaptic plasticity. This protein kinase is one of the two known calmodulin-sensitive protein kinases which phosphorylate synapsin I (Kennedy and Greengard, 1981; Nestler and Greengard, 1984). CaM K II has been identified in various animal species, e.g. rat, *Aplysia californica* (Schulman et al., 1985), *Loligo pealii* (Llinás et al., 1985) and in various organs of the rat (Schulman et al., 1985). This protein kinase is a multifunctional kinase, phosphorylating numerous substrates (Yamamoto et al., 1985; Schulman et al., 1985). Most investigators have purified CaM K II from rat brain cytosol (Goldenring et al., 1983; Bennett et al., 1983; Kuret and Schulman, 1985; Fukanaga et al., 1982, Kennedy et al., 1983a). However, the kinase has also been purified from membrane fractions (Kennedy et al., 1983a), postsynaptic densities (Kennedy et al., 1983b), cytoskeletal elements (Sahyoun et al., 1985), synaptic junctions (Rostas et al., 1983; Shields et al., 1984), cold-stable microtubules (Larson et al., 1985) and tubulin (Goldenring et al., 1984). The protein used to monitor the purification of CaM K II and the source used to isolate the kinase seem to determine its substrate specificity (compare Goldenring et al., 1983 to McGuinness et al., 1985 and Bennett et al., 1985). Thus, it seems that the isolated CaM K IIs are very similar in terms of autophosphorylation, relative amounts of subunits, IEP, etc., whereas their substrate specificity varies. The relative composition of the holoenzyme with respect to amounts of 50- and 58/60-kDa subunits present in it also varies over different brain regions (McGuinness et al., 1985).

Both subunits of CaM K II are autophosphorylated by an intramolecular mechanism (Kuret and Schulman, 1985; Shields et al., 1984) and even the separated subunits are capable of autophosphorylation (Kuret and Schulman, 1985). The effects of autophosphorylation of the kinase on its activity are controversial. Shields et al. (1984) have reported that autophosphorylation increases the amount of calmodulin bound to the subunits and that concomitantly the activity towards synapsin I is increased. The activity of the kinase towards α-casein and microtubule-associated protein-2 (MAP-2), however, is reduced by autophosphorylation (Yamauchi and Fujisawa, 1985).

Although our data (see above) and those of others (Wasterlain and Farber, 1982, 1984; Goldenring et al., 1986) suggest an involvement of CaM K II in epileptogenesis, a causal relationship between CaM K II phosphorylation and epileptogenesis has yet to be established.

Concluding remarks

Calcium plays a pivotal role in both synaptic transmission and membrane protein phosphorylation (see Introduction). The purpose of our studies was in the first place to correlate changes in synaptosomal protein phosphorylation on the one hand with changes in synaptic plasticity as measured electrophysiologically on the other hand. After establishing the correlation between the two processes, the next step was to identify the phosphorylation systems involved in synaptic plasticity. The results of our studies are summarized in Table II. We have identified three different classes of protein kinases to be involved in synaptic plasticity: calcium-dependent, phospholipid-sensitive kinases (B-50 kinase), calcium-/calmodulin-dependent protein kinases (50-kDa

TABLE II

Summary of the effects on protein phosphorylation after tetanization (LTP) and during epileptogenesis (4-AP)[a]

	LTP	4-AP
B-50	+	−
52 kDa	+	0
50 kDa	0	+

[a] +, stimulation; 0, no effect; −, inhibition.

protein auto-phosphorylation) and calcium-independent protein kinases (52-kDa protein kinase) employing two different model systems (LTP and 4-AP) in the hippocampus to study synaptic plasticity.

After application of a tetanus to the hippocampal slice two effects in the B-50/PPI system were observed. The phosphorylation of B-50 was stimulated at short intervals after tetanization concomitant with a decrease in the labeling of PIP_2. At longer time-intervals, the incorporation of label into PIP_2 was increased, whereas no concomitant changes could be observed in the degree of phosphorylation of B-50. Routtenberg and coworkers found more long-lasting effects on F1 (B-50) phosphorylation after in vivo tetanization (Lovinger et al., 1985). The phosphorylation of B-50 also seems to be involved in the induction of epileptiform activity in the hippocampal slice with the convulsant 4-AP. Whether PPI metabolism is also changed after 4-AP treatment in the slice is still subject to investigation.

The changes seen in pp50 phosphorylation after tetanization of the perforant path and in CaM K II autophosphorylation after induction of epileptiform activity with 4-AP in the hippocampal slice system are combined in the model presented in Fig. 7. The model is based on the observations presented in this chapter and on the experiments described by Greengard and coworkers (Nestler and Greengard, 1984; Chapter 25; Llinás et al., 1985) and Pauloin (Chapter 21). Llinás et al., (1985) have elegantly shown that

254

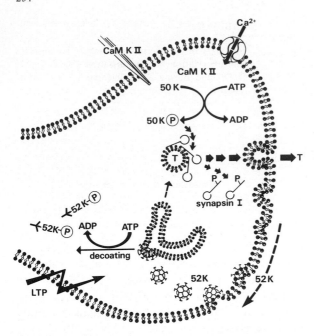

Fig. 7. Schematic representation of phosphorylation processes at the presynaptic terminal during neurotransmission. For explanation of the figure, see text.

intraterminal pressure injection of CaM K II in the squid giant synapse increases the rate of rise and amplitude of the postsynaptic potential (PSP) and decreases the latency of rise of the PSP. The effects were observed 24 min after injection, and the changes in electrophysiology observed resemble those of LTP in the central nervous system. Pressure injection of dephosphosynapsin I resulted in a decrease of the amplitude and rate of rise of the PSP. The authors (Llinás et al., 1985) suggest that after entrance of calcium, the activity of CaM K II is increased leading to the phosphorylation of synapsin I, which is subsequently dissociated from the synaptic vesicle. The removal of this constraint from the synaptic vesicle is thought to facilitate the fusion of the vesicles with the synaptic membrane, thus enhancing synaptic transmission.

Enhanced synaptic transmission will lead to increased fusion of synaptic vesicles to the presynaptic membrane resulting in an increased amount of membrane material, thereby expanding the presynaptic membrane. This excess of

membrane material can be retrieved from the membrane via coated pits and coated vesicles (Heuser and Reese, 1973; Fried and Blaustein, 1976, 1978; Kadota and Kadota, 1982; Miller and Heuser, 1984; Chapter 21). The coated vesicle is thought to fuse with large intracellular cisterna, whereby the coat is removed from the coated vesicle (Heuser and Reese, 1973; Miller and Heuser, 1984). The process of decoating is probably accompanied and maybe initiated by the phosphorylation of pp50, the major phosphoprotein in coated vesicles.

In our LTP model we have observed an increase in the phosphorylation of a 52-kDa protein (pp50) in synaptic plasma membranes in a post-hoc phosphorylation assay. This means that pp50 is not only present in coated vesicles in its phosphorylated state, but also in SPM, probably in the form of coated pits. Whether the phosphorylation of pp50 in coated pits is involved in the formation of these structures remains to be determined.

In conclusion, we believe that in both models we employed to study the role of protein phosphorylation in synaptic plasticity both calcium-dependent and -independent processes may be involved.

Acknowledgements

The authors wish to acknowledge J.H. Brakkee for his skillful biotechnical assistance and E.D. Kluis for his excellent artwork. This research was supported by CLEO-TNO grants A42 and A47 and FUNGO grant 900-548-072 (formerly 13-31-72) of the Dutch Organization for the Advancement of Pure Reseach (ZWO).

References

Agoston, D., Hargattai, P. and Nagy, A. (1983) Effects of 4-aminopyridine in calcium and changes in membrane potential in pinched-off nerve terminals from rat cerebral cortex. *J. Neurochem.*, 41:745–751.

Aloyo, V.J., Zwiers, H. and Gispen, W.H. (1982) B-50 protein kinase and kinase C in rat brain. *Prog. Brain Res.*, 56:303–315.

Aloyo, V.J., Zwiers. H. and Gispen, W.H. (1983) Phosphorylation of B-50 protein by calcium-activated, phospholipid-dependent protein kinase and B-50 protein kinase. *J. Neurochem.*, 41:649–653.

Baimbridge, K.G. and Miller, J.J. (1981) Calcium uptake and retention during long-term potentiation of neuronal activity in the rat hippocampal slice preparation. *Brain Res.*, 221:299–305.

Bär, P.R., Schotman, P., Gispen, W.H., Lopes da Silva, F.H. and Tielen, A.M. (1980) Changes in synaptic membrane phosphorylation after tetanic stimulation in the dentate area of the rat hippocampal slice. *Brain Res.*, 198:478–484.

Bär, P.R., Tielen, A.M., Lopes da Silva, F.H., Zwiers, H. and Gispen, W.H. (1982) Membrane phosphoproteins of rat hippocampus: sensitivity to tetanic stimulation and enkephalin. *Brain Res.*, 245:69–79.

Bär, P.R., Wiegant, F., Lopes da Silva, F.H. and Gispen, W.H. (1984) Tetanic stimulation affects the metabolism of phosphoinositides in hippocampal slices. *Brain Res.*, 321:381–385.

Bennett, M.K., Erondu, N.E. and Kennedy, M.B. (1983) Purification and characterization of a calmodulin-dependent protein kinase that is highly concentrated in brain. *J. Biol. Chem.*, 258:12735–12744.

Berridge, M.J. and Irvine, R.F. (1984) Inositol trisphosphate, a novel second messenger in cellular signal transduction. *Nature*, 312:315–321.

Bliss, T.V.P. (1979) Synaptic plasticity in the hippocampus. *Trends Neurosci.*, 2:42–45.

Bliss, T.V.P. and Dolphin, A.C. (1982) What is the mechanism of long-term potentiation in the hippocampus? *Trends Neurosci.*, 5:289–290.

Buckle, P.J. and Haas, H.L. (1982) Enhancement of synaptic transmission by 4-aminopyridine in hippocampal slices of the rat. *J. Physiol.*, 326:109–122.

Campbell, C., Squicciarini, J., Shia, M., Pilch, P.F. and Fine, R.E. (1984) Identification of a protein kinase as an intrinsic component of rat liver coated vesicles. *Biochemistry*, 23:4420–4426.

Dolphin, A.C. (1985) Long-term potentiation at peripheral synapses. *Trends Neurosci.*, 8:376–378.

Dolphin, A.C., Errington, M.L. and Bliss, T.V.P. (1982) Long-term potentiation of the perforant path in vivo is associated with increased glutamate release. *Nature*, 297:496–498.

Dunwiddie, T.V. and Lynch, G. (1979) The relationship between extracellular calcium concentrations and the induction of long-term potentiation. *Brain Res.*, 169:103–110.

Eccles, J.C. (1983) Calcium in long-term potentiation as a model system for memory. *Neuroscience*, 10:1071–1081.

Fried, R.C. and Blaustein, M.P. (1976) Synaptic vesicle recycling in synaptosomes in vitro. *Nature*, 261:255–256.

Fried, R.C. and Blaustein, M.C. (1978) Retrieval and recycling of synaptic vesicle membrane in pinched-off nerve terminal (synaptosomes). *J. Cell Biol.*, 78:685–700.

Fukanaga, K., Yamamoto, H., Iwasa, Y., Higashi, K. and Miyamoto, E. (1982) Purification and characterization of a Ca^{2+}- and calmodulin-dependent protein kinase from rat brain. *J. Neurochem.*, 39:1607–1617.

Galvan, M., Grafe, P. and Ten Bruggecate, G. (1982) Convulsant actions of 4-aminopyridine on the guinea pig olfactory cortex slice. *Brain Res.*, 241:75–86.

Gispen, W.H., Leunissen, J.L.M., Oestreicher, A.B., Verkleij, A.J. and Zwiers, H. (1985a) Presynaptic localization of B-50 phosphoprotein: The ACTH-sensitive protein kinase substrate involved in rat brain polyphosphoinositide metabolism. *Brain Res.*, 328:381–385.

Gispen, W.H., Van Dongen, C.J., De Graan, P.N.E., Oestreicher, A.B. and Zwiers, H. (1985b) The role of phosphoprotein B-50 in polyphosphoinositide metabolism in brain synaptic plasma membranes. In J.E. Bleasdale, J. Eichberg and G. Hauser (Eds.), *Inositol and Phosphoinositides, Metabolism and Regulation*, Humana Press, New Jersey, pp. 399–414.

Goddard, G.V., McIntyre, P.C. and Leech, C.K. (1969) A permanent change in brain function resulting from daily electrical stimulation. *Exp. Neurol.*, 25:295–330.

Goldenring, J.R., Gonzalez, B., McGuire, J.S. and DeLorenzo, R.J. (1983) Purification and characterization of a calmodulin-dependent kinase from rat brain cytosol able to phosphorylate tubulin and microtubule-associated proteins. *J. Biol. Chem.*, 258:12632–12640.

Goldenring, J.R., Casanova, J.E. and DeLorenzo, R.J. (1984) Tubulin-associated calmodulin-dependent protein kinase: evidence for an endogenous complex of tubulin with a calcium-calmodulin-dependent kinase. *J. Neurochem.*, 43:1669–1679.

Goldenring, J.R., Wasterlain, C.G., Oestreicher, A.B., De Graan, P.N.E., Farber, D.B., Glaser, G. and DeLorenzo, R.J. (1986) Kindling induces a long-lasting change in the activity of a hippocampal membrane calmodulin-dependent protein kinase system. *Brain Res.* (in press).

Goldstein, J.L., Anderson, R.G.W. and Brown, M.S. (1979) Coated pits, coated vesicles and receptor-mediated endocytosis. *Nature*, 279:679–685.

Goldstein, J.L., Anderson, R.G.W. and Brown, M.S. (1982) Receptor-mediated endocytosis and the cellular uptake of low density lipoprotein. *Ciba Foundation Symp.*, 92:77–95.

Griffiths, T., Evans, M.C. and Meldrum, B.S. (1982) Intracellular sites of early calcium accumulation in the rat hippocampus during status epilepticus. *Neurosci. Lett.*, 30:329–344.

Gustafsson, B., Galvan, M., Grafe, P. and Wigstrom, H. (1982) A transient outward current in a mammalian central neuron blocked by 4-aminopyridine. *Nature*, 299:252–254.

Hermann, A. and Gorman, A.L.F. (1981) Effects of 4-aminopyridine on potassium currents in a molluscan neurone. *J. Gen. Physiol.*, 78:63–86.

Heuser, J. and Reese, T. (1973) Evidence for recycling of synaptic vesicle membrane during transmitter release at the frog neuromuscular junction. *J. Cell Biol.*, 57:315–344.

Hokin, M.R. and Hokin, L.E. (1954) Effects of acetylcholine on phospholipids in the pancreas. *J. Biol. Chem.*, 209:549–558.

Hokin, L.E. and Hokin, M.R. (1959) The mechanism of phosphate exchange in phosphatidic acid in response to acetylcholine, *J. Biol. Chem.*, 234:1387–1390.

Kadota, T. and Kadota, K. (1982) Membrane retrieval by

macropinocytosis in presynaptic terminals during transmitter relase in cat synaptic ganglia in situ. *J. Electron Microsc.*, 31:73–80.

Kadota, K., Usami, M. and Takahashi, A. (1982) A protein kinase and its substrate associated with the outer coat and inner core of coated vesicles from bovine brain. *Biomed. Res.*, 3:575–578.

Kennedy, M.B. and Greengard, P. (1981) Two calcium/calmodulin-dependent protein kinases, which are highly concentrated in brain phosphorylate protein I at distinct sites. *Proc. Natl. Acad. Sci. U.S.A.*, 78:1293–1297.

Kennedy, M.B., McGuinness, T. and Greengard, P. (1983a) A calcium/calmodulin-dependent protein kinase from mammalian brain that phosphorylates synapsin I: partial purification and characterization. *J. Neurosci.*, 3:818–831.

Kennedy, M.B., Bennett, M.K. and Erondu, N.E. (1983b) Biochemical evidence that the 'major post-synaptic density protein' is subunit of a calmodulin-dependent protein kinase. *Proc. Natl. Acad. Sci. U.S.A.*, 80:7357–7361.

Kristjansson, G.I., Zwiers, H., Oestreicher, A.B. and Gispen, W.H. (1982) Evidence that the synaptic phosphoprotein B-50 is localized exclusively in nervous tissue. *J. Neurochem.*, 39:371–378.

Kuhnt, U., Mihaly, A. and Joo, F. (1985) Increased binding of calcium in the hippocampal slice during long-term potentiation. *Neurosci. Lett.*, 53:149–154.

Kuret, J. and Schulman, H. (1985) Mechanism of autophosphorylation of the multifunctional Ca^{2+}/calmodulin-dependent protein kinase. *J. Biol. Chem.*, 260:6427–6433.

Larson, R.E., Goldenring, J.R., Vallano, M.L. and DeLorenzo, R.J. (1985) Identification of endogenous calmodulin-dependent kinase and calmodulin-binding proteins in cold-stable microtubule preparations from rat brain. *J. Neurochem.*, 44:1566–1574.

Llinás, R., Walton, K. and Bohr, V. (1976) Synaptic transmission in squid giant synapse after potassium conductance blockage with external 3- and 4-aminopyridine. *Biophys. J.*, 16:83–86.

Llinás, R., McGuinness, T.L., Leonard, C.S., Sugimori, M. and Greengard, P. (1985) Intraterminal injection of synapsin I or calcium/calmodulin-dependent protein kinase II alters neurotransmitter release at the squid giant synapse. *Proc. Natl. Acad. Sci. U.S.A.*, 82:3035–3039.

Lopes da Silva, F.H., Bär, P.R., Tielen, A.M. and Gispen, W.H. (1982a) Plasticity in synaptic transmission of membrane-bound protein phosphorylation. *Progr. Brain Res.*, 55:369–377.

Lopes da Silva, F.H., Bär, P.R., Tielen, A.M. and Gispen, W.H. (1982b) Changes in membrane phosphorylation correlated with long-lasting potentiation in rat hippocampal slices. *Progr. Brain Res.*, 56:339–347.

Lovinger, D.M., Akers, R.F., Nelson, R.B., Barnes, C.A., McNaughton, B.L. and Routtenberg, A. (1985) A selective increase in phosphorylation of protein F1, a protein kinase C substrate, directly related to three day growth of long-term synaptic enhancement. *Brain Res.*, 343:137–143

Lynch, G. and Baudry, M. (1984) The biochemistry of memory:
a new and specific hypothesis. *Science*, 224:1057–1063.

McGuinness, T.L., Lai, Y. and Greengard, P. (1985) Ca^{2+}/calmodulin-dependent protein kinase II. Isozymic forms from rat forebrain and cerebellum. *J. Biol. Chem.*, 260:1696–1704.

Michell, R.H. (1975) Inositol phospholipids and cell surface receptor function. *Biochim. Biophys. Acta* 415: 81–148.

Michell, R.H. (1979) Inositol phospholipids and membrane function. *Trends Biochem. Sci.*, 4:128–131.

Miller, R.J. (1985) Second messengers, phosphorylation and neurotransmitter release. *Trends Neurosci.*, 8:461–465.

Miller, T.M. and Heuser, J.E. (1984) Endocytosis of synaptic vesicle membrane at the frog neuromuscular junction. *J. Cell Biol.*, 98:685–689.

Nestler, E.J. and Greengard, P. (1984) *Protein Phosphorylation in the Nervous System*, John Wiley and Sons, New York.

Nicholson, C., Steinberg, R., Stockle, H. and Ten Bruggecate, G. (1976) Calcium decrease associated with 4-aminopyridine-induced potassium increase in cat cerebellum. *Neurosci. Lett.*, 3:315–319.

Nishizuka, Y. (1984a) The role of protein kinase C in cell surface signal transduction and tumor promotion. *Nature*, 308:693–697.

Nishizuka, Y. (1984b) Turnover of inositol phospholipids and signal transduction. *Science*, 225:1365–1370.

Palade, G.E. (1975) Intracellular aspects of the process of protein secretion. *Science*, 189:347–358.

Pant, H.C., Gallant, P.E., Cohen, R., Neary, J.T. and Gainer, H. (1983) Calcium-dependent 4-aminopyridine stimulation of protein phosphorylation in squid optic lobe synaptosomes. *Cell. Mol. Neurobiol.*, 3:223–238.

Pauloin, A. and Jollès, P. (1984) Internal control of the coated vesicle pp50-specific kinase complex. *Nature*, 311:265–267.

Pauloin, P., Bernier, I. and Jollès, P. (1982) Presence of cyclic nucleotide Ca^{2+}-independent protein kinase in bovine brain coated vesicles. *Nature*, 298:574–576.

Pauloin, P., Loeb, J. and Jollès, P. (1984) Protein kinase(s) in bovine brain coated vesicles. *Biochim. Biophys. Acta*, 799:238–245.

Pearse, B.M.F. and Robinson, M.S. (1984) Purification and properties of 100 kD proteins from coated vesicles and their reconstruction with clathrin. *EMBO J.*, 3:1951–1957.

Rostas, J.A.P., Brent, V.A. and Dunkley, P.R. (1983) The major calmodulin-stimulated phosphoprotein of synaptic junctions and the major post-synaptic density protein are distinct. *Neurosci. Lett.*, 43:161–165.

Rothman, J.E. and Fine, R.E. (1980) Coated vesicles transport newly synthesized membrane glycoproteins from endoplasmic reticulum to plasma membrane in two successive stages. *Proc. Natl. Acad. Sci. U.S.A.*, 77:780–784.

Rothman, J.E., Bursztyn-Pettegrew, H. and Fine, R.E. (1980) Transport of the membrane glycoprotein of vesicular stomatitis virus to the cell surface in two stages by clathrin-coated vesicles. *J. Cell Biol.*, 86:162–171.

Routtenberg, A. and Lovinger, D.M. (1985) Selective increase in phosphorylation of a 47 kDa protein (F1) directly related to long-term potentiation. *Behav. Neural. Biol.*, 43:3–11.

Sahyoun, N., LeVine, H., Bronson, D., Siegel-Greenstein, F. and Cuatrecasas, P. (1985). Cytoskeletal calmodulin-dependent protein kinase. Characterization, solubilization, and purification from rat brain. *J. Biol. Chem.*, 260:1230–1237.

Schmid, S.L., Braell, W.A., Schlossman, D.M. and Rothman, J.E. (1984) A role for clathrin light chains in the recogniation of clathrin cages by 'uncoating ATPase'. *Nature*, 311:228–231.

Schrama, L.H., De Graan, P.N.E., Eichberg, J. and Gispen, W.H. (1986) Feedback control of the inositol phospholipid response in rat brain is sensitive to ACTH. *Eur. J. Pharmacol.*, 121:403–404.

Schulman, H., Kuret, J., Jefferson, A.B., Nose, P.S. and Spitzer, K.H. (1985) Ca^{2+}/calmodulin-dependent microtubule-associated protein 2 kinase: broad substrate specificity and multifunctional potential in diverse tissues. *Biochemistry*, 24:5320–5329.

Shields, S.M., Vernon, P.J. and Kelly, P.T. (1984) Autophosphorylation of calmodulin-kinase II in synaptic junctions modulates endogenous kinase activity. *J. Neurochem.*, 43:1599–1609.

Steinman, R.M., Mellman, I.S., Muller, W.A. and Cohn, Z.A. (1983) Endocytosis and recycling of plasma membranes. *J. Cell Biol.*, 96:1–27.

Thesleff, S. (1980) Aminopyridines and synaptic transmission. *Neuroscience*, 5:1413–1419.

Tielen, A.M., Lopes da Silva, F.H. Bär, P.R. and Gispen, W.H. (1982) Long-lasting post-tetanic potentiation in the dentate area of rat hippocampal slices and correlated changes in synaptic membrane phosphorylation. In C. Ajmone Marsan and H. Matthies (Eds.), *Neuronal Plasticity and Memory Formation*, Raven Press, New York, pp. 239–254.

Tielen, A.M., De Graan, P.N.E., Mollevanger, W.J., Lopes da Silva, F.H. and Gispen, W.H. (1983) Quantitative relationship between post-tetanic biochemical and electrophysiological changes in rat hippocampal slices. *Brain Res.*, 277:189–192.

Van Dongen, C.J., Zwiers, H., De Graan, P.N.E. and Gispen, W.H. (1985) Modulation of the activity of purified phosphatidylinositol 4-phosphate kinase by phosphorylated and dephosphorylated B-50 protein. *Biochem. Biophys. Res. Commun.*, 128:1219–1227.

Wasterlain, C.G. and Farber, D.B. (1982) A lasting change in protein phosphorylation associated with septal kindling. *Brain Res.*, 247:191–194.

Wasterlain, C.G. and Farber, D.B. (1984) Kindling alters the calcium/calmodulin-dependent phosphorylation of synaptic plasma membrane proteins in rat hippocampus. *Proc. Natl. Acad. Sci. U.S.A.*, 81:1253–1257.

Yamamoto, H., Fukanaga, K. Goto, S., Tanaka, E. and Miyamoto, E. (1985) Ca^{2+}, calmodulin-dependent regulation of microtubule formation via phosphorylation of microtubule-associated protein 2, τ factor, and tubulin, and comparison with the cyclic AMP-dependent phosphorylation. *J. Neurochem.*, 44:759–768.

Yamauchi, T. and Fujisawa, H. (1985) Self-regulation of calmodulin-dependent protein kinase II and glycogen synthase kinase by autophosphorylation. *Biochem. Biophys. Res. Commun.*, 129:213–219.

Zwiers, H., Schotman, P. and Gispen, W.H. (1980) Purification and some characteristics of an ACTH-sensitive protein kinase and its substrate protein in rat brain membranes. *J. Neurochem.*, 34:1689–1699.

W.H. Gispen and A. Routtenberg (Eds.)
Progress in Brain Research, Vol. 69
© 1986 Elsevier Science Publishers B.V. (Biomedical Division)

CHAPTER 21

Phosphorylation/dephosphorylation mechanisms in coated vesicles

Alain Pauloin and Pierre Jollès

*Laboratoire des Protéines (Unité C.N.R.S. No 1188), Université de Paris V, 45 rue des Saints-Pères,
F-75270 Paris Cedex 06, France*

A major development in cell biology in the last few years has been the gradual realization of the magnitude of intracellular membrane traffic and the multiplicity of pathways for such traffic in various cells. These intracellular transfers of membranous proteins between discontinuous regions of membrane occur via populations of vesicles. These transient structures are presumed to bud off from a donor membrane compartment, to traverse the intervening cytoplasm and to fuse with a target membrane compartment. Considerable attention is focused on specialized vesicular structures, the coated vesicles (CV), in relation to this intracellular traffic.

Nature of coated vesicles

These vesicles were initially identified by Bessis and Breton-Gorius (1957) in erythroblasts and during the next decade they were shown to be present in many different cells and tissues from animals and plants. It is likely that they constitute an ubiquitous and unique organelle in essentially all eukaryotic cells (Fig. 1). Kanaseki and Kadota (1969) first described the hexagonal and pentagonal features of the coat. Subsequently more detailed electron microscopy studies of isolated CV led to the proposal that the coats are polyhedra which consist of a basic structure of 12 pentagons complemented by a variable number of hexagons (Crowther et al., 1976; Heuser, 1980). Pearse (1975) was the first who developed a reproducible

purification scheme to prepare CV from various sources in order to analyze their constituents (Fig. 2). She isolated a 180-kDa protein which constitutes 70% of the coat. She named this protein clathrin, which means 'basket' in Greek, because it

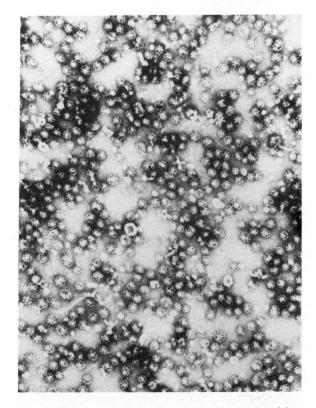

Fig. 1. Electron micrograph of bovine brain coated vesicles.

260

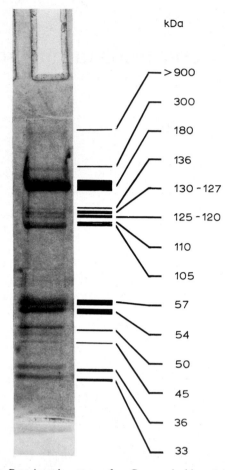

kDa
> 900
300
180
136
130 – 127
125 – 120
110
105
57
54
50
45
36
33

Fig. 2. **Protein gel pattern after Coomassie blue staining of** bovine brain coated vesicles.

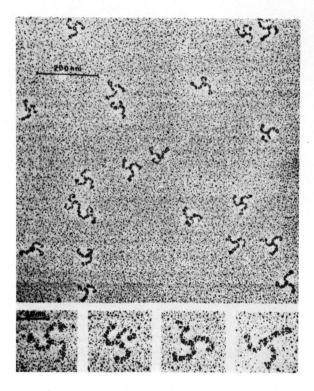

Fig. 3. Electron micrographs of 8.4 S clathrin triskelions after rotary shadowing. Reprinted by permission from *Nature*, Vol. 289, pp. 421, Copyright © 1981, Macmillan Journals Limited.

forms a regular geometric structure. There are two polypeptides (36 and 33 kDa), called the clathrin light chains, which co-purify with clathrin. Additional minor proteins of 110–100 kDa and 55–50 kDa have also been reported (Pearse, 1978; Rubenstein et al., 1981; Pfeffer and Kelly, 1981). Disruption and solubilization of the coats occur either in media of slightly alkaline pH devoid of divalent cations, in the presence of mild denaturants such as 2 M urea or at high concentrations of protonated amines (e.g. 0.5 M Tris) (Roth et al., 1977; Blitz et al., 1977; Keen et al., 1979). The solubilized coat subunits, called triskelions, sediment at 8 S and have a very characteristic shape when visualized by electron microscopy (Fig. 3)

(Ungewickell and Branton, 1981; Kirchhausen and Harrison, 1981). Triskelions are composed of three clathrin heavy chains found in non-covalent association with three randomly distributed light chains (Kirchhausen and Harrison, 1981; Kirchhausen et al., 1983). The latter were situated near the triskelion vertex and interacted with the proximal part of the clathrin heavy chains (Ungewickell et al., 1982; Ungewickell, 1983). Triskelions and the uncoated vesicles may be reassociated to form CV. The association triskelion–vesicles is a positively cooperative interaction mediated by the proximal part of the clathrin heavy chains (Hansal et al., 1984). Triskelions also can be repolymerized under defined conditions into cage-like structures that resemble the surface lattice of CV. This indicates that reassembly is not tightly dependent on the presence of membranes (Schook et al., 1979). Previous investigators have reported that coat reassembly was extremely pH dependent (Roth et al., 1977; Bloom et al., 1980b). Reassembly in low-salt buffers occurred only at pH 6.5 or below and could be reversed by raising the pH to 7.5. Nandi et al. (1981) reported increased rate of clathrin polymerization at more physiological pH, but only in the presence of high concentration of free divalent cations, certain polyamines or basic proteins. Keen et al (1979) have shown that Sepharose filtration of Tris-dissociated CV allowed separation of vesicles from a triskelion fraction and from another one called 'assembly polypeptides' (AP). Zaremba and Keen (1983) showed that in the absence of AP, coats formed from clathrin alone, under permissive buffer conditions, sediment in two broad bands on sucrose gradient (~ 200 and 400 S) as described by Jaarsfeld et al. (1981) and exhibit a wide range of diameters. In contrast, coats formed in the presence of AP, regardless of the buffer system employed, which sediment in a single band of 250 S, are uniform in size and have incorporated AP in the structure in addition of triskelions. Furthermore, it was recently shown that AP was very important for the binding of triskelions onto the uncoated vesicle to form CV (Prasad et al., 1985).

In order to construct pentagons and hexagons from triskelions, the latter must be placed at each vertex of the lattice and hinged joints on the three triskelion legs must exist to facilitate packing of triskelions into closed polyhedra (Crowther and Pearse, 1981). Since the distance between vertices in cages is 18.6 nm, the triskelion leg, which is 44 nm long, can easily extend along more than two edges, leading to an extensive overlap of four half-legs in each polyhedral edge. The kink in triskelion legs is located about 16 nm from the centerpoint, which demands that the legs should deviate before reaching the neighbouring vertex (Ungewickell and Branton, 1982).

The surface lattice of all CV characterized to date appear to be formed of triskelions, although there is a marked variation in size among CV. An early paper by Friend and Farquhar (1967) described two distinct populations in situ. One class, with a diameter >100 nm, was localized in the apical cytoplasm, and the other, with a smaller diameter of ~ 75 nm, was found primarily in the Golgi region. This size polymorphism may reflect the diversity in the functional role attributed to CV.

Basic functions of coated vesicles

Transfer of membranes and associated components between cellular compartments involves vesiculation of one membrane bilayer and further fusion of the vesicle with another one. CV are widely involved in the first of these steps. Formation of a lattice-like coat from clathrin and associated proteins accompanies vesiculation. (For more details, see the review of Fine and Ockleford (1984). Clathrin-coated vesicles have been found to be involved in the transport of membranes and/or proteins along major established pathways (Farquhar, 1983). These routes are:

(1) The endocytic pathway, where CV are involved in the uptake of adsorbed extracellular and plasma membrane proteins and in their subsequent delivery to lysosomes or other intracellular membrane compartments. It is the major route utilized in the receptor-mediated endocytosis (Goldstein et al., 1979, 1982). Over two dozen examples of high affinity binding sites which mediate the endocytosis of specific ligands are now known (Steinman et al., 1983).
(2) The transcellular route, which represents the major pathway for the transport of intact immunoglobulins across cells (Rodewald, 1973, 1980; Nagura et al., 1979; Renston et al., 1980).
(3) The exocytosis pathway, utilized in secretory cells for the discharge of secretory products, e.g. in pancreas and parotid salivary glands (Jamieson and Palade, 1971; Palade, 1975) or in cells infected with vesicular stomatitis virus, for the transport of the newly synthesized viral coat (G) protein (Rothman and Fine, 1980; Rothman et al., 1980).
(4) The plasmalemma to Golgi route, also highly developed in secretory cells, which is believed to be utilized for the recycling of secretory granule membranes (Herzog and Farquhar, 1977; Ottosen et al., 1980).
(5) The biosynthetic pathways for the transport of membrane proteins from the endoplasmic reticulum to the Golgi (Rothman et al., 1980) and the transport of lysosomal enzymes from the Golgi

complex to lysosomes (Holtzman et al., 1967; Nichols et al., 1971).

Functions of coated vesicles in nervous tissues

If CV are present in every cell types, they are particularly abundant in the nervous tissues. In order to elucidate the role of clathrin and CV, it is highly desirable to localize clathrin at cellular and subcellular levels. Indirect immunofluorescent labeling of cerebellar tissue sections with bovine brain clathrin antibodies exhibited profuse immunofluorescence in the granular layer, while dissociated cultures of neonatal rat cerebellar cells showed intense fluorescence in the cytoplasm and the processes of granule cell neurons (Bloom et al., 1980a). This may be related to the extensive formation and growth of dendrites by the granule cells, where growing dendrites in developing neuronal tissues are rich in CV (Rees et al., 1976). In cerebellar Purkinje and granule cell bodies, clathrin is localized on CV, on the budding areas from the Golgi-associated membrane and Golgi-associated vesicles. Furthermore, the membrane of the multivesicular body, the bound ribosomes, and the ground substances are also stained. In the myelinated axon, clathrin appears to be concentrated on certain segments and seems to fill the space between neurotubules and some vesicles. In certain synaptic terminals clathrin often seems attached to presynaptic vesicles and presynaptic and postsynaptic membranes (Bloom et al., 1980a).

In nervous tissues, CV assume nearly all the cellular functions precedently described, particularly those applied to the nervous mechanisms like the retrieval of synaptic membranes, axonal transport, nervous system development and the transport of opiate receptors.

The retrieval of synaptic membranes

The discovery of synaptic vesicles and the evidence for the quantal release of transmitter led to the hypothesis that transmitter release is accomplished by the exocytosis of synaptic vesicles. Secretion by exocytosis results in an increased surface area and it was proposed that a compensatory process of membrane retrieval must function to maintain a constant membrane surface. CV represent the mechanisms for retrieval of synaptic vesicle membranes from the plasmalemma because, during nerve stimulation, they proliferate at regions of the nerve terminals covered by Schwann cell processes and appear in various stages of coalescence with cisternae. In contrast, synaptic vesicles do not appear to return directly from the surface to form cisternae and the latter never appear to be directly connected to the surface. Thus it was postulated that CV shed their coats to become recycled synaptic vesicles (Heuser and Reese, 1973). Possible evidence for similar recycling events has been obtained from other synapses (Douglas et al., 1971; Nagasawa et al., 1971) and with synaptosomes (Fried and Blaustein, 1976, 1978). However, a controversy has arisen concerning membrane retrieval at the neuromuscular junction; some workers believe that retrieval is accomplished via endocytosis of uncoated vesicles at the active zone, where synaptic vesicle exocytosis normally occurs (Ceccarelli et al., 1973), while others argue that endocytosis of CV away from the active zone (and particularly beneath Schwann cell fingers) is the significant process (Heuser and Reese, 1973). To study membrane recycling at the neuromuscular junctions in more detail, Miller and Heuser (1984) quick-froze and freeze-fractured synapses at various times after a single electrical stimulus. They showed that the endocytic retrieval of the vesicle membranes back into the terminal occurs following two distinct types of endocytosis. The first few seconds after stimulation, relatively large uncoated vacuoles ($\sim 0.1\ \mu m$) are pinched off, both near to and far away from the active zone. The second endocytic process is slower, appeared at 1 s, reached a peak at 30 s and almost completely disappeared at 90 s. The endocytic structures are clathrin coated and this process first occurs by the formation of coated pits everywhere in the plasma membrane, except at the active zone. In one study utilizing turtle retina, Scheffer and Raviola (1978) showed the formation of CV in the cone cell endings during the period of stimulation. These CV are responsible for recycling of synaptic vesicle membranes in a fashion similar to other studies of neuronal endings. By indirect immunofluorescence clathrin has been localized in rat retina in regions containing synpatic endings in high density. This is indicative of active recycling of the synaptic membrane concomitant to neurotransmitter release and receptor molecule turnover (Bloom and Puszkin, 1983). In order to compare the biochemical composition of CV and synaptic vesicles, Kadota et al. (1983) attempted to develop a new method for purifying CV from bovine brain synaptosomes. This comparison showed that the synaptic vesicles differed from the CV by the presence of a 69-kDa protein and a Ca^{2+}/calmodulin-dependent protein kinase associated to its 39-kDa protein substrate (Kadota et al., 1984a). Thus if CV are converted into synaptic vesicles, an addition of proteins specific of the synaptic vesicles must take place during an intermediate stage (e.g. cisternae).

Axonal transport

The axon and its terminal depend on the continuous delivery of proteins synthesized in the cell body to maintain their structural and functional integrity. Axonal proteins leave the cell body as five separate groups, each different and moving at a distinct rate. Some of these proteins have been associated with specific structures in the axon, such as microtubules, neurofilaments, microfilaments and mitochondria. Thus the transport of proteins in the axon expresses the movement of complete subcellular structures rather than the movement of individual proteins (Tytell et al., 1981). Because CV are found in great quantities in axon terminals, and as the source of nearly all neuronal polypeptides is the neuron cell body, clathrin must be axonally transported to the terminal areas. In addition, the relative paucity of the CV form within the axon (Tsukita and Ishikawa, 1980) may be indirect evidence that clathrin travels as unassociated triskelion forms. In a first approach, Garner and Lasek (1981) showed that clathrin travels at a slow rate, associated to actin. Mori and Kurokawa (1981) agreed with the fact that clathrin is not a component of the fast axoplasmic transport, implying that the

polypeptide is not associated with agranular reticulum and vesiculotubular structures during its axonal transport. However a discrepancy appears when these authors suggest that clathrin and actin are not primarily associated during their migration. They postulate that clathrin is associated with such a delicate intraaxonal structure as the microtrabecular matrix and thereby is linked to mitochondria. Although clathrin does not undergo fast axonal transport, CV play a major, but not necessarily exclusive, role in the exit of fast-transported proteins from the Golgi cisternae (Stone et al., 1984). After CV bud off from Golgi cisternae in the cell body, coats must be shed in order to allow the incorporation of the proteins into the fast transport system. Since the most likely candidate for the fast transport vector is an elongated, smooth-membrane-bounded organelle (Ellisman and Lindsey, 1982), it is possible that this structure represents a fusion product of numerous decoated vesicles.

Nervous system development

Bastiani and Goodman (1984) have studied the factors that guide individual neuronal growth cones during embryonic development. They showed a highly specific interaction between developing growth cones in the grasshopper embryo. Numerous filopodia from an identified growth cone deeply insert within another identified growth cone, inducing the formation of coated pits and CV. This interaction is highly specific, since filopodia from other nearly related growth cones which contact the surface of the two interacting neurons neither penetrate them nor induce CV. At the same time, Bursztajn (1984) studied the formation of the neuromuscular junctions between ciliary neurons and cultured myotubes. He identified these synaptic contacts by the presence of acetylcholine receptors primarily confined to the postsynaptic sites beneath neuronal processes. The examination of these innervation sites on the ultrastructural level shows that the nerve terminals appear to protrude into the coated pits of the myoplasm. Numerous coated pits and CV were found beneath these early contacts.

Transport of opiate receptors

It was recently shown that purified CV from bovine forebrain contained high-affinity stereo-specific opiate alkaloid binding sites with characteristic opioid binding properties. It is therefore possible that opiate receptors either could be internalized via the coated pit–endosome pathway or could undergo exocytosis in this manner (Bennett et al., 1985).

Phosphorylation/dephosphorylation in coated vesicles

The repeated fusions and fissions of the clathrin-coated membranes and the diversity of the CV functions implicate selective processes for the choice of the proteins to be internalized and for the delivery of the latter to their final targets. Thus sophisticated mechanisms to control all the steps must exist. Protein phosphorylation is now recognized to be the major general mechanism by which intracellular events in mammalian tissues are controlled by external physiological stimuli (Cohen, 1982). We suspected that a phosphorylation event might be implicated and detected in CV. In order to investigate this further, we purified CV from bovine brain grey matter homogenate by two successive sucrose gradients (Keen et al., 1979) and incubated them at 37°C for 15 min in the presence of 12 mM Tris–HCl, pH 7.5, 32 mM KCl, 2 mM $MgCl_2$, 2.3 mM 2-mercaptoethanol and $[\gamma-^{32}P]ATP$. The polypeptide composition was analyzed by sodium dodecylsulfate polyacrylamide gel electrophoresis (SDS–PAGE) followed by autoradiography (Fig. 4). This experiment showed that a 50-kDa protein (called pp50) was clearly phosphorylated. This phosphorylation occurred without cAMP of cGMP, and the addition of these two cyclic nucleotides did not modify the ^{32}P incorporation. Likewise, Ca^{2+} and calmodulin had no effect on the pp50 phosphorylation. Because of the multiple roles played by CV, many previously described minor proteins were in fact some transported protein components. Thus these minor components reported by different authors vary quite widely, even when CV are isolated from the same source. Although this variability can be

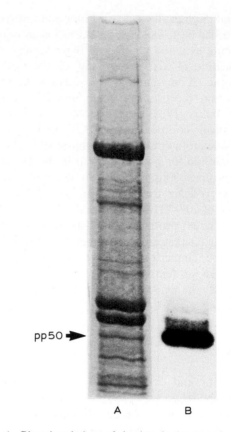

pp50 ➤

A   B

Fig. 4. Phosphorylation of bovine brain coated vesicles: Coomassie blue staining (A) and autoradiography (B).

explained partly by the various amounts of material analyzed on gels, it is also partly attributable to the presence of small amounts of contaminating membranes in the CV preparations. Smooth vesicles of approximately the same size could remain with CV. The fact that clathrin is negatively charged at pH 6.5 was utilized to purify CV near to homogeneity by agarose gel electrophoresis. Since contaminating smooth vesicles, devoid of clathrin, are less negatively charged and migrate more slowly than CV, they can thus be completely separated (Rubenstein et al., 1981). We used this method and showed not only the constant presence of the pp50 substrate with CV but also that the kinase activity is a constitutive part of CV (Pauloin et al., 1982). During the submission of our manuscript, Pfeffer and Kelly (1981) established the veritable minor component composition of bovine brain CV by use of permeation chromatography on a controlled pore glass column, and showed the peculiar presence of a 50-kDa protein in CV and nowhere else. Two independent laboratories confirmed all our results. Kadota et al. (1982) showed the presence of a cyclic nucleotides and Ca^{2+}/calmodulin-independent kinase activity in bovine brain which phosphorylated four proteins of 150, 120, 48 and 32 kDa. The 48-kDa component was strongly phosphorylated while the others were only slightly labeled. It is obvious that this 48-kDa protein corresponds to pp50. Moreover, Pfeffer et al (1983) also showed the strong labeling of pp50 in bovine brain CV and, in addition, detected six slightly radioactive bands of 140, 104, 72, 56, 54 and 35 kDa on overexposed films. When we demonstrated the presence of pp50 in CV, the phosphorylation of other bands was so slight that they were considered as background. The use of ATP of higher specific activity regularly resulted in the phosphorylation of 165- and 54-kDa proteins in addition to pp50. Occasionally, we also obtained slight labelling of ∼110- and 56-kDa proteins (Pauloin et al., 1984). Thus we practically obtained the same minor protein phosphorylation pattern as described by both the groups of Kadota and Pfeffer. The nature of the 165-kDa protein is not known. The latter is associated with the membrane core and is only detected after ^{32}P labeling; this fact seems to indicate that the 165-kDa protein is an internalized compound rather than an integral component of CV (Pauloin et al., 1984). The nature of the 54-kDa band was identified to the β-subunit of tubulin (Pfeffer et al., 1983; Wiedenman and Mimms, 1983; Kelly et al., 1983).

Comparative phosphorylation of several CV species showed that pp50 was present in every case, and was the most radioactive protein in all studied CV (Fig. 5). The phosphorylation pattern of CV minor proteins might reflect the membranous nature from which CV pinched off. Thus the fact that tubulin is a molecular component of CV must be restricted to the CV from brain and nervous tissues where tubulin is known to be a major component tightly associated with membrane, while tubulin is present only in trace amounts in both the adrenal gland and liver CV. The presence of multiple phosphorylated proteins

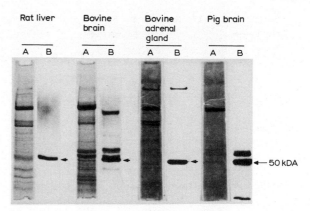

Fig. 5. Phosphorylation of coated vesicles from different origins. Comparison of the protein gel patterns after Coomassie blue staining (A) and autoradiography (B) from rat liver, bovine brain, bovine adrenal gland and pig brain.

in CV raises the question of the presence of multiple protein kinases. In spite of the absence of the purification and characterization of these putative kinases, which will constitute absolute proof of their existence, we showed indirectly that multiple kinases may occur in CV (Pauloin et al., 1984). Recently the presence of a casein kinase II, as described by Hathaway and Traugh (1983), has been reported in addition to the pp50 kinase in synaptosomal CV (Kadota et al., 1984b; Takahashi et al., 1985). Under standard phosphorylation conditions, neither clathrin heavy chain nor light chains were phosphorylated. However when a basic compound (histones, polylysine) was added to the incubation medium, the 33-kDa light chain was phosphorylated on a serine residue. The kinase responsible seemed to be the CV-casein kinase II (Usami et al., 1985; Schook et al., 1985).

Keen et al. (1979) showed that bovine brain CV are dissociated after treatment with protonated amines at neutral pH. Gel filtration of their CV–Tris extract allowed separation of the triskelion fraction from another one, described as the 'basket assembly factor', containing a 110-kDa protein and eluting in a volume corresponding to a molecular weight of 420 kDa. Recently Zaremba and Keen (1983) showed that this Tris fraction, recalled 'assembly polypeptides' (AP), contained several proteins of 110, 100 and ∼50 kDa, and was

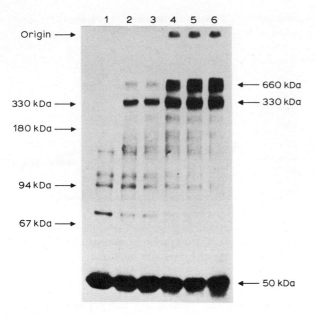

Fig. 6. Cross-linking by the bifunctional reagent dimethyladipimidate (DMA) of the ^{32}P-labeled assembly polypeptides. Lane 1, purified ^{32}P-labeled assembly polypeptides without DMA; lane 2–6, experiments carried out with DMA at 0.2, 0.4, 0.6, 0.8 and 1.0 mg/ml.

necessary for proper assembly of triskelions under physiological conditions. Pfeffer and co-workers (1983) also found that pp50 was associated with the 100-kDa protein group. We reported that, in addition to pp50, the whole kinase activity remained associated to AP. The enzymatic activity was stable. It was preserved for several months in a 0.5 M Tris–HCl buffer at 4°C or indefinitely at −30°C in 50% glycerol. Chemical cross-linking of the previously ^{32}P-labeled AP indicates that pp50 is closely associated with some proteins of the 100-kDa group, and forms a 330-kDa-^{32}P cross-linked complex (Fig. 6). No new bands of about 100 and 150 kDa appeared, which suggested the absence of pp50 dimer and trimer formation (Pauloin and Jollès, 1984). A few months later, two groups confirmed our results and presented additional data. Pearse and Robinson (1984) showed that further purification of Keen's fraction by a combination of gel filtration and chromatography on hydroxylapatite and DE-52 cellulose allowed the separation of two distinct fractions, one of which contained some of the 100-kDa proteins and the

other 100-kDa polypeptides associated to pp50. The latter appears to occur in a 1:1 molar ratio with the total of the 100-kDa polypeptides. After chemical cross-linking, the main product possesses an apparent molecular weight of 300 ± 50 kDa and appears to contain two 100-kDa polypeptides and two pp50 molecules. In the same way. Ungewickell (1984) also demonstrated the 100-kDa polypeptide–pp50 association and the presence of the pp50 kinase in the complex.

We studied the possible interaction of either the triskelions or the decoated vesicles with AP and its associated kinase. Increased amounts of triskelions had a stimulating effect on pp50 phosporylation and might enhance the labeling of the latter approximately 4-fold. The light chains seemed responsible for this stimulation, as clathrin heavy chains have only a very slight effect. Furthermore, decoated vesicles seemed to inhibit the pp50 phosphorylation, but lost their inhibiting effect when heated. This inhibition might be due either to the ATP consumption induced by the ATPases present in the decoated vesicles (Blitz et al., 1977; Stone et al., 1983; Forgac et al., 1983) or

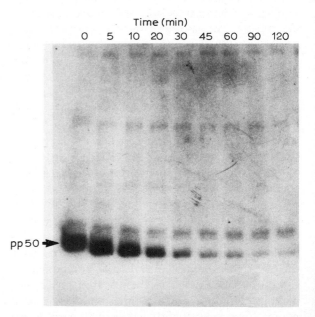

Fig. 7. Time course of pp50. ^{32}P-labeled coated vesicles were incubated for the indicated time in presence of 0.1 mM ATP, 1 mM MgCl$_2$ at 37°C, followed by SDS–PAGE and autoradiography.

to the presence of a pp50 phosphatase (Pauloin and Jollès, 1984). As we have shown that pp50 phosphorylation is under the position control of the light chains, a negative control by another part of the CV or by external stimuli might also exist. Indeed, we already suggested the presence of a pp50 phosphatase in CV. However the observed slow dephosphorylation raised the question concerning the presence of proteolytic activity or of the necessity of a phosphatase activator (Pauloin et al., 1984). We have since described the presence in bovine brain CV of a strong enzymatic activity which dephosphorylates pp50 (Fig. 7). This phosphoprotein phosphatase occurs under two interconvertible active and inactive forms. The activation process needs the simultaneous presence of Mg^{2+} and ATP or ADP. Unchelated ATP but not unchelated ADP inactivate this pp50 phosphatase which is associated with the vesicular core (Pauloin and Jollès, 1986).

Biochemical characterization of the pp50/kinase system

The biochemical characterization of this system is actually poorly documented. The main reason is the great difficulty of isolating pp50 and its kinase under native conditions, because of the strong interactions which take place in the 100/50-kDa complex. Hitherto, nobody has published the complete purification of either the active pp50 kinase or the phosphorylable pp50 substrate. Nevertheless some results are available.

pp50–kinase characteristics

We reported above that pp50 kinase is cyclic nucleotide and Ca^{2+}/calmodulin independent; only ATP may be used as phosphoryl donor and heparin has no action. Some other characteristics may be reported. Usami et al. (1984) showed that some divalent cations could be substituted for Mg^{2+} in order to activate the pp50 kinase according to the decreasing series $Mn^{2+} > Mg^{2+} > Co^{2+} > Ca^{2+} > Zn^{2+}$ for a constant 2 mM concentration. The dose-response studies of these divalent cations on the pp50 phosphorylation basically gave the same classification except

for Mg^{2+}, which was the most efficient (Pauloin, 1984). Contrary to casein and phosvitin, histones and protamine were not phosphorylated at all when they were added to CV. Furthermore, these exogenous basic substrates considerably reduced pp50 phosphorylation (Usami et al., 1984; Pauloin, 1984). It was shown that polyamines such as spermine and spermidine were able to stimulate some kinases. These two substances slightly enhanced the pp50 kinase activity. Optimum concentrations of spermine and spermidine were 1 and 2 mM, respectively (Pauloin, 1984). The 3 M urea treatment of CV allowed their separation into two sub-structural components, the clathrin coat and the vesicle core. The urea treatment approximately removed 30% of the 100/50-kDa complex, which appeared with the clathrin coat; the majority of the 100/50-kDa complex remained associated with the vesicle. The kinase activity was apparently found in the clathrin coat because the enzyme was poorly detected in the vesicle, irrespective of its high content of pp50. These results seemed to indicate that the kinase was related to the outer coat structures and its pp50 substrate to the inner vesicle (Kadota et al., 1982; Usami et al., 1984; Pauloin et al., 1984). However, recent evidence for the presence in the inner vesicle of the MgATP/ADP-dependent pp50-phosphatase might explain the absence of pp50 phosphorylation in the vesicle (Pauloin and Jollès, 1986). Recent evidence weakens the dichotomy between pp50-kinase and its substrate. Photolabeling of rat liver CV with 8-azido [α-^{32}P]ATP results in specific labeling of both the 53- and 51-kDa proteins. Preincubation with 10 mM N-ethylmaleimide inhibits kinase activity and concomitantly reduces photolabeling of the two substrates. Thus these data are consistent with the hypothesis that protein kinase activity resides in these two CV proteins and that they are catalyzing an autophosphorylation reaction (Campbell et al., 1984). Furthermore, when the partially purified AP was digested with elastase, the 100-kDa bands were rapidly degraded with little or no effect on either the pp50 integrity or the kinase activity (Zaremba and Keen, 1985). However, only purification of the kinase to homogeneity will prove this hypothesis.

Nature of the pp50 substrate

Pfeffer et al. (1983) made the first attempt to characterize the pp50 substrate. The latter appears to be related to brain microtubule-associated tau proteins since it can be specifically immunoprecipitated by an affinity-purified antiserum directed against these proteins. pp50 is distinct from the authentic 50-kDa tau protein since a comparable amount of pp50 binds less tau antiserum than the 50-kDa tau protein does, as detected by a solid-phase radioimmunoassay or immunoblotting procedures. Two-dimensional peptide mapping confirmed that the polypeptides were actually distinct, but revealed that pp50 shared common tryptic peptides with authentic tau proteins and may possess a common domain. In the same way, two-dimensional peptide mapping showed that pp50 was distinct from the 50-kDa subunit of a Ca^{2+}/calmodulin-dependent synapsin I kinase (Kennedy et al., 1983), previously known as the major postsynaptic density protein (Pfeffer and Kelly, 1983). The CV pp50 seems to be distinct from another about 50-kDa synaptic phosphoprotein, called B-50 by Gispen's group, since the latter is exclusively localized in nerve tissue (Kristjansson et al., 1982) whereas pp50 is also present in liver and adrenal gland at least (Pauloin et al., 1984).

Physiological functions of pp50 phosphorylation/ dephosphorylation

Numerous physiological phenomena necessary to cellular metabolism, motility and growth are regulated by reversible protein phosphorylation. At least a dozen steps in the working mechanism of CV may be theoretically regulated by pp50 phosphorylation/dephosphorylation. Nowadays the available data permit the expression of the two most likely mechanisms in which pp50 and its enzymatic system may be implicated: the intracytoplasmic traffic of free CV and the CV-coating/decoating processes.

Regulation of the intracytoplasmic traffic of free CV

The mechanism employed to direct a vesicle to any of the several potential intracellular sites is not understood. The presence of microtubule protein in CV suggests that these cytoskeletal elements may play a role in directing the transport of CV or CV-derived vesicles through the cytoplasm. To support this hypothesis, it was shown that MAP-2 can cross-link microtubules with CV (Sattilaro and Dentler, 1982) and triskelion centers were found to be attached to the microtubule 200-Å proteinaceous projection linkers (Imhof et al., 1983). Finally the recent identification of a 100-kDa protein associated with microtubules, intermediate filaments and CV in cultured cells by means of monoclonal antibodies directed against MAPs from bovine brain, added weight to the CV–microtubule relationship (Rodionov et al., 1985). The fact that tubulin antiserum precipitated pp50 even after complete disruption of CV with 0.5% SDS/1% Nonidet-P40, showed that tubulin polypeptides interact either directly with pp50 or with some other components tightly bound to pp50 (Pfeiffer et al., 1983). Furthermore pp50 appears to be related to a tau protein which is involved in the regulation of microtubule formation (Weingarten et al., 1975). These results seem to indicate that pp50 phosphorylation/dephosphorylation might regulate the anchorage of CV on the microtubules or trigger the CV migration along the latter.

Regulation of CV-coating/decoating process

Both coated pits and CV are highly dynamic structures, where the latter derive from the former by a kind of budding process that is accompanied by a rearrangement of the coat structure. Upon budding, CV rapidly shed their coats to allow them to fuse with their target membranes. The liberated triskelions are thought to return to the clathrin-coated membrane. The discovery in the bovine brain cytosol of a 70-kDa protein called 'uncoating protein', recently identified as an mammalian heat-shock protein (Ungewickell, 1985), and which, in the presence of ATP, is able to strip CV of a part of their coat, constitutes a first step in the knowledge of the clathrin cycle (Patzer et al., 1982; Schlossman et al., 1984). But the action of the 70-kDa protein is not sufficient to denude CV, as triskelions are also anchored by the means of 110-kDa proteins bound to the vesicle membrane itself (Unanue et al., 1981). The intriguing question is to know whether this 110-kDa anchorage protein corresponds to the ~100-kDa protein contained in the 100-kDa–pp50 complex (AP). When clathrin cages are reassembled with a saturating amount of 100-kDa–pp50 complex and studied by electron microscopy, the additional proteins appear to follow the underlying geometry of clathrin polyhedra, partially filling in the polygonal faces of the cage structures. Saturation appears to require about three 100-kDa molecules per triskelion (Pearse and Robinson, 1984). It was postulated that the 100-kDa–pp50 complex may increase the curvature of triskelion legs in order to generate smaller coats of uniform size (Zaremba and Keen, 1983) and that only the 100-kDa polypeptides were responsible of the reassembly activity (Zaremba and Keen, 1985). Preliminary experiments showed that pp50 phosphorylation did not seem to affect the binding of 100-kDa–pp50 to the triskelions (Ungewickell, 1984). Furthermore, reassociation of clathrin cages in the presence of AP takes place without ATP. Thus the pp50 role in the AP-mediated clathrin cage reassociation is not clear. However the introduction of a negatively charged phosphate group into pp50 could destabilize the interaction of the ternary complex 100-kDa–pp50–triskelion with the vesicle by charge repulsion if we consider that pp50 constitutes an interface between the vesicle and the ~100-kDa protein linked to the triskelion. In this regard, it is noteworthy that light chains act in the same way, first by enhancing the pp50 phosphorylation (Pauloin and Jollès, 1984) and secondly by allowing the release of clathrin from CV (Schmid et al., 1984). In vivo, coating and decoating processes must act very rapidly. The vesicular location of the pp50 phosphatase, the outer situation of the pp50 kinase and the fact that these two antagonistic enzymes need MgATP to be active may assure a fine steady-state responsible for either the maintenance or the rearrangement of the coat structure.

Conclusion

The kinase/phosphatase system associated to its specific pp50 substrate constitutes an extraordinary useful tool in order to study fundamental biochemical problems such as protein–protein interactions, enzymatic regulation and the molecular and physiological significance of protein phosphorylation. The different localization of the two antagonistic enzymatic activities amid the CV structure seems to indicate that pp50 plays an interface role between the membranous vesicle core and the clathrin coat. We are just at the beginning of these studies since we have only shown the presence of this CV-related enzymatic system. Clearly, many fascinating problems concerning the structure, organization, function and evolution of the pp50-kinase/phosphatase system remain open.

References

Bastiani, M.J. and Goodman, C.S. (1984) Neuronal growth cones: specific interactions mediated by filopodial insertion and induction of coated vesicles. *Proc. Natl. Acad. Sci. U.S.A.*, 81:1849–1853.

Bennett, D.B., Spain, J.W., Laskowski, M.B., Roth, B.L. and Coscia, C.J. (1985) Stereospecific opiate-binding sites occur in coated vesicles. *J. Neurosci.*, 5:3010–3015.

Bessis, M. and Breton Gorius, J. (1957) Iron particles in normal erythroblasts and normal and pathological erythrocytes. *J. Biophys. Biochem. Cytol.*, 3:503–505.

Blitz, A.A., Fine, R.E. and Tosselli, P.A. (1977) Evidence that coated vesicles isolated from brain are calcium-sequestering organelles resembling sarcoplasmic reticulum. *J. Cell. Biol.*,75:135–147.

Bloom, W.S., Fields, K.L., Yen, S.H., Haver, K., Schook, W. and Puszkin, S. (1980a) Brain clathrin: immunofluorescent patterns in cultured cells and tissues. *Proc. Natl. Acad. Sci. U.S.A.*, 77:5520–5524.

Bloom, W.S., Schook, W., Feagason, E., Ores, C. and Puszkin, S. (1980b) Brain clathrin: viscometric and turbidimetric properties of its ultrastructural assemblies. *Biochim. Biophys. Acta*, 598:447–455.

Bloom, W.S. and Puszkin, S. (1983) Brain clathrin. Immunofluorescent localization in rat retina. *J. Histochem. Cytochem.*, 31:46–52.

Bursztajn, S. (1984) Coated vesicles are associated with acetylcholine receptors at nerve-muscle contacts. *J. Neurocytol.*, 13:503–518.

Campbell, C., Squicciarini, J., Shia, M., Pilch, P.F. and Fine, R.E. (1984) Identification of a protein kinase as an intrinsic component of rat liver coated vesicles. *Biochemistry*, 23:4420–4426.

Ceccarelli, B., Hurlbut, W.P. and Mauro, A. (1973) Turnover of transmitter and synaptic vesicles at the frog neuromuscular junction. *J. Cell Biol.*, 57:499–524.

Cohen, P. (1982) The role of protein phosphorylation in neutral and hormonal control of cellular activity. *Nature*, 296:613–620.

Crowther, R.A., Finch, J.T. and Pearse, B.M.F. (1976) On the structure of coated vesicle. *J. Mol. Biol.*, 103:785–798.

Crowther, R.A. and Pearse, B.M.F. (1981) Assembly and packing of clathrin into coats. *J. Cell Biol.*, 91, 790–797.

Douglas, W.W., Nagasawa, J. and Schultz, R.A. (1971) Coated microvesicles in neurosecretory terminals of posterior pituitary glands shed their coats to become smooth 'synaptic' vesicles. *Nature*, 232:340–341.

Ellisman, M.H. and Lindsey, J.D. (1982) Organization of axoplasm–membranous and fibrillar components possibly involved in fast neuroplasmic tranport. In D.G. Weiss (Eds.), *Axoplasmic Transport*, Springer, New York, pp. 55–63.

Farquhar, M.G. (1983) Multiple pathways of exocytosis, endocytosis and membrane recycling: validation of a Golgi route. *Fed. Proc.*, 42:2407–2413.

Fine, R.E. and Ockleford, C.D. (1984) Supramolecular cytology of coated vesicles. *Int. Rev. Cytol.*, 91:1–43.

Forgac, M., Cantley, L., Wiedenmann, B., Altstiel, L. and Branton, D. (1983) Clathrin-coated vesicles contain and ATP-dependent proton pump. *Proc. Natl. Acad. Sci. U.S.A.*, 80:1300–1303.

Fried, R.C. and Blaustein, M.P. (1976) Synaptic vesicle recycling in synaptosomes in vitro. *Nature*, 261:255–256.

Fried, R.C. and Blaustein, M.P. (1978) Retrieval and recycling of synaptic vesicle membrane in pinched-off nerve terminal (synaptosomes). *J. Cell Biol.*, 78:685–700.

Friend, D.S. and Farquhar, M.G. (1967) Functions of coated vesicles during protein absorption in rat vas deferens. *J. Cell Biol.*, 35:357–376.

Garner, J.A. and Lasek, R.J. (1981) Clathrin is axonally transported as part of slow component b: the microfilament complex. *J. Cell Biol.*, 88:172–178.

Goldstein, J.L., Anderson, R.G.W. and Brown, M.S. (1979) Coated pits, coated vesicles, and receptor-mediated endocytosis. *Nature*, 279:679–685.

Goldstein, J.L., Anderson, R.G.W. and Brown, M.S. (1982) Receptor-mediated endocytosis and the cellular uptake of low density lipoprotein. *Ciba Found. Symp.*, 92:77–95.

Hanspal, M., Luna, E. and Branton, D. (1984) The association of clathrin fragments with coated vesicle membranes. *J. Biol. Chem.*, 259:11075–11082.

Hathaway, G.M. and Traugh, J.A. (1983) Casein kinase II. *Methods Enzymol.*, 99:317–331.

Herzog, V. and Farquhar, M.G. (1977) Luminal membrane retrieved after exocytosis reaches most Golgi cisternae in secretory cells. *Proc. Natl. Acad. Sci. U.S.A.*, 74:5073–5077.

Heuser, J.E. and Reese, T.S. (1973) Evidence for recycling of synaptic vesicle membrane during transmitter release at the frog neuromuscular junction. *J. Cell Biol.*, 57:315–344.

Heuser, J. (1980) Three-dimensional visualization of coated vesicle formation in fibroblasts. *J. Cell Biol.*, 84:560–583.

Holtzman, E., Novikoff, A.B. and Villaverde, H. (1967) Lysosomes and GERL in normal and chromatolytic neurons of the rat ganglion nodosum. *J. Cell Biol.*, 33:419–436.

Imhof, B.A., Marti, U., Boller, D., Frank, H. and Birchmeier, W. (1983) Association between coated vesicles and microtubules. *Exp. Cell. Res.*, 145:199–207.

Jaarsfeld, P.P., Nandi, P.U., Lippoldt, R.E., Sarroff, H. and Edelhoch, H. (1981) Polymerization of clathrin protomers into basket structures. *Biochemistry*, 20:4129–4136.

Jamieson, J.D. and Palade, G.E. (1971) Synthesis, intracellular transport and discharge of secretory proteins in stimulated pancreatic exocrine cells. *J. Cell Biol.*, 50:135–158.

Kadota, K., Usami, M. and Takahashi, A. (1982) A protein kinase and its substrate associated with the outer coat and the inner core of coated vesicles from bovine brain. *Biomed. Res.*, 3:575–578.

Kadota, K., Toyota, N., Miyazaki, N. and Kadota, T. (1983) Purification of coated vesicles from synaptosomes from bovine brain. *Biomed. Res.* 4:421–424.

Kadota, K., Toyota, N., Miyazaki, N. and Kadota, T. (1984a) Prerequisites for conversion of coated vesicles to synaptic vesicles. *Proc. Jpn. Acad. Sci. Ser. B*, 60:277–280.

Kadota, K., Toyota, N., Miyazaki, N. and Kadota, T. (1984b) Casein kinase II activity in coate ' vesicles prepared from synaptosomes from the bovine brain cortex. *Biomed. Res.*, 5:507–510.

Kanaseki, T. and Kadota, K. (1969) The vesicle in a basket. *J. Cell Biol.*, 42:202–220.

Keen, J.H., Willingham, M.C. and Pastan, I.H. (1979) Clathrin-coated vesicles: isolation, dissociation and factor-dependent reassociation of clathrin baskets. *Cell*, 16:303–312.

Kelly, W.G., Passaniti, A., Woods, J.W., Daiss, J.L. and Roth, T.F. (1983) Tubulin as a moleculur component of coated vesicles. *J. Cell Biol.*, 97:1191–1199.

Kennedy, M.B., Bennett, M.K. and Eronou, N.E. (1983) Biochemical and immunochemical evidence that the 'major postsynaptic density protein' is a subunit of a calmodulin-dependent protein kinase. *Proc. Natl. Acad. Sci. U.S.A.*, 80:7357–7361.

Kirchhausen, T. and Harrison, S.C. (1981) Protein organization in clathrin trimers. *Cell*, 23:755–761.

Kirchhausen, T., Harrison, S.C., Parham, P. and Brodsky, F.M. (1983) Location and distribution of the light chains in clathrin trimers. *Proc. Natl. Acad. Sci. U.S.A.*, 80:2481–2485.

Kristjansson, G.I., Zwiers, H., Oestreicher, A.B. and Gispen, W.H. (1982) Evidence that the synaptic phosphoprotein B-50 is localized exclusively in nerve tissue. *J. Neurochem.*, 39:371–378.

Miller, T.M. and Heuser, J.E. (1984) Endocytosis of synaptic vesicle membrane at the frog neuromuscular fonction. *J. Cell Biol.*, 98:685–689.

Mori, H. and Kurokawa, M. (1981) Intra-axonal transport of clathrin and actin. *Biomed. Res.*, 2:677–685.

Nagasawa, J., Douglas, W.W. and Schultz, R.A. (1971) Micropinocytotic origin of coated and smooth microvesicles ('synaptic vesicles') in neurosecretory terminals of posterior pituitary glands demonstrated by incorporation of horseradish peroxidase. *Nature*, 232:341–342.

Nagura, H., Nakane, P.K. and Brown, W.R. (1979) Translocation of dimeric IgA through neoplastic colon cells in vitro. *J. Immunol.*, 123:2359–2368.

Nandi, P.K., Van Jaarsveld, P.P., Lippoldt, R.E. and Edelhoch,

H. (1981) Effect of basic compounds on the polymerisation of clathrin. *Biochemistry*, 20:6706–6710.

Nichols, B.A., Bainton, D.F. and Farquhar, M.G. (1971) Differentiation of monocytes: origin, nature, and fate of their azurophil granules. *J. Cell Biol.*, 50:498–515.

Ottosen, P.D., Courtoy, P.J. and Farquhar, M.G. (1980) Pathways followed by membrane recovered from the surface of plasma cells and myeloma cells. *J. Exp. Med.*, 152:1–19.

Palade, G.E. (1975) Intracellular aspects of the process of protein secretion. *Science*, 189:347–358.

Patzer, E.J., Schlossman, D.M. and Rothman, J.E. (1982) Release of clathrin from coated vesicles dependent upon a nucleotide triphosphate and a cytosol fraction *J. Cell Biol.*, 93:230–236.

Pauloin, A., Bernier, I. and Jollès, P. (1982) Presence of a cyclic nucleotide/Ca^{2+}-independent protein kinase in bovine brain coated vesicles. *Nature*, 298:574–576.

Pauloin, A. (1984) Nature biochimique et fonctionnement du complexe protéine kinase-protéine substrat de 50 kDa spécifique d'une classe particulière de vésicules cytoplasmiques: les 'coated vesicles'. Thèse de Doctorat d'Etat. Université de Paris VI.

Pauloin, A. and Jollès, P. (1984) Internal control of the coated vesicle pp50-specific kinase complex. *Nature*, 311:265–267.

Pauloin, A. and Jollès, P. (1986) Presence of a MgATP/ADP-dependent pp50 phosphatase in bovine brain coated vesicles. *J. Biol. Chem.* (in press).

Pauloin, A., Loeb, J. and Jollès, P. (1984) Protein kinase(s) in bovine brain coated vesicles. *Biochim. Biophys. Acta*, 799:238–245.

Pearse, B.M.F. (1975) Coated vesicles from pig brain: purification and biochemical characterization. *J. Mol. Biol.*, 97:93–98.

Pearse, B.M.F. (1978) On the structural and functional components of coated vesicles. *J. Mol. Biol.*, 126:803–812.

Pearse, B.M.F. and Robinson, M.S. (1984) Purification and properties of 100-kd proteins from coated vesicles and their reconstitution with clathrin. *EMBO J.*, 3:1951–1957.

Pfeffer, S.R. and Kelly, R.B. (1981) Identification of minor components of coated vesicles by use of permeation chromatography. *J. Cell. Biol.*, 91:385–391.

Pfeffer, S.R. and Kelly, R.B. (1983) Identification of major, nontriskelion coated vesicle polypeptides. *J. Cell Biol.*, 97:174a.

Pfeffer, S.R., Drubin, D.G. and Kelly, R.B. (1983) Identification of three coated vesicle components as α- and β-tubulin linked to a phosphorylated 50,000-dalton polypeptide. *J. Cell Biol.*, 97:40–47.

Prasad, K., Lippoldt, R.E. and Edelhoch, H. (1985) Coat formation in coated vesicles. *Biochemistry*, 24:6421–6427.

Rees, R.P., Bunge, M.B. and Bunge, R.P. (1976) Morphological changes in the neuritic growth cone and target neuron during synaptic junction development in culture. *J. Cell Biol.*, 68:240–263.

Renston, R.H., Jones, A.L., Christiansen, W.D. and Hradek, G. (1980) Evidence for a vesicular transport mechanism in hepatocytes for biliary secretion of immunoglobulin A. *Science*, 208:1276–1278.

Rodewald, R. (1973) Intestinal transport of antibodies in the newborn rat. *J. Cell Biol.*, 58:189–211.

Rodewald, R. (1980) Distribution of immunoglobulin G receptors in the small intestine of the young rat. *J. Cell Biol.*, 85:18–32.

Rodionov, V.I., Nadezhdina, E.S., Leonova, E.V., Vaisberg, E.A., Kuznetsov, S.A. and Gelfand, V.I. (1985) Identification of a 100 kDa protein associated with microtubules, intermediate filaments and coated vesicles in cultured cells. *Exp. Cell Res.*, 159:377–387.

Roth, T.F., Woodward, M.P. and Wood, J. (1977) Comparison and selective dissociation of coated vesicles isolated from brain and oocytes. *J. Cell Biol.*, 75:372a.

Rothman, J.E. and Fine, R.E. (1980) Coated vesicles transport newly synthesized membrane glycoproteins from endoplasmic reticulum to plasma membrane in two successive stages. *Proc. Natl. Acad. Sci. U.S.A.*, 77:780–784.

Rothman, J.E., Bursztyn-Pettegrew, H. and Fine, R.E. (1980) Transport of the membrane glycoprotein of vesicular stomatitis virus to the cell surface in two stages by clathrin-coated vesicles. *J. Cell Biol.*, 86:162–171.

Rubenstein, J.L.R., Fine, R.E., Luskey, B.O. and Rothman, J.E. (1981) Purification of coated vesicles by agarose gel electrophoresis. *J. Cell Biol.*, 89:357–361.

Sattilaru, R.F. and Dentler, W.L. (1982) The association of MAP-2 with microtubules, actin filaments, and coated vesicles. In Sakai, H., Mohri, H. and Borisy, G. (Eds.), *Biological Functions of Microtubules and Related Structures*, Academic Press, New York, pp. 297–309.

Schaeffer, S. and Raviola, E. (1978) Membrane recycling in the cone cell endings of the turtle retina. *J. Cell Biol.*, 79:802–825.

Schlossman, D.M., Schmid, S.L., Braell, W.A. and Rothman, J.E. (1984) An enzyme that removes clathrin coat: purification of an uncoating ATPase. *J. Cell Biol.*, 99:723–733.

Schmid, S.L., Braell, W.A., Schlossman, D.M. and Rothman, J.E. (1984) A role for clathrin light chains in the recognition of clathrin cages by 'uncoating ATPase'. *Nature*, 311:228–231.

Schook, W., Puszkin, S., Bloom, W., Ores, C. and Kochwa, S. (1979) Mechanicochemical properties of brain clathrin: interaction with actin and α-actinin and polymerisation into basket like structures or filaments. *Proc. Natl. Acad. Sci. U.S.A.*, 76:116–120.

Schook, W.J. and Puszkin, S. (1985) Brain clathrin light chain 2 can be phosphorylated by a coated vesicle kinase. *Proc. Natl. Acad. Sci. U.S.A.*, 82:8039–8043.

Steineman, R.M., Mellman, I.S., Muller, W.A. and Cohn, Z.A. (1983) Endocytosis and recycling of plasma membrane. *J. Cell Biol.*, 96:1–27.

Stone, D.K., Xie, X.-S. and Racker, E. (1983) An ATP-driven proton pump in clathrin-coated vesicle. *J. Biol. Chem.*, 258:4059–4062.

Stone G.C., Hammerschlag, R. and Bobinski, J.A. (1984) Involvement of coated vesicles in the initiation of fast axonal transport. *Brain Res.*, 291:219–228.

272

Takahashi, A., Usami, M., Kadota, T. and Kadota, K. (1985) Properties of protein kinases in brain coated vesicles. *J. Biochem.*, 98:63–68.

Tsukita, S. and Ishikawa, S. (1980) The movement of membranous organelles in axons: electron microscopic identification of anterogradely and and retrogradely transported organelles. *J. Cell Biol.*, 84:513–530.

Tytell, M., Black, M.M., Garner, J.A. and Lasek, R.J. (1981) Axonal transport: each major rate component reflects the movement of distinct macromolecular complexes. *Science*, 214:179–181.

Unanue, E.R., Ungewickell, E. and Branton, D. (1981) The binding of clathrin triskelions to membrane from vesicles. *Cell*, 26:439–446.

Ungewickell, E. and Branton, D. (1981) Assembly units of clathrin coats. *Nature*, 289:420–422.

Ungewickell, E. and Branton, D. (1982) Triskelions: the building blocks of clathrin coats. *Trends Biochem. Sci.*, 7:358–361.

Ungewickell, E., Unanue, E.R. and Branton, D. (1982) Functional and structural studies on clathrin triskelions and baskets. *Cold Spring Harbor Symp.*, 57:723–731.

Ungewickell, E. (1983) Biochemical and immunological studies on clathrin light chains and their binding sites on clathrin triskelions. *EMBO J.*, 2:1401–1408.

Ungewickell, E. (1984) Characterization of clathrin and clathrin-associated proteins. *Biochem. Soc. Trans.*, 12:978–980.

Ungewickell, E. (1985) The 70-kD mammalian heat shock proteins are structurally and functionally related to the uncoating protein that releases clathrin triskelia from coated vesicles. *EMBO J.*, 4:3385–3391.

Usami, M., Takahashi, A. and Kadota, K. (1984) Protein kinase and its endogenous substrates in coated vesicles. *Biochim. Biophys. Acta*, 798:306–312.

Usami, M., Takahashi, A., Kadota, T. and Kadota, K. (1985) Phosphorylation of a clathrin light chain of coated vesicles in the presence of histones. *J. Biochem.*, 97:1819–1822.

Weingarten, M.D., Lockwood, A.H., Hwo, S. and Kirschner, M.W. (1975) A protein factor essential for microtubule assembly. *Proc. Natl. Acad. Sci. U.S.A.*, 72:1858–1862.

Wiedenmann, B. and Mimms, L.T. (1983) Tubulin is a major protein constituent of bovine brain coated vesicles. *Biochem. Biophys. Res. Commun.*, 115:303–311.

Zaremba, S. and Keen, J.H. (1983) Assembly polypeptides from coated vesicles mediate reassembly of unique clathrin coats. *J. Cell. Biol.*, 97:1339–1347.

Zaremba, S. and Keen, J.H. (1985) Limited proteolytic digestion of coated vesicle assembly polypeptides abolishes reassembly activity. *J. Cell. Biochem.*, 28:47–58.

W.H. Gispen and A. Routtenberg (Eds.)
Progress in Brain Research, Vol. 69,
© 1986 Elsevier Science Publishers B.V. (Biomedical Division)

CHAPTER 22

Depolarization-dependent protein phosphorylation in synaptosomes: mechanisms and significance

Peter R. Dunkley and Phillip J. Robinson*

The Neuroscience Group, Faculty of Medicine, The University of Newcastle, New South Wales 2308, Australia

Introduction

The release of neurotransmitters from nerve terminals is dependent upon calcium and ATP (Katz and Miledi, 1969; Blaustein, 1975; Bradford, 1975; Rasmussen and Goodman, 1977). A number of hypotheses have been developed to explain this dependency, but the molecular mechanism of neurotransmitter release is presently unknown.

The phosphorylation of proteins requires ATP and can be modulated by calcium (Dunkley, 1981; Rodnight, 1982; DeLorenzo et al., 1982; Nestler and Greengard, 1984). Activation of calcium-stimulated protein kinases has therefore been postulated to be the 'missing link' between the entry of calcium into nerve terminals and the release of neurotransmitters (Fig. 1; DeLorenzo et al., 1982; Nestler and Greengard, 1984).

Considerable indirect evidence supports the notion that calcium-stimulated protein phosphorylation may be involved in neurotransmitter release. Firstly, a number of calcium-dependent protein kinases are present in neuronal tissue (Kennedy and Greengard, 1981; Goldenring et al., 1983; Kennedy et al., 1983; Aloyo et al., 1983; Rostas et al., 1983b, 1986; Chapter 27) and many proteins are phosphorylated by these enzymes (Rodnight, 1982; DeLorenzo et al., 1982; Aloyo et al, 1983; Sorensen and Mahler, 1983; Walaas et al., 1983a,b; Akers and Routtenberg, 1985; Nestler and Greengard, 1984; Dunkley et al., 1986b).

Secondly, both the protein kinases and their substrates are present in subcellular locations consistent with a role in neurotransmitter release, including synaptic plasma membranes, synaptic vesicles, synaptic cytoskeleton and synaptoplasm (Rodnight, 1982; DeLorenzo et al., 1982; Nestler and Greengard, 1984; Sahyoun et al., 1985). Thirdly, depolarization of neuronal tissue causes a calcium- and ATP-dependent increase in the phosphorylation of a number of proteins, a phenomenon which has been observed in brain slices (Williams and Rodnight, 1977; Forn and Greengard, 1978) and intact neuronal cells (Novak-Hofer et al., 1985; DeRiemer et al., 1984; Saitoh and Schwartz, 1983, 1985). Finally, phosphorylation of nerve terminal-proteins has been observed in vivo (Julien and Mushynski, 1981; Mitrius et al., 1981; Berman et al., 1984; Rodnight et al., 1985; Lyn-Cook et al., 1985) and conditions that are known to alter neurotransmitter release in vivo also modify protein phosphorylation (Holmes et al., 1977; Dunkley et al., 1983; Williams and Clouet, 1982; Routtenberg et al., 1979, 1984, 1985).

A number of experimental systems have been used to investigate the role(s) of protein phosphorylation in neurotransmitter release (Nestler and Greengard, 1984) and of these, synaptosome preparations constitute an excellent model. These subcellular organelles have the particular advantage of being an in vitro nerve terminal preparation which retains the capacity to release neurotransmitters in a physiologically relevant manner (Bradford, 1975). They are relatively

---

*Present address: Merrell Dow Research Institute, Cincinnati, OH 45215, U.S.A.

274

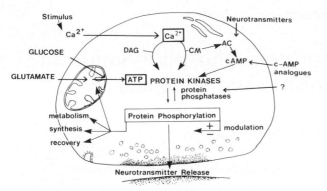

Fig. 1. A model for the phosphorylation of synaptosomal proteins. Entry of calcium (Ca^{2+}) into synaptosomes as a result of a stimulus such as depolarization can lead directly or indirectly to activation of diacyl glycerol (DAG) and hence protein kinase C and calmodulin (CM) or cyclic AMP (cAMP)-stimulated protein kinases. The extent of protein kinase activation can be altered by the environment of the synaptosome and the major factors operating here include the level of extrasynaptosomal calcium, the degree of activation of adenylate cyclase by neurotransmitters acting on presynaptic receptors, the availability of energy substrates such as glucose and glutamate for the provision of ATP and the extent of activation of protein phosphatases which provide vacant sites on proteins for protein kinases to label. The phosphorylation of various synaptosomal proteins can initiate their physiological effect, including neurotransmitter release, the recovery of synaptosomal energy, neurotransmitter and vesicle content and the metabolic status of the synaptosome.

homogeneous compared to neuronal cell cultures, which contain axons, cell bodies, dendrites and nuclei, and brain slices, which contain non-neuronal cells. Synaptosomes have the additional advantage that changes in protein phosphorylation can be measured directly, without the need for post hoc or back-phosphorylation procedures (Rodnight, 1982; Nestler and Greengard, 1984). This avoids the confounding effects of protein phosphatase activity which can occur during isolation of tissue and subsequent subcellular fractionation. Finally, synaptosomes can be studied in test-tube systems which allow a controlled environment to be maintained. This is especially useful when investigating the effects of drugs on protein phosphorylation and when neurotransmitter release needs to be measured in parallel (DeLorenzo et al., 1982).

A number of studies have documented changes

in protein phosphorylation following depolarization of synaptosomes which are dependent on exogenous calcium and endogenous ATP and which in general parallel the release of neurotransmitters (Krueger et al., 1977; Breithaupt and Babitch, 1979; DeLorenzo et al., 1979; Michaelson and Avissar, 1979; Michaelson et al., 1979; Wu et al., 1982; Robinson and Dunkley, 1983a,b,c, 1985; Nestler and Greengard, 1984; Robinson et al., 1984; Dunkley et al., 1986b). Assuming that these changes are not artefacts resulting from the in vitro conditions used it is likely that they are involved directly or indirectly in neurotransmitter release, as this is the primary function of nerve terminals.

The aims of this chapter are:

(a) To review the methods used to study synaptosomal protein phosphorylation in order to evaluate the limitations of the procedures and the likelihood of introducing in vitro artefacts.
(b) To describe the major synaptosomal phosphoproteins and the effect of depolarization on their labeling with $^{32}P_i$. Emphasis will be placed on phosphoproteins having molecular weights between 40 and 90 kDa, as these proteins have been extensively investigated in disrupted synaptic tissue.
(c) To propose mechanisms of protein kinase activation and control, which account for the observed phosphorylation of proteins before and after depolarization.
(d) To outline the possible functions of the major synaptosomal phosphoproteins in relation to neurotransmitter release.

What methods are used to investigate synaptosomal protein phosphorylation?

General procedures

The procedure generally used to investigate protein phosphorylation in intact synaptosomes was established by Krueger et al. (1977) and extensively developed in our laboratory (Robinson and Dunkley, 1983a, 1985; Dunkley et al., 1986b).

A subcellular fraction containing synaptosomes is isolated and incubated with $^{32}P_i$ for a suitable

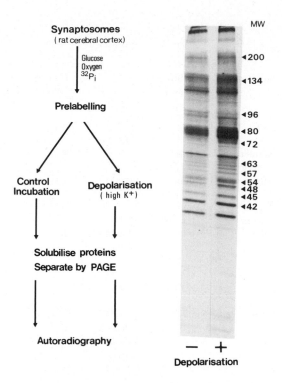

Fig. 2. The procedures used to investigate synaptosomal protein phosphorylation. A general outline of the steps involved is shown on the left. PAGE; polyacrylamide gel electrophoresis. Right: autoradiographs from a typical experiment (Robinson and Dunkley, 1983a) showing the synaptosomal phosphoproteins before and after depolarization. The apparent molecular weights of major phosphoproteins are indicated.

time in order to generate endogenous radiolabeled ATP ($[\gamma\text{-}^{32}P]ATP$) (Fig. 2). We refer to this incubation as the prelabeling period. Endogenous protein kinases use the $[\gamma\text{-}^{32}P]ATP$ and incorporate $^{32}P_i$ into serine and threonine residues in proteins that were made vacant by protein phosphatase activity. It should be noted here that many proteins will still contain phosphate which is not radiolabeled and it is assumed that the radiolabeled phosphate incorporation provides an accurate indication of what is occurring with all protein phosphorylation events. A depolarizing stimulus is applied to synaptosomes during a brief incubation period after which proteins are solubilized in sodium dodecylsulphate and fractionated by polyacrylamide gel electrophoresis. After drying the gels, auto-radiography reveals which phosphoproteins are labeled

during the prelabeling period and which are modulated by depolarization (Fig. 2). Most of the important variables in this procedure are discussed below and Table I summarizes the procedures used in other laboratories.

Tissue used to prepare synaptosomes

The most commonly used tissue for preparation of synaptosomes and investigation of depolarization-stimulated protein phosphorylation has been rat cerebral cortex (Table I). This tissue contains a large number of neurotransmitter types and thus the population of synaptosomes isolated is heterogeneous. The major phosphoproteins observed are likely to be present at a high concentration in most nerve terminals, be labeled rapidly or have a high molar ratio of $^{32}P_i$ to protein. The fact that most major phosphoproteins seen in rat cerebral cortex are also seen in other regions of the rat central nervous system (Walaas et al., 1983a, 1983b), in chicken brains (Breithaupt and Babitch, 1979; Rostas et al., 1983a) and in the brains of other species (Rodnight, 1982) supports this proposal. Michaelson et al. (1979) and Michaelson and Avissar (1979) have investigated synaptosomes obtained from *Torpedo* electric organ which contain a homogeneous population of cholinergic nerve terminals. The major phosphoproteins present were different from those found in the rat cortical synaptosomes and the proteins affected by dopolarization were also unique. Whether this reflects a species difference or an enrichment of cholinergic nerve terminal phosphoproteins is unknown.

Procedures used to prepare synaptosomes

The homogeneity of synaptosomes used to investigate the effects of depolarization of protein phosphorylation varies (Table 1). Most investigators have used the P2 fraction which contains, in addition to synaptosomes, mitochondria, myelin and a large population of unidentified membranous structures of both glial and neuronal origin. Use of this fraction is justified on two grounds. Firstly, the preparation is rapid, only a few steps are involved and the synaptosomes are not exposed to

TABLE I

The conditions used to study synaptosomal protein phosphorylation

Laboratory	Species	Fraction	Protein concn. (mg/ml)	Medium	Prelabeling		Time of depolarization
					Time	Calcium	
Krueger et al. (1977)	Rat (cortex)	P2	5.0	KRB[a]	30 min	0.1 mM EGTA	30 s
Clouet et al. (1978)	Rat (cortex)	P2B[b]	?	Isotonic medium	30 min	?	30 s
Huttner and Greengard (1979)	Rat (cortex)	P2	2.0	KRB	30 min	1.0 mM	30 s
DeLorenzo et al. (1979)	Rat (cortex)	P2B	10.0	Buffered saline	12 min	0	5 min
Michaelson and Avissar (1979)	Torpedo (electric organ)	P2B	1.8	KRB	30 min	0.1 mM EGTA	60 s
Breithaupt and Babitch (1979)	Chick (cortex)	P2B	2.0	KRB	15 s– 15 min	1.4 mM or 0	15 s
Sieghart (1981)	Rat (cortex)	P2	5.0	KRB	5 min	0.1 mM EGTA	5 min
Wu et al. (1982)	Rat (cortex)	P2	3.5	KRB	30 min	0.1 mM EGTA	30 s
Robinson and Dunkley (1983a, 1985)	Rat (cortex)	P2	2.5	KRB	45 min	0.1 mM	15 s

[a] Krebs–Ringer buffer.
[b] Purified synaptosomes.

hypertonic conditions; this significantly decreases the chances of loss of synaptosomal integrity by either chemical or mechanical damage. Secondly, a number of studies have indicated that during the prelabeling period the vast majority of phosphoproteins labeled with $^{32}P_i$, are those found within the synaptosomal portion of the P2 fraction (Krueger et al., 1977; Breithaupt and Babitch, 1979; Robinson and Dunkley, unpublished data). The results presented throughout this chapter were obtained using a crude synaptosomal (P2) fraction isolated from rat cerebral cortex.

Conditions used to prelabel synaptosomes

Radiolabeled ATP formation

Prelabeling synaptosomes leads to the uptake of radiolabeled phosphate and its incorporation into ATP (Fig. 3). This must occur primarily within mitochondria, as mitochondrial poisons dramatically inhibit subsequent protein phosphorylation (Krueger et al., 1977; Breithaupt and Babitch, 1979; Robinson et al., 1984). If the equilibrium between $^{32}P_i$ and $[\gamma^{-32}P]ATP$ is not reached before depolarization of synaptosomes, then any change in protein phosphorylation may simply reflect a change in the formation of radiolabeled ATP. Salamin et al. (1981) found that equilibrium between $^{32}P_i$ and $[\gamma^{-32}P]ATP$ did not occur in synaptosomes until 45 min. However, estimation of total ATP levels in the P2 fraction throughout an extended prelabeling period indicated that over 80% was lost by 180 min (Fig. 3) and any loss of total ATP is likely to lead to a decrease in synaptosomal viability. The prelabeling time chosen therefore reflects a balance between establishing an equilibrium for $^{32}P_i$ and maintenance of synaptosomal viability.

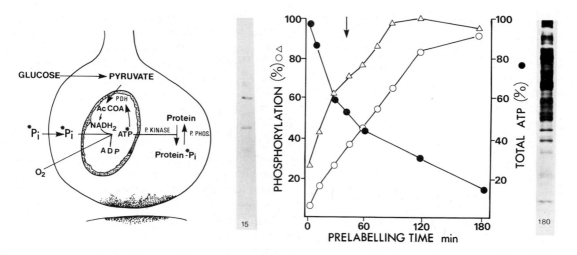

Fig. 3. The effect of prelabeling time on synaptosomal protein phosphorylation and ATP levels. The uptake of ^{32}P$_i$, its incorporation into ATP and transfer to protein is shown schematically on the left. Autoradiographs of synaptosomal phosphoproteins seen after prelabeling for 15 and 180 min are shown in the center and on the right. The incorporation of radiolabel into the mitochondrial enzyme pyruvate dehydrogenase (▲) and all synaptosomal phosphoproteins (○) is shown, together with the loss of total ATP (●), as measured by the luciferin–luciferase technique (Robinson et al., 1984). The arrow indicates the 45 min prelabeling point which is generally used in this laboratory.

Cold phosphate is not included during prelabeling as this competes with radiolabeled phosphate and drastically decreases the formation of radiolabeled ATP. Addition of inorganic phosphate did not modify the overall profile of labeled proteins (Robinson and Dunkley, unpublished data), but may affect other nerve terminal functions including neurotransmitter release.

The level and formation of radiolabeled ATP can be modified by the presence of substrates for mitochondrial ATP formation. Glucose, glutamate, succinate and 2-oxoglutarate all increase the phosphorylation of the α subunit of pyruvate dehydrogenase, a mitochondraial phosphoprotein, presumably by a metabolic effect on ATP formation (Sieghart, 1981; Robinson and Dunkley, unpublished data).

The concentration of synaptosomal protein used during prelabeling is another factor potentially able to modulate ATP formation. The higher the concentration of protein, the higher the requirements for glucose and oxygen, but Bradford (1975) found that synaptosomal beds maintained viability for longer periods than did dilute suspensions of synaptosomes.

Radiolabeled protein formation

Radiolabeled ATP is used by protein kinases to incorporate ^{32}P$_i$ into serine and threonine residues in proteins. Other protein kinases, such as tyrosine kinase (Gurd, 1985), will not be considered here. Incorporation can only occur into vacant sites and these are formed by protein phosphatase activity. Thus, the labeling of synaptosomal proteins is dependent on the level and specific activity of ATP, as well as on the relative activity of protein kinases and protein phosphatases. ^{32}P$_i$ incorporation into protein has three distinct phases (Fig. 3). In the first 10 min there is a very rapid incorporation of radiolabel, mainly into mitochondrial protein, such as the α subunit of pyruvate dehydrogenase. There is a subsequent period of up to 120 min in which the incorporation of ^{32}P$_i$ into protein is linear for almost all of the phosphoproteins labeled. There is then a decreased rate of incorporation from 120 min up to approximately 4 h (Robinson and Dunkley, 1983b), presumably because of decreased synaptosomal viability due to loss of ATP (Fig. 3).

In our laboratory 45 min is the usual period for prelabeling as this falls on the linear portion of the

278

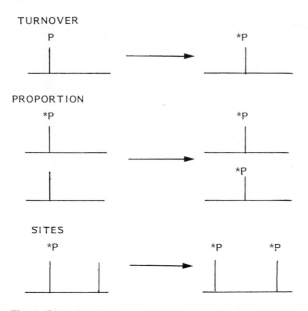

TURNOVER

PROPORTION

SITES

Fig. 4. Phosphate incorporation into synaptosomal protein. When the level of radiolabeled phosphate (*P) incorporated into protein is increased, three possible events could be occurring. Turnover reflects removal of unlabeled phosphate by protein phosphatases and its replacement by radiolabelled phosphate. This occurs during the prelabeling period and the rate of turnover may be increased on depolarization. No change in function occurs as a result of turnover. An increase in the proportion of total protein containing phosphate at a particular site will increase the activity of that protein or, if phosphorylation causes inhibition, the activity of the protein will be decreased. New sites can also be labeled which could allow a protein to undertake a new function as well as alter the level of existing function.

protein phosphorylation curve, and is the earliest time at which $^{32}P_i$ is likely to be in equilibrium with $[\gamma\text{-}^{32}P]ATP$. Others have used different times for prelabeling (Table I). It is clear that when synaptosomes are depolarized, even after 45 min prelabeling, equilibrium has not been established between labeled and unlabeled phosphate in protein, as basal incorporation continues to rise. It is possible therefore that some of the increased incorporation of radiolabel which occurs on depolarization may relate to increased turnover of radiolabeled for non-radiolabeled phosphate rather than phosphorylation of sites on proteins which were vacant before depolarization (Fig. 4). Turnover would not lead to a change in the

function of a protein as its phosphate content would be unaltered. This has not been investigated thoroughly for any synaptosomal phosphoprotein, although Krueger et al. (1977) claimed that increased phosphate incorporation rather than turnover occurred with synapsin I.

Incorporation of $^{32}P_i$ into vacant sites on proteins could reflect either a change in the number of sites labeled on a particular protein and/or a change in the proportion of that protein containing label (Fig. 4). Different physiological consequences could result from each type of change. Thus, a new site being labeled could reflect new or altered activity, while an increase in the proportion of phosphorylated to non-phosphorylated protein could only reflect an increase in the number of active (inactive) proteins. There is little information currently available on the stoichiometry of phosphorylation (mole of phosphate per mole of protein) of any protein within synaptosomes, although it is clear that many contain a number of phosphorylatable sites (see below).

Effects of calcium

The amount of calcium present in the prelabeling media varied from 0 to 2.5 mM between laboratories, and in a number of instances prelabeling was performed in the presence of EGTA (Table I). Calcium up to 0.1 mM increased basal phosphorylation while higher concentration inhibited phosphorylation (Robinson and Dunkley, 1985). It was found that addition of calcium alone to synaptosomes prelabeled in its absence markedly increased basal levels of protein phosphorylation and, hence, if the effects of depolarization are to be investigated, calcium should not be added with the depolarizing stimulus but the system should be in equilibrium with respect to calcium prior to depolarization.

Presynaptic effectors

Michaelson et al. (1979) have investigated synaptosomes isolated from *Torpedo* and found that acetylcholine, acting via a presynaptic receptor, modulates the degree of phosphorylation of proteins. Similar feedback mechanisms are likely to be operating in synaptosomes isolated from rat cerebral cortex, where a number of effectors will be released during the preincubation period. Thus, for example, released adenosine or other neurotransmitters with presynaptic receptors could act to modulate cyclic AMP or calcium levels within the synaptosomes and hence alter levels of protein phosphorylation (Fig. 1). To date, nobody has investigated the effects on protein phosphorylation of removing these neurotransmitters by superfusion or by the addition of specific antagonists.

Summary

The basal level of protein phosphorylation in synaptosomes depends on the tissue and the procedures used to prepare the synaptosomes. It also depends on the level and specific activity of radiolabeled ATP formed and the relative activity of protein kinases and protein phosphatases. These can be modulated by the amount of energy substrate, phosphate, protein, calcium and presynaptic effectors present during prelabeling and the length of the prelabeling period. Although these factors change the relative labeling of synaptosomal phosphoproteins, many of the labeled proteins have been found to be phosphoproteins in vivo (Rodnight et al., 1985; Lyn-Cook et al., 1985) and hence the incorporation of $^{32}P_i$ per se is not likely to be an artefact of the in vitro system. It remains for us to determine which in vitro condition most closely represents that occurring around nerve terminals in vivo but, for now at least, the optimum conditions and the limitations of the in vitro technique have been established.

Which synaptosomal phosphoproteins incorporate $^{32}P_i$ during the prelabeling period?

Previous studies using exogenous $[\gamma\text{-}^{32}P]ATP$ and lyzed synaptosomal tissue have identified a number of phosphoproteins, whose characteristics are known, including their molecular weight and pI values, which sites are labeled by specific protein kinases, the molecular weight of their phosphopeptides produced by protease digestion,

their solubility in acid, alkali and high ionic strength buffers, their subcellular distribution, their developmental profiles and, in some instances, their function (Rodnight, 1982; Mahler et al., 1982; Nestler and Greengard, 1984; Zwiers et al., 1985; Dunkley et al., 1986b). A number of the synaptosomal proteins labeled with $^{32}P_i$ during the prelabeling period have the same mobility as these previously well-characterized phosphoproteins (Fig. 5; Dunkley and Robinson. 1983; Robinson and Dunkley, 1983c; Dunkley et al., 1986b). Using a number of criteria, we established the identity of ten proteins labeled with $^{32}P_i$ in intact synaptosomes; phosphoprotein 83 is the 87K phosphoprotein; phosphoproteins 80 and 75 are synapsin Ia and Ib; phosphoproteins 72 and 57a are phosphoproteins IIIa and IIIb; phosphoproteins 63 and 48 are the calmodulin kinase subunits; phosphoprotein 57b is tubulin; phosphoprotein 45 is the B-50 protein; and phosphoprotein 42 is the α subunit of pyruvate dehydrogenase (Table II; Robinson and Dunkley, 1983b; Dunkley et al., 1986b). Only synapsin Ia and Ib (Krueger et al., 1977), the 87K phosphoprotein (Wu et al., 1982), and tubulin (DeLorenzo et al., 1982) had previously been identified as phosphoproteins in $^{32}P_i$-labeled synaptosomes. The most common name for these phosphoproteins will be used throughout the text rather than referring to them by the apparent molecular weight which we observe, as identity has been established (Table II).

The relative incorporation of $^{32}P_i$ into these synaptosomal proteins during the prelabeling period does not match that observed after exogenous ATP addition to lyzed synaptosomes, suggesting a unique pattern of protein kinase activation in the intact nerve terminal (Fig. 5). Synapsin Ia and Ib, and the α subunit of pyruvate dehydrogenase are major phosphoproteins, as is the unidentified phosphoprotein 65 (Fig. 5). The level of labeling of phosphoprotein 87, phosphoproteins IIIa and IIIb, the 63- and and 48-kDa calmodulin kinase subunits, tubulin and the B-50 protein is low compared to the level achieved under optimum conditions in lyzed synaptosomes (Dunkley et al., 1986b). One reason is the 45-min prelabeling time chosen, as increased labeling of some of these proteins occurs after 180 min (Fig.

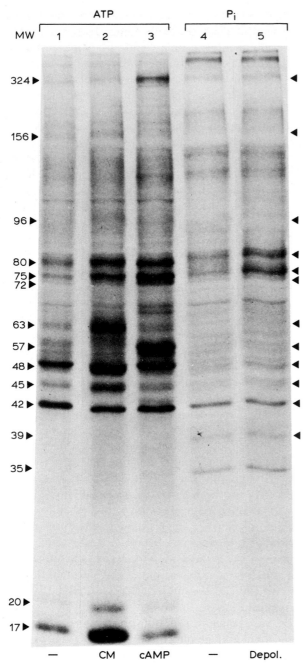

MW 1 2 3 4 5

ATP   P$_i$

324 ▶
156 ▶
96 ▶
80 ▶
75 ▶
72 ▶
63 ▶
57 ▶
48 ▶
45 ▶
42 ▶
39 ▶
35 ▶
20 ▶
17 ▶

— CM cAMP — Depol.

Fig. 5. Synaptosomal phosphoproteins labeled in lyzed tissue after incubation with [γ-^{32}P]ATP (tracks 1–3) or in intact tissue after incubation with ^{32}P$_i$ (tracks 4,5). ATP labeling was undertaken at 37°C for 30 s, with 40 μM ATP, 1.2 mM MgCl$_2$, 1.0 mM EGTA, 30 mM Tris-HCl (pH 7.4) and 1 mg of P2 protein per ml (-). Calmodulin (CM) was added to a final concentration of 0.1 μg/μl with 1.1 mM calcium and cyclic AMP (cAMP) was 50 μM (Dunkley and Robinson, 1981). P$_i$

3), suggesting that turnover of phosphate may be slower for this group of proteins. It should be remembered that the calmodulin kinase subunits and tubulin are localized on postsynaptic densities (Rostas et al., 1983b, 1986; Chapter 27) which remain attached to synaptosomes during tissue preparation and proteins in this location would not be accessible to the radiolabeled ATP formed within synaptosomes, but would be accessible to exogenous radiolabeled ATP. It is also possible that the protein kinases and protein phosphatases are not coupled to their substrates in the same way in intact synaptosomes, or that they are partially inactivated during the prelabeling period. Thus, actin is phosphorylated in lyzed synaptosomes by an endogenous cyclic AMP-stimulated protein kinase, but is hardly labeled in intact synaptosomes (Dunkley and Robinson, 1983; Dunkley et al., 1986b).

There are major differences in ^{32}P$_i$ incorporation into proteins in the high and low molecular weight regions of the polyacrylamide gel after the prelabeling period and after exogenous ATP is added to lyzed synaptosomes (Fig. 5). Some of these differences are currently being investigated.

Which protein kinases are active during prelabeling of intact synaptosomes?

Calmodulin kinase II, protein kinase C and the cyclic AMP-stimulated protein kinase are the major serine and threonine kinases present in synaptic tissue (Rodnight, 1982; Nestler and Greengard, 1984; Chapter 27); calmodulin kinase I was not detected in synaptosomes (Dunkley et al., 1986b). One approach to estimating the activity of these kinases in intact synaptosomes is to analyze the labeling of their specific substrates. As many proteins have more than one site phosphorylated

labeling was undertaken at 37°C for 45 min in buffer containing 143 mM Na, 4.7 mM K, 0.1 mM Ca, 1.2 mM Mg, 24.9 mM HCO$_3$, 126 mM Cl and 10 mM glucose and at a final protein concentration of 2.5 mg/ml (–). Depolarisation was for 15 s in the presence of 41 mM K (Depol; Robinson and Dunkley, 1985).

TABLE II

Synaptosomal phosphoproteins

MW[a,1]	pI[b,2]	Designations	ATP labeling[c] Kinase	P peptides[e]	Pi labeling[d] Identity[f]	P peptides[e]	Name
83–72 (77)	(4)	β2[6], 87[7]	C[1,7]	41 17 13[7], 15	S, P	41 17	P-protein
80	(10)	β3, 86, D_1[8]	CM[7] A[7] C[1]	65 41 35[7], 35 19 18 10[7], 10	N. P, A	65 41 32 19 17 10	Synapsin Ia
75	(10)	β4, 80, D_2	CM[7] A[7] C[1]	60 40 35[7], 32 19 18 10[7], 10	N, P, A	60 40 32 19 18 10	Synapsin Ib
72	7.1–7.6	β5, 74	A	28 21 7	N, P, A	21	Protein IIIa
65		66	–	26	P	26	P-protein 65
63 (60K)[5]	6.7–7.0	β6, 62, E	CM[5]	42	P?		CM kinase II
61	6.7–7.0	β7, 58	CM[5]	42	P?		CM kinase II
60			A[1]		P?		Reg subunit?
57a (59)[2]	6.5–7.3	γ2, 55	A[1]	21	N, P, A	21	Protein IIIb
57b (59)[2]	4.7, 5.0	γ2	CM[1], A[2]	19	P?		Tubulin
54		IIb	A[1]				Reg subunit?
53					P?		
50		γ3			P		Chapter 21
48 (50K)[5]	6.7–7.0[5]	γ4, 48, E_3, 52[9]. DPHM[9]	CM[5]	42 35	N, P?		CM kinase II
48–45 (46)[4]	4.2	γ5, 46, F_1, B-50[9]	C[1], ?	28[9], 27 15[9], 12		12	B-50
43 (44)[4]	5.2		A[2]	14	P?		Actin
42	6.9	F_2		32 17 13	P	32 17 13	Subunit PDH

[a] Apparent molecular weight[1]. Values in brackets are previous designations for the same phosphoprotein in our laboratory.

[b] Phosphoproteins 83, 80, 75 are estimates only [1]; phosphoprotein 72 showed two spots; phosphoprotein 57a showed five spots; phosphoprotein 57b was two spots, presumably α and β tubulin, phosphoproteins 63, 61 and 48 smeared to the origin[5].

[c] Incubation of lyzed synaptosomes with [γ-^{32}P] ATP.

[d] Incubation of intact synaptosomes with $^{32}P_i$.

[e] Apparent molecular weight of phosphopeptides obtained after *Staphylococcus aureus* protease digestion.

[f] This identification was made after measuring the mobility of the phosphoprotein on non-equilibrium pH gradient electrophoresis (N) and the mobility of phosphopeptides derived from it by protease digestion (P), before and after acid extraction (A) of labeled synaptosomes. S, present in P2 soluble fraction[5]. ?, probable identity.

Sources: 1, Dunkley et al. (1986b); 2, Robinson and Dunkley (1983a); 3, Robinson and Dunkley (1985); 4, Dunkley and Robinson (1983); 5, Rostas et al. (1986); 6, Rodnight (1982); 7. Walaas et al. (1983a, 1983b); 8, Routtenberg (1984); 9, Zwiers et al. (1985).

282

by more than one kinase, analysis of the labeling of whole proteins is inadequate and analysis of individual sites is required.

A method has been developed for proteolytic digestion of synaptosomal phosphoproteins within a large segment of polyacrylamide gel and subsequent fractionation of the phosphopeptides generated on a second polyacrylamide gel to form a phosphopeptide 'map' (Dunkley et al., 1986b). This procedure allowed the simultaneous analysis of $^{32}P_i$ -labeled phosphopeptides derived from all the synaptosomal phosphoproteins with molecular weights of between 40 and 90 kDa and increased the specificity of measuring protein kinase

activation. Typical phosphopeptide maps obtained after labeling lyzed synaptosomes with [γ-^{32}P]ATP under conditions which specifically activate cyclic AMP-, calcium- or calcium plus calmodulin-stimulated protein kinases are shown in Fig. 6. Activation of cyclic AMP-stimulated protein kinase increased $^{32}P_i$ incorporation into a number of phosphopeptides of approximately 20 kDa, while activation of calmodulin kinase increased incorporation into larger phosphopeptides. Comparison of the 'maps' obtained with calcium alone versus calcium plus calmodulin showed that calmodulin caused a marked decrease in the phosphorylation of at least four phospho-

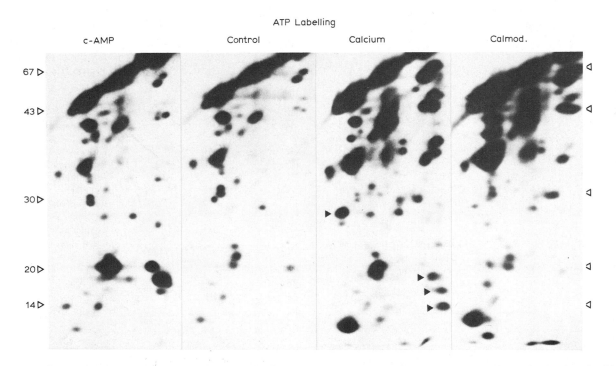

Fig. 6. Phosphopeptide 'maps' obtained after ATP labeling of lyzed synaptosomes. Lysed P2 fractions were incubated with [γ-^{32}P]ATP; phosphorylation was always in the presence of 1 mM EGTA (control), or with the addition of 50 μM cyclic AMP (cAMP), 1.1 mM calcium (calcium) or 1.1 mM calcium together with 0.1 μg/ul calmodulin (calmod). The labeled phosphoproteins were separated by PAGE as described in Fig. 5. The region of the polyacrylamide gel containing phosphoproteins of apparent molecular masses between 40 and 90 kDa was excised. This gel segment was then placed on the top of a second polyacrylamide gel (15% acrylamide) and the proteins within the segment were digested by adding Staphylococcus aureus V8 protease. After 30 min digestion, a current was applied to the second gel to separate the phosphopeptides produced by proteolysis. Phosphopeptides which had incorporated $^{32}P_i$ during incubation with radiolabeled ATP were detected by autoradiography of the polyacrylamide gel (Dunkley et al., 1986b). The top of the segment from the first gel which was digested with protease was placed on the right hand side of the second gel and the diagonal line of radiolabel seen across the top of each autoradiograph is undigested phosphoprotein. The apparent molecular weight of the radiolabeled phosphopeptides is indicated on the left. Phosphopeptides indicated with an arrow in the calcium autoradiograph showed decreased phosphorylation in the presence of calmodulin.

peptides (see arrows in Fig. 6). This is characteristic of the inhibition by calmodulin of protein kinase C (Wu et al., 1982; Albert et al., 1984), which was therefore assumed to have labeled these peptides. Using these 'maps', it is possible to identify phosphopeptides labeled specifically by each of the three major synaptosomal kinases. Some phosphopeptides are labeled by more than one kinase, while others are unaffected by activators or inhibitors of these enzymes (Fig. 6; Dunkley et al., 1986b).

Before using the peptide 'maps' to investigate the activity of specific protein kinases in intact synaptosomes, information was obtained about the proteins which, on digestion with protease, generated the labeled phosphopeptides. This was achieved by incubating lyzed synaptosomes with $[\gamma\text{-}^{32}P]ATP$, isolating the phosphoproteins by fractionation on two-dimensional gels or by acid extraction, and preparation of peptide 'maps' for individual phosphoproteins (Dunkley et al., 1986b). A number of results were obtained from these studies, including three which were unexpected. Firstly, phosphoprotein 87 and the B-50 protein are known substrates of protein kinase C and three of the peptides whose labeling was decreased in the presence of calmodulin are derived from these proteins, but in addition a phosphopeptide derived from synapsin Ia and Ib showed decreased labeling (Fig. 6). This suggests that synapsin I is a substrate for endogenous protein kinase C at the site usually labeled by cyclic AMP-stimulated protein kinase. The labeling of synapsin I and the B-50 protein by protein kinase C did not always occur when calcium was added alone, but the labeling of phosphoprotein 87 was very reproducible. Secondly, the B-50 protein was always labeled at a second site which was not inhibited by calmodulin. This suggests that the B-50 protein may be a substrate for a second protein kinase, or that not all of the actions of protein kinase C are inhibited by calmodulin. Thirdly, it was found that phosphoprotein IIIa was labeled by an endogenous calmodulin kinase at a site different to that labeled by the cyclic AMP kinase (Dunkley et al., 1986b).

When synaptosomes are prelabeled with $^{32}P_i$

and a 'map' is prepared, the majority of the phosphopeptides co-migrated with spots seen after ATP-labeling of lyzed synaptosomes, suggesting that cyclic AMP- and calmodulin-kinases and protein kinase C are all active (Fig. 7). Thus, the sites on synapsin Ia and Ib, phosphoprotein IIIa and IIIb labeled by cyclic AMP-stimulated protein kinases in lyzed synaptosomes were all labeled in intact synaptosomes. Similarly. the sites on synapsin Ia and Ib and phosphoprotein IIIa labeled by calmodulin kinase II, and the sites on phosphoprotein 87 labeled by protein kinase C in lyzed synaptosomes, were all labeled in intact synaptosomes. The B-50 protein was generally only labeled at one site (ca 12 kDa) in intact synaptosomes and that was the site not inhibited by the addition of calmodulin in lyzed synaptosomes. Very few new phosphopeptides were seen in intact synaptosomes, suggesting that calmodulin kinase II, cyclic AMP-stimulated kinase and protein kinase C account for most of the labeling in intact synaptosomes. The major exception has not been identified (Fig. 7; Dunkley et al., 1986b).

It is possible that in the intact synaptosome protein kinases could have altered access to substrates so that even though the peptide labeled in intact synaptosomes is the same as the peptide labeled in lyzed synaptosomes a different protein kinase could be responsible. It is difficult to prove that this is not occurring without some direct assay for protein kinase activation or means of specifically inhibiting particular protein kinases. However, the following results are consistent with the notion that protein kinase specificity remains essentially the same in intact synaptosomes as it is in lyzed synaptosomes. Firstly, when intact synaptosomes are prelabeled in the presence of dibutyryl cyclic AMP or theophylline, agents which increase cyclic AMP levels, there is a marked increase in labeling of synapsin Ia and Ib and phosphoprotein IIIa and IIIb at the sites labeled by the cyclic AMP-stimulated protein kinase in lyzed synaptosomes (Dunkley et al., 1986b). Few other phosphopeptides are affected. Thus, agents which increase cyclic AMP levels activate cyclic AMP-stimulated protein kinases in intact synaptosomes. Secondly, cyclic AMP-and calmodulin-stimulated

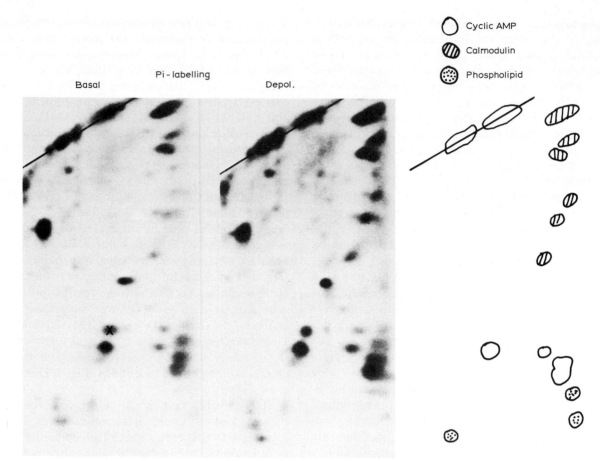

Fig. 7. Phosphopeptide 'maps' obtained after P$_i$ labeling of intact synaptosomes. An intact P2 fraction was incubated with ^{32}P$_i$ as described in the legend to Fig. 5. Before (basal) after (depol.) depolarization with 41 mM K for 15 s. The diagonal line of undigested protein is indicated on the right, as are the major phosphopeptides whose labeling was increased on depolarization. The protein kinase responsible for the major labeling of these phosphopeptides in lyzed synaptosomes (Fig. 5) is also indicated. The phosphopeptide labeled with a cross (×) was not observed to be labeled in lyzed synaptosomes incubated with [γ-^{32}P]ATP.

protein kinases are known to have little cross-reactivity in terms of peptide substrates (Fig. 6). Cross-reactivity occurs between cyclic AMP and protein kinase C (Vulliet et al., 1985) and it remains a possibility that protein kinase C could be responsible for some of the labeling of substrates, such as synapsin I in intact synaptosomes. However, no evidence was found for protein kinase C labeling of phosphoprotein IIIb, which was a major substrate for the cyclic AMP-stimulated protein kinase in lyzed synaptosomes and this substrate was heavily labeled in intact

synaptosomes at the same site (Figs. 6 and 7). Finally, decreasing the concentration of calcium during prelabeling inhibits the phosphorylation of the phosphopeptides labeled specifically by calmodulin-kinase and protein kinase C; although there was an inhibition of labeling of the peptides phosphorylated by cyclic AMP kinases, the extent of the decrease was less marked and was only complete in the presence of EGTA (Robinson and Dunkley, 1985, unpublished data). It is known that the activity of adenylate cyclase is dependent on calcium levels and a decrease in cyclic AMP levels at low calcium concentrations is not unexpected (Fig. 1).

What is the effect of depolarization on synaptosomal protein phosphorylation?

Depolarization increases the phosphorylation of a large number of synaptosomal phosphoproteins, including the 87K phosphoprotein, synapsin Ia and Ib, phosphoproteins IIIa and IIb and the B-50 proteins (Figs. 2 and 5). These changes are very reproducible and have been observed in a number of laboratories. In addition, there are smaller and more variable increases in the phosphorylation of a number of other synaptosomal phosphoproteins (Robinson and Dunkley, 1983b, 1985), including the 63- and 48-kDa subunits of the calmodulin kinase (Dunkley et al., 1986b).

Depolarization decreased the phosphorylation of some proteins and three types of dephosphorylation can be identified. Firstly, phosphoprotein 96 shows an immediate and dramatic loss of radiolabel on depolarization (Fig. 2) that is dependent on the presence of calcium (Robinson and Dunkley, 1983a, 1985). Secondly, the α subunit of pyruvate dehydrogenase is dephosphorylated at a slow rate and this is presumably due to activation of its specific calcium-activated phosphatase (Robinson and Dunkley, 1985). Finally, depolarization of synaptosomes for longer than 15 s leads to extensive dephosphorylation of most phosphoproteins (Robinson and Dunkley, 1983b, 1985; see Fig. 8 and below). This is presumed to be due to activation of protein phosphatases and possibly a concomitant inactivation of protein kinases (Robinson and Dunkley, 1985).

Which protein kinases are activated on depolarization?

Analysis of the phosphopeptide 'maps' obtained after depolarization of synaptosomes provides information on the protein kinases likely to be activated (Fig. 7; Dunkley et al., 1986b). Perhaps the most important result obtained is that no new phosphopeptide is observed after depolarization relative to the phosphopeptide 'maps' obtained after prelabeling. This suggests that no new

protein kinase that labels a different site becomes activated and no rearrangement or exposure of new sites on substrates occurs. Thus, even though there are likely to be redistributions of substrates and/or enzymes on depolarization (see below), only increased labeling of sites is occurring and no changed function of phosphoproteins is likely (Fig. 4). Whether the increased labeling reflects an increased proportion of phosphoproteins labeled or simply turnover of labeled for unlabeled phosphate (Fig. 4) has not been established, except for synapsin I where an increase in proportion of labeled protein occurred (Krueger et al., 1977).

A closer look at individual phosphopeptides indicates that calmodulin- and cyclic AMP-kinases and protein kinase C are all activated on depolarization. Thus, for example, the sites on synapsin I labeled by calmodulin- and cyclic AMP-kinases show increased phosphorylation. That the cyclic AMP-kinase is activated is supported by the increased labeling of phosphopeptides derived from phosphoproteins IIIa and IIIb. That the calmodulin kinase is activated is supported by the increase in labeling of phosphoprotein IIIa and the slight increase in autophosphorylation of phosphoprotein 48, the smaller subunit of calmodulin kinase II. Protein kinase C activation was clearcut and increased labeling of phosphoprotein 87 was always observed (Wu et al., 1982; Dunkley et al., 1986b). The increased activity of the cyclic AMP-kinase may be due to increased levels of cyclic AMP induced by calcium activation of adenylate cyclase, or feedback of released neurotransmitters acting via presynaptic receptors (Fig. 1; Dunkley et al., 1986b).

Antipsychotic drugs completely block the increases in protein phosphorylation observed on depolarization, presumably due to blockade of calcium binding to calmodulin (DeLorenzo et al., 1982; Robinson et al., 1984). Such an effect would inhibit calmodulin-stimulated protein kinases. An indirect inhibition of cyclic AMP-stimulated protein kinases (Fig. 1), and possibly an inhibition of protein kinase C, also occurs (Albert et al., 1984). This and other data suggest that the changes in protein phosphorylation which occur on depolarization are all dependent on calcium (Robinson and Dunkley, 1985). A summary of

286

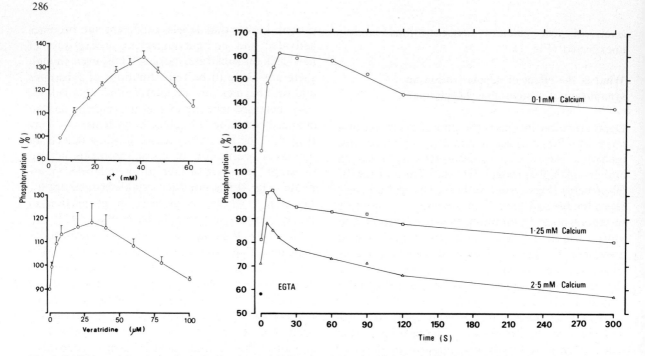

Fig. 8. Inhibition of depolarization-stimulated protein phosphorylation by high levels of calcium. Left: A P2 fraction was labeled with $^{32}P_i$ and depolarized in the presence of various concentrations of high K for 5 s or veratridine for 15 s (Robinson and Dunkley, 1983a). Right: A P2 fraction was labeled with $^{32}P_i$ and depolarized for the times indicated with 41 mM K buffer after prelabeling in the presence of EGTA (●), 0.1 mM calcium (○), 1.25 mM calcium (□) or 2.5 mM calcium (△). The results are for the labeling of all phosphoproteins relative to that observed when the P2 fraction was incubated for 45 min in the absence of exogenous calcium set at 100%.

some of the effects of calcium are shown in Fig. 8. Increasing the depolarizing agents K and veratridine initially, increases calcium entry into synaptosomes (Blaustein, 1975) but there is an optimum level for observing maximum depolarization-stimulated protein phosphorylation. Similarly, increasing the level of calcium added to non-depolarized synaptosomes initially increases and then decreases the extent of the protein phosphorylation (zero time, Fig. 8), while cytosolic calcium continues to rise (Nachshen, 1985). On depolarization for 5 s in the presence of EGTA virtually no increase in total protein phosphorylation is observed (Robinson and Dunkley, 1985); the largest increase is seen at 0.1 mM calcium, while even higher levels of calcium diminish the effect of depolarization (Fig. 8). Finally, as the period of depolarization is prolonged and more calcium enters the synaptosome, the rate of decrease in the levels of protein phosphoryla-

tion are again dependent on calcium, with the highest dephosphorylation rates being at 2.5 mM calcium (Fig. 8). The balance between protein kinase and protein phosphatase activity is therefore delicately controlled by calcium levels and once the increase in protein phosphorylation has been achieved it is reversed by protein phosphatase activation. This possibly assists in restoring nerve terminal proteins to their basal levels of phosphorylation prior to the next impulse.

What are the possible roles of the synaptosomal phosphoproteins in relation to neurotransmitter release?

The function of nerve terminals is to release neurotransmitters in response to a depolarizing signal coming from the axon. Synaptosomes represent a population of nerve terminals which retain the function of neurotransmitter release, but now do so in response to chemical depolarization (Bradford, 1975). All of the changes in synaptosomal protein phosphorylation which occur on depolarization are likely to be directly or indirectly involved in neurotransmitter release. Neurotransmission can be divided into four phases: activation, modulation, initiation and recovery. Activation represents the entry of calcium into nerve terminals, modulation of the effects of calcium depend on the state of the nerve terminal at the time of depolarization, initiation is the phase of vesicle fusion with the plasma membrane and the beginning of neurotransmitter release, and recovery is necessary to prepare the nerve terminal for the next depolarizing event. These phases are not sequential, but overlap in time and some events can be classified in more than one phase. A relationship between neurotransmitter release and synaptosomal protein phosphorylation could occur in any or all of these phases. The possible role of protein phosphorylation in each phase will now be discussed.

Activation

The first phase of neurotransmitter release involves a depolarization-stimulated change in ion permeability leading to calcium entry into nerve terminals. A number of ion channels in neuronal tissue have been identified as phosphoproteins, including sodium (Reichart and Kelly, 1983) and potassium (Goldin et al., 1983; Levitan et al., 1983; Novak-Hofer et al., 1985) channels, but only the α subunit of the sodium channel (260 kDa) has been identified as a phosphoprotein in synaptosomes (Costa et al., 1982). The role of phosphorylation of these ion channels and the effects of depolarization and subsequent calcium entry on their phosphorylation is unknown.

During this phase of depolarization-stimulated calcium entry, a number of events are likely to occur leading to activation of protein kinases. These include increased phosphoinositide metabolism, calcium binding to calmodulin and the redistribution of calmodulin, protein kinases and substrates within and between plasma membranes, cytoskeleton and cytosol.

Activation of phosphoinositide metabolism leads to diacylglycerol production and activation of protein kinase C (Nishizuka, 1983). Protein kinase C is present mainly in the cytosol and its distribution changes from cytosol to membranes on activation of other stimulus–secretion coupling systems (Drust and Martin, 1985; Hirota et al., 1985). Phosphoprotein 87 is a substrate for protein kinase C and its labeling increases on depolarization of synaptosomes (Wu et al., 1982; Dunkley et al., 1986b). The other major neuronal substrate of protein kinase C is the membrane-bound B-50 protein (Aloyo et al., 1983; Zwiers et al., 1985; Akers and Routtenberg, 1985; Routtenberg et al., 1985), whose phosphorylation is increased on depolarization. The B-50 protein shows increased phosphorylation in parallel with inactivation of diphosphoinositol kinase (Jolles et al., 1980; Oestreicher et al., 1983), but the exact relationship between the kinase and the B-50 protein is unknown. Protein kinase C may have other substrates at locations accessible to the cytosol, including synapsin I which is located on synaptic vesicles.

Some of the calcium which enters a nerve terminal binds to calmodulin and in other stimulus–secretion coupling systems this leads to increased calmodulin binding to membranes (Hikita et al., 1985). There, calmodulin is able to modulate the activity of calmodulin-stimulated protein kinases and possibly cyclic AMP-stimulated protein kinase (Fig. 1; Nestler and Greengard, 1984) and protein kinase C (Albert et al., 1984). The major calmodulin kinase in neurons is calmodulin kinase II (Kennedy et al., 1983) and the incorporation of $^{32}P_i$ into its 63- and 48-kDa subunits was only slightly increased by depolarization. The role of autophosphorylation of these subunits may involve their affinity for calmodulin (Shields et al., 1984; Levine et al., 1985), their binding to substrates, or their activation (Saitoh and Schwartz, 1985). The calmodulin-kinase is present in both membranes and cytosol, where it is associated with cytoskeletal proteins such as tubulin (Goldenring et al., 1984) and synapsin I (Nestler and Greengard, 1984). The effect of depolarization on its distribution is unknown, although in *Aplysia* there was a change in location from the cytoskeleton to the soluble fraction during stimulus–secretion coupling (Saitoh and Schwartz, 1985).

The regulatory subunits of the cyclic AMP-stimulated kinase are minor labeled proteins in intact synaptosomes and the effect of depolarization on their phosphorylation is uncertain (Dunkley et al., 1986b). However, in other systems the catalytic subunit of the kinase is released from membranes into the cytosol during activation (Williams and Rodnight, 1977).

Modulation

A second phase of neurotransmitter release involves modulation of the number of vesicles able to be released by a single depolarizing event. This will depend on the environment of the nerve terminal and will be affected by supply of energy substrates, the size and shape of the terminal, the frequency of depolarization and the presence of active presynaptic receptors (Cunnane, 1984). Modulation is likely to involve control of basal cytosolic calcium levels and/or control of the effects of raised intraterminal calcium.

Basal calcium levels are controlled by calcium ATPase activity on the plasma and synaptic vesicle membranes, sodium/calcium exchange mechanisms, and mitochondrial uptake of calcium (Blaustein, 1975; Nachshen, 1985) and these can potentially be controlled by protein phosphorylation. Thus, synaptic plasma membrane calcium ATPase is modulated by calmodulin (Ross and Cardenas, 1983), and the synaptic vesicles from *Torpedo* also have a calcium ATPase (Michaelson and Ophir, 1980). Phosphorylation of the α subunit of pyruvate dehydrogenase modulates calcium entry into mitochondria (Browning et al., 1982). The sodium/calcium exchange protein has not been identified.

Many neurotransmitter receptors have now been identified as phosphoproteins and, as some of these receptors are presynaptic, their activation could modulate the effects of calcium entry into nerve terminals (Fig. 1; Nestler and Greengard, 1984).

Increased protein phosphatase activity leads to a greater number of sites available for protein kinases to phosphorylate and hence the activity of these enzymes prior to depolarization could modulate the effects of calcium entry. The mechanisms which control protein phosphatases have been investigated (Cohen, 1982) and a number of protein inhibitors have been identified, including darp 32 and the G substrate which are both active when phosphorylated (Nestler and Greengard, 1984).

Initiation

A third phase is the initiation of fusion of vesicles with the plasma membrane and the beginning of neurotransmitter release. A number of vesicles are likely to be 'docked' at the plasma membrane waiting to fuse and, to date, the synaptic vesicle binding proteins in the plasma membrane have not been identified and the mechanism of fusion has not been established. It is possible that vesicle swelling will be a necessary prerequisite for fusion of synaptic vesicles with presynaptic terminals as has been found in other systems (Zimmerberg and Whitaker, 1985). Swelling is likely to involve translocation of ions or protein from the cytosol into the vesicle. The initiation phase may occur very rapidly, but a subsequent translocation of vesicles to the plasma membrane for release during either the current or a subsequent depolarizing event must also occur. Translocation in other stimulus–secretion coupling systems begins by freeing the vesicle from the cytoskeletal network which holds it in position (Trifaro, 1977). Synaptic vesicle membranes contain a number of protein kinases and phosphoproteins (DeLorenzo et al., 1979; Huttner et al., 1983; Moskowitz et al., 1983). The phosphoproteins identified include a number of cytoskeletal proteins, such as synapsin Ia and Ib, tubulin and actin. Microtubule associated protein (MAP) and fodrin (the neuronal form of spectrin) may also be present (Walaas et al., 1983a, Sobue et al., 1982). Synapsin I has recently been identified as being a neuronal form of the red blood cell protein 4.1, which is known to bind to actin and spectrin, forming cytoskeletal networks which assist in maintaining red blood cell shape (Baines and Bennett, 1985). Phosphoproteins IIIa and IIIb are structurally and antigenically similar to synapsin I and these proteins are likely to serve similar functions (Nestler and Greengard, 1984). Phosphorylation of synapsin I by a calcium-stimulated protein kinase causes it to fall off synaptic vesicles and presumably free vesicles from actin/fodrin networks (Huttner et al., 1983). Phosphorylation of tubulin (Larson et al., 1985) decreases polymerization and presumably allows vesicles to penetrate microtubule networks, some of which are known to be present around the periphery of nerve terminal cytoplasm (Gray, 1975). Thus, protein phosphorylation of major nerve terminal phosphoproteins is very likely to be involved in vesicle translocation prior to fusion and neurotransmitter release. The movement of vesicles may be further facilitated by myosin/actin interactions (Berl, 1975) and myosin is a phosphoprotein present in neurons (Nestler and Greengard, 1984).

Recovery

The final phase of neurotransmission is the recovery of energy, neurotransmitter content, synaptic vesicle protein and the metabolic status of the nerve terminal in preparation for the next depolarization. Neuronal tissue depends on glucose for its ATP and a crucial enzyme is pyruvate dehydrogenase. The α subunit of this enzyme is a phosphoprotein whose activity is inhibited when phosphorylated. A calcium-stimulated phosphatase specific to this enzyme is activated on depolarization of synaptosomes and this would lead to increased ATP synthesis necessary for recovery of the nerve (Robinson and Dunkley, 1983b, 1985). It is noteworthy that decreases in protein phosphorylation may be as important physiologically as increases. Depolarization also activates the resynthesis of neurotransmitters by activating the phosphorylation of enzymes such as tyrosine and tryptophan hydroxylase (Nestler and Greengard, 1984).

Future directions?

All the changes in synaptosomal protein phosphorylation observed on depolarization seem to have direct or indirect functional significance in neurotransmission. It is noteworthy that most of the major synaptosomal phosphoproteins involved are also found in non-neuronal tissue, or have non-neuronal counterparts that are closely related in structure, suggesting that they are not phosphoproteins specifically evolved for neurotransmitter release. In the future, it will be necessary to characterize the other major synaptosomal phosphoproteins that have not yet been extensively studied, especially those in the high molecular weight region of gels, whose phosphorylation is altered on depolarization. There are also many minor, but perhaps physiologically important, phosphoproteins that will need to be investigated in systems such as synaptosomes. Whether turnover or the proportion of labeled proteins is increased on depolarization, as well as the number of sites on individual proteins, must be determined before the observed changes in labeling of phosphoproteins on depolarization are proven to be physiologically meaningful. The protein kinases which phosphorylate proteins in synaptosomes have been identified but more information on their location, specificity and autophosphorylation subsequent to depolarization is required. The role of protein phosphatases in synaptosomes has hardly been studied. Further work is also required on the relationships between neurotransmitter release and protein phosphorylation, and especially their relative time courses after electrical stimulation of synaptosomes (Rodnight, 1982), and their responses to agents such as barium, which appears to inactivate protein phosphorylation but stimulate neurotransmitter release (Robinson and Dunkley, 1983c).

A number of techniques have recently been developed which will allow significant progress to be made in the near future. These include the development of techniques to permeabilize and transfer proteins across plasma membranes (Knight and Baker, 1983; Kenigsberg et al., 1985) and to study protein phosphorylation in vivo (Rodnight et al., 1985). Finally, a new technique has been developed to prepare synaptosomes using Percoll gradients (Dunkley et al., 1986a, 1986c). This procedure has the major advantages over traditional methods that it is rapid (taking less than 1 h), has fewer steps (as an S1 fraction can be applied to the gradient rather than a P2 fraction), maintains isotonic conditions throughout, and requires smaller samples, allowing more specific brain regions to be investigated. Furthermore, the Percoll procedure not only removes myelin and extrasynaptosomal mitochondria, but also leaky synaptosomes and synaptic plasma membranes. This unique feature makes the Percoll procedure the method of choice for future studies on synaptosomal protein phosphorylation. Investigation of the Percoll-isolated synaptosomes has shown that they are metabolically viable, in that they take up $^{32}P_i$ and phosphorylate proteins and take up calcium and release neurotransmitters in the normal way upon depolarization (Robinson et al., 1985; Dunkley et al., 1986a, 1986c). Furthermore, various populations of synaptosomes were separated on the Percoll gradient and each appears to have different morphology, phosphoprotein content and proportions of the neurotransmitters dopamine and serotonin (Robinson and Lovenberg, 1986; Dunkley et al., 1986a, 1986c). These sub-populations will be of special value in future studies on the role of synaptosomal protein phosphorylation in the release of particular neurotransmitters.

Acknowledgements

This work was supported by the National Health and Medical Research Council of Australia. Mrs. P. Jarvie and Ms. C. Baker are thanked for research assistance and Dr. J. Rostas is thanked for helpful discussions. Mrs. E. Fitzsimmons is thanked for typing the manuscript.

References

Akers, R.F. and Routtenberg, A. (1985) Protein kinase phosphorylates a 47 kDa protein directly related to synaptic plasticity. Brain Res., 334:147–151.

Albert, K.A., Wu, W.C.-S., Nairn, A.C, and Greengard, P. (1984) Inhibition by calmodulin of calcium/phospholipid-dependent protein phosphorylation. Proc. Natl. Acad. Sci. U.S.A., 81:3622–3625.

Aloyo, V.J., Zwiers, H. and Gispen, W.H. (1983) Phosphorylation of B-50 protein by calcium-activated phospholipid-dependent protein kinase and B-50 protein kinase. J. Neurochem., 41:649–653.

Baines, A.J. and Bennet, V. (1985) Synapsin I is a spectrin-binding protein immunologically related to erythrocyte protein 4.1. Nature, 315:410–413.

Berman, R.F., Hullihan, J.P., Kinnier, W.J. and Wilson, J.E. (1984) In vivo phosphorylation of postsynaptic density proteins. Neuroscience, 13:965–971.

Berl, S. (1975) Actomyosin-like protein in brain. In B.W. Agranoff and M.H. Aprison (Eds.) Advances in Neurochemistry. Vol. 1, Plenum Press, New York, pp. 157–191.

Blaustein M.P. (1975) Effects of potassium, veratradine and scorpion venon on calcium accumulation and transmitter release by nerve terminals in vitro. J. Physiol., 247:617–655.

Bradford, H.F. (1975) Isolated nerve terminals as an in vitro preparation for the study of dynamic aspects of transmitter release and metabolism. In L. Iverson, S. Iverson and S. Snyder (Eds.) Handbook of Psychopharmacology, Vol. I. Plenum Press, New York, pp. 191–252.

Breithaupt, T.B. and Babitch, J.A. (1979) Autophosphorylation of chick brain synaptic polypeptides. Phosphorylation of proteins during incubation of intact synaptosomes with $^{32}PO_4$. J. Neurobiol., 10:169–177.

Browning, M., Baudry, M. and Lynch, G. (1982) Evidence that high frequency stimulation influences the phosphorylation of pyruvate dehydrogenase and that the activity of this enzyme is linked to mitochondrial calcium sequestration. Prog. Brain Res., 56:317–338.

Clouet, D.H., O'Callaghan, J.P. and Williams, N. (1978) The effects of opiates on calcium-stimulated phosphorylation of synaptic membranes in intact synaptosomes from rat striatum. In J. Van Ree and L. Terenius (Eds.), Characteristics and Functions of Opioids, Elsevier, Amsterdam, pp. 351–352.

Cohen P. (1982) The role of protein phosphorylation in neural and hormonal control of cellular activity. Nature, 296:613–620.

Costa, M., Casnelli, J. and Catterall, W. (1982) Selective phosphorylation of the alpha subunit of the sodium channel by cAMP-dependent protein kinase. J. Biol. Chem., 257:7918–7921.

Cunnane, T.C. (1984) The mechanism of neurotransmitter release from sympathetic nerves. Trends Neurosci., 7:248–253.

DeLorenzo, R.J., Freedman, S.D., Yohe, W.B. and Maurer, S.C. (1979) Stimulation of Ca^{2+}-dependent neurotransmitter release and presynaptic nerve terminal protein phosphorylation by calmodulin and a calmodulin-like protein isolated from synaptic vesicles. Proc. Natl. Acad. Sci. U.S.A., 76:1838–1842.

DeLorenzo, R.J., Gonzalez, B., Goldenring, J.R., Bowling, A. and Jacobson, R. (1982) Calcium-calmodulin tubulin kinase system and its role in mediating the calcium signal in brain. Prog. Brain Res., 56:255–286.

DeRiemer, S.A., Kaczmarek, L.K., Lai, Y., McGuinness, T.L. and Greengard, P. (1984) Calcium/calmodulin-dependent protein phosphorylation in the nervous system of Aplysia. J. Neurosci., 4:1618–1625.

Drust, D.S. and Martin, T.F.J. (1985) Protein kinase C translocates from cytosol to membrane upon hormone activation: Effects of thyrotropin-releasing hormone in GH$_3$ cells. *Biochem. Biophys. Res. Commun.*, 128:531–537.

Dunkley, P.R. (1981) Phosphorylation of synaptosomal membrane proteins and evaluation of nerve cell function. In A.D. Kidman, J.K. Tomkins and R.A. Westerman (Eds.) *New Approaches to Nerve and Muscle Disorders*, Excerpta Medica, Amsterdam, pp. 38–51.

Dunkley, P.R. and Robinson, P.J. (1981) Calcium-stimulated protein kinases from rat cerebral cortex are inactivated by preincubation. *Biochem. Biophys. Res. Commun.*, 102:1196–1202.

Dunkley, P.R. and Robinson, P.J. (1983) The in vitro phosphorylation of actin from rat cerbral cortex. *Neurochem. Res.*, 8:865–871.

Dunkley, P.R., Cockburn, J., Power, P. and King, M.G. (1983) The effect of stress on CNS protein phosphorylation and cyclic AMP. In T. Kidman, J.K. Tomkins, C.A. Morris and N. Cooper (Eds.) *Molecular Pathology of Nerve and Muscle*, Humana Press, NJ, pp. 297–312.

Dunkley, P.R., Jarvie, P.E., Heath, J.W., Kidd, G.J. and Rostas, J.A.P. (1986a) A rapid method for isolation of synaptosomes on Percoll gradients. *Brain Res.*, 372:115–129.

Dunkley, P.R., Baker, C.M. and Robinson, P.J. (1986b) Depolarization-dependent protein phosphorylation in rat cortical synaptosomes: characterization of active protein kinases by phosphopeptide analysis of substrates. *J. Neurochem.*, 46:1692–1703.

Dunkley, P.R., Rostas, J.A.P., Heath, J.W. and Powis, D.A. (1986c) The preparation of and use of synaptosomes for studying secretion of catecholamines. In A. Poisner and J.M. Trifaro, *In Vitro Methods for Studying Secretion*. Elsevier, Amsterdam.

Forn, J. and Greengard, P. (1978) Depolarizing agents and cyclic nucleotides regulate the phosphorylation of specific neuronal proteins in rat cerebral cortex slices. *Proc. Natl. Acad. Sci. U.S.A.*, 75:5195–5199.

Goldenring, J.R., Gonzalez, B., McGuire, J.S. and DeLorenzo, R.J. (1983) Purification and characterization of a calmodulin-dependent tubulin kinase from rat brain cytosol able to phosphorylate tubulin and microtubule-associated proteins. *J. Biol. Chem.*, 258:12632–12640.

Goldenring, J.R., Casanova, J.E. and DeLorenzo, R.J. (1984) Tubulin-associated calmodulin-dependent kinase: Evidence for an endogenous complex of tubulin with a calcium-calmodulin-dependent kinase. *J. Neurochem.*, 43:1669–1679.

Goldin, S.M., Moczydlowski, E.G. and Papazian, D.M. (1983) Isolation and reconstitution of neuronal ion transport proteins. *Annu. Rev. Neurosci.*, 6:419–446.

Gray, E.G. (1975) Presynaptic microtubules and their association with synaptic vesicles. *Proc. Roy. Soc. London Ser. B*, 190:3690372.

Gurd, J.W. (1985) Phosphorylation of the postsynaptic density glycoprotein gp180 by endogenous tyrosine kinase. *Brain Res.*, 333:385–388.

Hirota, K., Hirota, T., Aguilera, G. and Catt, K. (1985) Hormone-induced redistribution of calcium-activated phospholipid-dependent protein kinase in pituitary gonadot-rophs. *J. Biol. Chem.*, 260:3243–3246.

Holmes, H., Rodnight, R. and Kapoor, R. (1977) Effects of electroshock and drugs administered in vivo on protein kinase activity in rat brain. *Pharmacol. Biochem. Behav.*, 6:415–419.

Hikita, T., Bader, M.F. and Trifaro, J.M. (1985) Adrenal chromaffin cell calmodulin: its subcellular distribution and binding to chromaffin granule membrane proteins. *J. Neurochem.*, 43:1087–1097.

Huttner, W.B. and Greengard, P. (1979) Multiple phosphorylation sites in protein I and their differential regulation by cyclic AMP and calcium. *Proc. Natl. Acad. Sci. U.S.A.*, 76:5402–5406.

Huttner, W.B., Scheibler, W., Greengard, P. and DeCamilli, P. (1983) Synapsin I, a nerve terminal specific phosphoprotein. III. Its association with synaptic vesicles studied in a highly purified synaptic vesicle preparation. *J. Cell Biol.*, 96:1374–1388.

Jolles, J., Zwiers, H., Van Dongen, C., Schotman, P., Wirtz, K.W.A. and Gispen, W.H. (1980) Modulation of brain polyphosphoinositide metabolism by ACTH-sensitive protein phosphorylation. *Nature*, 286:623–625.

Julien, J.-P. and Mushynski, W.E. (1981) A comparison of in vitro- and in vivo-phosphorylated neurofilament polypeptides. *J. Neurochem.*, 37:1579–1585.

Katz, B. and Miledi, R. (1969) Spontaneous and evoked activity of motro nerve endings in calcium ringer. *J. Physiol.*, 203:689–706.

Kenigsberg, R.L. and Trifaro, J.M. (1985) Microinjection of calmodulin antibodies into cultured chromaffin cells blocks catecholamine release in response to stimulation. *J. Neurosci.*, 14:335–347.

Kennedy, M.B. and Greengard, P. (1981) Two calcium/calmodulin-dependent protein kinases, which are highly concentrated in brain, phosphorylate protein I at distinct sites. *Proc. Natl. Acad. Sci. U.S.A.*, 78:1293–1297.

Kennedy, M.B., Bennett, M.K. and Erondu, N.E. (1983) Biochemical and immunochemical evidence that the 'major postsynaptic density protein' is a subunit of a calmodulin-dependent protein kinase. *Proc. Natl. Acad. Sci. U.S.A.*, 80:7457–7361.

Knight, D.E. and Baker, P.F. (1983) Stimulus–secretion coupling in isolated bovine adrenal medullary cells. *Q. J. Exp. Physiol.*, 68:123–143.

Krueger, B.K., Forn, J. and Greengard, P. (1977) Depolarization-induced phosphorylation of specific proteins, mediated by calcium ion influx, in rat brain synaptosomes. *J. Biol. Chem.*, 252:2764–2773.

Larson, R.E., Goldenring, J.R., Vallana, M.L. and DeLorenzo, R.J. (1985) Identification of endogenous calmodulin-dependent kinase and calmodulin-binding proteins in cold-stable microtubule preparations from rat brain. *J. Neurochem.*, 44:1566–1574.

LeVine H. III, Sahyoun, N.E. and Cuatrecasas, P. (1985) Calmodulin binding to the cytoskeletal neuronal calmodulin-dependent protein kinase is regulated by autophosphorylation. *Proc. Natl. Acad. Sci. U.S.A.*, 82:287–291.

292

Levitan, I.B., Adams, W.B., Lemos, J.R. and Novak-Hofer, I. (1983) A role for protein phosphorylation in the regulation of electrical activity of an identified nerve cell. *Prog. Brain Res.*, 58:71–76.

Lyn-Cook, B.D., Ruder, F.J. and Wilson, J.E. (1985) Regulation of phosphate incorporation into four brain phosphoproteins that are affected by experience. *J. Neurochem.*, 44:552–559.

Mahler, H.R., Kleine, L.P., Ratner, N. and Sorensen, R.G. (1982) Identification and topography of synaptic phosphoproteins. *Prog. Brain Res.*, 56:27–48.

Michaelson, D.M. and Avissar, S. (1979) Ca^{2+}-dependent protein phosphorylation of purely cholinergic *Torpedo* synaptosomes. *J. Biol. Chem.*, 254:12542–12546.

Michaelson, D.M. and Ophir, I. (1980) Sidedness of (calcium, magnesium) adenosine triphosphatase of purified *torpedo* synaptic vesicles. *J. Neurochem.*, 34:1483–1490.

Michaelson, D.M., Avissar, S., Kloos, Y. and Sokolovsky, M. (1979) Mechanism of acetylcholine release: possible involvement of presynaptic muscarinic receptors in regulation of acetylcholine release and protein phosphorylation. *Proc. Natl. Acad. Sci., U.S.A.*, 76:6336–6340.

Mitrius, J.C., Morgan, D.G. and Routtenberg, A. (1981) In vivo phosphorylation following ^{32}P-orthophosphate injection into neostriatum or hippocampus: Selective and rapid labelling of electrophoretically separated brain proteins. *Brain Res.*, 212:67–81.

Moskowitz, N., Glassman, A., Ores, C., Schook, W. and Puszkin, S. (1983) Phosphorylation of brain synaptic and coated vesicle proteins by endogenous Ca^{2+}/calmodulin- and cAMP-dependent protein kinases. *J. Neurochem.*, 40:711–718.

Nachshen, D.A. (1985) Regulation of cytosolic calcium concentration in presynaptic nerve endings isolated from rat brain. *J. Physiol.*, 363:87–101.

Nestler, E.J. and Greengard, P. (1984) Protein phosphorylation. In *The Nervous System.* John Wiley and Sons, New York.

Nishizuka, Y. (1983) Phospholipid degradation and signal translation for protein phosphorylation. *Trends Biochem. Sci.*, 8:13–16.

Novak-Hofer, I., Lemos, J.R., Villermain, M. and Levitan, I.B. (1985) Calcium- and cyclic nucleotide-dependent protein kinases and their substrates in the *Aplysia* nervous system. *J. Neurosci.*, 5:151–159.

Oestreicher, A.B., VanDongen, C.J., Zwiers, H. and Gispen, W.H. (1983) Affinity-purified anti-B-50 protein antibody: Interference with the function of the phosphoprotein B-50 in synaptic plasma membranes. *J. Neurochem.*, 41:331–340.

Rassmussen, H. and Goodman, D.B.P. (1977) Relationships between calcium and cyclic nucleotides in cell activation. *Physiol. Rev.*, 57:421–509.

Reichardt, L.F. and Kelly, R.B. (1983) A molecular description of nerve terminal function. *Annu. Rev. Biochem.*, 52:871–926.

Robinson, P.J. and Dunkley, P.R. (1983a) Depolarisation-dependent protein phosphorylation in rat cortical synaptosomes: factors determining the magnitude of the response. *J. Neurochem.*, 41:909–918.

Robinson, P.J. and Dunkley, P.R. (1983b) The role of protein phosphorylation in nerve cell function. In Austin L. and Jeffrey P.L. (Eds.) *Molecular Aspects of Neurological Disorders.* Academic Press, Sydney, pp. 345–348.

Robinson, P.J. and Dunkley, P.R. (1983c) Depolarisation-dependent protein phosphorylation in rat cortical synaptosomes: the effects of calcium, strontium and barium. *Neurosci. Lett.*, 43:85–90.

Robinson, P.J. and Dunkley, P.R. (1985) Depolarisation-dependent protein phosphorylation and dephosphorylation in rat cortical synaptosomes is modulated by calcium. *J. Neurochem.*, 44:338–348.

Robinson, P.J. and Lovenberg, W. (1986) Dopamine and serotonin in two populations of synaptosomes isolated by Percoll gradient centrifugation. *Neurochem. Int.* (in press).

Robinson, P.J., Jarvie, P. and Dunkley, P.R. (1984) Depolarisation-dependent protein phosphorylation in rat cortical synaptosomes is inhibited by fluphenazine at a step after calcium entry, *J. Neurochem.*, 43:659–667.

Rodnight, R. (1982) Aspects of protein phosphorylation in the nervous system with particular reference to synaptic transmission. *Prog. Brain Res.*, 56:1–25.

Rodnight, R., Trotta, E.F. and Perrett, C. (1985) A simple and economical method for studying protein phosphorylation in vivo in the rat brain. *J. Neurosci. Methods*, 13:87–95.

Ross, D.H. and Cardenas, H.L. (1983) Calmodulin stimulation of Ca^{2+}-dependent ATP hydrolysis and ATP-dependent Ca^{2+} transport in synaptic membranes. *J. Neurochem.*, 41:161–171.

Rostas, J.A.P., Guldner, F. and Dunkley, P.R. (1983a) Maturation of the post-synaptic density in the CNS. In T. Kidman, J.K. Tomnkins, C.A. Morris and N. Cooper (Eds.) *Molecular Pathology of Nerve and Muscle*, Humana Press, pp. 67–79.

Rostas, J.A.P., Brent, V.A. and Dunkley, P.R. (1983b) The major calmodulin-stimulated phosphoprotein of synaptic junctions and the major post-synaptic density protein are distinct. *Neurosci. Lett.*, 43:161–165.

Rostas, J.A.P., Brent, V.A., Heath, J.W., Neame, R.L.B., Powis, D.A., Weinberger, R.P. and Dunkley, P.R. (1986) The subcellular distribution of a membrane-bound calmodulin-stimulated protein kinase. *Neurochem. Res.*, 11:253–268.

Routtenberg, A. (1979) Anatomical localisation of phospho-protein and glycoprotein substrates of memory. *Prog. Neurobiol.*, 12:85–113.

Routtenberg, A. (1984) Phosphoprotein regulation of memory formation: Enhancement and control of synaptic plasticity by protein kinase C and protein Fl. Ann. N. Y. Acad. Sci.

Routtenberg, A., Lovinger, D.M. and Steward, O. (1985) Selective increase in phosphorylation state of a 47 kDa protein (F1) directly related to long term potentiation. *Behav. Neurol. Biol.*, 43:3–11.

Sahyoun, N., LeVine H. III, Bronson, D., Siegel-Greenstein, F. and Cuatrecasas, P. (1985) Cytoskeletal calmodulin-dependent portein kinase. Characterization, solubilization and purification from rat brain. *J. Biol. Cehm.*, 260:1230–1237.

Saitoh, T. and Schwartz, J.H. (1983) Serotonin alters the subcellular distribution of a Ca²⁺/calmodulin-binding protein in neurons of *Aplysia. Proc. Natl. Acad. Sci. U.S.A.*, 180:6708–6712.

Saitoh, T. and Schwarz, J.H. (1985) Phosphorylation-dependent subcellular translocation of a Ca²⁺/calmodulin-dependent protein kinase produces an autonomous enzyme in *Aplysia* neurons. *J. Cell Biol.*, 100:835–842.

Salamin, A., Deshusses, J. and Straub, R.W. (1981) Phosphate ion transport in rabbit brain synaptosomes. *J. Neurochem.*, 37:1419–1424.

Shields, S.M., Vernon, P.J. and Kelly, P.T. (1984) Autophosphorylation of calmodulin-kinase II in synaptic junctions modulates endogenous kinase activity. *J. Neurochem.*, 43:1599–1609.

Sieghart, W. (1981) Glutamate-stimulated phosphorylation of a specific protein in P2 fractions of rat cerebral cortex. *J. Neurochem.*, 37:1116–1124.

Sobue, K., Kanda, K., Yamagami, K. and Kakiuchi, S. (1982) Calcium- and calmodulin-dependent phosphorylation of calspectin (spectrin-like calmodulin binding protein, fodrin) by protein kinase systems in synaptosomal cytosol and membranes. *Biomed. Res.*, 3:561–570.

Sorenson, R.G. and Mahler, H.R. (1983) Calcium-stimulated protein phosphorylated in synaptic membranes. *J. Neurochem.*, 40:1349–1365.

Trifaro, J.M. (1977) Common mechanisms of hormone secretion. *Annu. Rev. Pharmacol. Toxicol.*, 17:27–47.

Vulliet, P.R., Woodgett, J.R., Ferrari, S. and Hardie, D.G. (1985) Characterisation of the sites phosphorylated on tyrosine hydroxylase by Ca- and phospholipid-dependent protein kinase, calmodulin-dependent multiprotein kinase and cyclic AMP-dependent protein kinase. *FEBS Lett.*, 182:335–339.

Walaas, S.I., Nairn, A.C. and Greengard, P. (1983a) Regional distribution of calcium- and cyclic adenosine 3′5′-monophosphate-regulated protein phosphorylation systems in mammalian brain. I. Particulate systems. *J. Neurosci.*, 3:291–301.

Walaas, S.I. Nairn, A.C. and Greengard, P. (1983b) Regional distribution of calcium- and cyclic adenosine 3′5′-monophosphate-regulated protein phosphorylation systems in mammalian brain. II. Soluble systems. *J. Neurosci.*, 3:302–311.

Williams, N. and Clouet, D.H. (1982) The effect of acute opioid administration on the phosphorylation of rat striatal synaptic membrane proteins. *J. Pharmacol. Exp. Ther.*, 220:278–286.

Williams, M. and Rodnight, R. (1977) Protein phosphorylation in nervous tissue: Possible involvement in nervous tissue function and relationship to cyclic nucleotide metabolism. *Prog. Neurol.*, 8:183–250.

Wu, W.C.-S., Walaas, W.I., Nairn, A.C. and Greengard, P. (1982) Calcium/phospholipid regulates phosphorylation of a M_r '87K' substrate protein in brain synaptosomes. *Proc. Natl. Acad. Sci. U.S.A.*, 79:5249–5253.

Zimmerberg, J. and Whitaker, M. (1985) Irreversible swelling of secretory granules during exocytosis caused by calcium. *Nature*, 315:581–584.

Zwiers, H., Verhaagen, J., van Dongen, C.J., de Graan, P.N.E. and Gispen, W.H. (1985) Resolution of rat brain synaptic phosphoprotein B-50 into multiple forms by two-dimensional electrophoresis: Evidence for multisite phosphorylation. *J. Neurochem.*, 44:1083–1090.

W.H. Gispen and A. Routtenberg (Eds.)
Progress in Brain Research, Vol. 69
© 1986 Elsevier Science Publishers B.V. (Biomedical Division)

CHAPTER 23

Cyclic nucleotide- and calcium-dependent protein phosphorylation in rat pineal gland: physiological and pharmacological regulation

Fabio Benfenati[1], Mauro Cimino[2]*, Costanza Farabegoli[1], Flaminio Cattabeni[2] and Luigi F. Agnati[1]

[1]*Department of Human Physiology, University of Modena, Via Campi 287, 41100 Modena and* [2]*Department of Pharmacology and Pharmacognosy, University of Urbino, Via S. Chiara 27, 61029 Urbino, Italy*

Introduction

The pineal gland attracted the attention and the imagination of many scientists since the third century B.C. and, from time to time, it was considered as a sphincter regulating the flow of thought in the liquoral spaces, the seat of the soul, the third eye or even, more empirically, as a simple lymph node (Kappers, 1979).

In the last 50 years, systematic anatomical and physiological studies led to the idea of the pineal gland as a neuroendocrine transducer converting neural and environmental information into a hormonal response, namely the secretion of melatonin. The pineal gland lies outside the blood–brain barrier and thus it is sensitive to several kinds of stimuli coming from the periphery, including gonadal hormones and drugs which do not enter the brain (Axelrod, 1974; Tamarkin et al., 1985).

Although derived from neural tissue and often described as a part of the epithalamus, the adult mammalian pineal gland is innervated by the peripheral autonomic system. In many vertebrate classes, mammals included, the pineal complex acts as a biological clock converting information about environmental lighting into a specific hormonal output (Brown et al., 1981).

The glands of reptiles and amphibians are directly photosensitive (Menaker et al., 1978) but, during the phylogenesis, the pineal has been transformed into a pure neuroendocrine organ which receives lighting information from the eyes through a complex neuronal pathway, schematically shown in Fig. 1A. Nerve impulses, stimulated by light impinging on the retinas and carrying the coded photic information, travel via the optic nerve, optic chiasm and following decussation to the hypothalamic suprachiasmatic nucleus (retino–hypothalamic tract), a structure which seems to represent the main autonomous oscillator generating circadian rhythmicity. Projections from this nucleus synapse in the paraventricular nucleus and reach the sympathetic preganglionic nuclei located in the inter-mediolateral column of the spinal cord. Impulses are then conveyed by preganglionic fibres to the superior cervical ganglia and finally post-ganglionic adrenergic fibres reach the pineal via the two nervi conarii. Although this sympathetic innervation provides the major regulatory input to the gland, also a parasympathetic input has been observed in mammals (Kappers, 1960; Moore and Klein, 1974; Rusak and Zucker, 1979; Kappers, 1982).

Melatonin, the pineal hormone, is an indole-

---

*To whom correspondence should be sent.

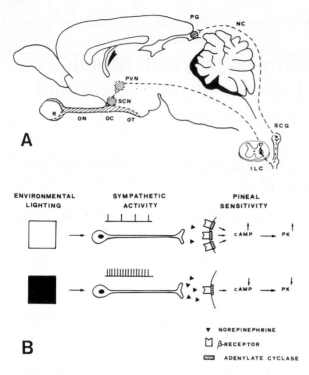

A

B

ENVIRONMENTAL LIGHTING · SYMPATHETIC ACTIVITY · PINEAL SENSITIVITY

cAMP → PK

▼ NOREPINEPHRINE
☐ β-RECEPTOR
▨ ADENYLATE CYCLASE

Fig. 1. A: Schematic representation of the neuroanatomical pathways innervating the rat pineal gland (R, retina; ON, optic nerve; OC, optic chiasm; OT, optic tract; SCN, suprachiasmatic nucleus; PVN, paraventricular nucleus; ILC, intermediolateral column of the spinal cord; SCG, superior cervical ganglion; NC, nervi conarii; PG, pineal gland). B. Schematic diagram of the light-induced changes in sympathetic activity and compensatory biochemical mechanisms in the pineal gland.

amine with powerful physiological effects changing from a species to another. In amphibians, it controls the color of the skin, in birds it regulates circadian rhythms, in mammals it affects reproductive cycles and maturation mediating the effects of light on the sexual sphere (Menaker et al., 1978).

The synthesis of melatonin starts from serotonin which is transformed in *N*-acetyl-serotonin by the enzyme serotonin-*N*-acetyltransferase (SNAT) and subsequently *O*-methylated by hydroxyindole-*O*-methyltransferase (HIOMT) to form 5-methoxy-*N*-acetyltryptamine or melatonin (Weissback et al., 1960; Axelrod and Weissback, 1961).

The effects of environmental lighting on pineal

indoleamine metabolism and melatonin biosynthesis result from a light-induced decrease and a dark-induced increase in the firing rate of the adrenergic fibres innervating the gland (Fig. 1B) (Taylor and Wilson, 1970). These activity changes are able to affect melatonin synthesis through a number of neurochemical steps which link the environmental inputs to the hormonal output.

Biochemical and functional aspects of the adrenergic regulation of rat pineal gland

The β-adrenergic system

The daily dark–light cycle and environmental light have profound effects on the stimulation of the pineal gland by the sympathetic nerves. Under an ordinary dark–light cycle, there is a decreased release of norepinephrine from the terminals during the light period, as a consequence of the concomitant low activity of the adrenergic innervation. The release of norepinephrine and the sympathetic activity, on the other hand, are increased in the darkness (Taylor and Wilson, 1970; Brownstein and Axelrod, 1974). This diurnal variation exerts its action on the different molecular components of the adrenergic system at the postsynaptic level. Thus, the density of the β-adrenergic receptors is higher during the day, reaching its maximum at the end of the light period, and declines during the night showing the lowest level after 12 hours of darkness (Fig. 1B) (Romero and Axelrod, 1974; Romero et al., 1975; Kebabian et al., 1975). These compensatory receptor changes, which apparently tend to compensate the system fluctuations linked to circadian rhythmicity, actually enhance pineal sensitivity to the phasic dark-induced sympathetic activation.

On the other hand, constant light induces a supersensitive state of β-receptors while a subsensitivity is observed for intact animals kept in constant darkness. In particular, glands taken from animals exposed to light for 24 hours have 70% more β-adrenergic binding sites than do glands taken from animals at the end of their 12-hour dark period (Kebabian et al., 1975). Alterations in the sensitivity of β-receptors to adrenergic stimulation can be achieved also by pharmacological manipulations and lesion studies. In fact, an increased density of β-adrenergic receptors in the pineal gland has been reported in animals treated with reserpine, 6-hydroxy-dopamine or ganglionectomy, whereas the chronic administration of the antidepressant drug desimipramine induces a reduction in the number of these receptors (Deguchi and Axelrod, 1972, 1973a, 1973b; Strada and Weiss, 1974; Moyer et al., 1979).

The first evidence for a catecholamine-stimulated adenylate cyclase activity in pineal homogenate was reported by Weiss and Costa (1967). The pharmacological characterization showed that this enzyme is functionally coupled to a β-adrenergic receptor (Weiss and Costa, 1968; Strada et al., 1972). Therefore, the induced receptor changes correlate with variations in adenylate cyclase activity and cyclic AMP (cAMP) accumulation. Thus, as described for the β-receptor, there is a light–dark difference in the adenylate cyclase activity and cAMP accumulation in the pineal gland after stimulation with the β-adrenergic agonist isoproterenol, with a maximal response at the end of the 12-hour light period which progressively declines in the dark (Kebabian et al., 1975; Romero et al., 1975). Supersensitive glands, obtained either by exposing the animals to constant light for 24 hours or by denervation procedures, display a higher basal and catecholamine-stimulated adenylate cyclase activity (Weiss and Costa, 1967; Kebabian et al., 1975). On the other hand, a subsensitive state of the β-adrenergic receptor and adenylate cyclase similar to that reported after darkness can be pharmacologically induced by treatment with isoproterenol or with the noradrenaline re-uptake inhibitor desimipramine (Kebabian et al., 1975; Moyer et al., 1979). All these data suggest that changes in the β-adrenergic stimulation induce fast compensatory mechanisms which are an expression of the high degree of plasticity of the system.

These changes in the mechanisms regulating cAMP accumulation and evidence that the pineal is rich in cAMP-depend protein kinase led researchers to investigate the role of this enzyme in pineal function and its regulation by the same agents and manipulations used to study the β-adrenergic receptor system. Thus, it has been reported that animals exposed for 24 hours to constant light show a 50% increase in cAMP-dependent protein kinase activity as compared to the activity of the enzyme at the end of the dark period. This enhanced activity was ascribed to an increase in the enzyme V_{max} rather than to an increased protein synthesis. Protein kinase activity is also raised in denervated glands or in glands taken from reserpinized animals, suggesting that protein kinase and its specific substrates may play a key role in the biochemical and functional effects of adrenergic agonists and in the regulation of gland sensitivity to adrenergic stimulation (Fontana and Lovenberg, 1971; Zatz and O'Dea, 1976).

Functional correlates

The activity of SNAT, the key enzyme for melatonin synthesis, is controlled by the pineal sympathetic innervation. Therefore the activity of SNAT also shows a light–dark cycle with a maximal activity in the night when the β-adrenergic stimulation is increased (Klein and Weller, 1970).

The induction of SNAT activity by sympathetic stimulation has been extensively studied and documented by a large number of scientific reports. In vitro studies showed that the addition of norepinephrine or isoproterenol to cultured pineals cause an increase in SNAT activity, an effect which can be antagonized by the presence of propranolol (Klein and Berg, 1970; Deguchi and Axelrod, 1972b; Deguchi, 1973). These data have also been confirmed in in vivo studies (Deguchi and Axelrod, 1972a). cAMP is one of the major candidates for SNAT induction (Klein and Weller, 1973). In fact cholera toxin, an irreversible activator of adenylate cyclase, and dibutyryl cAMP markedly increase the enzyme activity. However it is not yet completely understood which is the exact molecular mechanism involved in SNAT activation and which molecualr component of the β-adrenergic system is responsible for such an activation (Klein et al., 1970; Minneman and Iversen, 1976).

Recent studies aimed to establish a correlation between induction of SNAT activity and cAMP-dependent protein kinase stimulation showed that this latter enzyme can be stimulated by agents, such as cholera toxin and isoproterenol, which also induce SNAT activity, suggesting a possible role of cAMP-dependent protein phosphorylation in pineal function (Zatz and O'Dea, 1976; Zatz, 1977).

The α-adrenergic system

α_1-Adrenergic receptors have demonstrated in rat pineal gland (Sugden and Klein, 1984). Using the high-affinity ligand [^{125}I]iodo-2-[β-(4-hydroxyphenyl)ethylaminomethyl] tetralone ([^{125}I]-HEAT) to label these receptors, Sugden and Klein (1985) found that, in contrast to the β_1-adrenergic receptors, the binding sites labeled by this ligand do not show a circadian rhythm. Furthermore the acute or chronic administration of α_1-adrenoreceptor agonists failed to change the number of specific binding sites. However, these authors demonstrated that pineal α_1-adrenoreceptors are indeed under neuronal control, since an increase in the number of [^{125}I]HEAT binding sites after ganglionectomy or 3-week constant light exposure was observed.

Concerning the role of the biochemical events occurring in the pineal following adrenergic stimulation, it has been reported that the activation of the α_1-adrenergic receptors induces changes in phosphatidylinositol turnover (Houser et al., 1974; Nijjar et al., 1980). There is not yet convincing evidence on the functional role of these α_1-receptors since it has been reported that the β-adrenergic stimulation of pineal SNAT can be potentiated either by α_1-specific agonists or antagonists (Alphs and Lovenberg, 1974; Sugden et al., 1984). Thus, although an effect of α-adrenergic drugs on SNAT induction has been found, it is not clear whether it is mediated by α- or β-receptors. These observations indicate that the α-receptors of the pineal gland have different regulatory mechanisms with respect to the β-receptors and that probably they mediate some functional aspects of pineal activity through different biochemical mechanisms.

Protein phosphorylation in rat pineal homogenate

Cyclic nucleotide-dependent protein phosphorylation

The cAMP-dependent protein kinase from rat and bovine pineal gland has been purified and characterized by Fontana and Lovenberg (1971). The gland is a rich source of this enzyme with an activity higher than that reported in brain tissue. As mentioned before, there is now evidence for a role of cAMP-dependent protein kinase in pineal function, namely in the induction of SNAT activity. However a detailed study of endogenous protein substrates has never been carried out. Recently, the phosphorylation of a specific nuclear protein with a molecular weight of 34 000 during SNAT induction (Winters et al., 1977), and a diurnal variation in the content of pineal synapsin I (Nestler et al., 1982), an endogenous substrate for both cAMP- and calcium/calmodulin-dependent protein kinases (Ueda and Greengard, 1977; Krueger et al., 1977), have been reported.

In the present study, the state of phosphorylation of endogenous substrate proteins in vitro in the presence of increasing concentrations of cyclic nucleotides has been evaluated (Fig. 2). cAMP added to pineal homogenate induces an increase in the phosphorylation of three major protein bands of apparent molecular weight 59 000 (59K), 56 000 (56K) and 35 000 (35K) (Fig. 2, left lanes). An induction of phosphorylation is also present in proteins of higher molecular weight but less pronounced. The effect of cAMP is dose-dependent, reaching its maximum at a cAMP concentration of 1 µM for the 59K, whereas for 56K and 35K a concentration of the cyclic nucleotide as high as 10 µM does not yet induce the maximal effect (Fig. 3A). At this concentration the degree of ^{32}P incorporation into the 59K protein is twice that found for the 56K and 35K, indicating that the cAMP-stimulated bands display different sensitivity to the cyclic nucleotide-activated protein kinase and/or that the substrate proteins may be present in different amounts within the pinealocytes. This suggests that, in vitro, the 59K protein can be considered the most prominent endogenous substrate for the cAMP-dependent

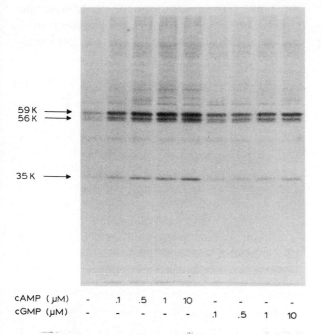

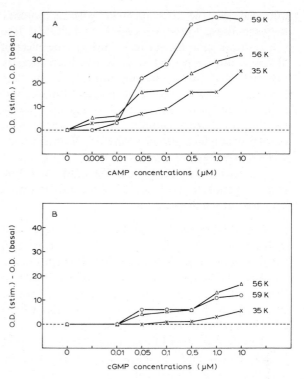

Fig. 2. Gel autoradiographs showing the response of protein phosphorylation in rat pineal gland to increasing concentrations of cyclic nucleotides. The endogenous phosphorylation was determined using 250 μg wet weight of pineal homogenate in 50 mM HEPES buffer, pH 7.4, containing 0.1 mM EGTA, 5 mM MgCl₂, 1 mM dithiothreitol (DTT) and 0.5 mM 3-isobuthyl-l-methylxantine (IBMX) in the absence or presence of increasing concentrations of either cAMP or cGMP ranging from 0.1 to 10 μM. Samples were preincubated at 30°C for 2 min and the phosphorylation reaction was started by the addition of $[\gamma$-^{32}P]ATP (3–5 μCi/sample, 4 μM final concentration). After incubation at 30°C for 10 s, the reaction was terminated by the addition of an equal volume of a stop solution containing 4% sodium dodecylsulfate (SDS), 10% 2-mercaptoethanol, 20% glycerol and 0.002% bromophenol blue in 0.12 M TRIS–HCl, pH 6.8. Samples were then boiled for 2 min and subjected to SDS–polyacrylamide gel electrophoresis (SDS–PAGE, 10% acrylamide in the separating gel) according to the procedure of Laemmli (1970). Autoradiography of the dried gel was performed using Ilford X-ray film. Arrows indicate the apparent molecular weight of the major phosphoproteins analyzed.

Fig. 3. Microdensitometrical analysis of ^{32}P incorporation into the 59K, 56K and 35K protein bands stimulated by increasing concentrations of cAMP (A) or cGMP (B). On the X-axis the final concentrations of cyclic nucleotides ranging from 0.005 to 10 μM are shown; on the Y-axis the differences between optical density (O.D.) of protein bands in stimulated and basal conditions are reported in arbitrary units.

protein kinase with respect to the 56K and 35K proteins.

The role of cGMP in pineal function has not yet been entirely elucidated, although it is responsive to stimulation of the rat pineal. In fact, in vitro exposure of glands to norepinephrine or to depolarizing concentrations of potassium increases cGMP levels (O'Dea and Zatz, 1976). These observations led us to investigate also the effects of exogenous cGMP addition on pineal protein phosphorylation. Fig. 2 (right lanes) shows that the addition of cGMP also stimulates the ^{32}P incorporation into the same protein bands observed for cAMP. However, this cyclic nucleotide displays a lower potency and selectivity in the induction of protein phosphorylation than cAMP. In fact, less ^{32}P is incorporated by the three protein bands and this incorporation, in contrast with that observed in presence of cAMP, is of the same entity for the 59K and the 56K with an even higher phosphorylation for the latter (Fig. 3B).

Cyclic inosine monophosphate (cIMP) is also able to enhance protein phosphorylation in pineal gland homogenate. Its effect is much more pronounced on the 59K protein with a potency between those found for cAMP and cGMP (see the autoradiography of Fig. 5, lane 7). The effect of cIMP is not surprising since it has been already reported that this cyclic nucleotide does not act through a cIMP-dependent protein kinase, but rather it elicits its biochemical effects by binding to the regulatory subunit of the cAMP- and cGMP-dependent protein kinases (Walter et al., 1977; Casnellie et al., 1978).

The sensitivity of the same 59K, 56K and 35K protein bands to both cAMP and cGMP opens up three possibilities, namely:

(*a*) A cGMP-dependent protein kinase does exist in the pineal and it is active on the same protein substrates of the cAMP dependent protein kinase.
(*b*) A cGMP-dependent protein kinase exists in the pineal and it phosphorylates its own protein substrates with a molecular weight similar to the cAMP-dependent protein kinase substrates.
(*c*) A cGMP-protein kinase activity does not exist in the pineal and the effect of cGMP may be ascribed to a non-specific stimulation of the cAMP-dependent protein kinase for the rather low selectivity of the cAMP binding site in the regulatory subunit.

Due to the narrow substrate specificity of the cGMP-dependent protein kinase, there is no evidence in the literature for the existence of endogenous substrates for both cAMP- and cGMP-dependent protein kinases in the brain, with the exception of histones and some peptides (Nestler and Greengard, 1984; Nairn et al., 1985). Moreover, in mammalian brain only one specific substrate, called G-substrate, has been found (Nairn and Greengard, 1983). Thus, it is likely that the effect of cGMP observed on pineal phosphoproteins could mainly be ascribed to a non-specific action of the guanine nucleotide on the cAMP-dependent protein kinase. However, in order to test the above mentioned hypotheses, we used the following experimental approaches:

(*a*) We performed two-dimensional gel electrophoresis of the phosphorylated pineal homogenate proteins after stimulation with either cAMP or cGMP in order to show whether these cyclic nucleotides enhance the phsophorylation of the same protein substrates or of different substrates that comigrate in the same position in the sodium dodecylsulfate polyacrylamide gel electrophoresis (SDS–PAGE) system.

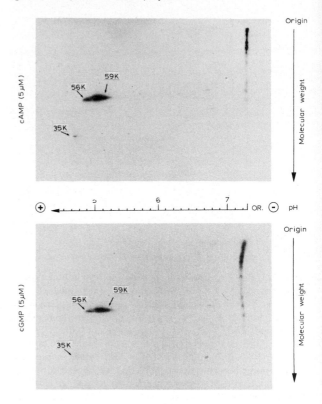

Fig. 4. Autoradiography of the two-dimensional separation of pineal phosphoproteins stimulated by cAMP (upper gel) or cGMP (lower gel). The two-dimensional gel electrophoresis was carried out according to O'Farrell (1975). Following the phosphorylation assay, the reaction was stopped by immersion in liquid nitrogen and lyophilization of the samples. The lyophilized samples, containing the equivalent homogenate of one pineal gland, were resuspended in 100 µl lysis buffer. In the first dimension, isoelectric focussing (IEF) was accomplished in tube gels (127.5 mm × 2.5 mm i.d.) containing 4.75% acrylamide with 8 M urea and a 4:1 ratio of (pH 5–7) and (pH 3–10) ampholines at a final concentration of 2%. Proteins were focussed overnight for 20 h. Upon completion, gels were gently extruded from the glass tubes and allowed to equilibrate for 30 minutes in a solution containing 10% glycerol, 2% SDS, 5% 2-mercaptoethanol and 0.625 M TRIS, pH 6.8. To separate the proteins in the second dimension, the IEF gels were placed on the top of a 10% SDS–polyacrylamide slab gel. Electrophoresis and autoradiography were accomplished as described above. The pH range of the IEF run is indicated in the figure together with the apparent molecular weight of the three major phosphoproteins (arrows). The concentration of the cyclic nucleotides used in the assay was 5 µM.

(b) We tested the specificity of the cyclic nucleotide-induced phosphorylation by using the specific inhibitor of the cAMP-dependent protein kinase, which seems to bind to the active site of the catalytic subunit, inducing a competitive inhibition of the enzyme (Walsh et al., 1971).

In Fig. 4 the phosphoproteins present in pineal homogenate were resolved on two-dimensional isoelectric focussing (IEF)/SDS−PAGE (O'Farrell, 1975). The similar autoradiographic pattern demonstrates that cAMP and cGMP stimulate the phosphorylation of the same 59K, 56K and 35K porteins of isoelectric point ranging from 5.5 to 4.5 and that the possibility of different comigrating proteins can be ruled out. However, these results suggest that both cyclic nucleotides induced the phosphorylation of the same substrates through the activation of a cyclic nucleotide-dependent protein kinase, but do not exclude

the existence of a cGMP-dependent enzyme. The evidence for the non-specific effect elicited by cGMP and cIMP on protein phosphorylation is given in Fig. 5. The addition of the specific cAMP-dependent protein kinase inhibitor (Walsh inhibitor) dramatically reduces the cAMP-, cGMP- and cIMP-dependent stimulation of 59K protein phosphorylation, indicating that both cGMP and cIMP exert their effects by acting on the pineal cAMP-dependent protein kinase. The different potencies of the various cyclic nucleotides in inducing phosphorylation of the above-mentioned protein bands can be explained by a lower affinity for the binding site in the regulatory subunit of the cAMP-dependent enzyme or by a possible different sensitivity to phosphodiesterase breakdown. The activity of this enzyme, however, is kept at very low levels by the addition of the phosphodiesterase inhibitor isobuthylmethylxantine (IBMX, 0.5 mM).

Calcium/calmodulin- and calcium/phosphatidylserine-dependent phosphorylation

Recently calmodulin activity has also been found in the pineal gland (Zhou et al., 1985). This enzyme activator greatly enhances the activity of calcium/calmodulin-dependent protein kinases in brain tissue (Nairn et al., 1985). Therefore we have investigated the possibility that one or more of these enzymes could exist in the pineal gland and could phosphorylate specific substrates. The exogenous addition of calcium to pineal homogenate does not induce by itself a marked enhancement of ^{32}P incorporation in protein bands. The major substrate appears to be a 46-kDa protein, whose phosphorylation shows a dose dependency with a peak effect at 0.2 mM calcium concentration (Fig. 6, left panel; Fig. 7A). Few other bands of higher molecular weight also appear to be sensitive to calcium stimulation, but to a lesser extent. Further studies were aimed to determine whether the low phosphorylation observed after the addition of exogenous calcium was due to the low pineal content of either calmodulin or the enzyme.

Since calcium exerts its effects on protein phosphorylation by stimulating either a calcium/calmodulin (Ca/CM)- or a calcium/phosphatidylserine (Ca/Ps)-protein kinase, we wished to know

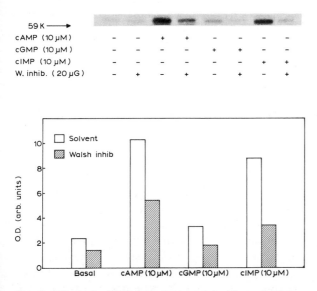

Fig. 5. Effect of cAMP-dependent protein kinase inhibitor (Walsh inhibitor) on the phosphorylation of the 59K protein stimulated by cAMP, cGMP and cIMP. The concentration of each cyclic nucleotide used in the incubation mixture was 10 μM. Before the addition of cyclic nucleotides, pineal homogenates were preincubated at 30°C for 5 min in the absence or presence of 20 μg/sample Walsh inhibitor (upper panel). The phosphorylation procedure was carried out as described in legend to Fig. 2. The lower panel shows the semiquantitative evaluation of ^{32}P incorporation in the absence (open columns) or presence (dashed columns) of Walsh inhibitor. In the Y-axis optical density (O.D.) values are reported in arbitrary units.

302

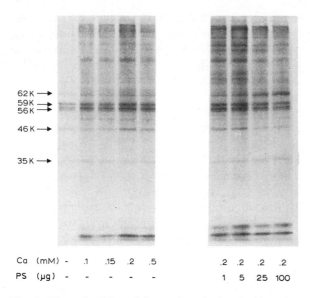

Ca (mM) -   .1   .15   .2   .5   .2   .2   .2   .2
PS (µg) -   -   -   -   -   1   5   25   100

Fig. 6. Effect of calcium (left panel) and phosphatidylserine (right panel) on protein phosphorylation in rat pineal homogenate. The assay was carried out after the addition of increasing concentrations of exogenous calcium (Ca, 0.1–0.5 mM) or of phosphatidylserine (PS, 1–100 µg/sample) in presence of 0.2 mM calcium. Arrows indicate the apparent molecular weight of the phosphoproteins investigated.

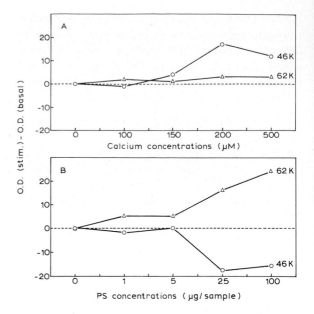

Fig. 7. Semiquantitative analysis of the changes in the phosphorylation state of the 62K and 46K proteins induced by the presence of increasing concentrations of calcium (Ca, upper panel) and phosphatidylserine (PS, lower panel). For further details see legend to Fig. 3 and 6.

whether the 46K protein is phosphorylated by one or both these enzymes. The possible involvement of Ca/PS-protein kinase in pineal function comes from recent reports concerning the biological role of α-receptor sites present in the pineal gland. The occupation of the α-adrenergic receptors by agonist appears not only to potentiate the β-adrenergic stimulation of SNAT activity, but also to mediate an increase in phosphatidylinositol turnover (Nijjar et al., 1980; Sugden et al., 1984). Two products (diacylglycerol and inositol triphosphate) formed from the phosphoinositide breakdown have been reported to regulate the Ca/PS-protein kinase (protein kinase C) activity and the mobilization of intracellular calcium (Nishizuka, 1984). The effects of the addition of increasing concentrations of exogenous phosphatidylserine in the presence of 0.2 mM calcium are illustrated in Fig. 6 (right panel). A dose-dependent increase of the ^{32}P incorporation into a 62-kDa protein band is observed. The phosphorylation of this protein, rather weak after

the addition of calcium alone, increases linearly along with phosphatidylserine concentrations up to 100 µg/sample. This concentration, however, is quite high and exerts some inhibitory effects on other phosphoproteins, namely the calcium-sensitive 46K protein band (Fig. 7B).

The effect of endogenous calcium on pineal phosphorylation has been counteracted by using EGTA. In fact the addition of this chelating agent (0.1 mM) to the incubation mixture reduces the ^{32}P incorporation in the high molecular weight region of the gel (Fig. 8, first two lanes). In this experimental condition the 46K band is not phosphorylated and it becomes apparent only after the addition of calcium. In the presence of exogenous calmodulin, an enhanced phosphorylation in the 62K and 52K regions is observed. As discussed before, phosphatidylserine is also able to induce a dose-dependent increase in the ^{32}P incorporation into the 62K protein. The increased phosphorylation elicited by both calmodulin and phosphatidylserine is strongly antagonized by trifluoperazine (Fig. 8). Since this antipsychotic

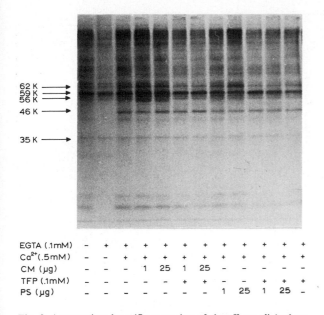

EGTA (.1mM)	−	+	+	+	+	+	+	+	+	+	+	+
Ca²⁺(.5mM)	−	−	+	+	+	+	+	+	+	+	+	+
CM (μg)	−	−	−	1	25	1	25	−	−	−	−	−
TFP (.1mM)	−	−	−	−	−	+	+	−	−	+	+	+
PS (μg)	−	−	−	−	−	−	−	1	25	1	25	−

Fig. 8. Antagonism by trifluoperazine of the effects elicited on protein phosphorylation by the exogenous addition of either calmodulin or phosphatidylserine. The phosphorylation assay was carried out in the absence and presence of 0.5 mM calcium. The amounts of calmodulin (CM) and phosphatidylserine (PS) were 1 and 25 μg/sample for each activator. The samples, containing 250 μg (wet weight) of pineal homogenate, were preincubated for 2 min at 30°C in presence of either CM and PS alone or the activators plus 0.1 mM trifluoperazine (TFP). Phosphorylation was started by the addition of [γ-³²P]ATP and stopped after 10 s at 30°C. The arrows indicate the apparent molecular weight of the phosphoproteins described in the text.

phenotiazine has been reported to inhibit the activity of both Ca/CM- and Ca/PS-protein kinases (Wrenn et al., 1981), these results suggest that the observed phosphorylation in pineal homogenate can be mediated by these enzymes and that the 62K protein may represent a good substrate for both of them. However, the calcium-stimulated 46K phosphoprotein which, from its electrophoretical mobility, could resemble the F1 protein or the B-50 protein reported by Erlich and Routtenberg (1974) and Zwiers et al. (1976), is not affected by the exogenous addition of either calmodulin or phosphatidylserine and its state of phosphorylation is not modified by trifluoperazine. This indicates that the 46K protein may not represent a specific substrate for the Ca/CM- or

Ca/PS-protein kinases, and it suggests that its phosphorylation could be regulated by a different protein kinase present in the pineal gland such as, for example, the calcium-dependent protease-activated protein kinase I reported by Tuazon et al. (1984).

Regulation of pineal protein phosphorylation by environmental lighting and adrenergic drugs

As discussed before, exposure of experimental animals to constant light for 18 hours induces a supersensitive state of the β-receptor system, whereas the same period in the dark leads to its down-regulation. Under these experimental conditions, a change in the basal and cAMP-stimulated activity of the protein kinase has been reported, suggesting that a possible alteration in the state of phosphorylation of previously described substrate proteins may occur (Zatz and O'Dea, 1976). Fig. 9 shows a representative autoradiograph of the protein phosphorylation pattern in pineal homogenates from rats exposed for 18 hours to constant light or dark conditions and killed 15 minutes after the subcutaneous administration of either saline or (−)isoproterenol (5 mg/kg). In saline-treated animals the autoradiographic pattern did not show any difference in the ³²P incorporation in the 59K, 56K and 46K protein bands in both light- and dark-exposed rats. Following (−)isoproterenol administration, a clear-cut enhancement in the phosphorylation of the 56K and 59K proteins is observed only in the light-exposed animals.

A more detailed microdensitometrical analysis of the 46K calcium-sensitive and the three major cAMP-sensitive proteins (59K, 56K and 35K) is reported in Figs. 10 and 11. As described above, after β-adrenergic receptor stimulation the 59K and 56K proteins can be highly phosphorylated in vitro. However, the 35K protein, which is phosphorylated in the presence of exogenous cAMP, is not affected by the administration of the adrenergic agonist. The addition of cAMP (1 μM) to the incubation mixture does not further enhance the isoproterenol-induced phosphorylation of the 59K and 56K proteins, indicating that the endogeneous levels of cAMP after the

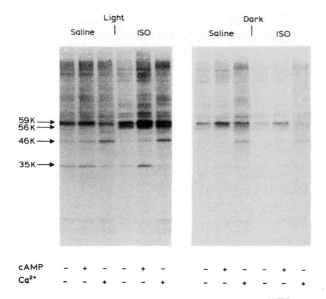

cAMP   − + −   − + −   − + −   − + −

Ca²⁺   − − +   − − +   − − +   − − +

Fig. 9. Effect of constant light and dark exposure on pineal protein phosphorylation in saline- and (−)isoproterenol (ISO)-treated rats. To animals kept in constant light or darkness for 18 hours, either saline or (−)isoproterenol (5 mg/kg body weight) was administered subcutaneously 15 minutes before killing. The pineals were rapidly removed and homogenized in 50 mM HEPES buffer pH 7.4, 0.1 mM EGTA, 5 mM MgCl₂, 1 mM DTT and 0.5 mM IBMX. The in vitro phosphorylation assay was performed on aliquots of homogenate in the absence and presence of either cAMP (1 µM) or calcium (0.5 mM) as reported in lenged to Fig. 2. Phosphorylated proteins were separated by SDS–PAGE and ³²P incorporation visualized by autoradiography. The molecular wieghts of the proteins of interest are indicated by the arrows.

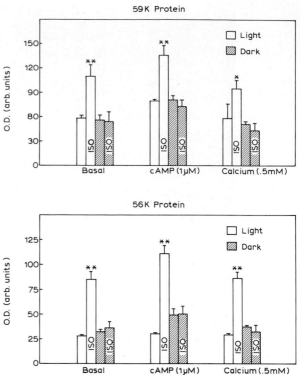

Fig. 10. Semiquantitative analysis of the ³²P incorporation in the cAMP-sensitive bands 59K and 56K proteins in light- (open columns) and dark- (dashed columns) exposed rats after subcutaneous administration of saline or (−)isoproterenol (ISO). The drug administration schedule and the experimental procedure are described in legend to Fig. 9. The results obtained from the densitometrical analysis of the autoradiograms are expressed as optical density (O.D., arbitrary units). The columns in the plot represent the mean ± SEM of five independent replications. The statistical analysis was carried out by using the Duncan's multiple comparison test (* $p < 0.05$, ** $p < 0.01$ versus the respective light- or dark-exposed saline groups) (Rocchetti and Recchia, 1982).

administration of the drug are already high enough to maximally stimulate the cAMP-dependent protein kinase. Once again, the phosphorylating pattern of the 35K protein appears to be different since the addition of 1 µM exogenous cAMP does induce an increase in ³²P incorporation in this protein not observed after (−) isoproterenol alone.

We were not able, in our experimental conditions, to determine whether the 35K protein may represent the nuclear phosphoprotein reported by Winters et al. (1977); however, if this is the case, the lack of phosphorylation 15 minutes after isoproterenol can be explained by considering that this time is not sufficient to allow the translocation of the protein kinase catalytic subunit from the cytoplasm to the nucleus. Then the uneven compartmentalization of the above-mentioned substrate proteins for the cAMP-dependent protein kinase can explain the different phosphorylation observed in our experimental conditions. Alternatively, since the 35K band seems to be the only cAMP-dependent phosphoprotein sensitive to the light–dark cycle in basal conditions, it is possible that in vivo this protein is differentially regulated by the cAMP-dependent protein kinase compared with the 59K and 56K

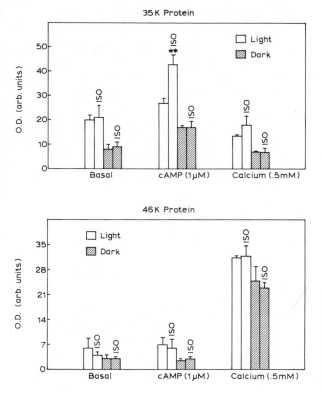

Fig. 11. Semiquantitative analysis of the 32P incorporation in the cAMP-sensitive (35K) and calcium-sensitive (46K) proteins in light- (open columns) and dark- (dashed columns) exposed rats after the subcutaneous administration of saline or (−)isoproterenol (ISO). For further details see legend to Fig. 10.

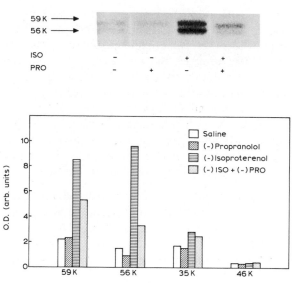

Fig. 12. Effects of β-adrenergic drugs on pineal protein phosphorylation in rats exposed for 18 hours to constant light. ^{32}P incorporation was evaluated after subcutaneous administration of (−)isoproterenol (5 mg/kg, 15 min before killing), (−)propranolol (29 mg/kg, 45 min before killing), or (−)propranolol plus (−)isoproterenol. A representative autoradiography of ^{32}P incorporation in 59K and 56K proteins is illustrated in the upper panel. The microdensitometrical analysis of the phosphorylation of the 59K, 56K and 35K cAMP-sensitive and the 46K calcium-sensitive bands after the different pharmacological treatments is reported in the lower panel.

phosphoproteins, suggesting a possible involvement in different biological processes.

As expected, in presence of exogenous calcium (0.5 mM), the phosphorylation pattern of the 59K, 56K and 35K cAMP-sensitive proteins is quite similar to that observed in basal conditions. On the contrary, the ^{32}P incorporation into the 46K calcium-sensitive band (Fig. 11) appears to be completely unaffected by both environmental lighting and β-receptor activation but highly stimulated only after the addition of exogenous calcium.

Taken together, these data indicate that the observed variations in the phosphorylation state of the cAMP-sensitive proteins are related to the β-adrenergic system in vivo. This hypothesis is further strengthened by the observation that the β-

adrenergic antagonist propranolol (20 mg/kg), injected 30 minutes before isoproterenol administration, partially prevented the isoproterenol stimulating effect on the 59K and 56K proteins but did not change by itself the state of phosphorylation of these proteins (Fig. 12). Then the changes occurring in pineal β-receptors and catecholamine-sensitive adenylate cyclase during supersensitivity development seem to be accompanied also by variations in cAMP-dependent protein kinase activity and phosphorylation of substrate proteins.

Conclusions

In this study we report the presence of specific protein substrates for the cAMP-, Ca/CM- and Ca/PS-dependent protein kinases in the pineal gland. Three major proteins of 59, 56 and 35 kDa are phosphorylated by the cAMP-dependent enzyme. They are also sensitive, though to a lesser extent, to other cyclic nucleotides such as cGMP or cIMP; however, the results indicate that this effect is mediated by the cAMP-sensitive protein kinase and that the existence in the pineal gland of a cGMP-dependent enzyme can be ruled out.

On the other hand, calcium is also able to affect pineal protein phosphorylation, although with a weaker effect. Calcium may exert its action through the following possible mechanisms:

(a) by stimulating a calcium/calmodulin-dependent protein kinase and increasing the phosphorylation of protein bands in the 52–62 kDa range;
(b) by stimulating a calcium/phosphatidylserine-dependent protein kinase and increasing ^{32}P incorporation in a 62-kDa protein;
(c) by stimulating by itself the phosphorylation of a 46-kDa protein through the activation of a not yet characterized protein kinase.

Experiments designed to study protein phosphorylation in different physiological and pharmacological conditions affecting the adrenergic system show that changes in pineal function can be reflected by changes in the state of phosphorylation of substrate proteins. In fact, increases in β-adrenergic receptor sensitivity achieved by exposing animals to constant light can induce an increase in the phosphorylation of some cAMP-dependent protein kinase substrates following isoproterenol stimulation; however, such an effect is not observed in subsensitive conditions.

Then the sensitivity of the pineal gland to β-adrenergic stimulation seems to be modulated at different levels of the recognition and transduction mechanisms. The observed results prove that the variations in cAMP-dependent protein kinase activity are mediated by β-adrenergic receptors since the stimulating effect induced by isoproterenol can be blocked by the β-receptor antagonist propranolol. On the contrary, the calcium-dependent protein kinase activity seems to be unaffected by environmental lighting and β-adrenergic receptor manipulations. Thus, the cAMP- and calcium-dependent phosphorylating processes may be involved in different aspects of pineal function.

Acknowledgements

This work was supported by a grant of MPI 60% and by an international grant from the Italian National Research Council (CNR). We thank Dr. W.H. Gispen, Division of Molecular Neurobiology, Rudolph Magnus Institute for Pharmacology, Utrecht University, The Netherlands for the fruitful discussion and Dr. M. Zoli, Department of Human Physiology, Modena University, Italy for the careful revision of the manuscript.

References

Alphs, L. and Lovenberg, W. (1984) Modulation of rat pineal acetyl-Co A: arylamine N-acetyltransferase induction by alpha adrenergic drugs. J. Pharmacol. Exp Ther., 230:431–437.

Axelrod, J. (1974) The pineal gland: a neurochemical transducer. Science, 184:1341–1348.

Axelrod, J. and Weissach. H. (1961) Purification and properties of hydroxyindole-O-methyltransferase. J. Biol. Chem., 236:211–213.

Brown, G., Grota, L. Bubenik, G., Niles. L. and Tsui, H. (1981) Physiologic regulation of melatonin. In N. Birau and W. Schlott (Eds.), Melatonin – Current Status and Perspectives. Advances in The Biosciences, Vol. 29, Pergamon Press, Oxford, pp. 95–112.

Brownstein, M.J. and Axelrod, J. (1974) Pineal gland: a 24-h rhythm in norepinephrine turnover. Science, 184:163–165.

Casnellie, J.E., Schlichter, D.J., Walter, U. and Greengard, P. (1978) Photoaffinity labeling of a guanosine 3':5'-monophosphate-dependent protein kinase from vascular smooth muscle. J. Biol. Chem., 253:4771–4776.

Deguchi, T. (1973) Role of the β-adrenergic receptor in the elevation of adenosine cyclic 3'.5'-monophosphate and induction of serotonin N-acetyltransferase in rat pineal glands. Mol. Pharmacol., 9:184–190.

Deguchi, T. and Axelrod, J. (1972a) Induction and superinduction of serotonin N-acetyltransferase by adrenergic drugs and denervation in the rat pineal gland. Proc. Natl. Acad. Sci. U.S.A., 69: 2208–2211.

Deguchi, T. and Axelrod, J. (1972b) Control of circadian change of serotonin N-acetyltransferase in pineal organ of the β-adrenergic receptor. Proc. Natl. Acad. Sci. U.S.A., 69:2547–2550.

Deguchi, T. and Axelrod, J. (1973a) Supersensitivity and subsensitivity of the β-adrenergic receptor in pineal gland regulated by catecholamine transmitter. Proc. Natl. Acad. Sci. U.S.A., 70:2411–2414.

Deguchi, T. and Axelrod, J. (1973b) Superinduction of serotonin N-acetyltransferase and supersensitivity of adenylate cylcase to catecholamine in denervated pineal gland. Mol. Pharmacol., 9:612–618.

Erlich, Y.H. and Routtenberg, A. (1974) Cyclic AMP regulates phosphorylation of three protein components of rat cerebral cortex membranes for thirty minutes. *FEBS Lett.*, 45:237–243.

Fontana, J.A. and Lovenberg, W. (1971) A cyclic AMP-dependent protein kinase of the bovine pineal gland. *Proc. Natl. Acad. Sci. U.S.A.*, 68:2787–2790.

Hauser, G., Shein, H.M. and Eichberg, J. (1974) Relationship of α-adrenergic receptors in rat pineal gland to drug-induced stimulation of phospholipid metabolism. *Nature*, 252:482–483.

Kappers, J.A. (1960) The development, topographical relations and innervation of the epiphysis cerebri in the albino rat. *Z. Zellforsch. Mikrosk. Anat.*, 52:163–215.

Kappers, J.A. (1979) Short history of pineal discovery and research. In J.A. Kappers and P. Pevet (Eds.). *The Pineal Gland of Vertebrates Including Man, Progress in Brain Research, Vol. 52*, Elsevier, Amsterdam, pp. 3–22.

Kappers, J.A. (1982) Innervation of the vertebrate pineal organ. In J. Axelrod, F. Fraschini and G.P. Velo (Eds.). *The Pineal Gland and its Endocrine Role*, Plenum Press, New York, pp. 87–112.

Kebabian, J.W., Zatz, M., Romero, J.A. and Axelrod, J. (1975) Rapid changes in rat pineal β-adrenergic receptor: alterations in ^{3}H-alprenolol binding and adenylate cyclase. *Proc. Natl. Acad. Sci. U.S.A.*, 72:3735–3739.

Klein, D.C. and Berg, G.R. (1970) Pineal gland: stimulation of melatonin production by norepinephrine involves cyclic AMP-mediated stimulation of N-acetyltransferase. *Adv. Biochem. Psychopharmacol.*, 3:241–263.

Klein, D.C. and Weller, J. (1970) Indole metabolism in the pineal gland: a circadian rhythm in N-acetyltransferase. *Science.* 169:1093–1095.

Klein, D.C. and Weller, J. (1973) Adrenergic adenosine 3′,5′-monophosphate regulation of serotonin N-acetyltransferase activity and the temporal relationship of serotonin N-acetyltransferase activity to synthesis of ^{3}H-N-acetylserotonin and ^{3}H-melatonin in cultured rat pineal. *J. Pharmacol. Exp. Ther.*, 186:516–527.

Klein, D.C., Berg, G.R. and Weller, J. (1970) Melatonin synthesis: adenosine 3′,5′-monophosphate and norepinephrine stimulate N-acetyltransferase. *Science*, 168:979–980.

Krueger, B.K., Forn, J. and Greengard, P. (1977) Depolarization-induced phosphorylation of specific proteins, mediated by calcium ion influx, in rat brain synaptosomes. *J. Biol. Chem.*, 252:2764–2773.

Laemmli, U.K. (1970) Cleavage of structural proteins during the assembly of the head of bacteriophage T4. *Nature*, 227:680–685.

Menaker, M., Takahashi, J.S. and Eskin, A. (1978) The physiology of circadian pacemakers. *Annu. Rev. Physiol.*, 40:501–526.

Minneman, K.P. and Iversen, L.L. (1976) Cholera toxin induces pineal enzymes in culture. *Science*, 192:803–805.

Moore, R.Y. and Klein, D.C. (1974) Visual pathways and central neural control of a circadian rhythm in pineal serotonin N-acetyltransferase activity. *Brain Res.*, 71:17–33.

Moyer, J.A., Greenberg, L.H., Frazer, A., Brunswick, D.J., Mendels, J. and Weiss, B. (1979) Opposite effects of acute and repeated administration of desmethylimipramine on adrenergic responsiveness in rat pineal gland. *Life Sci.*, 24:2237–2244.

Nairn, A.C. and Greengard, P. (1983) Cyclic GMP-dependent protein phosphorylation in mammalian brain. *Fed. Proc.*, 42:3107–3113.

Nairn, A.C., Hemmings, H.C. Jr. and Greengard, P. (1985) Protein kinases in the brain. *Annu. Rev. Biochem.*, 54:931–976.

Nestler, E.J. and Greengard, P. (1984) *Protein Phosphorylation in The Nervous System*, John Wiley & Sons, New York.

Nestler, E.J., Zatz, M. and Greengard, P. (1982) A diurnal rhythm in pineal protein I content mediated by β-adrenergic neurotransmission. *Science*, 217:357–359.

Nishizuka, Y. (1984) Turnover of inositol phospholipids and signal transduction. *Science*, 225:1365–1370.

Nijjar, M.S., Smith, T.L. and Hauser, G. (1980) Evidence against dopaminergic and further support for α-adrenergic receptor involvement in the pineal phosphatidylinositol effect. *J. Neurochem.*, 34:813–821.

O'Dea, R.F. and Zatz, M. (1976) Catecholamine-stimulated cyclic GMP accumulation in the rat pineal: Apparent presynaptic site of action. *Proc. Natl. Acad. Sci. U.S.A.*, 73:3398–3402.

O'Farrell, P.H. (1975) High resolution two-dimensional electrophoresis of proteins. *J. Biol. Chem.*, 250:4007–4021.

Rocchetti, M. and Recchia, M. (1982) SPBS: statistical programs for biological sciences. Mini computer software for applying routine biostatistical methods. *Comput. Progr. Biomed.*, 14:7–20.

Romero, J.A. and Axelrod, J. (1974) Pineal β-adrenergic receptor: diurnal variation in sensitivity. *Science*, 184:1091–1092.

Romero, J.A., Zatz, M., Kebabian, J.W. and Axelrod, J. (1975) Circadian cycles in binding of ^{3}H-alprenolol to β-adrenergic receptor sites in pineal. *Nature*, 258:435–436.

Rusak, B. and Zucker, I. (1979) Neural regulation of circadian rhythms. *Physiol. Rev.*, 59:449–526.

Strada, S.J. and Weiss, B. (1974) Increased response to catecholamines of the cyclic AMP system of rat pineal gland induced by decreased sympathetic activity. *Arch. Biochem. Biophys.*, 160:197–204.

Strada, S., Klein, D.C., Weller, J. and Weiss B. (1972) Norepinephrine stimulation of cyclic adenosine monophosphate in cultured pineal glands. *Endocrinology*, 90:1470–1475.

Sugden, D. and Klein, D.C. (1984) Rat pineal α₁-adrenoceptors: identification and characterization using [^{125}I] iodo-2-[β-(4-hydroxyphenyl)-ethylaminomethyl]-tetralone ([^{125}I]HEAT). *Endocrinology*, 114:435–440.

Sugden, D. and Klein, D.C. (1985) Regulation of rat pineal α₁-adrenoceptors. *J. Neurochem.*, 44:63–67.

Sugden, D., Weller, J.L., Klein, D.C., Kirk, K.L. and Creveling, C.R. (1984) Alpha-adrenergic potentiation of beta-adrenergic stimulation of rat pineal N-acetyltransferase. Studies using cirazoline and fluorine analogs of norepinephrine. *Biochem. Pharmacol.*, 33:3947–3950.

Tamarkin, L., Baird, C.J. and Almeida, O.F.X. (1985) Melatonin: a coordinating signal for mammalian reproduction? *Science*, 227:714–720.

Taylor, A.N. and Wilson, R.W. (1970) Electrophysiological evidence for the action of light on the pineal gland in the rat. *Experientia*, 26:267–269.

Tuazon, P.T. and Traugh, J.A. (1984) Activation of actin-activated ATPase in smooth muscle by phosphorylation of myosin light chain with protease-activated kinase I. *J. Biol. Chem.*, 259:541–546.

Ueda, T. and Greengard, P. (1977) Adenosine 3′:5′-monophosphate-regulated phosphoprotein system of neuronal membranes. I. Solubilization, purification, and some properties of an endogenous phosphoprotein. *J.Biol. Chem.*, 252:5155–5163.

Walsh, D.A., Ashby, C.D., Gonzales, C., Calkins, D., Fischer, E. and Krebs, E.G. (1971) Purification and characterization of a protein kinase inhibitor of adenosine 3′,5′-monophosphate-dependent protein kinases. *J. Biol. Chem.*, 246:1977–1985.

Walter, U., Uno, I., Liu, A.Y.-C. and Greengard, P. (1977) Identification, characterization, and quantitative measurements of cyclic AMP receptor proteins in cytosol of various tissues using a photoaffinity ligand. *J. Biol. Chem.*, 252:6494–6500.

Weiss, B. and Costa, E. (1967) Adenyl cyclase activity in rat pineal gland: effects of chronic denervation and norepinephrine. Science, 156:1750–1752.

Weiss, B. and Costa, E. (1968) Selective stimulation of adenyl cyclase activity in rat pineal by pharmacologically active catecholamines. *J. Pharmacol. Exp. Ther.*, 161:310–319.

Weissbach, H., Redfield, B.G. and Axelrod, J. (1960) Biosynthesis of melatonin: enzymic conversion of serotonin to *N*-acetylserotonin. *Biochim. Biophys. Acta*, 43:352–353.

Winters, K.E., Morrissey, J.J., Loos, P.J. and Lovenberg, W. (1977) Pineal protein phosphorylation during serotonin *N*-acetyltransferase induction. *Proc. Natl. Acad. Sci. U.S.A.*, 74:1928–1931.

Wrenn, R.W., Katoh, N., Schatzman, R.C. and Kuo, J.F. (1981) Inhibition by phenothiazine antipsychotic drugs of calcium-dependent phosphorylation of cerebral cortex proteins regulated by phospholipid or calmodulin. *Life Sci.*, 29:725–733.

Zatz, M. (1977) Effects of cholera tocin on supersensitive and subsensitive rat pineal glands: regulation of sensitivity at multiple sites. *Life Sci.*, 21:1267–1276.

Zatz, M. and O'Dea, R.F. (1976) Regulation of protein kinase in rat pineal: increased V_{max} in supersensitive glands. *J. Cyclic Nucleotide Res.*, 2:427-439.

Zhou, L.W., Mayer, J.A., Muth, E.A., Clark, B., Palkovits, M. and Weiss, B. (1985) Regional distribution of calmodulin activity in rat brain. *J. Neurochem.*, 44:1657–1662.

Zwiers, H., Veldhuis, H.D., Schotman, P. and Gispen, W.H. (1976) ACTH, cyclic nucleotides, and brain protein phosphorylation in vitro. *Neurochem. Res.*, 1:669–677.

W.H. Gispen and A. Routtenberg (Eds.)
Progress in Brain Research, Vol. 69
© 1986 Elsevier Science Publishers B.V. (Biomedical Division)

CHAPTER 24

Drosophila mutants with memory deficits

Peter Friedrich[1], Piroska Dévay[1], Viktor Dombrádi[3], Zoltán Kiss[2], Ildikó Láng[1], Marianna Pintér[1] and Magda Solti[1]

[1]*Institute of Enzymology and* [2]*Institute of Biochemistry, Biological Research Center, Hungarian Academy of Sciences, P.O.Box 7, H-1502 Budapest, and* [3]*Institute of Medical Chemistry, University Medical School of Debrecen, Hungary*

Introduction

Insects are undoubtedly the most successful class of animals. They far outnumber the rest of animal kingdom, in respect of the number of both species and individuals. This unique abundance must stem from a close and multifarious adaptation to the earth's biosphere. It may look somewhat odd, if not disquieting, that this evolutionary success has been achieved by organisms thought to be governed solely by genetically determined, fixed behavioral patterns, i.e. by behavioral automatons.

It has lately been shown, however, that insects are not mere automatons, but display behavioral plasticity: they possess the faculties of learning and memory. This has been convincingly demonstrated with dipterans (flies), an order of insects including the fruit fly *Drosphila melanogaster*, the blowfly *Phormia regina* and the house fly *Musca domestica* (cf. McGuire, 1984). Although generalizations may be premature since dipterans count more than 80 000 species, it is impressive that all three flies tested exhibited some types of learning. Moreover, the learning ability of *Drosophila* has been found to parallel evolutionary fitness (Hewitt et al., 1983).

Fruit flies are attractive organisms for the study of learning and memory. They are easy to maintain in the laboratory, even in mass culture, their generation time is short and their nervous system is fairly simple. Behaviorally, flies are quite entertaining. Above all, the ease of producing mutants renders them suitable for the genetic dissection of the learning and memory processes. This holds true particularly for *Drosophila melanogaster*, the much investigated object of classical genetics. In addition to the vast amount of information available about its genome, it lends itself readily to molecular genetic manipulations.

Genetic dissection offers the unique possibility to knock out, in principle, any macromolecule along a reaction sequence, be it an enzyme, a receptor, a structural protein or something else. The techniques of molecular genetics allow one to produce these proteins, however rare, in reasonable amounts for detailed structure–function studies. These potential advantages compensate for the undeniable drawback, from a biochemist's viewpoint, that the fruit fly's brain is definitely smaller than that of, say, an ox.

At present there are half a dozen mutations known to affect conditioning in *Drosophila*. Importantly, the biochemical lesion in all those characterized so far is somehow related to cAMP metabolism. The *dunce* strains (6 alleles available) have a crippled cAMP-specific phosphodiesterase (PDE-II), with consequentially elevated overall cAMP levels (Dudai et al., 1976; Byers et al., 1981; Davis and Kiger, 1981). There is strong evidence that the mutation is located in the structural gene of this enzyme (Kauvar, 1982; Shotwell, 1983). The *rutabaga* flies are impaired in a Ca^{2+}/calmodulin-activated adenylate cyclase catalytic subunit (Dudai et al., 1983, 1984; Livingstone et al., 1984), resulting in overall cAMP levels slightly below normal. The mutant turnip seems to be affected in the stimulatory GTP-binding protein of adenylate cyclase (cf. Tully, 1984). *Ddc* (dopa decarboxylase deficient) is a temperature-sensitive mutation; such flies are unable to synthesize dopamine and serotonin at restrictive temperatures and completely fail to learn under the same condition (Livingstone and Tempel, 1983; Tempel et al., 1984). The biochemical background in mutants *cabbage* and *amnesiac* is under investigation.

Behavior studies indicate that *dunce*, *rutabaga*, *amnesiac* and probably *cabbage* are, in fact, able to acquire a labile form of memory, but this rapidly wanes (Dudai, 1979, 1983; Quinn et al., 1979; Duerr and Quinn, 1982; Dudai et al., 1984). Hence, they are regarded as memory mutants. In contrast, *Ddc* appears to be affected in the phase of acquisition rather than memory storage (Tempel et al., 1983).

As the biochemical anomaly centers around cAMP metabolism, one tends to think that protein phosphorylation is altered in these mutants. This is an almost inevitable assumption, in view of the generally accepted role of cAMP in eukaryotic cells. Indeed, protein phosphorylation has been shown to play a pivotal role in both non-associative and associative learning of mollusks (Kandel and Schwartz, 1982; Hawkins et al., 1983; Shuster et al., 1985; Neary and Alkon, 1983; Alkon, 1984). It would therefore be rather surprising if protein phosphorylation eventually turned out not to be involved in the memory process of *Drosophila*.

The question is how to approach protein phosphorylation in *Drosophila* from this viewpoint. Unfortunately, the central nervous system of *Drosophila* is much less suitable for electrophysiological studies than that of mollusks. Neurons are small and the neural circuits involved in the various learning processes have not been identified. Hence, doing biochemistry at the single cell level, as done with *Aplysia* (Levitan et al., 1983; and references therein) and *Hermissenda* (Alkon, 1984; Acosta-Urquidi et al., 1984) has so far been out of reach with the fruit fly. To gain insight into the protein phosphorylation processes of *Drosophila* we have conducted comparative studies on a variety of aspects in wild type Canton-S and the memory mutant *dunce* strains.

Activation of *Drosophila*\glycogen phosphorylase

In mammals, glycogen phosphorylase is regulated via phosphorylation and dephosphorylation catalyzed by the respective kinase and phosphatase, which are part of the cascade starting with hormone-sensitive adenylate cyclase. In an attempt to assess the metabolic consequences of the high cAMP level present in *dunce* mutants, we examined the phosphorylation of glycogen phosphorylase in the different strains.

We purified the enzyme from whole flies to homogeneity and characterized some of its properties (Dombrádi et al., 1985). The *Drosophila* enzyme proved to be rather similar to its mammalian counterparts. It was activated by phosphorylation and deactivated by dephosphorylation. These reactions could equally be catalyzed in vitro by rabbit muscle or *Drosophila* phosphorylase kinase and phosphatase, respectively. The phosphorylation in vivo of glycogen phosphorylase could also be demonstrated in fruit flies (Dombrádi et al., 1986).

The comparison of phosphorylase-a (the phosphorylated form) level gave the following values: Canton-S, $20 \pm 5\%$; *dunce*^{M11}, $34 \pm 5\%$ of total phosphorylase (Dombrádi, unpublished). Since *dunce*^{M11} is an allele amorphic with respect to PDE-II, it has 4 to 6 times as high a cAMP level as the normal (Davis and Kiger, 1981). It seems that the elevated cAMP raised, though only moderately, the phosphorylase-a level in the mutant. The mechanism of this enhancement is not clear, because cAMP apparently had no effect on phosphorylase kinase in crude *Drosophila* homogenate or in surviving larval brain (Dombrádi, Erdődi, Risnik, Friedrich and Bot, unpublished), suggesting that cAMP-dependent protein kinase is not involved in the phosphorylase cascade in the same manner as with mammals. It is possible, however, that cAMP acts via inhibition of phosphorylase phosphatase by phosphorylating the phosphatase inhibitor-1.

Phosphorylase is unlikely to be directly involved in the learning and memory processes of

Drosophila. Nevertheless, it has been claimed that in certain mammalian neurons the level of phosphorylase-a reflects the firing activity of the cell (Woolf et al., 1984). In *Drosophila* brain glycogen granules can be seen by electron microscopy (Technau and Heisenberg, 1982) and fairly high phosphorylase activity can be measured in larval brain homogenate (Risnik and Friedrich, unpublished).

Search for differences in protein phosphorylation between wild type and *dunce* strains

The protein phosphorylation patterns of different *Drosophila* strains were studied by labeling both in vivo and in vitro (Dévay et al., 1984). In the in vivo experiments flies were fed [^{32}P]orthophosphate and then harvested; the heads were dislodged by sonication in liquid nitrogen. The head homogenates were immediately subjected to sodium dodecylsulfate–polyacrylamide gel electrophoresis (SDS–PAGE) followed by autoradiography. Fig. 1 shows the densitometric tracing obtained with Canton-S, *dunce^2* and *dunce^{M11}* heads. (The *dunce^2* mutant is hypomorphic with respect to PDE-II and has cAMP levels intermediate between Canton-S and *dunce^{M11}* (Byers et al., 1981; Davis and Kiger, 1981). It is seen that peaks corresponding to apparent $M_r \geqslant 120$ kDa are gradually increasing in the order Canton-S $<$ *dunce^2* $<$ *dunce^{M11}*. Owing to the poor resolution this experiment only indicates that there is indeed some enhancement of protein phosphorylation in the *dunce* strains. Work is underway to analyze the protein pattern by two-dimensional electrophoresis.

In the in vitro experiment fresh head homogenates were incubated with [γ-^{32}P]ATP for short periods of time (0.5 to 3 min). The only consistently occurring difference between Canton-S and *dunce^{M11}* was in a band of apparent $M_r \approx 53$ kDa, which was present in the mutant but was absent in the wild type. Even in the mutant, this band could be detected only in fresh (2 min-old) homogenate; the band rapidly waned when the homogenate was further incubated and practically disappeared around 5 min. However, this 53-kDa band was markedly increased if, prior to labeled ATP,

cAMP ($\sim 3 \mu$M) was added to the homogenate. cAMP was much less effective and Ca^{2+}/calmodulin had no effect at all. These data suggested that the 53-kDa protein was a substrate of cAMP-dependent protein kinase.

Differential cAMP-induced dephosphorylation of the 53-kDa protein in wild type and *dunce* flies

During the course of characterization of the 53-kDa substrate protein we came upon a peculiar phenomenon (Dévay et al., 1986). Studying the cAMP concentration dependence of labeling of the 53-kDa band in Canton-S and *dunce^{M11}* head homogenates, there was a characteristic difference between the two strains: while in Canton-S labeling became fairly constant above 3μM cAMP added, the same curve for *dunce^{M11}* showed a sharp maximum at about the same cAMP concentration and the label dramatically decreased toward higher nucleotide concentrations (Fig. 2). The time course of labeling (Fig. 3) indicated that the diminution of label in *dunce* was due to dephosphorylation rather than inhibited phosphorylation: while the label was nearly constant in Canton-S, it decreased in *dunce* from the earliest time (30 s) onward. This differential sensitivity to added cAMP could be traced back to the dissimilar PDE activities of the two strains: it should be recalled that *dunce^{M11}* does not contain PDE-II, which constitutes about two-thirds of total cAMP-splitting activity in wild type (Davis and Kiger, 1981). The evidence for this came from the experiment when 10 mM theophylline, a PDE inhibitor, was also added to Canton-S homogenate along with cAMP (Fig. 3): the *dunce*-type dephosphorylation was then 'phonecopied'. Apparently, a sustained critical cAMP level is to be maintained in order for dephosphorylation to occur.

Identification of the 53-kDa protein as the regulatory (R) subunit of cAMP-dependent protein kinase

In a preliminary characterization of protein phosphatases in *Drosophila* (Dombrádi, Bot and Friedrich, unpublished) we found at least one type

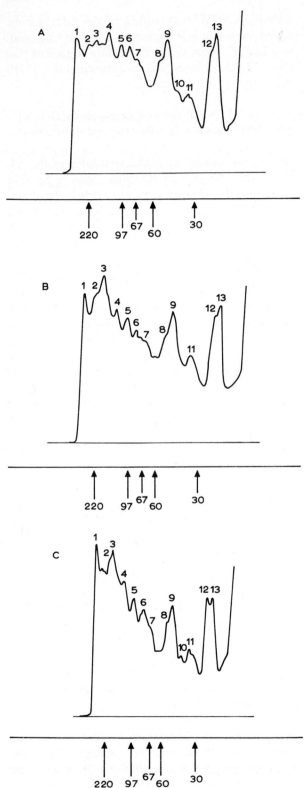

1 and one type 2 protein phosphatase, according to the terminology adopted for mammalian enzymes (Ingebritsen and Cohen, 1983), on the basis of inhibition by heat-stable protein inhibitors 1 and 2 from rabbit muscle. However, neither of these enzymes seemed to be activated by cAMP.

The explanation for cAMP-induced dephosphorylation of the 53-kDa protein came from 'chase' experiments (Fig. 4). Namely, when after labeling in Canton-S head homogenate according to the standard protocol we added a large excess of cold ATP, the label in the 53-kDa band remained constant. This finding suggests that the stable level of labeling is not due to a dynamic phosphorylation–dephosphorylation equilibrium. In contrast, if instead of cold ATP, cAMP was added to the mixture, the label in the 53-kDa band decreased. This can be interpreted only by assuming that the 53-kDa protein is identical with the R subunit of cAMP-dependent protein kinase.

What then occurs in our experimental setup is autophosphorylation of cAMP-dependent protein kinase. When cAMP is repeatedly added, the holoenzyme dissociates and the R subunit is dephosphorylated by endogenous protein phosphatases. In fact, the analogous phenomenon has been demonstrated for cAMP-dependent kinases purified from other sources (Uno, 1980; Gomes et al., 1983).

We provided the following evidence for the identity of 53-kDa protein and R subunit:

(a) Labeling of the 53-kDa band was unaffected by the heat-stable (Walsh) inhibitor (cf. Rangel-Aldao and Rosen, 1976a).
(b) Labeling was diminished by cAMP if Zn^{2+} was used instead of Mg^{2+} (Walter et al., 1977).
(c) Affinity sorption on cAMP–agarose selectively removed the 53-kDa band, indicating that the corresponding protein is a cAMP-binding species.

Fig. 1. Protein phosphorylation patterns of *Drosophila* heads after labeling with $^{32}P_i$ in vivo. The densitometric tracings of autoradiographic films made of SDS–PAGE slabs are seen. A, Canton-S; B, *dunce²*; C, *dunce^{M11}* Molecular mass markers are indicated in kDa. In *dunce* flies labeling around peak 3 is increased. From Dévay et al. (1984).

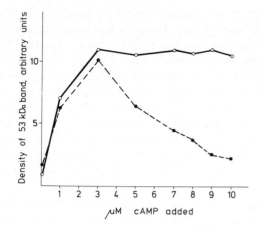

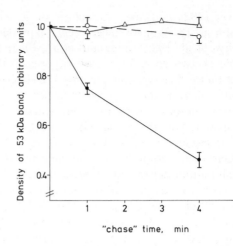

Fig. 2. Effect of cAMP on the labeling of 53-kDa protein in *Drosophila* head homogenate with $[\gamma\text{-}^{32}P]ATP$. Phosphorylation time: 3 min at 0°C. Labeling was evaluated by densitometry of autoradiographic films made of SDS–PAGE slabs, ○, Canton-S; ●, *dunce*^{M11}. From Dévay et al. (1986).

Fig. 4. Effect of 'chase' with cold ATP and with cAMP on the labeling of 53-kDa protein. Phosphorylation was made as in Fig. 2, with 3 μM cAMP added for 1 min; then 1 mM unlabeled ATP (△) or 3 μM cAMP (●) or H_2O (○) was added to the homogenate. These additions were made at 0 time on the abscissa. Density values at 0 time were taken as unity. From Dévay et al. (1986).

Furthermore, *Drosophila* cAMP-dependent protein kinase has recently been purified and characterized (Foster et al., 1984); the R-II subunit has and apparent M_r between 52 and 58 kDa on SDS–PAGE depending on the state of phosphorylation, and a propensity for autophosphorylation like its mammalian counterpart. '

All these data leave little doubt that the 53-kDa protein is indeed identical with the R subunit of cAMP-dependent protein kinase.

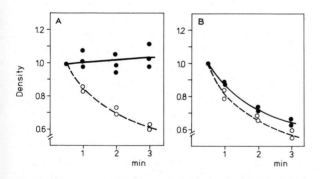

Fig. 3. Time course of labeling of 53-kDa protein. Phosphorylation was carried out as in Fig. 2, with 10 μM cAMP added. The density obtained at 30 s was taken as unity. A, Canton-S heads; B, *dunce*^{M11} heads. ●, without theophylline; ○, with 10 mM theophylline. From Dévay et al. (1986).

Possible consequences of altered autophosphorylation of cAMP-dependent protein kinase in *dunce* flies

One can only speculate about the possible involvement of altered autophosphorylation in the memory deficit of *dunce* flies. It has been shown in mammals that autophosphorylation of the R subunit slows down its reassociation with the catalytic subunit (Rangel-Aldao and Rosen, 1976b). The elevated cAMP level in *dunce* may shift the state of phosphorylation of the R subunit toward dephosphorylation, which in turn would favor reformation of the holoenzyme and repeated autophosphorylation of R. Phosphorylated R, at the sustained high cAMP level, would leave the holoenzyme, and the whole process starts over again. This postulated enhanced phosphorylation turnover in R is of unknown significance.

The R subunit can interact with cellular elements other than the catalytic subunit (cf. Lohmann et al., 1984), which may be influenced by the state of phosphorylation of R. The association of R with the cell membrane has been invoked in the long-term memory of *Aplysia* (Kandel and

Schwartz, 1982) and the interaction of R with chromatin is thought to affect gene expression (Nesterova et al., 1982; Jungmann et al., 1983). In fact, gene expression is likely to be altered in the brain of *dunce* flies, as suggested by the different sensitivity of Kenyon-cell fiber number in the mushroom bodies (corpora pedunculata) to environmental stimuli in the wild type and the mutant (Heisenberg, 1984; Technau, 1984). The subcellular distribution in *Aplysia* neurons of a Ca^{2+}/calmodulin-dependent protein kinase has been shown to be affected by phosphorylation (Saitoh and Schwartz, 1985). Thus the phosphorylation of R may likewise affect the distribution of cAMP-dependent protein kinase in *Drosophila* neurons, which can be relevant to the memory process.

Protein kinase C in wild type and *dunce* flies

We examined in fly head homogenate the effect of activators of protein kinase C on the protein phosphorylation pattern. As seen in Fig. 5, addition of phosphatidylserine and the tumor-promoting phorbol ester 12-*O*-tetradecanoylphorbol-13-acetate (TPA) increased the labeling of several proteins and also decreased the labeling of some others in wild-type Canton-S heads. In contrast, in *dunce*^{M11} head homogenate the above activators had hardly any effect. These preliminary data may reflect an important relationship. Nishizuka (1984) has pointed out that in some cells cAMP-dependent protein kinase and protein kinase C interact antagonistically in signal transduction. The predominance of the cAMP-dependent kinase in *dunce* may interfere with the functioning of protein kinase C. It remains to be seen what role, if any, protein kinase C plays in the processes of learning and memory of *Drosophila*.

Modulation of cAMP level in surviving larval brain

In an attempt to study cAMP-dependent protein phosphorylation in intact *Drosophila* nervous tissue we conducted experiments with surviving larval brains. We have earlier shown that the brain tissue of *dunce* larvae is deficient in PDE-II

(Solti et al., 1983). The importance of working with quasi-intact brain when studying protein phosphorylation has recently been emphasized by Rodnight et al. (1985). Larval brains are fairly easy to obtain by dissection of third instar larvae under a stereomicroscope. The dissected brains were placed in *Drosophila*–Ringer solution also containing 10 mM glucose and kept at 25°C. The ATP content of brains (12 ± 2 nmol/mg protein) practically did not change up to at least three hours, suggesting that cellular metabolism was largely intact.

Drosophila adenylate cyclase has been shown to be activated by the neurotransmitters octopamine, dopamine and serotonin (Uzzan and Dudai, 1982). Evidence has been presented that there are receptors for these agents in the membrain fraction of *Drosophila* heads (Dudai and Zvi, 1984a, 1984b). Furthermore, *Drosophila* adenylate cyclase is activated by the diterpene forskolin (Dudai et al., 1983; Livingstone et al., 1984), which acts directly on the catalytic subunit of the enzyme system in mammals (Seamon and Daly, 1981). In surviving larval brain octopamine increased cAMP level, but the effect was transient, probably owing to desensitization (Fig. 6). In the presence of theophylline the cAMP rise was more pronounced and decline was retarded. Dopamine and serotonin (1 mM) produced somewhat smaller cAMP increments (not shown). In contrast, forskolin induced a large increase in cAMP content in the absence of phosphodiesterase inhibitor (Fig. 7): under the conditions used the increase was about 15-fold in 20 min. In cell-free system forskolin has been reported to produce an approximately five-fold activation of *Drosophila* adenylate cyclase (Dudai et al., 1983, 1984; Livingstone et al., 1984). From Fig. 7 the extent of activation in the intact brain cannot be deduced, since such accumulation curves are the outcome of cAMP turnover (cf. Goka et al., 1983).

It is of interest to compare the catalytic potentials of adenylate cyclase and cAMP-phosphodiesterases in *Drosophila*. From the data of Uzzan and Dudai (1982) and Livingstone et al. (1984) on adenylate cyclase and of Davis and Kiger (1981) on cAMP-phosphodiesterase, the activity ratio PDE/adenylate cyclase is estimated to be in the

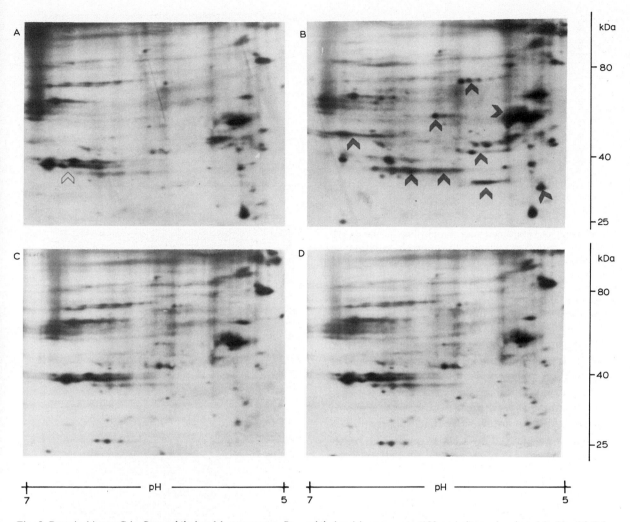

Fig. 5. Protein kinase C in *Drosophila* head homogenate. *Drosophila* head homogenate (100 mg/ml) was incubated in 20 mM Tris–HCl, pH 7.6, 1.3 mM MgCl$_2$, 50 µM CaCl$_2$ at 25°C with 25 µM [γ-^{32}P]ATP for 6 min. A and C: no additions. B and D: with 0.3 mg/ml phosphatidylserine + 0.1 µM 12-O-tetradecanoylphorbol-13-acetate. Isoelectric focussing and SDS–PAGE (12%) was followed by autoradiography. A and B: Canton-S. C and D: *dunce^{M11}*. Full and empty arrowheads mark major increase and decrease, respectively, in labeling of protein kinase C activation.

order of 10^2. The fact that a fewfold activation of adenylate cyclase leads to a very substantial accumulation of cAMP points to the spatial separation (compartmentation) of the two activities. Alternatively, protection against destruction is also provided by sequestration via binding; indeed, we have found that part of the 'extra' cAMP in *dunce^{M11}* flies is protein-bound, probably to the R subunit of cAMP-dependent protein kinase (Friedrich et al., 1984).

Protein phosphorylation in surviving larval brain

We examined the effect of cAMP-generating treatments on protein phosphorylation in larval brains. The brains were first incubated with carrier-free [^{32}P]orthophosphate included in the *Drosophila*–Ringer to label endogenous ATP for 2 hours, then various agents were added and after 30 min the brains were sonicated and analyzed by two-dimensional SDS-PAGE followed by autoradiography.

316

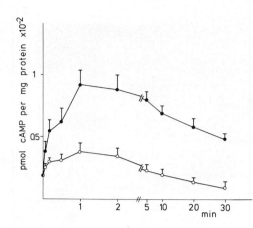

Fig. 6. Effect of octopamine and theophylline on the cAMP content of Canton-S larval brains. Brains freshly dissected from third instar larvae were incubated in Ringer containing 10 mM glucose at 25°C, with additions as below. At times two brains were removed and their cAMP content was determined by acetylation radio-immunoassay. ○, 1 mM octopamine; ●, 1 mM octopamine + 10 mM theophylline.

Some preliminary data are summarized in Fig. 8. Dibutyryl-cAMP and octopamine increased the label in three polypeptides of $M_r \sim 25$ kDa and pI 6.4–6.6. Forskolin had the same effect, whereas with dopamine the picture was somewhat different (not shown). It is noteworthy that apparently few proteins were affected by cAMP-generating treatments.

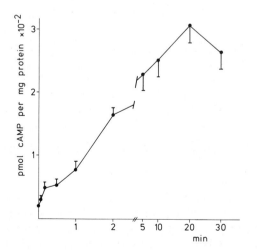

Fig. 7. Effect of forskolin (100 µM) on cAMP content of Canton-S larval brains. Brains were incubated and processed as in Fig. 6.

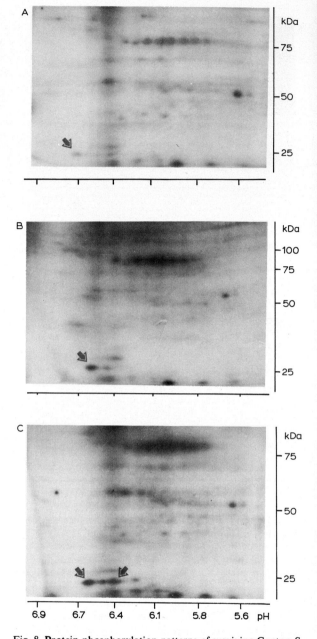

Fig. 8. **Protein phosphorylation patterns of surviving Canton-S larval brains.** Ten brains were incubated in Ringer solution containing 10 mM glucose and 4 MBq carrier-free [^{32}P]orthophosphate. After 2 hours the drugs indicated were added and the mixture was further incubated for 30 min. Brains were disrupted by sonication in the presence of 50 mM NaF, extracted with acetone and the precipitate was subjected to isoelectric focussing followed by gradient (4 to 12%) SDS–PAGE. Dried gels were autoradiographed. A, no addition; B, 1 mM octopamine; C, 0.9 mM dibutyryl-cAMP.

Genetic versus phenocopied mutants

The genetic dissection of a physiological process, such as learning and memory, via mutants offers various approaches to molecular mechanisms. First, the mutants themselves can be studied with the aim of finding the site of mutation and the protein affected, thereby recognizing a link in the chain of events making up that process. Once this achieved, the study of mutants leads to insights as to how the mutated organism reconciles life with the given defect. It follows that what we then study is no longer the normal physiological process but rather its handicapped version. While such investigations provide valuable information, it must be clear that, in a sense, they point away from the original direction. For example, if we want to understand the molecular mechanism of learning and memory in fruit flies and therefore set out to isolate mutants, such as *dunce* and *rutabaga*, we may conclude that a normally functioning PDE-II and Ca^{2+}/calmodulin-activated adenylate cyclase are likely to be needed for associative memory to persist. We can make the inference that a, probably Ca^{2+}-induced, cAMP pulse of the proper amplitude and duration is needed in certain neurons for the plastic change to occur. Furthermore, we may undertake to find the protein(s) whose over-phosphorylation or lack of dynamic phosphorylation–dephosphorylation results in the memory deficit.

On the other hand, the study of mutants proper has certain limitations. Namely, mutant populations tend to accumulate over many generations a number of compensatory changes that attenuate the mutant phenotype. Thus, *dunce* strains have been observed to gradually increase their A value (cf. Tully, 1984) or, in our experience, lower their initially high cAMP level. But even if this drift does not occur, in the case of the mutant our object of study is an organism adapted to the genetic defect, e.g. an enzyme deficiency, rather than an organism acutely faced with the dysfunction of the given enzyme. One cannot tell a priori whether the impaired physiological function is the immediate consequence of enzyme dysfunction or is due to secondary, compensatory processes.

This is where the second approach offered by genetic dissection, which capitalizes on the heuristic value of identified mutations, comes in. Namely, if the mutation hits an enzyme one may look for, or even devise, specific inhibitors for that enzyme and administer them to wild type animals in order to phenocopy the mutation. Phenocopying means the production of mutant phenotype without the actual genetic mutation. Phenocopying may be particularly suitable to distinguish short-term and long-term mutational effects. Furthermore, working with wild type animals one need not consider, in an unpredictable manner, the accumulated attenuating influences in the mutant.

Pharmacological phenocopying of memory mutations

With the above considerations in mind we initiated work on the phenocopy of various memory mutants of *Drosophila*. The *dunce* mutation can be mimicked by PDE inhibitors: caffeine lowers the learning index, A^{*}, of wild type flies (cf. ref. 24 in Byers et al., 1981). In our experience, 1-hour exposure to theophylline effected a dose-dependent reduction in A (Fig. 9). While caffeine and theophylline inhibit PDE isoenzymes rather indiscriminately, there is hope of finding inhibitors specific for PDE-I and PDE-II among the many potential phosphodiesterase inhibitors synthesized and tested by pharmaceutical research as antidepressants and cardiotonics. In fact, investigations along these lines are underway in several labor-

---

*The learning index, A, referred to in this paper has been determined by the shock–odour paradigm of Quinn et al (1974). In this system, perfect learning means $A = 1$, whereas total lack of learning is $A = 0$. Normal flies have a A value of 0.3–0.4 (e.g. Dudai et al., 1976; Byers et al., 1981). The Quinn et al. procedure has been criticized for its being a population rather than individual learning test and for the low value of normal flies, which raised the possibility of an intelligent subpopulation. However, Tully (1984) has shown that the procedure of Quinn et al. for the assessment of classical conditioning is conceptually correct, it is imperfect only in practical aspects; in an improved procedure the wild type flies' learning index approaches unity.

318

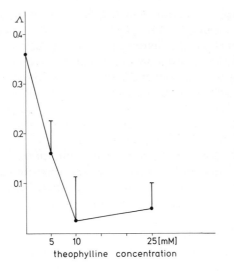

Fig. 9. Effect of theophylline on the learning index of Canton-S flies. Flies were fed theophylline, at the indicated concentration, in 2% sucrose for 1 hour at 25°C. Learning index was determined by the shock–odour paradigm of Quinn et al. (1974).

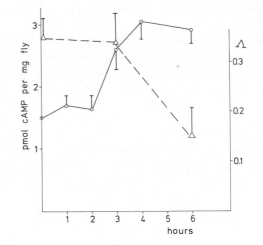

Fig. 10. Effect of forskolin on the cAMP content (○) and learning index (△) of Canton-S flies. Flies were fed 50 μM forskolin in 2% sucrose for the times indicated. cAMP was determined by radioimmunoassay (cf. Friedrich et al., 1984) and the learning index, Λ, as in Fig. 9.

atories (Byers and Gustafsson, 1985; Solti and Friedrich, unpublished).

When Canton-S flies were fed trifluoperazine (10 mg/ml in 2% sucrose) the learning index gradually decreased from 0.36 to 0.10 in 24 hours (Láng and Friedrich, unpublished result). While there is no evidence for the point of attack of trifluoperazine, a Ca^{2+}/calmodulin antagonist, in *Drosophila*, the treatment can tentatively be regarded as phenocopy of the *rutabaga* mutation.

The dramatic increase in cAMP content of larval brains on the effect of forskolin (cf. Fig. 7) prompted us to examine how forskolin affected associative learning (Fig. 10). Under the conditions adopted forskolin, fed to Canton-S flies, increased the overall cAMP level about 2-fold after 3 hours of exposure. The learning index, Λ, was unchanged at 3 hours and decreased only to one-half by 6 hours. The feature that draws attention here is that elevated cAMP does not immediately result in memory impairment. As a comparison, in *dunce¹* and *dunce²* the learning index is almost zero at cAMP levels found by us after 3 hours of forskolin treatment (Byers et al., 1981). This finding lends further support to the idea (Dudai 1985; Livingstone et al., 1984) that it is not the absolute level of cAMP but rather its appropriate dynamics that is needed for learning and memory storage.

How does the cAMP metabolic disorder in *Drosophila* lead to memory deficit?

The several lines of investigation conducted in our and other laboratories have not yet led to a coherent model of the memory mechanism of fruit flies. Most of the data described in this paper represent departures to, rather than arrival at, the preconceived destination. If we accept the reasonable working hypothesis that the various abnormalities of cAMP metabolism observed in the different mutants are responsible for the memory deficit, the question remains what the next links are in the chain of events.

As already pointed out above, cAMP levels per se are not decisive, since similar memory deficits are produced in *dunce* strains at elevated cAMP as in *rutabaga* with slightly lower than normal cAMP level, or in the double mutant dnc^{M11} rut/dnc^{M11} rut at intermediate cAMP levels (Livingstone et al., 1984). The *rutabaga* mutation has been suggested to fit models developed for *Aplysia* (Hawkins et al., 1983; Ocorr et al., 1985) inasmuch as convergent effects of neurotransmitter and Ca^{2+} on adenylate cyclase might be postulated to be the crux of the matter (Dudai et al., 1983; Livingstone et al., 1984). In the case of *dunce*, elevated cAMP has been implicated in creating a high noise level in neurons (Dudai, 1985) and/or promoting the erasure of memory trace, possibly via dephosphorylation (Dudai, 1985; Friedrich et al., 1985). It has recently been suggested that a bistable switch can be constructed from two protein kinases and a protein phosphatase (Lisman, 1985). However, there is no evidence for such a mechanism in *Drosophila*. The dephosphorylation observed by us at high cAMP concentration pertains to the R subunit of cAMP-dependent protein kinase, which is a special case of dephosphorylation enhancement. In mammalian systems the $ATP-Mg^{2+}$-dependent protein phosphatases were not affected by cAMP (Resink et al., 1983; Jurgensen et al., 1984). However, apparent activation of protein phosphatase by cAMP in S49 mouse lymphoma cells has recently been described (Kiss and Steinberg, 1985). Work is in progress in our laboratory to characterize *Drosophila* protein phosphatases and the potential role of cAMP in their regulation.

Our concepts about the *dunce* phenotype have gained a new dimension by the findings that experience effects the axon number of Kenyon cells in *Drosophila* brain (Technau and Heisenberg, 1982; Technau, 1984) and the experience-dependent increase in fiber number does not occur in *dunce* mutants (Heisenberg, 1984). If the wiring in the brain of *dunce* flies and larvae markedly differs from normal, then the memory deficit may simply be due, for example, to an insufficient sensory input caused by a decrease in the number of synapses. This would be a typically long-term effect of the mutation and would raise doubts about interpretations that invoke modulation of synaptic strength in an otherwise unchanged network. On the other hand, the fact that the learning index is decreased by a 1-hour exposure to PDE inhibitors argues for a short-term effect not involving network reorganization. However, it has not been established by behavioral analysis that the same type of memory deficit is produced by theophylline and by the *dunce* mutation.

The characterization and identification of proteins phosphorylated in *Drosophila* brain under the effect of cAMP-generating treatments may lead us further in the elucidation of the memory process. Careful analysis may reveal different phosphorylation effects for the various adenylate cyclase-activating neurotransmitters. In particular, dopamine and serotonin seem to be of special interest. Namely, the temperature-sensitive mutant Ddc^{ts1} (dopa decarboxylase deficient) cannot synthesize these monoamines (Livingstone and Tempel, 1983) and has $\Lambda = 0.00$ (Tempel et al., 1984) at restrictive temperatures. Importantly, octopamine synthesis is normal in *Ddc* flies. In contrast, the circadian rhythm mutant per^0 exhibits impaired octopamine synthesis and normal olfactory learning. Although these data indicate the participation of dopamine and/or serotonin in olfactory learning, the relevance of these neurotransmitters to *dunce* is questionable, because the *Ddc* mutation, unlike *dunce*, seems to affect learning (acquisition) rather than memory (Tempel et al., 1983). Clearly, studies on protein kinase C are also worth extending to this experimental system.

Finally, we may consider an intriguing possibility that pertains to the role of balanced cAMP pulse in the proper neurons, which is crucial for associative learning. According to current concepts this cAMP pulse induces protein phosphorylation. However, a cAMP pulse, i.e. a period of enhanced cAMP turnover, might also act in other ways. Goldberg et al. (1983) proposed that in phototransduction not the cGMP concentration but rather the increased cGMP turnover would be the mediator. The 'by-products' of cyclic nucleotide turnover are protons and pyrophosphate. If these species are liberated next to the membrane, they may influence membrane potential and Ca^{2+} mobility, thereby modulating synaptic transmission. One may speculate that the *rutabaga* and *dunce* mutations each block one of the two steps of this turnover. If elevated cAMP is produced not by enzyme inhibition but by activation, the decrease in Λ does not immediately take place (cf. Fig. 10). Perhaps the significance of cAMP turnover at synapses deserves more attention. This is not at all meant to question cAMP-dependent protein phosphorylation. But there is no reason to reject a priori that cAMP can do something useful during both its existence and decay.

References

Acosta-Urquidi, J., Alkon, D.L. and Neary, J.T. (1984) Ca^{2+}-dependent protein kinase injection in a photoreceptor mimics biophysical effects of associative learning. *Science*, 224:1254–1257.

Alkon, D.L. (1984) Calcium-mediated reduction of ionic currents: A biophysical memory trace. *Science*, 226:1037–1045.

Byers, D. and Gustafsson, C.A. (1985) Selective pharmacology of cyclic AMP phosphodiesterase I and II of *Drosophila melanogaster*. *Mol. Pharmacol.* (in press).

Byers, D., Davis, R.L. and Kiger, J.A. Jr. (1981) Defect in cyclic AMP phosphodiesterase due to the *dunce* mutation of learning in *Drosophila melanogaster*. *Nature*, 289:79–81.

Davis, R.L. and Kiger, J.A. Jr. (1981) *Dunce* mutants of *Drosophila melanogaster:* Mutants defective in the cyclic AMP phosphodiesterase enzyme system. *J.Cell Biol.*, 90:101–107.

Dévay, P., Solti, M., Kiss, I., Dombrádi, V. and Friedrich, P. (1984) Differences in protein phosphorylation in vivo and in vitro between wild type and *Dunce* mutant strains of *Drosophila melanogaster*. *Int. J. Biochem.*, 16:1401–1408.

Dévay, P., Pintér, M., Yalcin, A.S. and Friedrich, P. (1986) Altered autophosphorylation of cAMP-dependent protein kinase in the *dunce* memory mutant of *Drosophila melanogaster*. *Neuroscience*, 18:193–203.

Dombrádi, V., Hajdu, J., Friedrich, P. and Bot, G. (1985) Purification and characterization of glycogen phosphorylase from *Drosophila melanogaster*. *Insect Biochem.*, 15:403–410.

Dombrádi, V., Dévay, P., Friedrich, P. and Bot, G (1986) Regulation of glycogen phosphorylase in *Drosophila melanogaster:* Reversible phosphorylation dephosphorylation. *Insert Biochem.*, 16:557–566.

Dudai, Y. (1979) Behavioral plasticity in a *Drosophila* mutant, *dunce*^{DB276}. *J. Comp. Physiol.*, 130:271–275.

Dudai, Y. (1983) Mutations affect storage and use of memory differentially in *Drosophila*. *Proc. Natl. Acad. Sci. U.S.A.*, 80:5445–5448.

Dudai, Y. (1985) Genes, enzymes and learning in *Drosophila*. *Trends Neurosci.* 8:18–21.

Dudai, Y. and Zvi, S. (1984a) High-affinity [^{3}H]octopamine-binding sites in *Drosophila melanogaster:* Interaction with ligands and relationship to octopamine receptors. *Comp. Biochem. Physiol.*, 77C:145–151.

Dudai, Y. and Zvi, S. (1984b) [^{3}H]Serotonin binds to two classes of sites in *Drosophila* head homogenate. *Comp. Biochem. Physiol.*, 77C:305–309.

Dudai, Y., Jan, Y.-N., Byers, D., Quinn, W.G. and Benzer, S. (1976) *Dunce*, a mutant of *Drosophila* deficient in learning. *Proc. Natl. Acad. Sci. U.S.A.*, 73:1684–1688.

Dudai, Y., Uzzan, A. and Zvi, S. (1983) Abnormal activity of adenylate cyclase in the *Drosophila* memory mutant *rutabaga*. *Neurosci. Lett.*, 42:207–212.

Dudai, Y., Zvi, S. and Segel, S. (1984) A defective conditioned behavior and a defective adenylate cyclase in the *Drosophila* mutant *Rutabaga*. *J. Comp. Physiol. A*, 155:569–576.

Duerr, J.S. and Quinn, W.G. (1982) Three *Drosophila* mutations that block associative learning also affect habituation and sensitization. *Proc. Natl. Acad. Sci. U.S.A.*, 79:3646–3650.

Friedrich, P., Solti, M. and Gyurkovics, H. (1984) Microcompartmentation of cAMP in wild type and memory-mutant *dunce* strains of *Drosophila melanogaster*. *J. Cell. Biochem.*, 26:197–203.

Friedrich, P., Dévay, P., Solti, M. and Pintér, M. (1985) Protein phosphorylation in *dunce* memory-mutant *Drosophila*. *Acta Biochim. Biophys. Acad. Sci. Hung.* (in press).

Foster, J.L., Guttman, J.J., Hall, L.M. and Rosen, O.M. (1984) *Drosophila* cAMP-dependent protein kinase. *J. Biol. Chem.*, 259:13049–13055.

Goldberg, N.D., Ames, A., Gander, J.E. and Walseth, T.F. (1983) Magnitude of increase in retinal cGMP metabolic flux determined by ^{18}O incorporation into nucleotide α-phosphryls corresponds with intensity of photic stimulation. *J. Biol. Chem.*, 258:9213–9219.

Goka, T.J., Barker, R., Maxwell, B.L. and Butcher, R.W. (1983) Desensitization and cyclic AMP turnover in S49 cells. *J. Cycl. Nucl. Prot. Phosph. Res.*, 9:49–57.

Gomes, S.L., Juliani, M.H., Maia, J.C.C. and Rangel-Aldao, R. (1983) Autophosphorylation and rapid dephosphorylation of the cAMP-dependent protein kinase from *Blastocladiella emersonii* zoospores. *J. Biol. Chem.*, 258:6972–6978.

Hawkins, R.D., Abrams, T.W., Carew, T.J. and Kandel, E.R. (1983) A cellular mechanism of chemical conditioning in *Aplysia*: Activity-dependent amplification of presynaptic facilitation. *Science*, 219:400–405.

Heisenberg, M. (1984) *EMBO Drosophila Workshop*, Crete.

Hewitt, J.K., Fulker, D.W. and Hewitt, C.A. (1983) Genetic architecture of olfactory discriminative avoidance conditioning in *Drosophila melanogaster*. *J. Comp. Psychol.*, 97:52–58.

Ingebritsen, T.S. and Cohen, P. (1983) The protein phosphatases involved in cellular regulation. *Eur. J. Biochem.*, 132:255–261.

Jungmann, R.A., Kelley, D.C., Miles, M.F. and Milkowski, D.M. (1983) Cyclic AMP regulation of lactate dehydrogenase. Isoproterenol and N^6, O^2-dibutylryl cyclic AMP increase the rate of transcription and change the stability of lactate dehydrogenase A subunit messenger RNA in rat C6 glioma cells. *J. Biol. Chem.*, 258:5312–5318.

Jurgensen, S., Shackter, E., Huang, C.Y., Chock, P.B., Yang, S.D., Vandenheede, J.R. and Merlevede, W. (1984) On the mechanism of activation of ATP. Mg(II)-dependent phosphoprotein phosphatase by kinase F_6. *J. Biol. Chem.*, 259:5864–5870.

Kandel, E.R. and Schwartz, J.H. (1982) Molecular biology of learning: Modulation of transmitter release. *Science*, 218:433–443.

Kauvar, L.M. (1982) Defective cyclic adenosine 3':5'-monophosphate phosphodiesterase in the *Drosophila* memory mutant *dunce*. *J. Neurosci.*, 2:1347–1358.

Kiss, Z. and Steinberg, R.A. (1985) Cyclic AMP stimulates dephosphorylation of specific proteins in intact S49 mouse lymphoma cells. *FEBS Lett.*, 180:207–211.

Levitan, I.B., Lemos, J.R. and Novak-Hofer, I. (1983) Protein phosphorylation and the regulation of ion channels. *Trends Neurosci.* 6:496–499.

Lisman, J.E. (1985) A mechanism for memory storage insensitive to molecular turnover: A bistable autophosphorylating kinase. *Proc. Natl. Acad. Sci. U.S.A.*, 82:3055–3057.

Livingstone, M.S. and Tempel, B.L. (1983) Genetic dissection of monoamine transmitter synthesis in *Drosophila*. *Nature*, 303:67–70.

Livingstone, M.S., Sziber, P.P. and Quinn, W.G. (1984) Loss of calcium/calmodulin responsiveness in adenylate cyclase of *rutabaga*, a *Drosophila* learning mutant. *Cell*, 37:205–215.

Lohmann, S.M., DeCamilli, P., Einig, I. and Walter, U. (1984) High-affinity binding of the regulatory subunit (R_{II}) of cAMP-dependent protein kinase to microtubule-associated and other cellular proteins. *Proc. Natl. Acad. Sci. U.S.A.*, 81:6723–6727.

McGuire, T.R. (1984) Learning in three species of Diptera: The blow fly *Phormia regina*, the fruit fly *Drosophila melanagaster*, and the house fly *Musca domestica*. *Behav. Genet.*, 14:480–526.

Neary, J.T. and Alkon, D.L. (1983) Protein phosphorylation/dephosphorylation and the transient, voltage-dependent potassium conductance in *Hermissenda crassicornis*. *J. Biol. Chem.*, 258:8979–8983.

Nesterova, M.V., Glukhov, A.I. and Severin, E.S. (1982) Effect of the regulatory subunit of cAMP-dependent protein kinase on the genetic activity of eukaryotic cells. *Mol. Cell. Biochem.*, 49:53–61.

Nishizuka, Y. (1984) The role of protein kinase C in cell surface signal transduction and tumour promotion. *Nature*, 308:693–698.

Ocorr, K.A., Walters, E.T. and Byrne, J.H. (1985) Associative conditioning analog selectively increases cAMP levels of tail sensory neurons in *Aplysia*. *Proc. Natl. Acad. Sci. U.S.A.*, 82:2548–2552.

Quinn, W.G., Harris, W.A. and Benzer, S. (1974) Conditioned behavior in *Drosophila melanogaster*. *Proc. Natl. Acad. Sci. U.S.A.*, 71:708–712.

Quinn, W.G., Sziber, P.P. and Booker, R. (1979) The *Drosophila* memory mutant amnesiac. *Nature*, 277:212–214.

Rangel-Aldao, R. and Rosen, O.M. (1976a) Mechanism of self-phosphorylation of adenosine 3′:5′-monophosphate-dependent protein kinase from bovine cardiac muscle. *J. Biol. Chem.*, 251:7526–7529.

Rangel-Aldao, R. and Rosen, O.M. (1976b) Dissociation and reassociation of phosphorylated and nonphosphorylated forms of cAMP-dependent protein kinase from bovine cardiac muscle. *J. Biol. Chem.*, 251:3375–3380.

Resink, T.J., Hemming, B.A., Tung, H.Y.L. and Cohen, P. (1983) Characterization of a reconstituted Mg-ATP-dependent protein phosphatase. *Eur. J. Biochem.*, 133:455–461.

Rodnight, R., Trotta, E.E. and Perrett, C. (1985) A simple and economical method for studying protein phosphorylation in vivo in the rat brain. *J. Neurosci. Methods*, 13:87–95.

Saitoh, T. and Schwartz, J.H. (1985) Phosphorylation-dependent subcellular translocation of a Ca^{2+}/calmodulin-dependent protein kinase produces an autonomous enzyme in *Aplysia* neurons. *J. Cell Biol.*, 100:835–842.

Seamon, K.B. and Daly, J.W. (1981) Forskolin: A unique diterpene activator of cyclic AMP-generating systems. *J. Cycl. Nucl. Res.*, 7:201–224.

Shotwell, S.L. (1983) Cyclic adenosine 3′:5′-monophosphate phosphodiesterase and its role in learning in *Drosophila*. *J. Neurosci.*, 3:739–747.

Shuster, M.J., Camardo, J.S., Siegelbaum, S.A. and Kandel, E.R. (1985) Cyclic AMP-dependent protein kinase closes the serotonin-sensitive K^+ channels of *Aplysia* sensory neurones in cell-free membrane patches. *Nature*, 313:392–395.

Solti, M., Dévay, P., Kiss, I., Londesborough, J. and Friedrich, P. (1983) Cyclic nucleotide phosphodiesterases in larval brain of wild-type and *dunce* mutant strains of *Drosophila melanogaster*: Isoenzyme pattern and activation by Ca^{2+}/calmodulin. *Biochem. Biophys. Res. Commun.*, 111:652–658.

Technau, G.M. (1984) Fiber number in the mushroom bodies of adult *Drosophila melanogaster* depends on age, sex and experience. *J. Neurogenet.*, 1:113–126.

Technau, G. and Heisenberg, M. (1982) Neural reorganization during metamorphosis of the corpora pedunculata in *Drosophila melanogaster*. *Nature*, 295:405–407.

Tempel, B.L., Bonini, N., Dawson, D.R. and Quinn, W.G. (1983) Reward learning in normal and mutant *Drosophila*. *Proc. Natl. Acad. Sci. U.S.A.*, 80:1482–1486.

Tempel, B.L., Livingstone, M.S. and Quinn, W.G. (1984) Mutations in the dopa decarboxylase gene affect learning in *Drosophila*. *Proc. Natl. Acad. Sci. U.S.A.*, 81:3577–3581.

Tully, T. (1984) *Drosophila* learning: Behavior and biochemistry. *Behav. Genet.*, 14:527–557.

Uno, I. (1980) Phosphorylation and dephosphorylation of the regulatory subunit of cyclic 3′-5′-monophosphate-dependent protein kinase (type II) in vivo and in vitro. *Biochim. Biophys. Acta*, 631:59–69.

Uzzan, A. and Dudai, Y. (1982) Aminergic receptors in *Drosophila melanogaster*: Responsiveness of adenylate cyclase to putative neurotransmitters. *J. Neurochem.*, 38:1542–1550.

Walter, U., Uno, I., Liu, A.Y.-C. and Greengard, P. (1977) Study of autophosphorylation of isoenzymes of cyclic AMP-dependent protein kinases. *J. Biol. Chem.*, 252:6588–6590.

Woolf, C.J., Chong, M.S. and Ainsworth, A. (1984) Axotomy increases glycogen phosphorylase activity in motoneurones. *Neuroscience*, 12:1261–1269.

W.H. Gispen and A. Routtenberg (Eds.)
Progress in Brain Research, Vol. 69
© 1986 Elsevier Science Publishers B.V. (Biomedical Division)

CHAPTER 25

Synapsin I:
A review of its distribution and biological regulation

Eric J. Nestler[1] and Paul Greengard[2]

[1]*Department of Psychiatry, Yale University School of Medicine, New Haven, CT and* [2]*Laboratory of Molecular and Cellular Neuroscience, The Rockefeller University, New York, NY, U.S.A.*

Increasing evidence indicates that phosphorylation of cellular proteins, both inside and outside of the nervous system, represents a fundamental mechanism by which numerous physiological processes are regulated (Nestler and Greengard, 1984). According to this view, the identification of the specific phosphoprotein(s) involved in the regulation of a particular physiological process is crucial to the elucidation of the molecular pathway through which such regulation is achieved. One approach to the identification of these regulatory phosphoproteins is to search for previously unknown proteins by virtue of their phosphorylation in response to appropriate stimuli, and then to characterize these proteins with respect to their biochemical, anatomical, and physiological properties (Nestler and Greengard, 1983, 1984). One strength of this approach is that it is open-ended and has the potential for discovering new proteins involved in previously unsuspected regulatory pathways. One of the best characterized neuronal phosphoproteins discovered using this approach is Synapsin I. Consideration of Synapsin I shows the unique power of this experimental approach. Furthermore, Synapsin I can serve as a prototype for future studies in that its investigation illustrates the process by which new neuronal phosphoproteins can be discovered and characterized.

Synapsin I (previously termed Protein I) was first identified in 1972 in studies designed to search for phosphoproteins that might play a role in the regulation of synaptic transmission. In those studies, Synapsin I was shown to be a major endogenous substrate for cyclic AMP-dependent protein kinase in particulate synaptic fractions of brain (Johnson et al., 1972; Ueda et al., 1973). Subsequently, Synapsin I was shown to be a major endogenous substrate for calcium-dependent protein kinases in particulate synaptic fractions (Krueger et al., 1977; Sieghart et al., 1979). Fig. 1 illustrates the type of experiments that led to the identification of Synapsin I as a major endogenous substrate protein for both classes of protein kinases.

Since its original discovery more than 10 years ago, Synapsin I has been purified to homogeneity from bovine brain (Ueda and Greengard, 1977) and rat brain (Huttner et al., 1981) and has been extensively characterized. This paper reviews what is now known about the biochemical properties, distribution, and biological regulation of Synapsin I. The available evidence strongly supports the hypothesis that Synapsin I is part of the molecular machinery in nerve terminals that regulates neurotransmitter release.

Physicochemical properties and protein kinase specificity

Some of the physicochemical properties of Synapsin I are summarized in Table I. Synapsin I consists of two closely related proteins, Synapsin

Autoradiograph   PS

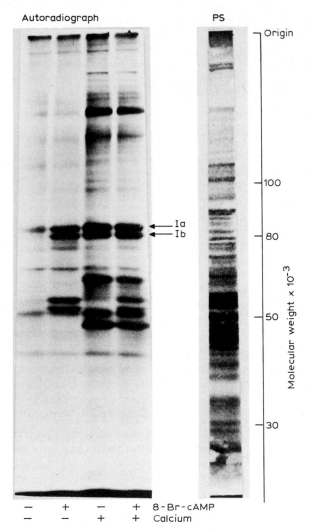

Origin

100

80 ← Ia
   ← Ib

50

30

Molecular weight × 10⁻³

−   +   −   +   8-Br-cAMP
−   −   +   +   Calcium

Fig. 1. Effect of cyclic AMP and calcium on endogenous protein phosphorylation in lyzed synaptosomes. Lyzed synaptosomes were phosphorylated with $[\gamma\text{-}^{32}P]ATP$, in the absence or presence of $10\,\mu M$ 8-bromo-cyclic AMP or 0.3 mM free $\cdot Ca^{2+}$. After termination of the phosphorylation reaction, samples were subjected to SDS–PAGE followed by protein staining (PS) and autoradiography. Arrows indicate positions of Synapsin Ia and Synapsin Ib. (From Huttner and Greengard, 1979.)

TABLE I

Some physicochemical properties of Synapsin I

Property	Synapsin Ia	Synapsin Ib
Molar proportion	1	2
Molecular weight	86 000	80 000
Isoelectric point	10.3	10.2
Stokes radius	59 Å	59 Å
Sedimentation coefficient	2.9 S	2.9 S
Frictional ratio	2.2	2.2
Acid soluble	yes	yes
Amino acid composition	rich in proline and glycine	
Other structural features	a collegenase-insensitive domain and a proline-rich collagenase-sensitive domain	

From Nestler and Greengard, 1984 (based on Ueda and Greengard, 1977).

genase-insensitive domain, and a proline-rich domain that is rapidly and specifically degraded by highly purified collagenase (Ueda and Greengard, 1977). Recently, the messenger RNA for Synapsin I has been isolated and it appears that distinct species of messenger RNA exist for Synapsin Ia and Ib (DeGennaro et al., 1983; Wallace et al., 1985).

The protein kinase specificity of Synapsin I is summarized in Table II. Synapsin I is an effective substrate protein for at least three distinct protein kinases in brain and undergoes multisite phosphorylation. Synapsin I contains one serine

TABLE II

Protein kinase specificity of Synapsin I

Synapsin I undergoes multisite phosphorylation.

(1) One serine residue (site 1) in the collagenase-insensitive domain is phosphorylated both by cyclic AMP-dependent protein kinase and by calcium/calmodulin-dependent protein kinase I.

(2) Two serine residues (sites 2 and 3) in the collagenase-sensitive domain are phosphorylated by calcium/calmodulin-dependent protein kinase II.

(3) Not an effective substrate for cyclic GMP-dependent protein kinase or for calcium/phosphatidylserine-dependent protein kinase (protein kinase C).

From Nestler and Greengard, 1984.

Ia and Synapsin Ib, with molecular weights of 86 000 and 80 000, respectively. Synapsin I is an extremely basic, highly elongated, and acid-soluble protein. A variety of physicochemical data indicate that Synapsin I consists of two domains, each representing roughly half of the molecule: a colla-

residue (site 1) in the collagenase-insensitive domain of the molecule that is phosphorylated both by cyclic AMP-dependent protein kinase and by calcium/calmodulin-dependent protein kinase I (Huttner et al., 1981; Kennedy and Greengard, 1981). Synapsin I also contains two serine residues (sites 2 and 3) in the collagenase-sensitive domain of the molecule that are phosphorylated by calcium/calmodulin-dependent protein kinase II (Huttner et al., 1981; Kennedy and Greengard, 1981; Kennedy et al., 1983). For each of these three protein kinases, Synapsin I is one of the best substrate proteins known.

Distribution

The distribution of Synapsin I has been studied by a variety of techniques, including radioimmunoassay and other immunochemical techniques, subcellular fractionation, and light and electron microscope immunocytochemistry. The results of such studies are summarized in Table III. Synapsin I is present only in the nervous system (Ueda and Greengard, 1977) and, within the nervous system, is present only in neurons (Sieghart et al., 1978; De Camilli et al., 1979, 1983a; Bloom et al., 1979; Fried et al., 1982). Synapsin I, measured by radioimmunoassay, represents approximately 0.4% of the total protein present in the cerebral cortex of each of five mammalian

TABLE III

Distribution of Synapsin I

(1) Present only in nervous system (both central and peripheral).
(2) Within nervous system, present only in neurons.
(3) Within neurons, concentrated in presynaptic terminals.
(4) Within terminals, associated with synaptic vesicles.
(5) Present at virtually all synapses.
(6) Not present in adrenal chromaffin cells or anterior pituitary, but present in pinealocytes and posterior pituitary.
(7) Appears simultaneously with synapse formation during development.
(8) Proteins related to Synapsin I present in nervous systems of species throughout the animal kingdom.

Modified from Nestler and Greengard, 1984.

species studied, indicating that Synapsin I is a major protein in mammalian brain (Goelz et al., 1981). The levels of Synapsin I in peripheral tissues were found to be much lower than those in cerebral cortex, results attributable to the fact that the density of synaptic elements in peripheral tissues is much lower than that in brain (Fried et al., 1982).

Several lines of evidence indicate that, within neurons, Synapsin I is concentrated in presynaptic nerve terminals and appears to be present in virtually all presynaptic nerve terminals throughout the nervous system. First, the immunocytochemical staining pattern of Synapsin I in hundreds of sections through numerous regions of the central and peripheral nervous system is consistent with a localization of Synapsin I to all nerve terminals: Synapsin I staining surrounds cell bodies and dendrites (which themselves are unstained) and leaves little space on the surface of the neurons to account for the presence of any unstained synapses (e.g., see Fig. 2) (De Camilli et al., 1983a; C. Ouimet and P. Greengard, unpublished observations). Second, electron microscope study of rat brain synaptosomes, using ferritin-labeled antibodies to Synapsin I, has demonstrated the presence of Synapsin I in close to 100% of all synaptosomes examined in hundreds of electron microscope sections (De Camilli et al., 1983b). Third, denervation of peripheral tissues, such as adrenal medulla, results in a virtually complete loss of Synapsin I content (Fried et al., 1982). Finally, Synapsin I has been shown to be present in nerve terminals of several different neurotransmitter types, including noradrenergic, cholinergic, dopaminergic, GABAergic, and glutamatergic nerve terminals (see Nestler and Greengard, 1984).

Within presynaptic nerve terminals, Synapsin I is associated primarily with synaptic vesicles, as shown by electron microscopy (e.g., see Fig. 3) (Bloom et al., 1979; De Camilli et al., 1983b) and by subcellular fractionation studies (Ueda et al., 1979; Fried et al., 1982; Huttner et al., 1983). In fact, Synapsin I appears to be a major protein of synaptic vesicles: it represents approximately 6% of the total protein present in highly purified vesicle preparations (Huttner et al., 1983). Recent

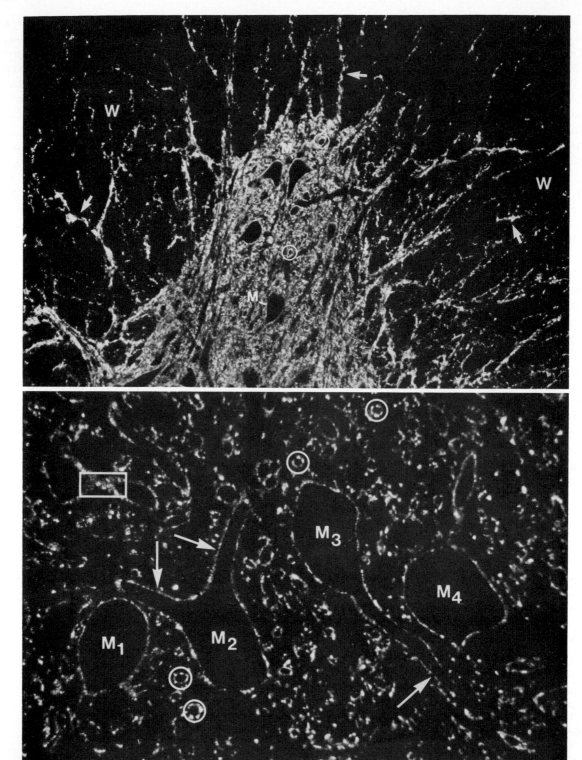

electron microscope studies have further suggested that Synapsin I is preferentially associated with small (40 to 60 nm) synaptic vesicles rather than large (greater than 60 nm) dense-core vesicles in nerve terminals of the bovine hypothalamus (Navone et al., 1984). Since the smaller vesicles appear to be restricted to nervous tissue, whereas the larger ones are present in many types of secretory cells in addition to neurons, this observation, if extended to other regions of the nervous system, may explain (Navone et al., 1984) why Synapsin I is present in nervous tissue but absent from non-nervous cells – including even those, such as adrenal chromaffin cells, that are developmentally related to neurons and serve a secretory function.

A variety of biochemical studies have demonstrated, in agreement with electron microscope observations (see Fig. 3), that Synapsin I is located on the outer or cytoplasmic surface of synaptic vesicle membranes (Huttner et al., 1983). The collagenase-sensitive domain of Synapsin I appears to be the region of the molecule that binds to synaptic vesicles, and phosphorylation of Synapsin I in this domain (i.e., at sites 2 and 3) by calcium/calmodulin-dependent protein kinase II decreases its ability to bind to synaptic vesicles, at least under some experimental conditions (Huttner et al., 1983; Schiebler et al., 1986). Synaptic vesicles appear to contain a specific, saturable, and high-affinity ($K_d = 10$ nM) binding site for Synapsin I (Schiebler et al., 1983; 1986). Possibly the collagenase-insensitive domain of Synapsin I binds to some other component of the nerve terminal, such as the cytoskeleton or plasma membrane, with the phosphorylation of this domain regulating this interaction. If this is so, then Synapsin I could be viewed as forming a physical bridge between synaptic vesicles and the cytoskeleton or plasma membrane, with the integrity of this bridge regulated by the multisite phosphorylation of Synapsin I. This idea, illustrated schematically in Fig. 4, represents one molecular mechanism through which Synapsin I might regulate synaptic vesicle availability and neurotransmitter release, as discussed below. Studies are now under way to identify the element of the cytoskeleton or plasma membrane that binds the collagenase-insensitive domain of Synapsin I in the nerve terminal. In this regard it should be noted that Baines and Bennett (1985) have recently reported that Synapsin I is a spectrin-binding protein in vitro. It will be important to determine in future studies which domain of Synapsin I is involved, whether the phosphorylation of that domain regulates its binding to spectrin, and whether such binding is physiologically significant.

The specific localization of Synapsin I to synaptic vesicles suggests that assay of this protein can provide a direct measure of the amount of synaptic vesicles in a given region of the nervous system, and thereby provide a measure of the density of nerve terminals (size of individual nerve terminals × number of nerve terminals) in that region (Goelz et al., 1981). Such an approach should be of considerable value, because a detailed morphometric examination of the regional distribution of nerve terminals in the central and peripheral nervous systems, an enormously difficult and tedious undertaking, has not been carried out. The validity of using Synapsin I levels as an indicator of synaptic density is supported by several lines of evidence (see Nestler and Greengard, 1984). Most recently, consistent with the observation that senile dementia of the Alzheimer's type is associated with a loss of presynaptic nerve terminals in the hippocampus, it has been found that Synapsin I levels in hippo-

Fig. 2. Fluorescence micrograph illustrating distribution of Synapsin I immunoreactivity in the anterior horn of the rat spinal cord. Top: 10 µM thick frozen transverse section. Immunoreactivity is visible in the gray matter and in its radiations into the white matter (arrows), but not in the white matter (W). The dark images of unstained motor neuron cell bodies (M) and their dendrites are sharply outlined by rows of fluorescent synapses. Bottom: 1-µM thick plastic transverse section. The profiles of the perikarya of four motor neurons ($M_1 - M_4$) outlined by fluorescent synapses on their surfaces are visible. Arrows indicate dendrites emerging from M_2 and M_3. The white rectangle indicates a region where the section has been cut tangentially to the surface of a large dendrite so that synapses on this dendrite are seen 'en face'. Cross-sections of dendrites surrounded by fluorescent synapses are indicated by white circles. (Top × 119; Bottom × 481; from De Camilli et al., 1983a.)

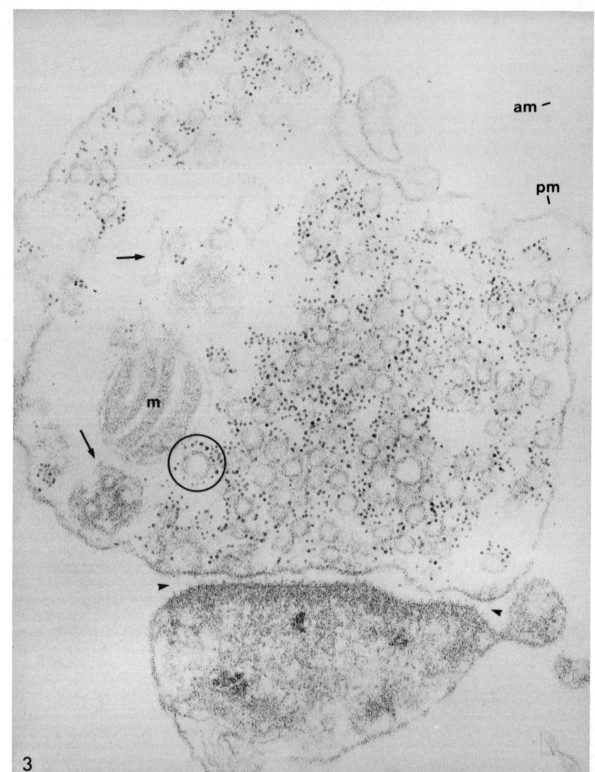

am

pm

m

3

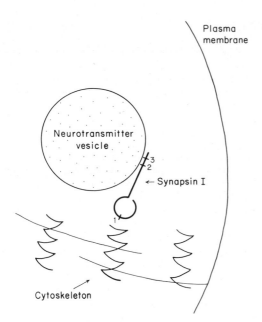

campi from patients with senile dementia of the Alzheimer's type are significantly lower than the levels in hippocampi from patients with multi-infarct dementia or from control patients (Perdahl et al., 1984). It should be emphasized that differences observed in Synapsin I levels between different samples of nervous tissue can reflect differences in (a) the number of nerve terminals, (b) the number of synaptic vesicles per nerve terminal, and/or (c) the amount of Synapsin I per synaptic vesicle.

Synapsin I appears in brain during development at about the time of synaptogenesis (Lohmann et al., 1978). Recent studies have shown that this appearance is associated with a concomitant appearance of messenger RNA for Synapsin I (DeGennaro et al., 1983; Wallace et al., 1985). The association of synaptogenesis with the appearance of both Synapsin I and messenger RNA for Synapsin I has been observed in several brain regions and in brains of several mammalian species (DeGennaro et al., 1983). The mechanism underlying the expression of Synapsin I at the time of synaptogenesis remains unknown. Further research is needed to distinguish between two possible interpretations of the data: firstly that the initiation of Synapsin I synthesis occurs in the innervating neuron as a result of some interaction between the innervating neuron and its target neuron and secondly that the initiation of Synapsin I synthesis in the innervating neuron does not require this cell–cell interaction, but, rather, is an event that is genetically programmed to occur at roughly the same time as the formation of synaptic contacts with target neurons. Recent observations by Ellis et al. (1985) that Synapsin I is present in growth cones isolated from fetal rat brain support the latter interpretation by indicating that Synapsin I is already present in brain during axonal sprouting. Nevertheless, the specific temporal association of Synapsin I expression

Fig. 4. Schematic diagram of the proposed localization of Synapsin I in the nerve terminal. The figure shows the binding of the collagenase-sensitive domain of Synapsin 1 to a neurotransmitter vesicle and the speculated binding of the collagenase-insensitive domain to the cytoskeleton. Alternatively, the collagenase-insensitive domain might bind to the plasma membrane or some other element of the nerve terminal. 1, 2, and 3 represent phosphorylation sites 1, 2, and 3 of Synapsin I. Phosphorylation of the collagenase-sensitive domain (sites 2 and 3) has been shown to decrease the binding of Synapsin I to synaptic vesicles. It is suggested that phosphorylation of the collagenase-insensitive domain (site 1) may alter the binding of Synapsin I to the cytoskeleton or plasma membrane. According to this scheme, Synapsin I serves as a physical bridge between synaptic vesicles and the cytoskeleton or plasma membrane, with the state of phosphorylation of Synapsin I determining the integrity of this bridge at each end. The function of the bridge (and of Synapsin I phosphorylation) would be to regulate the processes of translocation (the movement of the vesicle toward the plasma membrane) and/or of prefusion (the docking of the vesicle with the plasma membrane) (see also Fig. 9). In this manner, Synapsin I phosphorylation would mediate the effects of certain physiological stimuli on neurotransmitter release.

Fig. 3. Electron micrograph of a synaptosomal preparation embedded in agarose and labeled for Synapsin I by immunoferritin. The large majority of ferritin particles are associated with synaptic vesicles. Ferritin particles can be seen forming a corona around a vesicle (circled). Mitochondria (m), plasma membranes (pm) and vesicular structures other than synaptic vesicles (arrows) are unlabeled by the ferritin particles. At least some of the ferritin particles apparently not contiguous to synaptic vesicles might be associated with vesicles out of the plane of the section. am = agarose matrix. Synaptic clefts are indicated by arrowheads (× 95 000; from De Camilli et al., 1983b.)

with the onset of synaptogenesis has made it possible to use Synapsin I as a convenient indicator for synaptogenesis in developmental studies of the nervous system (e.g., see Levitt et al., 1984).

Phylogenetic studies of Synapsin I have revealed that it is a highly conserved protein. The Synapsin I molecules in brains of several mammalian species, including human brain, are immunochemically indistinguishable and exhibit similar biochemical and physicochemical properties (Goelz et al., 1981). In addition, proteins that cross-react immunologically with mammalian Synapsin I have been identified in the nervous systems of species throughout the animal kingdom, including all other vertebrate classes (bird, reptile, amphibian, and fish) and three invertebrate phyla (echinodermata, arthropoda, and mollusca) (Sorensen and Babitch, 1984; Goelz et al., 1985; Llinas et al., 1985). The proteins present in nonmammalian species exhibit different molecular weights from mammalian Synapsin I, but resemble it in a number of other ways. For example, four proteins present in fish brain that cross-react with Synapsin I antisera and enriched in synaptic fractions of fish brain, are acid soluble, are digested by collagenase, and are substrates for endogenous protein kinases (Goelz et al., 1985). As another example, proteins in *Manduca* moths that cross-react with Synapsin I appear in moth head ganglia as the adult moths emerge from pupation, the time during which synaptogenesis occurs (Goelz et al., 1985). The early evolutionary appearance of Synapsin I-like proteins and the highly conserved nature of Synapsin I in mammals suggests that the protein plays a vital role in neuronal function.

Regulation of state of phosphorylation by physiological and pharmacological stimuli

Regulation of the state of phosphorylation of Synapsin I has been studied in a variety of nervous tissue preparations. The results of such studies are summarized in Table IV. Consistent with the observations that Synapsin I is phosphorylated by cyclic AMP-dependent and calcium-dependent protein kinases in vitro, the state of phosphorylation of Synapsin I is stimulated in intact neuronal preparations by a variety of man-

TABLE IV

Physiological and pharmacological regulation of Synapsin I

(1) In synaptosomes and in slices of nervous tissue, depolarizing agents and cyclic AMP increase state of phosphorylation.

(2) In specific anatomical regions of central and peripheral nervous system, the relevant neurotransmitters increase state of phosphorylation:
  (a) serotonin and adenosine in facial motor nucleus
  (b) dopamine in superior cervical ganglion, posterior pituitary, caudatoputamen, and substantia nigra
  (c) norepinephrine in frontal cortex.

(3) In isolated superior cervical ganglion and in posterior pituitary, impulse conduction under physiological conditions increases state of phosphorylation.

(4) In whole animals, convulsants increase and depressants decrease state of phosphorylation in cerebrum

(5) In whole animals, neurotransmitters and hormones increase total amount in specific brain regions:
  (a) norepinephrine in pinealocytes
  (b) corticosterone in hippocampus
  (c) opiates in striatum

Modified from Nestler and Greengard, 1984.

ipulations that increase cyclic AMP or calcium levels in neurons. In synaptosomes (Krueger et al., 1977; Huttner and Greengard, 1979) and slices (Forn and Greengard, 1978) of nervous tissue, depolarizing agents, which increase the flux of calcium into nerve terminals, stimulate a calcium-dependent phosphorylation of Synapsin I. In these same preparations, phosphodiesterase inhibitors, which increase the levels of cyclic AMP, and cyclic AMP analogs stimulate a calcium-independent phosphorylation of Synapsin I.

Synapsin I phosphorylation is regulated by a number of specific neurotransmitters in well-defined, relatively homogenous regions of the nervous system. Serotonin and adenosine have been shown to increase the state of phosphorylation of Synapsin I in rat facial motor nucleus (Dolphin and Greengard, 1981a, 1981b), dopamine has been shown to increase the state of phosphorylation of Synapsin I in bovine and rabbit superior cervical ganglion (Nestler and Greengard, 1980, 1982b), in rat posterior pituitary (Tsou and Greengard, 1982), and in rat caudatoputamen and substantia nigra (S.I. Walaas and P. Greengard, unpublished observations); and norepinephrine has been shown to increase the state of phosphorylation of Synapsin I in rat frontal cortex (Mobley and Greengard, 1985). In each of these regions, the respective neurotransmitter appears to stimulate the phosphorylation of Synapsin I in the presynaptic nerve terminals via an increase in cyclic AMP levels and the activation of cyclic AMP-dependent protein kinase.

Since the state of phosphorylation of Synapsin I is regulated in nerve terminals by neurotransmitters acting on presynaptic receptors, investigation of Synapsin I phosphorylation can be used to study presynaptic receptors in the nervous system. Indeed, in all of the regions so far examined, study of Synapsin I phosphorylation has either revealed the existence of previously unidentified presynaptic receptors, or confirmed the existence of presynaptic receptors that had been identified by other methods. In most cases, it was found that receptors for the same type of neurotransmitter are present on presynaptic nerve terminals and on postsynaptic cell bodies and dendrites (see Fig. 5), suggesting that a dual action of neurotransmitter at a single synapse is a common synaptic mechanism. According to this idea, at many synapses, a given neurotransmitter acts both on presynaptic nerve terminals, where it regulates the amount of a second neurotransmitter released in response to nerve impulses, and on postsynaptic cell bodies and dendrites, where it regulates the responsiveness of the postsynaptic element to that second neurotransmitter (Nestler and Greengard, 1983, 1984).

Study of Synapsin I phosphorylation can also be used to estimate the percentage of nerve terminals in a given region of the nervous system that possesses certain classes of presynaptic receptors. For example, norepinephrine, acting at β-adrenergic receptors, has been found to stimulate the phosphorylation of roughly one-third of the Synapsin I present in the frontal cortex (Mobley and Greengard, 1985). These results indicate that at least one-third of all of the nerve terminals in this brain region possess presynaptic β-adrenergic receptors. Moreover, since it has been estimated that only a very small fraction of nerve terminals

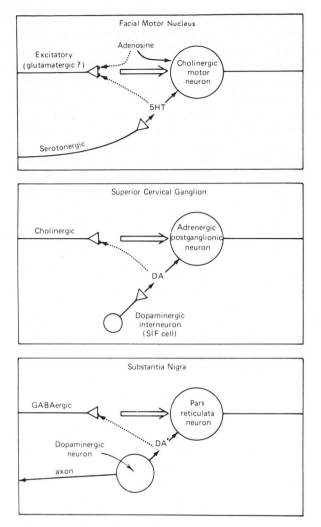

Fig. 5. Schematic diagram of the synaptic organization of rat facial motor nucleus (top panel), rabbit or cow superior cervical ganglion (middle panel) and rat substantia nigra (bottom panel). The study of Synapsin I phosphorylation in these three regions of the nervous system has revealed or confirmed the existence of types of neurotransmitter receptors on presynaptic nerve terminals that had previously been shown to exist on postsynaptic neurons. For simplicity, pathways representing the cholinergic innervation of dopaminergic interneurons in the superior cervical ganglion and the GABAergic innervation of dopaminergic neurons in the substantia nigra are omitted. It should be noted that, in the substantia nigra, dopamine is released from the dendrites, rather than from the axons, of dopaminergic neurons. Open arrows, main synaptic pathway; solid arrows, previously identified actions of neurotransmitter; dotted arrows, actions detected or verified by studies of Synapsin I. 5HT, serotonin; DA, dopamine; SIF cell, small intensely fluorescent cell; GABA, γ-aminobutyric acid. (From Nestler and Greengard, 1984).

332

in the cortex is noradrenergic, these studies of Synapsin I phosphorylation support the possibility that a substantial percentage of all nerve terminals in the cortex respond physiologically to norepinephrine released by distant noradrenergic nerve terminals. The results support the proposal (see Reader et al., 1979) that noradrenergic nerve terminals function in the cortex in a paracrine manner. Thus, study of Synapsin I phosphorylation has provided a unique method for detecting and characterizing presynaptic receptors directly, as well as for elucidating their role in synaptic transmission.

Brief periods of impulse conduction, under physiological conditions, have been shown to increase the state of phosphorylation of Synapsin I in nerve terminals of the rabbit superior cervical ganglion (Nestler and Greengard, 1982a, 1982b) and rat posterior pituitary (Tsou and Greengard, 1982). In the ganglion it was found that as few as 20 nerve impulses significantly stimulated Synapsin I phosphorylation. The amount of Synapsin I phosphorylated in response to preganglionic nerve stimulation was approximately 2% of the total presynaptic Synaptic I per nerve impulse. Furthermore, the changes in the phosphorylation of site 1 of Synapsin I, elicited by nerve impulse conduction, were found to be nearly stoichiometric: preganglionic nerve stimulation resulted in the conversion of roughly 80% of presynaptic Synapsin I from the dephosphorylated to the phosphorylated form (Nestler and Greengard, 1982b). Fig. 6 shows the change in dephospho-Synapsin I, measured by 'back phosphorylation,' observed in response to 5 s of preganglionic nerve stimulation at 10 Hz, as a function of the time after initiation of nerve stimulation. Since the total amount of Synapsin I, measured by radioimmunoassay, was not altered by nerve stimulation, the decreases observed in the amount of dephospho-Synapsin I (Fig. 6) reflect increases in the state of phosphorylation of Synapsin I in response to nerve impulse conduction. An increase in the state of phosphorylation of Synapsin I was first observed within 20 s after initiation of nerve stimulation and appeared to be maximal at 30 to 60 s, after which time the state of phosphorylation returned to control levels (Nestler and Greengard,

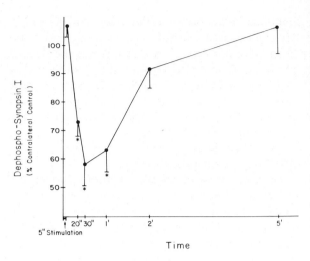

Fig. 6. Effect of a brief period (5 s) of impulse conduction on amount of dephospho-Synapsin I in rabbit superior cervical ganglion, as a function of time after stimulation. The preganglionic nerve supplying one ganglion of each rabbit was stimulated via a suction electrode at 10 Hz for 5 s; stimulated and contralateral control ganglia were homogenized in 1% SDS at various times afterwards. Dephospho-Synapsin I was determined by back phosphorylation, and the amount in the stimulated ganglion compared with that in the contralateral control ganglion. Values shown are means ±S.E.M. The number of pairs of ganglia used ranged from 3 to 7. *Significantly different from control ($p < 0.05$) by two-tailed t-test. (From Nestler and Greengard, 1982a.)

1982a). The data shown in Fig. 6 reflect the state of phosphorylation of both the collagenase-insensitive and collagenase-sensitive domains of Synapsin I. Other data (Nestler and Greengard, 1982a, 1982b) indicate that the state of phosphorylation of the individual domains (i.e., site 1 and sites 2/3) changes with similar time courses.

Further studies on the rabbit superior cervical ganglion were performed to determine whether the changes observed in Synapsin I phosphorylation in response to nerve impulse conduction or to dopamine occurred presynaptically or postsynaptically (Nestler and Greengard, 1982b). These studies, summarized in Fig. 7, revealed that the ganglion contains two 'pools' of Synapsin I. One pool, representing about 60% of total ganglion Synapsin I, is located in presynaptic nerve terminals. This preganglionic pool disappears on surgical denervation of the ganglion, is unaffected by brief exposure to the protein synthesis inhibitor

THE RABBIT SUPERIOR CERVICAL GANGLION CONTAINS TWO POOLS OF SYNAPSIN I,
ONE PRESYNAPTIC AND ONE POSTSYNAPTIC, WITH DIFFERENT CHARACTERISTICS

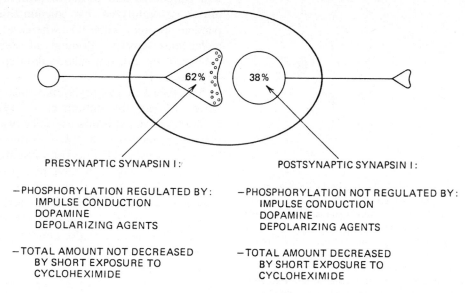

PRESYNAPTIC SYNAPSIN I:

—PHOSPHORYLATION REGULATED BY:
 IMPULSE CONDUCTION
 DOPAMINE
 DEPOLARIZING AGENTS

—TOTAL AMOUNT NOT DECREASED
 BY SHORT EXPOSURE TO
 CYCLOHEXIMIDE

POSTSYNAPTIC SYNAPSIN I:

—PHOSPHORYLATION NOT REGULATED BY:
 IMPULSE CONDUCTION
 DOPAMINE
 DEPOLARIZING AGENTS

—TOTAL AMOUNT DECREASED
 BY SHORT EXPOSURE TO
 CYCLOHEXIMIDE

Fig. 7. Schematic diagram of the distribution and regulation of Synapsin I in the rabbit superior cervical ganglion. (From Nestler and Greengard, 1982b.)

cycloheximide, and undergoes phosphorylation in response to nerve impulses, dopamine, or high potassium concentration (which depolarizes neuronal membranes). The other pool, representing about 40% of total ganglion Synapsin I, is located in the cell bodies of ganglionic neurons. This postsynaptic pool is unaffected by denervation, is decreased by brief exposure to cycloheximide, and does not undergo phosphorylation in response to a variety of physiological and pharmacological stimuli. Rather, postsynaptic Synapsin I appears to represent newly synthesized Synapsin I, presumably en route to the nerve terminals arising from the ganglionic cell bodies where it will serve its physiological function.

Study of the rabbit superior cervical ganglion and rat posterior pituitary has indicated that two first messengers regulate Synapsin I phosphorylation in nerve terminals of these tissues: the nerve impulse itself and the neurotransmitter dopamine (see Fig. 8). Evidence indicates that these first messengers regulate Synapsin I phosphorylation via different mechanisms: impulse conduction in-

creases Synapsin I phosphorylation through the activation of calcium-dependent protein kinases, and dopamine increases Synapsin I phosphorylation through the activation of cyclic AMP-dependent protein kinase. First, the effects of nerve impulse conduction and of high potassium concentration on Synapsin I phosphorylation are dependent on extracellular calcium, whereas those of dopamine and of cyclic AMP analogs are not (Nestler and Greengard, 1982a, 1982b). Second, nerve impulse conduction and high potassium concentration stimulate the phosphorylation of Synapsin I both in the collagenase-insensitive and in the collagenase-sensitive domains of the molecule, observations consistent with the expectation, based on studies with purified Synapsin I and protein kinases, that activation of calcium-dependent protein kinases would increase the state of phosphorylation of both regions of Synapsin I. In contrast, dopamine, cyclic AMP analogs, and forskolin (which activates adenylate cyclase) stimulate the phosphorylation only of the collagenase-insensitive region of Synapsin I, observations consistent with the

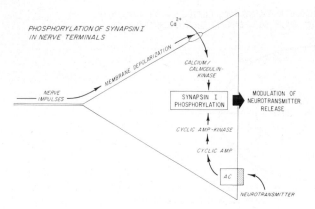

Fig. 8. Schematic diagram of the regulation of Synapsin I phosphorylation in nerve terminals by two first messengers. One first messenger, nerve impulse conduction, stimulates Synapsin I phosphorylation through the depolarization of the nerve terminal plasma membrane, an increase in free calcium levels, and the activation of calcium-dependent protein kinases. We propose that such phosphorylation of Synapsin I is involved in various calcium-dependent mechanisms of regulation of neurotransmitter release, including the phenomenon of post-tetanic potentiation. The other first messenger, a neurotransmitter, stimulates Synapsin I phosphorylation through the activation of its presynaptic receptor and of adenylate cyclase (AC), an increase in cyclic AMP levels, and the activation of cyclic AMP-dependent protein kinase. We propose that such phosphorylation of Synapsin I is involved in cyclic AMP-dependent mechanisms by which several neurotransmitters acting on presynaptic receptors of axon terminals regulate neurotransmitter release. Nerve impulse conduction would be expected to stimulate Synapsin I phosphorylation in all nerve terminals throughout the nervous system. In contrast, only some neurotransmitters would be expected to stimulate Synapsin I phosphorylation, and only in certain nerve terminals. This is because, for any given nerve terminal, Synapsin I phosphorylation would be stimulated only by those neurotransmitters for which there are appropriate receptors on the presynaptic nerve terminal plasma membrane. Other neurotransmitters, acting on other presynaptic receptors (not shown in the figure), alter calcium levels in the nerve terminal and thereby would be expected to regulate Synapsin I phosphorylation and neurotransmitter release.

expectation, based on studies with purified Synapsin I and protein kinases, that activation of cyclic AMP-dependent protein kinase would increase the state of phosphorylation of Synapsin I only in this region (Nestler and Greengard, 1982b; Tsou and Greengard, 1982). Based on studies with cell-free preparations of brain tissue, we hypothesize that the calcium-dependent phosphorylation

of the collagenase-insensitive domain of Synapsin I in ganglionic and posterior pituitary nerve terminals is catalyzed by calcium/calmodulin-dependent protein kinase I, wherease that of the collagenase-sensitive domain of Synapsin I is catalyzed by calcium/calmodulin-dependent protein kinase II.

Synapsin I phosphorylation is also regulated in whole animals (Strombom et al., 1979). Administration of convulsants to mice was found to increase Synapsin I phosphorylation, whereas administration of central nervous system depressants was found to decrease such phosphorylation, in whole cerebrum. Because convulsants increase and depressants decrease neuronal activity in the brain, these results are consistent with the observations that nerve impulse conduction stimulates Synapsin I phosphorylation in isolated intact nervous tissue.

Regulation of total amount by physiological and pharmacological stimuli

A number of studies have shown that not only the state of phosphorylation, but also the total amount, of Synapsin I is regulated in the nervous system (see Table IV). First, norepinephrine, apparently acting through the activation of β-adrenergic receptors and increases in cellular cyclic AMP levels, has been shown to increase the total amount of Synapsin I in rat pinealocytes (Nestler et al., 1982). Second, corticosterone has been shown to increase the total amount of Synapsin I in rat hippocampus, a brain region rich in corticosterone receptors, but not in other brain regions that contain few such receptors (Nestler et al., 1981). Finally, morphine has been shown to increase the total amount of Synapsin I in rat striatum, a brain region rich in opiate receptors, but not in other brain regions that contain few such receptors (T. Tsou, E. Perdahl, and P. Greengard, unpublished observations). Whereas regulation of the state of phosphorylation of Synapsin I is presumably involved in mediating dynamic and readily reversible changes in neuronal function, regulation of the total amount of Synapsin I in these systems may be involved in mediating longer-term changes.

Direct evidence for a role of Synapsin I in neuronal function

Direct evidence for a role of Synapsin I in neurotransmitter release has recently been obtained in studies of the squid giant synapse (Llinas et al., 1985). In these studies neurotransmitter release was determined by measuring the amplitude, rate of rise, and latency of the postsynaptic potential generated in response to presynaptic depolarizing steps under voltage clamp conditions. Injection of purified dephosphorylated Synapsin I into nerve terminals at the synapse was found to decrease the amplitude and rate of rise of the postsynaptic potential. In contrast, injection of purified Synapsin I that had been phosphorylated on its collagenase-sensitive domain (sites 2 and 3) by calcium/calmodulin-dependent protein kinase II, as well as injection of heat-denatured dephospho-Synapsin I, had no effect on these parameters of neurotransmitter release. Injection of purified calcium/calmodulin-dependent protein kinase II into nerve terminals increased the amplitude and rate of rise, and decreased the latency, of the postsynaptic potential. The effects of dephospho-Synapsin I and of calcium/calmodulin-dependent protein kinase II on the postsynaptic potential occurred in the absence of any detectable changes in presynaptic calcium current. These results provide support for the idea that neurotransmitter release can be modulated by biochemical mechanisms and that Synapsin I phosphorylation is involved in such modulation.

Speculation regarding the role of Synapsin I in neuronal function

Synapsin I appears to be present at high concentration in most, and probably in all, presynaptic nerve terminals in virtually all neurons throughout the nervous system, where it is associated with neurotransmitter vesicles. This distribution, and the recent demonstration that the injection of dephospho-Synapsin I into nerve terminals decreases neurotransmitter release from those terminals, support the hypothesis that Synapsin I plays some role in regulating the process by which neurotransmitter is released from the nerve terminal. In contrast to the ubiquity of Synapsin I in nervous tissue, it is virtually absent from non-nervous tissues, including even those with a secretory function. This pattern of distribution of Synapsin I suggests that it may play a role in a neuron-specific regulation of the release process, rather than in the release process per se. Several questions can be asked regarding possible roles of Synapsin I in neurotransmitter release (see Nestler and Greengard, 1984).

Does phosphorylation of Synapsin I promote or inhibit neurotransmitter release? Two lines of evidence suggest that the phosphorylation of Synapsin I is associated with the promotion of neurotransmitter release. First, studies on the squid giant synapse, in which the injection of dephospho-Synapsin I decreases release and that of calcium/calmodulin-dependent protein kinase II increases release, have provided direct evidence that the phosphorylation of Synapsin I at its collagenase-sensitive domain leads to the facilitation of neurotransmitter release.

The second line of evidence is correlative. An elevation either in calcium or in cyclic AMP potentiates the release of neurotransmitter from various nerve terminals under a variety of experimental conditions. For example, brief periods of impulse conduction, apparently acting through calcium, increase the amount of neurotransmitter released in response to a single nerve impulse in numerous types of neuronal preparations, a process known as 'post-tetanic potentiation' (Rosenthal, 1969; Zengel et al., 1980). Similarly, cyclic AMP, and several neurotransmitters that appear to act through cyclic AMP, increase the amount of neurotransmitter released in response to a single nerve impulse in several types of neuronal preparations (see Dunwiddie and Hoffer, 1982), including nerve terminals at the neuromuscular junction (Miyamoto and Breckenridge, 1974), innervated nerve terminals at axoaxonic synapses (Kandel and Schwartz, 1982), nerve terminals in sympathetic ganglia (Kuba et al., 1981), and nerve terminals in the central nervous system (Reubi et al., 1977; Cheramy et al., 1981). Interestingly, brief periods of impulse conduction, apparently acting through calcium, and several neurotransmitters, apparently acting through cyclic AMP, stimulate the phosphorylation of Synapsin I in a variety of neuronal preparations (Fig. 8). In fact, the time course of changes in Synapsin I phosphorylation in the superior cervical ganglion in response to impulse conduction (at both domains of the molecule) or to dopamine (at the collagenase-insensitive domain of the molecule) is consistent with the time courses according to which neurotransmitter release is regulated by either stimulus in sympathetic ganglia (see Fig. 6 and Zengel et al., 1980; Kuba et al., 1981). Moreover, cyclic AMP-dependent protein kinase and calcium/calmodulin-dependent protein kinase I phosphorylate Synapsin I on the same individual serine residue (site 1). It is possible, therefore, that an increase in the state of phosphorylation of Synapsin I in the collagenase-insensitive domain represents a common molecular pathway through which brief periods of impulse conduction and certain neurotransmitters facilitate neurotransmitter release at the synapse.

Is phospho-Synapsin I or dephospho-Synapsin I the 'active' form of the molecule? If, as seems likely, an increase in the state of phosphorylation of Synapsin I leads to enhancement of neurotransmitter release, then either of two models is feasible. According to one model, phospho-Synapsin I would be the active form of the molecule and would promote neurotransmitter release; dephospho-Synapsin I would be the inactive form of the molecule and would have no biological activity. In this case, conversion of dephospho-Synapsin I to phospho-Synapsin I would increase neurotransmitter release by increasing the level of the active form. According to the second model, dephospho-Synapsin I would be the active form of the molecule and would inhibit neurotransmitter release; phospho-Synapsin I would be the inactive form of the molecule and would have no biological activity. In this case, conversion of dephospho-Synapsin I to phospho-Synapsin I would increase neurotransmitter release by decreasing the level of the active (inhibitory) form of Synapsin I, that is by de-inhibiting the release process. The injection studies in the squid giant synapse suggest that, with respect to the collagenase-sensitive domain of Synapsin I, the dephospho-form is the active form of the molecule. Further work is needed to determine whether the other domain of

Synapsin I is active in its phosphorylated or dephosphorylated state.

At which of the various stages in the life cycle of the neurotransmitter vesicle does Synapsin I become phosphorylated, and what is the molecular effect of its phosphorylation? An understanding of the detailed role of Synapsin I in the regulation of neurotransmitter release from nerve terminals is limited by lack of knowledge of the cell biology of the release process. However, one possible sequence of events by which neurotransmitter release from nerve terminals might occur is shown schematically in Fig. 9. One can imagine two priming steps that occur prior to the release process per se. In the first such step, the vesicle would undergo translocation from a position some distance away from the plasma membrane to the immediate vicinity of the plasma membrane. In the second step, the vesicle and plasma membrane would undergo some process of prefusion or 'docking.' Then, when a nerve impulse arrives at the plasma membrane of the nerve terminal, the resulting wave of depolarization and calcium entry would lead to the fusion–release process. The purpose of the priming steps would be to poise the vesicles in a 'fusion-ready' state. Regulation of the priming steps would alter the number of vesicles in that fusion-ready state. If one assumes that the probability of an individual vesicle fusing with the plasma membrane is independent of the number of

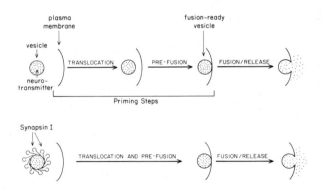

Fig. 9. Schematic diagram of regulation of neurotransmitter release from synaptic vesicles. The purpose of the diagram is to distinguish between the relatively slow priming steps (in which Synapsin I is hypothesized to play a role) and the more rapid fusion–release process. (Modified from Greengard, 1981).

vesicles in the fusion-ready state, then changes in the number of vesicles in that state would lead to changes in the number of fusion events, and therefore in the amount of neurotransmitter released, per nerve impulse. Regulation of these priming steps might represent some of the mechanisms by which physiological stimuli, through Synapsin I phosphorylation, control neurotransmitter release. Alternatively or in addition, it is possible that Synapsin I is involved in regulating some aspect of the process by which small synaptic vesicles are retrieved from the plasma membrane and prepared for subsequent fusion–release.

We currently hypothesize that phosphorylation of Synapsin I is involved in one or both of the two priming steps, rather than in the fusion–release process per se. One can imagine a number of mechanisms by which phosphorylation of Synapsin I at either domain might alter one of these two priming steps and thereby enhance neurotransmitter release (see Figs. 4 and 9). For example, it is possible that phosphorylation of Synapsin I, at its collagenase-insensitive domain, might alter its interaction with some element of the cytoskeleton and thereby promote translocation of the neurotransmitter vesicle toward the plasma membrane. Alternatively, it is possible that phosphorylation of this domain of Synapsin I alters the interaction of the translocated vesicle with the plasma membrane, that is, alters some prefusion step. By either mechanism, phosphorylation would increase the number of vesicles in the fusion-ready state and would thereby increase the amount of neurotransmitter released in response to a nerve impulse.

Phosphorylation of the collagenase-sensitive domain of Synapsin I could also regulate one or both of the priming steps of the release process. The phosphorylation of Synapsin I in this domain appears to promote the detachment of the protein from neurotransmitter vesicles. Furthermore, in studies on the squid giant synapse, injection of dephospho-Synapsin I decreased neurotransmitter release, whereas the injection of Synapsin I phosphorylated on its collagenase-sensitive domain had no detectable effect. The results are compatible with the following working model regarding the molecular action of Synapsin I via its collagen-ase-sensitive domain. Dephospho-Synapsin I is the active form of that domain of the molecule. In the resting state, dephospho-Synapsin I binds to the cytoplasmic surface of neurotransmitter vesicles and thereby decreases the ability of the vesicles to move towards and/or fuse with the plasma membrane. In the stimulated state, the phosphorylation of Synapsin I in the collagenase-sensitive domain in response to physiological stimuli could be visualized as triggering the detachment of Synapsin I from the vesicle, thereby allowing the vesicle to attain a fusion-ready state.

Conclusions

For many years, chemical and electrical stimuli have been known to regulate neurotransmitter release from nerve terminals. Cyclic AMP and calcium have been implicated as second messengers in these regulatory processes. However, virtually no information has been available concerning the molecular mechanisms through which such regulation is achieved. It is now apparent that the investigation of protein phosphorylation systems represents a powerful approach with which to study these mechanisms. This approach has made possible the discovery of Synapsin I, a major phosphoprotein of synaptic vesicles. The evidence presented in this review supports the hypothesis that Synapsin I represents part of the basic molecular machinery through which physiological stimuli regulate the amount of neurotransmitter released from nerve terminals throughout the nervous system.

References

Baines, A.J. and Bennett, V. (1985) Synapsin I is a spectrin-binding protein immunologically related to erythrocyte protein 4.1 *Nature*, 315:410–413.

Bloom, F.E., Ueda, T., Battenberg, E. and Greengard, P. (1979) Immunocytochemical localization in synapses of Protein I, an endogenous substrate for protein kinases in mammalian brain. *Proc. Natl. Acad. Sci. U.S.A.*, 76:5982–5986.

Cheramy, A., Leviel, V. and Glowinski, J. (1981) Dendritic release of dopamine in the substantia nigra. *Nature*, 289: 537–542.

De Camilli, P., Ueda, T., Bloom, F.E., Battenberg, E. and Greengard, P. (1979) Widespread distribution of Protein I in

338

the central and peripheral nervous system. *Proc. Natl. Acad. Sci. U.S.A.*, 76:5977–5981.

De Camilli, P., Cameron, R. and Greengard, P. (1983a) Synapsin I (Protein I), a nerve terminal-specific phosphoprotein. I. Its general distribution in synapses of the central and peripheral nervous system demonstrated by immunofluorescence in frozen and plastic sections. *J. Cell Biol.*, 96:1337–1354.

De Camilli, P., Harris, S.M., Huttner, W.B. and Greengard, P. (1983b) Synapsin I (Protein I), a nerve terminal-specific phosphoprotein. II. Its specific association with synaptic vesicles demonstrated by immunocytochemistry in agarose-embedded synaptosomes. *J. Cell Biol.*, 96:1355–1373.

DeGennaro, L.J., Kanazir, S.D., Wallace, W.C., Lewis, R.M. and Greengard, P. (1983) Neuron-specific phosphoproteins as models for neuronal gene expression. *Cold Spring Harbor Symp. Quant. Biol.*, 48:337–345.

Dolphin, A.C. and Greengard, P. (1981a) Serotonin stimulates phosphorylation of Protein I in the facial motor nucleus of rat brain. *Nature*, 289:76–79.

Dolphin, A.C. and Greengard, P. (1981b) Neurotransmitter and neuromodulator-dependent alterations in phosphorylation of Protein I in slices of rat facial nucleus. *J. Neurosci.*, 1:192–203.

Dunwiddie, T.V. and Hoffer, B.J. (1982) The role of cyclic nucleotides in the nervous system. *Hand. Exp. Pharmacol.*, 58(Part 2):389–463.

Ellis, L., Katz, F. and Pfenninger, K.H. (1985) Nerve growth cones isolated from fetal rat brain. II. Cyclic adenosine 3':5'-monophosphate (cAMP)-binding proteins and cAMP-dependent protein phosphorylation. *J. Neurosci.*, 5:1393–1401.

Fried, G., Nestler, E.J., De Camilli, P., Stjärne, L., Olson, L., Lundberg, J.M., Hökfelt, T., Ouimet, C.C. and Greengard, P. (1982) Cellular and subcellular localization of Protein I in the peripheral nervous system. *Proc. Natl. Acad. Sci. U.S.A.*, 79:2717–2721.

Goelz, S.E., Nestler, E.J., Chehrazi, B. and Greengard, P. (1981) Distribution of Protein I in mammalian brain as determined by a detergent-based radioimmunoassay. *Proc. Natl. Acad. Sci. U.S.A.*, 78:2130–2134.

Goelz, S.E., Nestler, E.J. and Greengard, P. (1985) Phylogenetic survey of proteins related to Synapsin I and biochemical analysis of four such proteins from fish brain. *J. Neurochem.*, 45:63–72.

Greengard, P. (1981) Receptors coupled to intracellular messengers. In L. Stjarne, P. Hedqvist, A. Wennmalm, and H. Lagercrantz (Eds.), *Chemical Neurotransmission-75 Years*, Academic Press, New York, pp. 377–384.

Huttner, W.B. and Greengard, P. (1979) Multiple phosphorylation sites in Protein I and their differential regulation by cyclic AMP and calcium. *Proc. Natl. Acad. Sci. U.S.A.*, 75:5402–5406.

Huttner, W.B., DeGennaro, L.J. and Greengard, P. (1981) Differential phosphorylation of multiple sites in purified Protein I by cyclic AMP-dependent and calcium-dependent protein kinases. *J. Biol. Chem.*, 256:1482–1488.

Huttner, W.B., Schiebler, W., Greengard, P. and De Camilli, P. (1983) Synapsin I (Protein I), a nerve terminal-specific phosphoprotein. III. Its association with synaptic vesicles studied in a highly-purified synaptic vesicle preparation. *J. Cell Biol.*, 96:1374–1388.

Johnson, E.M., Ueda, T., Maeno, H. and Greengard, P. (1972) Adenosine 3',5'-monophosphate-dependent phosphorylation of a specific protein in synaptic membrane fractions from rat cerebrum. *J. Biol. Chem.*, 247:5650–5652.

Kandel, E.R. and Schwartz, J.H. (1982) Molecular biology of learning: Modulation of transmitter release. *Science*, 218:433–442.

Kennedy, M.B. and Greengard, P. (1981) Two calcium/calmodulin-dependent protein kinases, which are highly concentrated in brain, phosphorylate Protein I at distinct sites. *Proc. Natl. Acad. Sci. U.S.A.*, 78:1293–1297.

Kennedy, M.B., McGuinness, T. and Greengard, P. (1983) A calcium/calmodulin-dependent protein kinase activity from mammalian brain that phosphorylates Synapsin I: Partial purification and characterization. *J. Neurosci.*, 3:818–831.

Krueger, B.K., Forn, J. and Greengard, P. (1977) Depolarization-induced phosphorylation of specific proteins, mediated by calcium ion influx, in rat brain synaptosomes. *J. Biol. Chem.* 252:2764–2773.

Kuba, K., Kato, E., Kumamoto, E., Koketsu, K. and Hirai, K. (1981) Sustained potentiation of transmitter release by adrenaline and dibutyryl cyclic AMP in sympathetic ganglia. *Nature*, 291:654–656.

Levitt, P., Rakic, P., De Camilli, P. and Greengard, P. (1984) Emergence of cyclic guanosine 3':5'-monophosphate-dependent protein kinase immunoreactivity in developing Rhesus monkey cerebellum: Correlative immunocytochemical and electron microscopic analysis. *J. Neurosci.*, 4:2553–2564.

Llinas, R., McGuinness, T.L., Leonard, C.S., Sugimori, M. and Greengard, P. (1985) Intraterminal injection of Synapsin I or calcium/calmodulin-dependent protein kinase II alters neurotransmitter release at the squid giant synapse. *Proc. Natl. Acad. Sci. U.S.A.*, 82:3035–3039.

Lohmann, S.M., Ueda, T. and Greengard, P. (1978) Ontogeny of synaptic phosphoproteins in brain. *Proc. Natl. Acad. Sci. U.S.A.*, 75:4037–4041.

Miyamoto, M.D. and Breckenridge, B.M. (1974) A cyclic adenosine monophosphate link in the catecholamine enhancement of transmitter release at the neuromuscular junction. *J. Gen. Physiol.*, 63:609–624.

Mobley, P. and Greengard, P. (1985) Evidence for widespread effects of noradrenaline on axon terminals in the rat frontal cortex. *Proc. Natl. Acad. Sci. U.S.A.*, 82:945–947.

Navone, F., Greengard, P. and De Camilli, P. (1984) Synapsin I in nerve terminals: Selective association with small synaptic vesicles. *Science*, 226:1209–1211.

Nestler, E.J. and Greengard, P. (1980) Dopamine and depolarizing agents regulate the state of phosphorylation of Protein I in mammalian superior cervical sumpathetic ganglion. *Proc. Natl. Acad. Sci. U.S.A.*, 77:7479–7483.

Nestler, E.J. and Greengard, P. (1982a) Nerve impulses increase the state of phosphorylation of Protein I in the rabbit superior cervical ganglion. *Nature*, 296:452–454.

Nestler, E.J. and Greengard, P. (1982b) Distribution of Protein I and regulation of its state of phosphorylation in the rabbit superior cervical ganglion. *J. Neurosci.*, 2:1011–1023.

Nestler, E.J. and Greengard, P. (1983) Protein phosphorylation in the brain. *Nature*, 305:583–588.

Nestler, E.J. and Greengard, P. (1984) *Protein phosphorylation in the Nervous System*, Wiley, New York.

Nestler, E.J., Rainbow, T.C., McEwen, B.S. and Greengard, P. (1981) Corticosterone increases the level of Protein I, a neuron-specific phosphoprotein, in rat hippocampus. *Science*, 212:1162–1164.

Nestler, E.J., Zatz, M. and Greengard, P. (1982) A diurnal rhythm in pineal Protein I levels mediated by β-adrenergic neurotransmission. *Science*, 217:357–359.

Perdahl, E., Adolfsson, R., Alafuzoff, I., Albert, K.A., Nestler, E.J., Greengard, P. and Winblad, B. (1984) Synapsin I (Protein I) in different brain regions in senile dementia of Alzheimer type and multi-infarct dementia. *J. Neural Transmission*, 60:133–141.

Reader, T.A., Ferron, A., Descarries, L. and Jasper, H.H. (1979) Modulatory role for biogenic amines in the cerebral cortex. Microiontophoretic studies. *Brain Res.*, 160:217–229.

Reubi, J.-C., Iversen, L.L. and Jessell, T.M. (1977) Dopamine selectively increases ^{3}H-GABA release from slices of rat substantia nigra in vitro. *Nature*, 268:652–654.

Rosenthal, J. (1969) Post-tetanic potentiation at the neuromuscular junction of the frog. *J. Physiol.*, 203:121–133.

Schiebler, W., Rothlein, J., Jahn, R., Doucet, J.P. and Greengard, P. (1983) Synapsin I (Protein I) binds specifically and with high affinity to highly purified synaptic vesicles from rat brain. *Soc. Neurosci. Abstr.*, 9:882.

Schiebler, W., Jahn, R., Doncet, J.-P., Rothlein, J. and Greengard, P. (1982) Characterization of Synapsin I binding to small synaptic vesicles. *J. Biol. Chem.*, 261:8383–8390.

Sieghart, W., Forn, J., Schwarcz, R., Coyle, J.T. and Greengard, P. (1978) Neuronal localization of specific brain phosphoproteins. *Brain Res.*, 156:345–350.

Sieghart, W., Forn, J. and Greengard, P. (1979) Ca^{2+} and cyclic AMP regulate phosphorylation of same two membrane-associated proteins specific to nervous tissue. *Proc. Natl. Acad. Sci. U.S.A.*, 76:2475–2479.

Sorensen, R.G. and Babitch, J.A. (1984) Identification and comparison of Protein I in chick and rat forebrain. *J. Neurochem.*, 42:705–710.

Tsou, K. and Greengard, P. (1982) Regulation of phosphorylation of Proteins I, IIIa, and IIIb in rat neurophophysis in vitro by electrical stimulation and by neuroactive agents. *Proc Natl. Acad. Sci. U.S.A.*, 79:6075–6079.

Ueda, T. and Greengard, P. (1977) Adenosine 3':5'-monophosphate-regulated phosphoprotein system of neuronal membranes. I. Solubilization, purification, and some properties of an endogenous phosphoprotein. *J. Biol. Chem.*, 252:5155–5163.

Ueda, T., Maeno, H. and Greengard, P. (1973) Regulation of endogenous phosphorylation of specific proteins in synaptic membrane fractions from rat brain by adenosine 3':5'-monophosphate. *J. Biol. Chem.*, 248:8295–8305.

Ueda, T., Greengard, P., Berzins, K., Cohen, R.S., Blomberg, F., Grab, D.J. and Siekevitz, P. (1979) Subcellular distribution in cerebral cortex of two proteins phosphorylated by a cAMP-dependent protein kinase. *J. Cell Biol.*, 83:308–319.

Wallace, W.C., Lewis, R.M., Kanazir, S., DeGennaro, L.J. and Greengard, P. (1985) Neuron-specific phosphoproteins as models for neuron gene expression. In W.A. Walker and C. Zomzely-Neurath (Eds.), *Gene Expression in Brain*, Wiley, New York, pp. 99–124.

Zengel, J.E., Magleby, K.L., Horn, J.P., McAfee, D.A. and Yarowsky, P.J. (1980) Facilitation, augmentation, and potentiation of synaptic transmission at the superior cervical ganglion of the rabbit. *J. Gen. Physiol.*, 76:213–231.

W.H. Gispen and A. Routtenberg (Eds.)
Progress in Brain Research, Vol. 69
© 1986 Elsevier Science Publishers B.V. (Biomedical Division)

CHAPTER 26

Association of calmodulin-dependent kinase II and its substrate proteins with neuronal cytoskeleton

James R. Goldenring,[1]* Mary Lou Vallano,[1]** Robert S. Lasher,[2] Tetsufumi Ueda[3] and Robert J. DeLorenzo[1]***

[1]*Department of Neurology, Yale University School of Medicine, New Haven, CT 06510, [2]Department of Anatomy, University of Colorado Medical School, Denver, CO 80262 and [3]Departments of Pharmacology and Psychiatry, Mental Health Research Institute, University of Michigan, U.S.A.*

Introduction

The neuronal cytoplasm contains a diverse array of interconnecting filamentous and tubular elements. While early views of cellular contents obtained through the use of transmission electron microscopy pictured a relatively sparse intracellular milieu, recent investigations of neurons with deep freeze etch techniques have revealed the complexity of the dense cellular matrix (Gulley and Reese, 1981; Schnapp and Reese, 1982; Landis and Reese, 1983; Hirokawa et al., 1984, 1985). The maintenance and dynamic alteration of this trabecular meshwork of filaments and microtubules are critical processes in the integration of cellular function. Increasing evidence suggests that the second messenger-dependent phosphorylation systems activated by calcium ions and cyclic AMP are important regulators of the neuronal cytoskeleton (Rasmussen, 1981). In this chapter, we will review recent work in our own and other laboratories which indicates that phosphorylation of cytoskeletal proteins may mediate many of the physiological responses to calcium influx.

Calmodulin-dependent kinase in brain

The importance of calmodulin-dependent kinase activities in regulating cytoskeletal dynamics has been recognized for some time in the well-characterized case of myosin light chain kinase in smooth muscle (Adelstein et al., 1980). In the smooth muscle enzyme system, phosphorylation of myosin light chains following the influx of calcium ions into the cell stimulates actin–myosin interactions and thereby induces contraction. No such contractile process has been observed with calmodulin-dependent kinase activity in brain but recent evidence has demonstrated the association of brain calmodulin-dependent kinases with the neuronal cytoskeleton (Oiumet et al., 1984; Vallano et al., 1985a, 1985b 1985c).

Calmodulin-dependent kinases have recently been purified from rat forebrain by a number of groups. At least two types of calmodulin-dependent kinases exist in rat forebrain (Miyamoto et al., 1981). The major form, now designated as calmodulin kinase II (CAMK II), has been extensively studied in recent years (Goldenring et al., 1983; Bennett et al., 1983; Schulman, 1984a; McGuinness et al., 1985; Fukunaga et al., 1982; Yamauchi and Fujisawa,

Present addresses: *Surgical Service (112), West Haven Veterans Administration Medical Center, West Spring Street, West Haven, CT 06516. **Department of Pharmacology, State University Hospital of the Upstate Medical Center, 750 E. Adams Street, Syracuse, NY 13210. ***Department of Neurology, Medical College of Virginia, MCV Station 599, Richmond, VA 23298.

342

1983). The kinase exists as a large holoenzyme complex of approximately 600–650 kDa consisting of nine 52-kDa α and three 63 kDa β subunits (Bennett et al., 1983) (previously referred to by our laboratory as ρ and σ respectively). The subunits display an apparent isoelectric point near neutrality. Both of the subunits appear to possess calmodulin-binding sites and both autophosphorylate in the presence of calmodulin (Fig. 1).

While CAMK II activity was purified by different groups utilizing various substrates including tubulin (Goldenring et al., 1983), synapsin I (Bennett et al., 1983; McGuinness et al., 1983), microtubule-associated protein 2 (MAP-2) (Goldenring et al., 1983; Schulman, 1984a), myosin light chains (Fukunaga et al., 1982) and tryptophan monooxygenase (Yamauchi and Fujisawa, 1983). it is now clear that synapsin I and MAP-2 demonstrate the highest levels of phosphate incorporation per mole of protein in in vitro assays. We originally reported that synapsin I was not a substrate for the calmodulin-dependent kinase. However, recently we have determined that this observation resulted from the presence of a low molecular weight inhibitor substance which is variably present in preparations of synapsin I purified by the method of Ueda and Greengard (1977). Similarly, while some investigators have been unable to observe calmodulin-dependent phosphorylation of tubulin (Bennett et al., 1983), this finding has recently been confirmed (Yamamoto et al., 1985a). Indeed, the investigation of CAMK II phosphorylation of various substrates including synapsin I, tubulin and glycogen synthase (Bennett et al., 1983), has demonstrated that substrate phosphorylation in vitro may be highly dependent on the preparation and native state of substrate proteins.

Several recent investigations have suggested that CAMK II exists in isozymic forms, not only in peripheral tissues but in different brain regions. McGuinness et al. (1985) have shown that CAMK II isolated from cerebellum has similar kinetic properties and substrate profiles with CAMK II from forebrain, but the ratio of the subunits is inverted with a molar ratio of one α to four β subunits. These results are consistent with the hypothesis that all of the subunits of the kinase

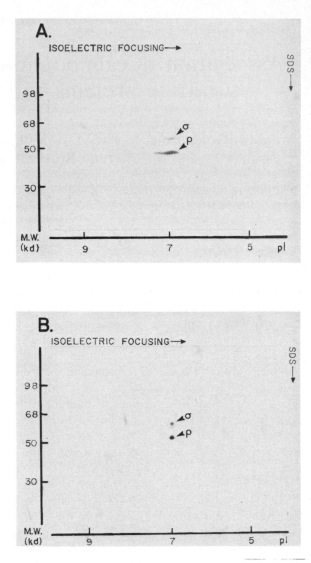

Fig. 1. CAMK II resolved on 2-dimensional gels. A: CAMK II purified by the method of Goldenring et al. (1983) was resolved by 2-dimensional isoelectric focussing/SDS–PAGE (O'Farrell et al., 1977). The gel was then processed for ^{125}I-calmodulin overlay by a modification of the method of Carlin et al. (1981). The bottom 2 cm of the gel were removed immediately following resolution in the second dimension in order to remove ampholytes which might bind calmodulin (Goldenring et al., 1983). The autoradiograph shows the two calmodulin-binding subunits, ρ (now designated α) and σ (now designated β) focussed at neutrality. B: CAMK II was autophosphorylated in the presence of 1 μg of calmodulin, 100 μM Ca^{2+}, and 10 μM ATP and then resolved in 2-dimensional electrophoresis. The autoradiograph demonstrates that both of the CAMK II subunits autophosphorylate, focussing near neturality.

may be catalytic. Whether specific subunits of the kinase may have more specificity for particular substrates has not been determined since the brain enzymes have been refractory to subunit separation attempts. Calmodulin-dependent kinases in peripheral tissues including glycogen synthase kinase from muscle (McGuinness et al., 1983) and ribosomal protein S6 kinase from pancreas (Gorelick et al., 1983) have been shown to be homologous with the forebrain CAMK II. These reports suggest that CAMK II isozymes exist as a family of homologous multifunctional calmodulin-dependent kinases in many tissues.

Association of calmodulin-dependent kinase with cytoskeleton

Postsynaptic density

Grab et al. (1981) first reported that the post-synaptic density (PSD) of rat forebrain was highly enriched for calmodulin-dependent kinase activity and calmodulin-binding proteins (Carlin et al., 1981). The major calmodulin-binding protein in PSDs was shown to be the major PSD protein (mPSDp) which comprises up to 50% of the protein in PSD preparations (Kelly and Cotman, 1978). Three groups, including our own, have now demonstrated that the mPSDp is the α subunit of CAMK II in PSDs (kennedy et al., 1983; Goldenring et al., 1984; Kelly, et al., 1984). These data suggest that CAMK II exists as the major insoluble matrix component of the PSD. The explanation for the presence of a calmodulin-dependent kinase as a major structural component of the PSD remains unclear. However, one hypothesis proposes that the fixation of CAMK II beneath the postsynaptic membrane in a specific orientation may confer greater speed in response following influx of calcium ion.

The filamentous structure of the PSD has received considerable attention as a possible location for cytoskeletal alterations that could be involved with memory (Siekevitz, 1985). In addition to mPSDp, PSDs contain tubulin, actin (Kelly and Cotman, 1978), microtubule-associated proteins, synapsin I (Ueda et al., 1979) and the calmodulin and actin-binding protein fodrin (Carlin et al., 1983). Phosphorylation of these substrates by CAMK II or autophosphorylation may provide a rapid biochemical response to calcium influx. Nevertheless, the exact role of CAMK II in PSD function is unknown, as are the identities of physiological endogenous PSD substrates.

Protein kinase in microtubule preparations

The presence of cyclic AMP-dependent protein kinase in microtubule preparations has been documented by Vallee and his coworkers (Vallee, 1980; Vallee et al., 1984; Theurkauf and Vallee, 1982). Cyclic AMP-dependent protein kinase is directly complexed with a portion of the MAP-2 molecules in microtubule preparations (Theurkauf and Vallee, 1983). Fig. 2 shows the pattern of cyclic AMP-stimulated phosphorylation in twice-polymerized microtubule preparations, with prominent phosphorylation of MAP-2 and several other phosphoproteins including a 80-kDa doublet. While the presence of cyclic AMP-dependent kinase has been recognized for some time, the presence of calmodulin-dependent kinase has not been documented until recently (Vallano et al., 1985b; Larson et al., 1985). Calmodulin-dependent kinase activity is especially difficult to stabilize in crude preparations, necessitating rapid preparation times (Juskevich et al., 1982; Goldenring et al., 1983). Through the utilization of more stringent preparation techniques with rapid sacrifice and homogenization in chelator and protease inhibitors, we have been able to demonstrate calmodulin-dependent phosphorylation in in vitro microtubule preparations (Fig. 2). Calmodulin-dependent kinase activity in microtubules phosphorylates endogenous MAP-2 and several 50–60-kDa proteins which have been identified as α and β tubulin and the autophosphorylating subunits of CAMK II. The calmodulin-dependent kinase in microtubule preparations was identical to CAMK II by all criteria studied including:

(a) apparent molecular weights of component subunits,
(b) isoelectric points of autophosphorylating subunits,
(c) phosphopeptide maps of autophosphorylated subunits,

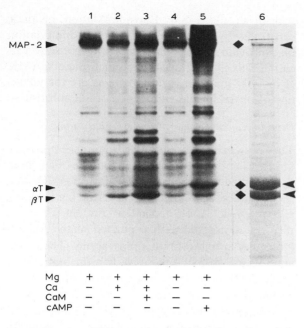

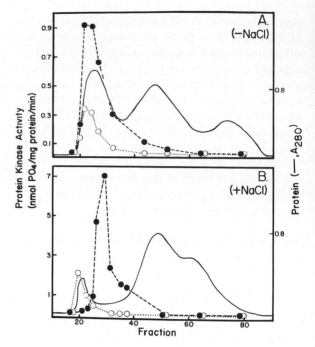

Fig. 2. Kinase activities associated with in vitro microtubule preparations. Cold-labile microtubules were prepared by two cycles of temperature-dependent assembly/disassembly (Shelanski et al., 1973) with modifications to preserve kinase activites (Vallano et al., 1985b). The protein staining pattern (lane 6) and autoradiograph (lanes 1–5) is shown for phosphorylated twice-cycled microtubule protein resolved in 1-dimensional SDS–PAGE. Microtubule protein was incubated for 1 min in the presence of 7 µM ATP, 20 mM MES, pH 6.7 at 35°C in a 100-µl reaction volume containing 4 mM Mg^{2+} (Mg), 50 µM Ca^{2+} (Ca), 1 µg calmodulin (CaM) and 10 µM cyclic AMP (cAMP). The positions of α tubulin (α T), β tubulin (βT) and MAP-2 are indicated. (From Vallano et al., 1985b.)

Fig. 3. Separation of calmodulin-dependent and cyclic AMP-dependent kinase activities in microtubule preparations. A: Chromatography in the absence of NaCl. Twice cycled microtubule protein was chromatographed on Bio-Gel A-15m and phosphorylated under standard conditions (as in Fig. 2). Fractions were assayed for calmodulin-dependent MAP-2 phosphorylation (○) and cyclic AMP-dependent MAP-2 phosphorylation (●). The ordinate values represent the total kinase activity in each corresponding fraction. The elution of protein was monitored at 280 nm (solid line). Column buffer contained 10 mM MES (pH 6.75) and 0.1 mM MgCl$_2$ B: Chromatography in the presence of NaCl. Experimental procedure was as described in A, except that the column buffer and the microtubule protein sample contained 500 mM NaCl. (From Vallano et al., 1985b.)

(*d*) calmodulin-binding properties of enzyme subunits,

(*e*) phosphotreonine phosphorylation on β tubulin, and

(*f*) phosphopeptide phosphorylation pattern of MAP-2 (see below).

In addition to its presence in cold-labile microtubules, CAMK II was highly enriched in cold-stable microtubule preparations (Larson et al., 1985). As in the cold-labile microtubules, CAMK II in cold-stable microtubules phosphorylated MAP-2 and tubulin as well as a 80-kDa phosphoprotein doublet.

We have recently demonstrated that cyclic AMP-dependent and calmodulin-dependent kinase activities can be separated in microtubule preparations (Vallano et al., 1985b). When microtubule protein was chromatographed over Bio-Gel A-15m resin in the absence of salt, the vast majority of both cyclic AMP-dependent and calmodulin-dependent kinase activity eluted in the void fraction (Figs. 3A and 4A). However, when chromatography was performed in the presence of 500 mM NaCl, conditions under which microtubule oligomers depolymerize into their component 6S tubulin and MAP-2 (Vallee, 1980;

Weingarten et al., 1974; Vallee and Borisy, 1978), the two kinase activities were separated (Figs. 3B and 4B). While cyclic AMP-dependent phosphory-

lation of an endogenous population of MAP-2 partitioned into the included fractions, the majority of the calmodulin-dependent phosphorylation of a separate population of endogenous MAP-2 eluted in the void fraction. These results indicate that there are two populations of MAP-2 in microtubule preparations, one associated with cyclic AMP-dependent kinase and the other associated with calmodulin-dependent kinase.

The void fraction prepared from microtubule preparations chromatographed in the presence of 500 mM NaCl is also highly enriched for neurofilaments (Berkowitz et al., 1977; Vallano et al., 1985c) which, unlike microtubules, are stable in high ionic strength solutions. The calmodulin-dependent kinase present in the neurofilament fraction from Bio-Gel A15m chromatography was identical to CAMK II by all of the biochemical criteria utilized above. Similar results were obtained when cold-stable microtubule preparations were chromatographed on Bio-Gel A15m (Vallano et al., 1985c).

Characterization of endogenous substrates for CAMK II in microtubule preparations

Microtubule-associated protein 2

Microtubule-associated protein 2 (MAP-2) is a high molecular weight microtubule-associated protein which decorates microtubules at periodic intervals (Kim et al., 1979). MAP-2 is highly phosphorylated endogenously (Vallee, 1980; Theurkauf and Vallee, 1983). Theurkauf and Vallee have demonstrated that MAP-2 is phosphorylated on 20–22 sites, 8–13 of which can be phosphorylated by cyclic AMP-dependent kinase. We have previously shown that cyclic AMP-dependent kinase and CAMK II have different phosphoamino acid preferences in MAP-2, with the former phosphorylating only serine residues while the latter phosphorylates both serine and threonine (Goldenring et al., 1983). Schulman (1984b) showed, using limited proteolytic digestion (Cleveland et al., 1977), that the two kinases elicited markedly different phosphopeptide patterns. We have recently extended this observation with total tryptic two-dimensional peptide maps

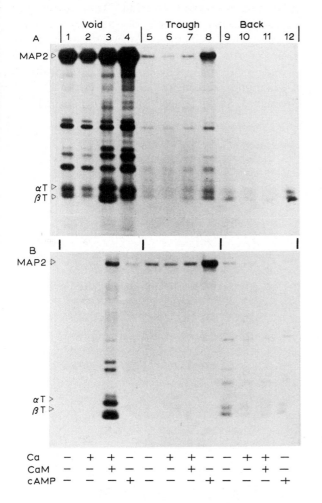

Fig. 4. Phosphorylation of microtubule protein by endogenous calmodulin-dependent and cyclic AMP-dependent protein kinase activities in microtubules. A: Autoradiograph of phosphorylation of microtubule protein separated on Bio-Gel A-15m corresponding to samples from the profile in Fig. 3A. Void = fraction 24; Trough = fraction 32; Back = fraction 44. B: Autoradiograph of microtubule protein separated on Bio-Gel A15m in the presence of 500 mM NaCl corresponding to samples from the elution profile in Fig. 3B. Void ('neurofilament fraction') = fraction 22; Trough = fraction 34; Back = fraction 52. All samples were phosphorylated under standard conditions in the presence of the additions indicated and were subsequently resolved on 7% SDS–PAGE gels. (From Vallano et al., 1985b.)

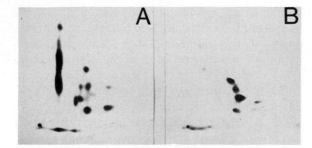

Fig. 5. Phosphopeptide mapping of MAP-2 phosphorylation by cyclic AMP-dependent and calmodulin-dependent kinase endogenous to microtubules. Twice-cycled microtubule protein was incubated in the presence of Mg^{2+} and 10 μM cyclic AMP (A) or Mg^{2+}, Ca^{2+}, and calmodulin (B) under standard conditions and subsequently resolved on SDS–PAGE. MAP-2 was excised from the gels, digested to completion with trypsin, and phosphopeptides were resolved on 2-dimensional electrophoresis/chromatography by a modification of the method of Axelrod (Axelrod, 1978; Goldenring et al., 1985b). Electrophoresis was from left to right, and chromatography was from the bottom to the top. (Modified from Vallano et al., 1985b.)

of MAP-2 phosphorylation (Vallano et al., 1985c; Goldenring et al., 1985b). Fig. 5 shows the patterns from MAP-2 phosphorylated by endogenous microtubule-associated cyclic AMP-dependent kinase (Fig. 5A) and CAMK II (Fig. 5B). The endogenous cyclic AMP-dependent kinase phosphorylated 11 major phosphopeptides all on serine residues, while CAMK II phosphorylated MAP-2 on 5 major phosphopeptides on both serine and threonine residues (Goldenring et al., 1985a). Since three of the calmodulin-dependent phosphopeptides contained both serine and threonine, a total of at least 8 sites for CAMK II phosphorylation must exist according to this method of analysis. In addition, CAMK II purified from forebrain cytosal phosphorylated MAP-2 with a phosphopeptide pattern identical to that for MAP-2 phosphorylated by CAMK II endogenous to microtubule preparations, indicating its potential utility in reconstitution studies.

Identification of a 80-kDa phosphoprotein in microtubule preparations as synapsin I

Fig. 2 and 4 clearly demonstrate that both cyclic AMP-dependent and calmodulin-dependent kinases phosphorylated a 80-kDa phosphoprotein

(pp80) which partitioned with CAMK II into the neurofilament fraction. This 80-kDa phosphoprotein was observed in both cold-labile and cold-stable microtubules (Larson et al., 1985) as well as in the neurofilament fraction. This pattern of phosphorylation by both of the major kinase systems as well as its molecular weight were reminiscent of the characteristics of the well-characterized neuronal phosphoprotein, synapsin I (Ueda and Greengard, 1977; Huttner and Greengard, 1979). Indeed, purified synapsin I co-

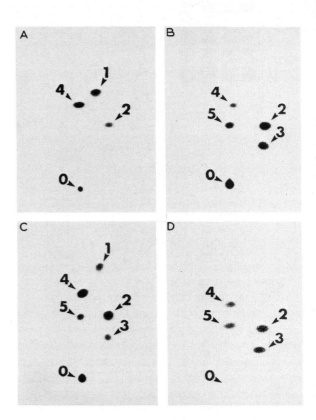

Fig. 6. Two-dimensional phosphopeptide mapping of complete tryptic digests of pp80 and synapsin I. Phosphorylated proteins were excised from SDS–PAGE gels and processed for 2-dimensional phosphopeptide mapping by the method of Axelrod (1978). Electrophoresis was from left to right and chromatography was from bottom to top. A: Phosphopeptide digest corresponding to cyclic AMP-dependent phosphorylation of pp80 in microtubule preparations. B: Phosphopeptide digest of calmodulin-dependent phosphorylation of pp80 in microtubule preparations. C: Comigration of digests in A and B. D: Phosphopeptide digest of purified synapsin I phosphorylated by purified CAMK II.

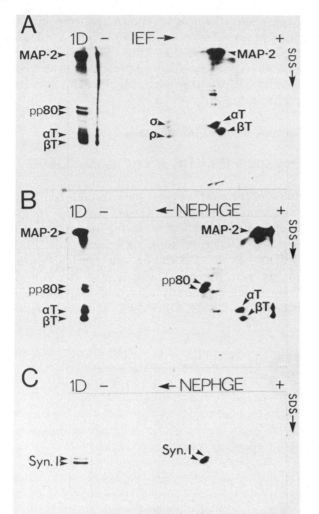

Fig. 7. Calmodulin-dependent kinase activity in neurofilament fraction resolved in two dimensions. A: Autoradiograph of calmodulin-dependent phosphorylation of neurofilament fraction protein resolved in isoelectric focussing/SDS–PAGE gels. The corresponding one-dimensional phosphorylation pattern shows that pp80 phosphorylation failed to focus. B: Calmodulin-dependent phosphorylation of neurofilament fraction protein resolved in NEPHGE/SDS–PAGE gels. The corresponding one-dimensional phosphorylation pattern at the left demonstrates that pp80 phosphorylation was qunatitatively recovered as a rapidly migrating basic phosphoprotein doublet on NEPHGE. C: Purified synapsin I phosphorylated by catalytic subunit of cyclic AMP-dependent kinase resolved in NEPHGE/SDS–PAGE gels with the corresponding one-dimensional pattern on left. Positions of α tubulin (αT), β tubulin (βT), the ρ(α) subunit of CAMK II (ρ), the σ (β) subunit of CAMK II (σ), pp80 and MAP-2 are indicated.

migrated on 1-dimensional SDS-PAGE with the protein staining and phosphorylation of pp80.

In order to further investigate the identity of pp80, 2-dimensional phosphopeptide mapping was performed (Fig. 6). The results revealed that cyclic AMP-dependent kinase phosphorylated pp80 on three tryptic peptides while calmodulin-dependent kinase phosphorylated pp80 on four peptides. Two of the four peptides were phosphorylated by both kinases (Fig. 6C). Purified synapsin I phosphorylated by purified CAMK II demonstrated a phosphopeptide pattern that was identical to that for pp80 phosphorylation by endogenous microtubule-associated CAMK II. These phosphopeptide maps were consistent with those of Huttner et al. (1981) for synapsin I. The pp80 also showed limited proteolytic peptide maps that were identical to those of synapsin I.

In order to characterize pp80 further, calmodulin-dependent kinase phosphorylation of neurofilament fraction protein was resolved on 2-dimensional isoelectric focussing/SDS–PAGE gels. This technique clearly resolved the phosphorylation of MAP-2. α and β tubulin, and the ρ and σ (α and β) subunits of CAMK II (Fig. 7A). The phosphorylation of pp80, however, did not enter the isoelectric focussing gel. Thus, in order to investigate the possibility that pp80, like synapsin I, was a highly basic protein, the same sample was resolved on non-equilibrium pH gradient electrophoresis (NEPHGE; Fig. 7B) (O'Farrell et al., 1977). The autoradiograph demonstrates that pp80 was resolved as a rapidly migrating, highly basic phosphoprotein doublet on NEPHGE. The pp80 co-migrated with purified synapsin I phosphorylated by the catalytic subunit of cyclic AMP-dependent kinase, as well as the protein staining of purified synapsin I added to the sample prior to electrophoresis. Thus, by all of these criteria, pp80 was shown to be identical to synapsin I. These results suggest that one of the functions of synapsin I involves interaction with neuronal cytoskeleton.

Other microtubule-associated substrates for CAMK II

We have previously reported that tubulin is a

substrate of CAMK II (Goldenring et al., 1983), and this observation has been confirmed by others (Yamamoto et al., 1985a). Figs. 2 and 7 demonstrate that α and β tubulin are substrates for CAMK II in both microtubule preparations and the neurofilament fraction. Tubulin exists in the neurofilament fraction as an extensive decoration of neurofilaments. The specific activity of tubulin phosphorylation is approximately one tenth that for synapsin I and MAP-2 in the preparations.

We have recently shown that neurofilament proteins are also substrates for CAMK II, incorporating approximately one mole of phosphate per mole of each of the neurofilament triplet proteins (Vallano et al., 1985a). Preliminary results suggest that the neurofilament triplet proteins isolated in the neurofilament fraction from microtubule preparations may be extensively phosphorylated endogenously. Indeed, Julien and

Myshynski (1982) have shown that the neurofilament proteins isolated from spinal cord are highly phosphorylated. Thus, CAMK II may phosphorylate neurofilament proteins with a higher specific activity than that observed in in vitro preparations.

Immunochemical investigations

Association of CAMK II with the cytoskeleton

Immunochemical studies have established that monoclonal antibodies against CAMK II are specifically associated with the neuronal cytoskeleton (Oiumet et al., 1984; Lasher et al., 1985; Vallano et al., 1985c). In situ labeling experiments were performed with a monoclonal antibody which specifically recognizes only the $\alpha(\rho)$ subunit of CAMK II (MAB 37:10:3). Fig. 8

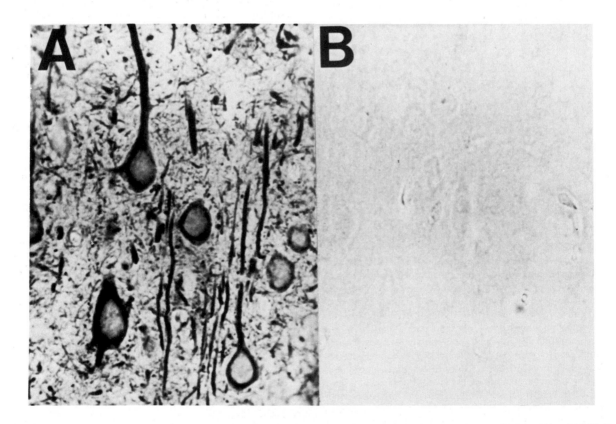

Fig. 8. Light micrographs of sections of rat cerebral cortex. A: Sections labeled with IgM monoclonal antibody against CAMK II (MAB 37:10:3). B: Section labeled with MOPC 104E, a non-specific mouse IgM myeloma. Sections were not counterstained. Magnification = 685 ×.

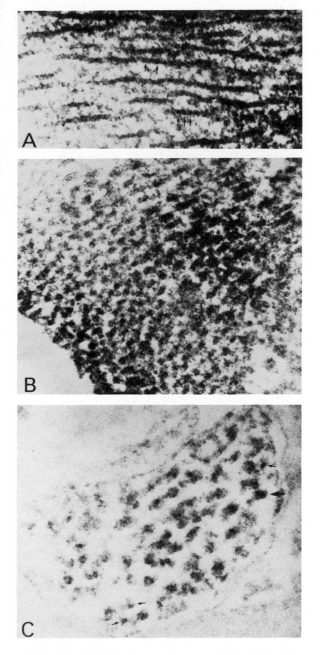

Fig. 9. Electron micrographs of thin sections through a dendrite from the superficial layer of rat cerebral cortex. A: Longitudinal section labeled with IgM monoclonal antibody against CAMK II with labeling of microtubules (Magnification = 72 320 ×). B: Cross to oblique section (Magnification = 72 320 ×).C: Cross section of a small dendrite in the hippocampus with labeling of both microtubules (large arrow) and neurofilaments (small arrows). Magnification = 133 900 ×. No label was observed in control sections. Thin sections were not counterstained.

demonstrates the labeling of cortical cells with anti-CAMK II antibody. The antibody labeled the perikarya and dendritic processes of cortical cells. The sections also demonstrated punctate staining in a synaptic distribution. Fig. 9 shows electron micrographs of antibody labeling of neurofilaments and microtubules in cortical dendrites. Electron microscopy also revealed heavy labeling of PSDs. Preliminary results indicate that there is an apparent periodicity in the binding to microtubules of the antibodies against CAMK II. The spherical aggregates of the reaction product have a center-to-center spacing of approximately 30 to 36 nm, similar to that seen for MAP-2 (Job et al., 1981). Microtubules and neurofilaments prepared in vitro also labeled specifically with MAB 37:10:3.

Ouimet et al. (1984) have also raised a monoclonal antibody to CAMK II which recognizes both of the subunits of the kinase. Their work in tissue sections demonstrates labeling with CAMK II antibody beneath the plasmalemma, on the surface of mitochondria and synaptic vesicles, on microtubules and in the PSDs. Overall, staining was more intense in the dendritic and perikaryonal cytoplasm with less staining in the axons. The results of the immunocytochemical studies indicate that CAMK II is highly localized to neuronal cytoskeletal elements, in proximitiy to its best substrate proteins.

Association of synapsin I with the cytoskeleton

Recent studies have indicated that synapsin I is immunologically homologous with erythrocyte protein 4.1, which is an important component of the erythrocyte cytoskeleton (Baines and Bennett, 1984, 1985). These results suggested that synapsin I might be representative of a more general class of cytoskeletal proteins. Our biochemical investigations of in vitro microtubule and neurofilament preparations suggest an association of synapsin I with the cytoskeleton. Indeed, using an affinity-purified rabbit IgG against synapsin I (Bloom et al., 1979), we have determined that synapsin I is enriched approximately 20-fold in the neurofilament fraction as compared with brain homogenate. Synapsin I-like immunoreactivity was observed in in vitro preparations of neurofilaments. In situ, synapsin I-like immuno-reactivity was observed associated with micro-tubules and neurofilaments as well as with synaptic vesicles and PSDs (Goldenring et al., 1986). All of these results indicate that synapsin I is associated with the neuronal cytoskeleton, suggesting that it may serve as a substrate for cytoskeletally associated CAMK II.

Phosphorylation and the regulation of neuronal cytoskeleton

Microtubules, neurofilaments and microfilaments are all linked by a dense network of cross-bridges (Hirokawa et al., 1984, 1985; Wuerker, 1970; Ellisman and Porter, 1980). If these cytoskeletal elements are viewed as sets of semi-rigid structures or cables, the possible dynamics of their inter-actions can be simplified to a case of fixed and mobile elements. Each cytoskeletal element contains its cable-like core with arm-like structures projecting from their surfaces. These projections could then interact with each other, directly with another cable core, with proteins on membrane surfaces or directly with membranes themselves. Thus, two major groups of cytoskeletal proteins can be identified: one group consists of proteins which comprise the cable core: tubulin, actin and 70-kDa neurofilament protein. A second group consists of the projection proteins: MAP-2, MAP-1 and possibly synapsin I. An intermediate group, comprised of proteins which contain core as well as projection domains, also exists, as in the case of 140-kDa and 210-kDa neurofilament proteins.

In this simplified model, the cable cores can be thought of as relatively fixed structures, even though it is clear that microtubules, for example, may be constantly assembled and disassembled from opposite ends (Julien and Myshynski, 1982). The projection proteins and the cross-linkages they form, however, may be relatively labile, accounting for rapid changes in the interaction of the main cable structures with each other and with membrane surfaces. Thus, one can hypothesize that long-term changes might be mediated by covalent modification of the cable core components, while short-term dynamic changes would be mediated by modifications of projection proteins.

In this article we have reviewed evidence for CAMK II phosphorylation of both core and projection proteins. The main cytoskeletally associated projection protein, MAP-2, is phosphorylated by both cyclic AMP-dependent and calmodulin-dependent kinases. A role for MAP-2 in microtubule dynamics has been suggested by several studies. MAP-2 enhances the rate of microtubule formation in vitro (Herzog and Weber, 1978). Phosphorylation of MAP-2 by either cyclic AMP-dependent kinase (Jameson et al., 1980) or calmodulin-dependent kinase (Yamamoto et al., 1983, 1985b Yamauchi and Fujisawa, 1982) decreases the ability of MAP-2 to promote microtubule polymerization. In addition, MAP-2 has recently been implicated in the interaction of microtubules with neurofilaments (Leterrier et al., 1982; Aamodt and Williams, 1984). MAP-2 immunoreactivity has also been documented in PSDs and in dendritic spines devoid of microtubules (Caceres et al., 1984). These results indicate that MAP-2 may serve a more general role as a projection protein cross-linking a number of different cytoskeletal elements. Recent work suggests that MAP-2 itself is a calmodulin-binding protein (Lee and Wolff, 1984). Whether cyclic AMP-dependent or calmodulin-dependent kinase phosphorylation of MAP-2 alters its calmodulin-binding properties as well as the function of its interaction with calmodulin in vivo remains to be determined.

Synapsin I has been extensively characterized by Greengard and his colleagues as a neuron- and synaptic vesicle-specific phosphoprotein (Greengard, 1981; Nestler and Greengard, 1984). Synapsin I phosphorylation has been temporally correlated with calcium influx into synaptosomes (Krueger et al., 1977; Robinson and Dunkley, 1985). Greengard (1981) has suggested that phosphorylation of synapsin I by CAMK II following influx of calcium ions into the nerve terminal might facilitate vesicle fusion with the plasma membrane. Huttner et al. (1983) have provided evidence that phosphorylation of synapsin I on its collagenase-sensitive tail region disassociates the protein from the synaptic vesicle membrane. Llinas et al. (1985) have recently provided corroberative evidence for this theory through studies in squid axon where microinjection of dephospho-synapsin I, but not synapsin I phosphorylated by CAMK II, decreased neurotransmission. Our results demonstrating the association of synapsin I with cytoskeletal elements suggest that synapsin I may be the link between the cytoskeleton and the synaptic vesicle membrane. Our results indicate that synapsin I is tightly bound to neurofilaments. Thus, neurofilaments might serve as the anchor for synapsin I as it binds to and releases from synaptic vesicles. Whether phosphorylation of synapsin I alters its interaction with neurofilaments remains to be determined.

Our results further suggest a more general cellular distribution of synapsin I in association with neurofilaments and microtubules. Evidence for the presence of synapsin I in PSDs is controversial (Bloom et al., 1979; De Camilli et al., 1983a, 1983b; Navone et al., 1984). The data indicate a more general role of synapsin I as a crosslinker of the cytoskeleton.

Recent evidence suggests that synapsin I is immunologically homologous with erythrocyte protein 4.1 (Goodman et al., 1984; Baines and Bennett, 1985). Protein 4.1 exists in a complex with actin and spectrin (Cohen and Foley, 1984; Cohen and Langley, 1984). The PSD is rich in fodrin, the spectrin analog in non-erythrocyte tissues (Carlin et al., 1983). Thus, it is tempting to hypothesize that synapsin I may be associated with fodrin in PSDs, the presynaptic grid and on synaptic vesicles. The exact identity of 'brain 4.1' and its relationship with synapsin I will require further elucidation. Nevertheless, the localization of synapsin I on neurofilaments indicates that the protein might serve a more general role as a mediator of interactions between actin filaments, neurofilaments, microtubules and membrane surfaces.

Thus, as in the case of MAP-2, synapsin I may be a projection protein mediating the interactions among a number of cytoskeletal elements as well as between the cytoskeleton and membrane surfaces. In the light of the possible role of these proteins in mediating dynamic changes in cytoskeletal structure, it is important to note that both MAP-2 and synapsin I are tightly associated with neurofilaments and microtubules in close proximity with CAMK II. Such a configuration places CAMK II in a key position to exert major effects on the cytoskeleton in response to increases in intracellular calcium ion concentration. Transient alterations in intracellular calcium ion concentration may elicit global changes in the cytoskeletal matrix through calmodulin-dependent phosphorylation of projection proteins.

Acknowledgements

The research detailed here was supported by USPHS grant NS 13532, RCDA 5-KOA NS-245 from NINCDS and AFOSR grant AFOSR-82-0284 to RJD; and USPHS grand NS 15113 to TU. JRG is a recipient of a Medical Scientist Training Program Fellowship.

References

Aamodt, E.J. and Williams, R.C. (1984) Microtubule-associated proteins connect microtubules and neurofilaments in vitro. *Biochemistry*, 23:6023–6031.

Adelstein, R.S., Conti, M.A. and Pato, M.D. (1980) Regulation of myosin light chain kinase by reversible phosphorylation and calcium-calmodulin. *Ann. N.Y. Acad. Sci.*, 356:142–150.

Axelrod, N. (1978) Phosphoprotein of adenovirus 2. *Virology*, 87:366–383.

Baines, A.J. and Bennett, V. (1984) Pig brain 4.1: Identification and purification. *J. Cell Biol.*, 99:300a.

Baines, A.J. and Bennett, V. (1985) Synapsin I is a spectrin-binding protein immunologically related to erythrocyte protein 4.1. *Nature*, 315:410–413.

Bennett, M.K., Erondu, N.E. and Kennedy, M.B. (1983) Purification and characterization of a calmodulin-dependent kinase that is highly concentrated in brain. *J. Biol. Chem.*, 258:12735–12744.

Berkowitz, S.A., Katagiri, J., Binder, H.K. and Williams, R.C. (1977) Separation and characterization of microtubule proteins from calf brain. *Biochemistry*, 16:5610–5617.

Bloom, F.E., Ueda, T., Battenberg, E. and Greengard, P. (1979) Immunocytochemical localization, in synapses, of protein I, an endogenous substrate for protein kinases in mammalian brain. *Proc. Natl. Acad. Sci. U.S.A.*, 76, 5982–5986.

Caceres, A., Binder, L.I., Payne, M.R., Bender, P., Rebhun, L. and Steward, O. (1984) Differential subcellular localization of tubulin and the microtubule-associated protein MAP2 in brain tissue as revealed by immunocytochemistry with monoclonal hybridoma antibodies. *J. Neurosci.*, 4:394–410.

Carlin, R.K., Grab, D.J. and Siekevitz, P. (1981) Function of calmodulin in postsynaptic density. III. Calmodulin binding proteins of the postsynaptic density. *J. Cell Biol.*, 89:449–455.

352

Carlin, R.K., Bartelt, D.C. and Siekevitz, P. (1983) Identification of fodrin as a major calmodulin-binding protein in postsynaptic density preparations. *J. Cell Biol.*, 96:443–448.

Cleveland, D.W., Fischer, S.G., Kirschner, M.W. and Laemmli, U.K. (1977) Peptide mapping by limited proteolysis in sodium dodecyl sulfate and analysis by gel electrophoresis. *J. Biol. Chem.*, 252:1102–1106.

Cohen, C.M. and Foley, S.F. (1984) Biochemical characterization of complex formation by human erythrocyte spectrin, protein 4.1, and actin. *Biochemistry*, 23:6091–6098.

Cohen, C.M. and Langley, R.C. (1984) Functional characterization of human erythrocyte spectrin alpha and beta chains: Association with actin and erythrocyte protein 4.1. *Biochemistry*, 23:4488–4495.

De Camilli, P., Cameron, R. and Greengard, P. (1983a) Synapsin I (Protein I), a nerve terminal-specific phosphoprotein. I. Its general distribution in synapses of the central and peripheral nervous system demonstrated by immunoflourescence in frozen and plastic sections. *J. Cell. Biol.*, 96:1337–1354.

De Camilli, P., Harris, S.M., Huttner, W.B. and Greengard, P. (1983b) Synapsin I (Protein I) a nerve terminal-specific phosphoprotein. II. Its specific association with synaptic vesicles demonstrated by immunocytochemistry in agarose-embedded synaptosomes. *J. Cell. Biol.*, 96;1355–1373.

Ellisman, M.H. and Porter, K.R. (1980) Microtrabecular structure of the axoplasmic matrix: Visualization of crosslinking structures and their distribution. *J. Cell Biol.*, 87:464–479.

Fukunga, K., Yamamoto, H., Matsui, K., Higashi, K. and Miyamoto, E. (1982) Purification and characterization of a calcium and calmodulin-dependent protein kinase from rat brain. *J. Neurochem.*, 39:1607–1617.

Goldenring, J.R., Gonzalez, B., McGuire, J.S. and DeLorenzo, R.J. (1983) Purification and characterization of a calmodulin-dependent kinase from rat brain cytosol able to phosphorylate tubulin and microtubule-associated proteins. *J. Biol. Chem.*, 258:12632–12640.

Goldenring, J.R., McGuire, J.S. and DeLorenzo, R.J. (1984) Identification of the major postsynaptic density protein as homologous with the major calmodulin-binding subunit of a calmodulin-dependent protein kinase. *J. Neurochem.*, 42:1077–1084.

Goldenring, J.R., Vallano, M.L. and DeLorenzo, R.J. (1985) Phosphorylation of microtubule associated protein 2 at distinct sites by calmodulin-dependent and cyclic AMP-dependent kinase. *J. Neurochem.*, 45:900–905.

Goldenring, J.R., Lasher, R.S., Vallano, M.L., Ueda, T., Naito, S., Sternberger, N.H., Sternberger, L.A. and DeLorenzo, R.J. (1986) Association of Synapsin I with neuronal cytoskeleton. Identification of cytoskeletal preparations in vitro and immunocytochemical localization in brain of Synapsin I. *J. Biol. Chem.*, 261:8495–8504.

Goodman, S.R., Casoria, L.A. and Coleman, D.B. (1984) Identification and location of brain protein 4.1. *Science*, 224:1433–1436.

Gorelick, F.S., Cohn, J.A., Freedman, S.D., Delahunt, N.G., Gershoni, J.M. and Jamieson, J.D. (1983) Calmodulin-stimulated protein kinase activity from rat pancreas. *J. Cell Biol.*, 97:1294–1298.

Grab, D.J., Carlin, R.K. and Siekevitz, P. (1981) Function of calmodulin in postsynaptic density. II. Presence of calmodulin-activatable protein kinase activity. *J. Cell Biol.*, 89:440–448.

Greengard, P. (1981) Intracellular signals in the brain. *Harvey Lect.*, 75:277–331.

Gulley, R.L. and Reese, T.S. (1981) Cytoskeletol organization of the postsynaptic complex. *J. Cell. Biol.*, 91:298–302.

Herzog, W. and Weber, K. (1978) Fractionation of brain microtubule-associated proteins: Isolation of two different proteins which stimulate tubulin polymerization in vitro. *Eur. J. Biochem.*, 92:1–8.

Hirokawa, N., Glicksman, M.A. and Willard, M.B. (1984) Organization of mammalian neurofilament polypeptides within the neuronal cytoskeleton. *J. Cell. Biol.*, 98:1532–1536.

Hirokawa, N., Bloom, G.S. and Vallee, R.B. (1985) Cytoskeletal architecture and immunocytochemical localization of microtubule-associated proteins in regions of axons associated with rapid axonal transport: The β,β'-iminodipropionitrile-intoxicated axon as a model system. *J. Cell Biol.*, 101:227–239.

Huttner, W.B. and Greengard, P. (1979) Multiple phosphorylation sites on Protein I and their differential regulation by cyclic AMP and calcium. *Proc. Natl. Acad. Sci. U.S.A.*, 76:5402–5406.

Huttner, W.B., DeGennaro, L.J. and Greengard, P. (1981) Differential phosphorylation of multiple sites in purified protein I by cyclic AMP-dependent and calcium-dependent protein kinases. *J. Biol. Chem.*, 256:1482–1488.

Huttner, W.B., Schiebler, W., Greengard, P. and De Camilli, P. (1983) Synapsin I (Protein I), a nerve terminal-specific phosphoprotein. III. Its association with synaptic vesicles studied in a highly purified synaptic vesicle preparation. *J. Cell Biol..*, 96:1374–1388.

Jameson, L., Frey, T., Zeeberg, B., Dalldorf, F. and Caplow, M. (1980) Inhibition of microtubule assembly by phosphorylation of microtubule-associated proteins. *Biochemistry*, 19:2472–2479.

Job, D., Fischer, E.H. and Margolis, R.L. (1981) Rapid disassembly of cold-stable microtubules by calmodulin. *Proc. Natl. Acad. Sci. U.S.A.*, 78:4679–4682.

Julien, J.-P. and Myshynski, W.E. (1982) A comparison of in vitro and in vivo phosphorylated neurofilament polypeptides. *J. Neurochem.*, 37;579–585.

Juskevich, J.C., Kuhn, D.M. and Lovenberg, W. (1982) Calcium-enhanced inactivation of calmodulin-dependent kinase from synaptosomes. *Biochem. Biophys. Res. Commun.*, 108:24–30.

Kelly, P.T. and Cotman, C.W. (1978) Synaptic protein: Characterization of tubulin and actin and identification of a distinct postsynaptic density polypeptide. *J. Cell Biol.*, 79:173–183.

Kelly, P.T., McGuinness, T.L. and Greengard, P. (1984) Evidence that the major postsynaptic density protein is a component of a calcium/calmodulin-dependent protein kinase. *Proc. Natl. Acad. Sci. U.S.A.*, 81:945–949.

Kennedy, M.B., McGuinness, T. and Greengard, P. (1983) A calcium/calmodulin-dependent protein kinase from mammalian brain that phosphorylates synapsin I: Partial purification and characterization. *J. Neurosci.*, 3:818–831.

Kim, H., Binder, L.I. and Rosenbaum, J.L. (1979) The periodic association of MAP 2 with brain microtubules in vitro. *J. Cell Biol.*, 80:266–276.

Krueger, B.K., Forn, J. and Greengard, P. (1977) Depolarization-induced phosphorylation of specific proteins, mediated by calcium ion influx, in rat brain synaptosomes. *J. Biol. Chem.*, 252:2764–2773.

Landis, D.M.D. and Reese, T.S. (1983) Cytoplasmic organization in cerebellar dendritic spines. *J. Cell Biol.*, 97:1169–1178.

Larson, R.E., Goldenring, J.R., Vallano, M.L. and DeLorenzo, R.J. (1985) Identification of endogenous calmodulin-dependent kinase and calmodulin-binding proteins in cold-stable microtubule preparations from brain. *J. Neurochem.*, 44:1566–1574.

Lasher, R.S., Goldenring, J.R. and DeLorenzo, R.J. (1985) Immunocytochemical localization of calcium/calmodulin-dependent protein kinase II in rat brain. *Anat. Rec.*, 211:105A.

Lee, Y.C. and Wolff, J. (1984) The calmodulin-binding domain of microtubule-associated protein 2. *J. Biol. Chem.*, 259:8041–8044.

Leterrier, J.-F., Liem, R.K.H. and Shelanski, M.L. (1982) Interactions between neurofilaments and microtubule-associated proteins: A possible mechanism for intraorganellar bridging. *J. Cell Biol.*, 95:982–986.

Llinas, R., McGuinness, T.L., Leonard, C.S., Sugimori, M. and Greengard, P. (1985) Intraterminal injection of synapsin I of calcium/calmodulin-dependent protein kinase II alters neurotransmitter release at the squid giant synapse. *Proc. Natl. Acad. Sci. U.S.A.*, 82:3035–3039.

McGuinness, T.L., Lai, Y., Greengard, P., Woodgett, J.R. and Cohen, P. (1983) A multifunctional calmodulin-dependent protein kinase: Similarities between skeletal muscle glycogen synthase kinase and a brain synapsin I kinase. *FEBS Lett.*, 163:329–334.

McGuinness, T.L., Lai, Y. and Greengard, P. (1985) Calcium/calmodulin-dependent protein kinase II: Isozymic forms from rat forebrain and cerebellum. *J. Biol. Chem.*, 260:1696–1704.

Miyamoto, E., Fukunaga, K., Matsui, K. and Iwasa, Y. (1981) Occurence of two types of calcium-dependent protein kinases in the cytosol fraction of the brain. *J. Neurochem.*, 37:1324–1330.

Navone, F., Greengard, P. and DeCamilli, P. (1984) Synapsin I in nerve terminals: Selective association with small synaptic vesicles. *Science*, 226:810–812.

Nestler, E.J. and Greengard, P. (1984) *Protein Phosphorylation in the Nervous System*, Wiley, New York.

O'Farrell, P.Z., Goodman, H.W. and O'Farrell, P.H. (1977) High resolution two-dimensional electrophoresis of basic as well as acidic proteins. *Cell*, 12:1133–1142.

Oiumet, C.C., McGuinness, T.L. and Greengard, P. (1984) Immunocytochemical localization of calcium/calmodulin-dependent protein kinase II in rat brain. *Proc. Natl. Acad. Sci. U.S.A.*, 81:5604–5608.

Rasmussen, H. (1981) *Calcium and cAMP as Synarchic Messengers*, Wiley, New York.

Robinson, P.J. and Dunkley, P.R. (1985) Depolarisation-dependent protein phosphorylation and dephosphorylation in rat cortical synaptosomes is modulated by calcium. *J. Neurochem.*, 44:338–348.

Schnapp, B.J. and Reese, T.S. (1982) Cytoplasmic structure in rapid-frozen axons. *J. Cell Biol.*, 94:667–679.

Schulman, H. (1984a) Phosphorylation of microtubule-associated proteins by a calcium/calmodulin-dependent protein kinase. *J. Cell Biol.*, 99:11–19.

Schulman, H. (1984b) Differential phosphorylation of MAP-2 stimulated by calcium-calmodulin and cyclic AMP. *Mol. Cell. Biol.*, 4:1175–1178.

Shelanski, M.L., Gaskin, R. and Cantor, C.R. (1973) Microtubule assembly in the absence of added nucleotides. *Proc. Natl. Acad. Sci. U.S.A.*, 70, 765–768.

Siekevitz, P. (1985) The postsynaptic density: A possible role in long-lasting effects in the central nervous system. *Proc. Natl. Acad. Sci. U.S.A.*, 82, 3494–3498.

Theurkauf, W.E. and Vallee, R.B. (1982) Molecular characterization of the cAMP-dependent protein kinase bound to microtubule-associated protein 2. *J. Biol. Chem.*, 257:3284–3290.

Theurkauf, W.C. and Vallee, R.B. (1983) Extensive cAMP-dependent and cAMP-independent phosphorylation of microtubule-associated protein 2. *J. Biol. Chem.*, 258:7883–7886.

Ueda, T. and Greengard, P. (1977) Adenosine 3':5'-monophosphate-regulated phosphoprotein system of neural membranes. I. Solubilization, purification, and some properties of an endogenous phosphoprotein. *J. Biol. Chem.*, 252:5155–5163.

Ueda, T., Greengard, P., Berzins, K., Cohen, R.S., Blomber, F., Grab, D.J. and Siekevitz, P. (1979) Subcellular distribution in cerebral cortex of two proteins phosphorylated by a cAMP-dependent protein kinase. *J. Cell Biol.*, 83:308–319.

Vallano, M.L., Buckholz, T.M. and DeLorenzo, R.J. (1985a) Phosphorylation of neurofilament proteins by endogenous calcium/calmodulin-dependent protein kinase. *Biochem. Biophys. Res. Commun.*, 130:957–963.

Vallano, M.L., Goldenring, J.R., Buckholz, T.M., Larson, R.E. and DeLorenzo, R.J. (1985b) Separation of endogenous calmodulin- and cAMP-dependent kinases from microtubule preparations. *Proc. Natl. Acad. Sci. U.S.A.*, 82:3202–3206.

Vallano, M.L., Goldenring, J.R., Lasher, R.S. and DeLorenzo, R.J. (1985c) Association of calcium/calmodulin-dependent kinase with cytoskeletal preparations: Phosphorylation of tubulin, neurofilament and microtubule-associated proteins. *Ann. N.Y. Acad. Sci.*, 466:357–374.

Vallee, R.B. (1980) Structure and phosphorylation of microtubule-associated protein 2 (MAP 2). *Proc. Natl. Acad. Sci. U.S.A.*, 77, 3206–3210.

Vallee, R.B. and Borisy, G.G. (1978) The non-tubulin component of microtubule protein oligomers: Effect on self-

354

association and hydrodynamic properties. *J. Biol. Chem.*, 253:2834–2845.

Vallee, R.B., Bloom, G.S. and Theurkauf, W.E. (1984) Microtubule-associated proteins: Subunits of the cytomatrix. *J. Cell Biol.*, 99:38s–44s.

Weingarten, M.D., Suter, M.M., Littman, D.R. and Kirschner, M.W. (1974) Properties of the polymerization products of microtubules from mammalian brain. *Biochemistry*, 13:5529–5537.

Wuerker, R. (1970) Neurofilaments and glial filaments. *Tissue Cell*, 2:1–19.

Yamamoto, H., Fukunaga, K., Tanaka, E. and Miyamoto, E. (1983) Calcium and calmodulin-dependent phosphorylation of microtubule-associated protein 2 and tau factor, and inhibition of microtubules assembly. *J. Neurochem.*, 41:1119–1125.

Yamamoto, H., Fukunaga, K., Goto, S., Tanaka, E. and Miyamoto, E. (1985a) Calcium, calmodulin-dependent re-gulation of microtubule formation via phosphorylation of microtubule-associated protein 2, tau factor, and tubulin, and comparison with cyclic AMP-dependent phosphory-lation. *J. Neurochem.*, 44:759–768.

Yamamoto, H., Fukunaga, K., Goto, S., Tanaka, E. and Miyamoto, E. (1985b) Calcium, calmodulin-dependent re-gulation of microtubule formation via phosphorylation of microtubule-associated protein 2, tau factor and tubulin, and comparison with the cyclic AMP-dependent phosphory-lation. *J. Neurochem.*, 44:759–768.

Yamauchi, T. and Fujisawa, H. (1982) Phosphorylation of microtubule-associated protein 2 by calmodulin-dependent protein kinase (Kinase II) which occurs only in brain tissues. *Biochem. Biophys. Res. Commun.*, 109:975–981.

Yamauchi, T. and Fujisawa, H. (1983) Purification and charac-terization of the brain calmodulin-dependent protein kinase (Kinase II) which is involved in the activation of tryptophan 5-monooxygenase. *Eur. J. Biochem.*, 132:15–21.

W.H. Gispen and A. Routtenberg (Eds.)
Progress in Brain Research, Vol. 69
© 1986 Elsevier Science Publishers B.V. (Biomedical Division)

CHAPTER 27

Multiple pools and multiple forms of calmodulin-stimulated protein kinase during development: relationship to postsynaptic densities

John A.P. Rostas, Ron P. Weinberger and Peter R. Dunkley

The Neuroscience Group, Faculty of Medicine, University of Newcastle, N.S.W. 2308, Australia

Introduction

The postsynaptic density (PSD)

The PSD is a protein-rich regulatory structure present in the postsynaptic neuron on the cytoplasmic surface of the postsynaptic membrane at most CNS synapses, irrespective of neurotransmitter. The PSD has been much studied morphologically since it is easy to identify by electron microscopy and can be selectively stained (Bloom and Aghajanian, 1966). It can also be isolated by subcellular fractionation techniques in good yield and purity allowing extensive biochemical analysis (Cotman and Kelly, 1980; Gurd, 1982). The PSD is believed to be contiguous with the cytoskeleton and has been proposed to develop as a specialization of it (Gulley and Reese, 1981). It also appears to be tightly bound to a number of protein components of the postsynaptic membrane which protrude into the synaptic cleft (Cotman and Taylor, 1974; Kelly et al., 1976; Gurd, 1977; Foster et al., 1981; Matus et al., 1981; Gordon-Weeks and Harding, 1983). It is believed that the major ways in which the PSD regulates synaptic function are by altering the arrangement of postsynaptic membrane components and restricting their mobility (Kelly et al., 1976; Matus and Walters, 1976) and by modifying the shape of the postsynaptic membrane surface and/or dendritic spine (Crick, 1982). Thus the PSD is regarded as a critical structure

and ideal control point linking the apparatus for reception of synaptic signals to the apparatus for propagating them.

Morphological studies have shown that the PSD is a dynamic structure which alters its shape and size during normal development (Blue and Parnavelas, 1983) and in response to learning (Stewart et al., 1984), long-term potentiation (Desmond and Levy, 1983), anesthesia (Devon and Jones, 1981), lesion-induced synaptogensis and synaptic reorganization (Hoff et al., 1981) and sensory stimulation (Güldner and Ingham, 1979; Rees et al., 1985). It has been proposed that these changes in the morphology of the PSD are an index of the changing properties of the synapse (Nieto-Sampedro et al., 1982b; Carlin and Siekevitz, 1983).

Molecular composition of the PSD

The molecular composition of fractions enriched in PSDs is remarkably constant between different species and within different regions of forebrain (Rostas et al., 1979; Nieto-Sampedro et al., 1982), although cerebellar fractions have a different composition (Carlin et al., 1980; Flanagan et al., 1982; Gordon-Weeks and Harding, 1983; Groswald et al., 1983; Aoki et al., 1985). Biochemical analysis is consistent with the view that the PSD is a specialization of the cytoskeleton: tubulin, actin, calmodulin and fodrin are all major protein components of fractions enriched in SJs and PSDs. Myosin, intermediate filament proteins, micro-tubule-associated proteins and Synapsin I have been identified in these fractions (Kelly and Cotman, 1978; Cotman and Kelly, 1980; Beach et al., 1981; Gurd, 1982; Groswald and Kelly, 1983) although myelin basic protein and glial fibrillary acidic protein, which are obviously contaminants, are also present in considerable quantity (Matus et al., 1980). The presence of most of the cyto-skeletal proteins in PSDs in vivo has been sup-ported by immunohistochemistry or independent biochemical investigations (Wood et al., 1980; Matus et al., 1982; Ratner and Mahler, 1983; Caceres et al., 1983, 1984; Aoki et al., 1985). A recent study on the rates of synthesis of the major proteins in synaptic junctions (SJs) (Sedman et al., 1985) showed that the junctional tubulin and actin had a much slower rate of turnover than the same molecules associated with the cytosol or non-junctional membranes. Therefore, these cyto-skeletal proteins are not only present in PSDs but they behave as a separate metabolic pool at the PSD and may have specialized functions there.

The major protein component of the PSD isolated from adult cerebral cortex is largely deter-gent insoluble, has an apparent molecular weight of 50 000 and was initially known as the major PSD protein or mPSDp. This protein is highly conserved during evolution (Rostas et al., 1979; Nieto-Sampedro et al., 1982). During development there is a large increase in the concentration of the mPSDp while the concentrations of the other major proteins change very little (Kelly and Cotman, 1981; Fu et al., 1981; Rostas et al., 1981). This increase occurs after the main period of synaptogenesis and is probably an index of syn-apse maturation. The increase in the mPSDp cor-relates with an increase in the thickness of the PSDs, but is accompanied by little change in the length of the active zone (Rostas et al., 1984). In the chicken, the rate of this increase, though not the final level of mPSDp, is able to be influenced by changes in hormone levels (Rostas and Jeffrey 1981), although the exact nature of the endocrine effect is not known. Because of the close correla-tion between the thickness of the PSD and the concentration of the mPSDp during development,

it is reasonable to assume that the changes in the PSD thickness, which are thought to be the mor-phological evidence of a structural plasticity in the nervous system, are occurring due to a change in the amount of bound mPSDp. Apart from prelim-inary chemical analysis, and a demonstration that the mPSDp was not related to any known fibrous cytoskeletal protein (Kelly and Cotman, 1977), very little was known about the identity and function of the mPSDp. Until 1983, the mPSDp was believed to be an insoluble membrane-bound protein specifically located at PSDs and not present in other subcellular compartments (Kelly and Montgomery, 1982). This view has now radically changed.

Calmodulin-stimulated protein kinase in the PSD and its relationship to the major PSD protein (mPSDp)

In 1981, Grab, Carlin and Siekevitz reported that isolated PSDs contained a calmodulin-stimulated protein kinase activity which led to the phos-phorylation of many proteins, the most prominent of which had apparent molecular masses of 50 kDa (50K) and 60 kDa (60K). They also de-monstrated that when polyacrylamide gels con-taining PSD fractions were incubated with ^{125}I-calmodulin, most of the binding occurred to the 50K and 60K region (Carlin et al., 1981). Shortly thereafter, a number of groups purified cal-modulin-stimulated protein kinases from rat cere-bral cortex (Fukunaga et al., 1982; Goldenring et al., 1982; Kennedy et al., 1983) and showed that they contained a 50K and 60K subunit*, both of which underwent autophosphorylation and bound calmodulin. Prompted by these results, we com-pared the properties of the 50K subunit of the

---

*In this paper, we refer to the subunits of the cal-modulin-stimulated protein kinase II as having ap-parent molecular masses of 50 kDa and 60 kDa (Rostas et al., 1986). Other investigators (Kennedy and Green-gard, 1981; Fukunga et al., 1982; Goldenring et al., 1983; Bennett et al., 1983) have assigned apparent molecular weights of 48–52 kDa and 60–63 kDa. In our modified gel electrophoresis system, we find that the subunits migrate at 53 and 63 kDa (Weinberger et al., 1986).

soluble enzyme and the mPSDp in different tissues and subcellular fractions and during development. We found that, while they were very similar, they appeared to be distinct by a number of criteria (Rostas et al., 1983). The major differences were the solubilities of the two proteins and the fact that the mPSDp exhibited heterogeneity in that a small proportion underwent autophosphorylation just like the soluble subunit, but the majority was not autophosphorylated (Fig. 1). We refer to the

TABLE I

The relationship between the 50K subunit of the soluble calmodulin-stimulated protein kinase II and the major PSD protein

Similarities	Purified kinase subunit and mPSDp have the same apparent molecular weight and isoelectric point. (1–3)
	Antibodies raised against soluble kinase or mPSDp recognize both proteins in vitro. (1, 2, 4)
	Two-dimensional tryptic peptide maps and V8 phosphopeptide maps of kinase and mPSDp are almost identical. (1–3)
Differences	mPSDp is highly insoluble. (5)
	Most of the mPSDp does not undergo autophosphorylation. (6, 7)
	Antibodies raised against soluble kinase and mPSDp show selectivity for their parent antigen in situ: by immunohistochemistry soluble kinase antibody preferentially stains neuronal cytoplasm with weaker staining of PSDs (8) whereas mPSDp antibody preferentially stains PSDs with little staining of neuronal cytoplasm(4).

1. Kennedy et al., 1983; 2, Kelly et al., 1984; 3, Goldenring et al., 1984; 4, P. Kelly and O. Steward, personal communications; 5, Kelly and Cotman, 1978; 6, Rostas et al., 1983; 7, Rostas et al., 1986; 8, Ouimet et al., 1984.

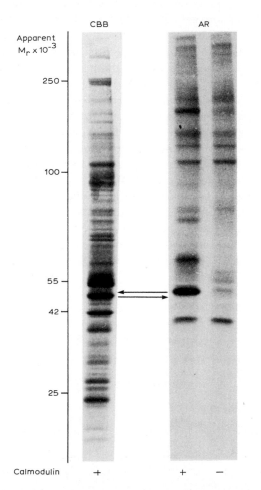

Fig. 1. Protein and phosphoprotein patterns obtained after labeling a synaptic junction fraction in the presence or absence of calcium and calmodulin as described in Rostas et al (1983). AR, autoradiogram; CBB, protein stain obtained with Coomassie brilliant blue. The relative mobilities of the labeled 50K subunit of the kinase and the unlabeled 50K subunit (mPSDp) are indicated by the arrows.

latter as the inactive form of the mPSDp. Even extending the time of incubation to as long as 30 min with periodic ATP supplementation left the majority of the mPSDp unlabeled, whereas the soluble kinase subunit was all labeled and converted to the lower mobility form in 5 min (Kennedy et al., 1983; Bennett et al., 1983; Rostas et al., 1986). Based on these results, we proposed that the inactive mPSDp and the 50K subunit of the soluble enzyme were either different gene products or slightly modified forms of the same protein (Rostas et al., 1983). With access to purified enzyme and antibodies to the kinase, Kennedy et al. (1983), Kelly et al. (1984) and Goldenring et al. (1984) independently demonstrated the great similarity between the mPSDp and the 50K subunit. It is now generally accepted that the majority of the mPSDp probably represents a modified form of the 50K subunit which no longer has autophosphorylation activity and is tightly associated with the PSD. The possible nature of this modification will be discussed later in this chapter. In the absence of a direct demonstration of this modification, however, the possibility of the majority of the mPSDp being a different gene product cannot yet be discarded. The similarities and differences between these proteins are summarized in Table I.

Properties of calmodulin-stimulated protein kinase II

The most abundant calmodulin-dependent protein kinase in brain, and the one which has been most thoroughly studied, is known as calmodulin-stimulated protein kinase II, because it was one of two enzymes originally purified based on their ability to phosphorylate synapsin I (Kennedy and Greengard, 1981; Kennedy et al., 1983). A number of calmodulin-stimulated protein kinases have been purified from rat brain based on their abilities to phosphorylate other proteins including tubulin (Goldenring et al., 1983), smooth muscle myosin light chain (Fukunaga et al., 1982), tryptophan 5-monooxygenase (Yamauchi and Fujisawa, 1983) and casein (Kuret and Schulman, 1984). Based on the physicochemical properties of the enzymes and their subunits, these are probably all the same enzyme and the different substrate specificities probably reflect different methods of preparation of the substrates (McGuinness et al., 1985). The enzyme is believed to have a broad substrate specificity which is dictated in vivo by the availability of substrates in its immediate environment (Kuret and Schulman, 1984; McGuinness et al., 1985).

The purified cytosolic holoenzyme from adult rat forebrain has an apparent molecular weight of 550K and is composed of subunits of 50K and 60K in a ratio of 3:1 (Bennett et al., 1983; Kennedy et al., 1983). All three subunits bind calmodulin and are autophosphorylated. A minor subunit of 58K also exists which is thought to be produced from the 60K subunit by proteolysis (Bennett et al., 1983; McGuinness et al., 1985). The cerebellum has a different form of this enzyme in which the 50K:60K subunit ratio is 1:4 and the 58K subunit is more prominent (McGuinness et al., 1985).

The enzyme appears to be preferentially localized to neurons (Ouimet et al., 1984) and is widely distributed in soluble and membrane-bound forms and associated with the nuclear matrix (Sahyoun et al., 1984a,), neuronal cytoskeleton (Sahyoun et al., 1985) and microtubules (Goldenring et al., 1984). The enzyme

TABLE II

Quantitative distribution of radioactivity in subcellular fractions after labeling INT-treated P2 membrane in the presence of calmodulin

	Protein (mg)	Acid-stable radioactivity (O.D.)[a]			
		Total (per 55 µg)	50 K (per 55 µg)	50 K (per fraction)	%50 K (per fraction)
P2 Memb/INT	16.3	1 170	260	76 170	100
M0.8	3.3	830	100	6 180	8
M1.0	4.0	1 690	320	22 910	30
SPM	2.0	3 640	1 060	38 400	50
Mp	2.0	660	150	5 460	7
SJ[b]	0.16	5 840	2 000	5 850	8
PSD[b]	0.04	6 380	2 380	1 680	2

[a] Arbitrary optical density units scanned at the optimum exposure for each sample and normalized.
[b] Values scaled up as if all the SPM fraction would have been used to prepare the SJ or PSD fraction.

activity towards exogenous substrates is equally distributed between the two forms in adult forebrain (Kennedy et al., 1983). The majority of the membrane-bound enzyme activity can be extracted in solutions of low ionic strength and, when solubilized in this way, has properties indistinguishable from that of the cytosolic enzyme (Kennedy et al., 1983). In cerebellum, the majority of the kinase activity towards exogenous substrates is membrane-bound (McGuinness et al., 1985). The mode of binding of the solubilizable enzyme to membranes and the proportion present in different cellular locations (i.e. plasma membrane: presynaptic, postsynaptic or nonsynaptic, synaptic vesicles, other organelle membranes or PSD) is unknown. The form and properties of the portion of the membrane-bound kinase which is not extractable has not been extensively investigated and, while it is generally assumed to be located at the PSD, this has not been demonstrated.

Subcellular distribution of membrane-bound calmodulin-stimulated protein kinase II in adult rat cerebral cortex

We have utilized the fact that the subunits of the calmodulin-stimulated kinase undergo autophosphorylation in the presence of calcium and calmodulin to investigate the distribution of the enzyme among membrane fractions from cerebral cortex. For the quantitative determination of distribution it is not possible to prepare subcellular fractions and then phosphorylate each under a standard set of conditions. This is because the incorporation depends on the net balance of kinase and phosphatase activities and these enzymes may be differently distributed or differentially extracted by the detergents used in the preparation of synaptic junction (SJ) and PSD fractions. In order to overcome this problem, we labeled the crude synaptic membrane fraction (P2-M) (Fig. 2) after treatment with p-iodonitrotetrazolium violet (INT) (Davis and Bloom, 1973) and then purified individual membrane populations from this mixture by the methods of Cotman and Taylor (1972) and Cotman et al. (1974). The autophosphorylation was quantitated from the auto-

radiograms of one-dimensional gels. This approach was possible because we were able to show, by a combination of biochemical techniques, that in all the membrane and soluble fractions from adult cortex the only significantly phosphorylated protein at 50K was the subunit of this kinase (Rostas et al., 1986). While the 60K subunit accounted for the majority of the radioactivity at 60K, other phosphoproteins were also present. Other workers (Kennedy et al., 1983; Kelly et al., 1984; Goldenring et al., 1984) have further shown that the kinase subunits account for virtually all the protein at 50K and 60K in SJ and PSD fractions.

To control for the effects of phosphatase activity, all samples were kept on ice until the end of the experiment and then all frozen at the same time. To measure the phosphatase activity occurring during this experiment one aliquot of the crude membrane fraction was frozen at time zero and another was kept on ice for the duration of the experiment. The left hand panel of Fig. 3 shows that there was very little phosphatase activity under these conditions and that the small activity present was directed evenly against all the phosphoprotein bands. Only 15% of the radioactivity in the 50K subunit was lost during the 4 h at 4°C compared with 50% lost in 30 s at 37°C in the same fraction not treated with INT (Table III). Thus INT treatment results in a significant inhibition of phosphatase activity.

All the calmodulin-stimulated phosphoproteins, including the 50K subunit, were distributed among the subcellular fractions (Fig. 3, Table II) in a way that paralleled the distribution of PSDs and markers for synaptic plasma membranes (Cotman and Taylor, 1972; Davis and Bloom, 1973): relatively depleted in $M_{0.8}$ and Mp (fractions enriched in myelin and mitochondria respectively) and relatively enriched in $M_{1.0}$ and SPM (fractions enriched in synaptic plasma membranes and PSDs). The preparation of SJ and PSD fractions from the SPM fraction produced a further enrichment in all these calmodulin-stimulated phosphoproteins. Thus, under these in vitro labeling conditions, the substrates for calmodulin-stimulated protein kinases are all proteins present in the same membrane fragments as the subunits

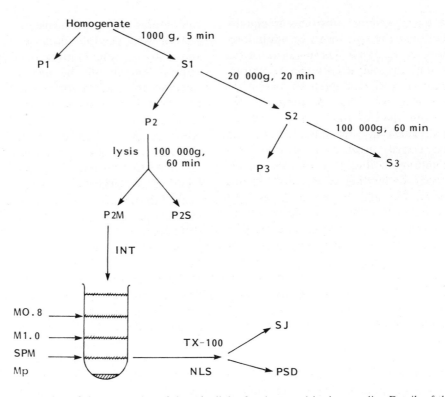

Fig. 2. Schematic representation of the preparation of the subcellular fractions used in these studies. Details of the procedure for preparing SJ (synaptic junction) and PSD (postsynaptic density) fractions from INT (ρ-iodonitrotetrazolium)-treated membranes can be found in Rostas et al. (1986). The major constituents of the four crude fractions are well characterized in adult brain: S3, general cytosol from both neurons and glia; P2-S, predominantly neuronal presynaptic cytosol plus some loosely bound membrane material released by osmotic lysis; P2-M, crude synaptic membranes plus organelles such as mitochondria, myelin, lysosomes; P3, small membrane fragments of diverse origin but largely endoplasmic reticulum with some plasma membranes. The composition of these fractions from developing brain is less well defined.

of the calmodulin-stimulated protein kinase. This suggests that at least the majority are probably so associated in vivo and they may well be substrates of the kinase. However, the possibility of changed location following phosphorylation or some arte-factual association as a result of homogenization cannot be ignored (Matus et al., 1980).

When the SPM fraction was extracted with detergents to produce an SJ or a PSD fraction, the majority of the labeled kinase was solubilized. This was not unexpected as 50–90% of the fore-brain particulate kinase can be solubilized in low ionic strength solution (Kennedy et al., 1983). It therefore appears that the bulk of the rapidly autophosphorylated membrane-bound calmodulin kinase is not tightly bound, but its exact location

is unknown. The detergent-insoluble and extract-able pools could be due to multiple pools within the PSD (which exist in vivo or have been created during subfractionation) or they could represent the PSD-associated and non-PSD membrane-as-sociated enzyme pools respectively. This data cannot distinguish between these two possibilities. It is noteworthy that the ratio of label in the 50K and 60K bands was constant (2.7 ± 0.2) in all membrane fractions and in both detergent-soluble and -insoluble pools, suggesting that the subunits exist as a stable multimer.

The autophosphorylated 50K subunit of the kinase was enriched in both the SJ and PSD fractions by a factor of about two. By contrast, the mPSDp was enriched in the SJ and PSD fractions

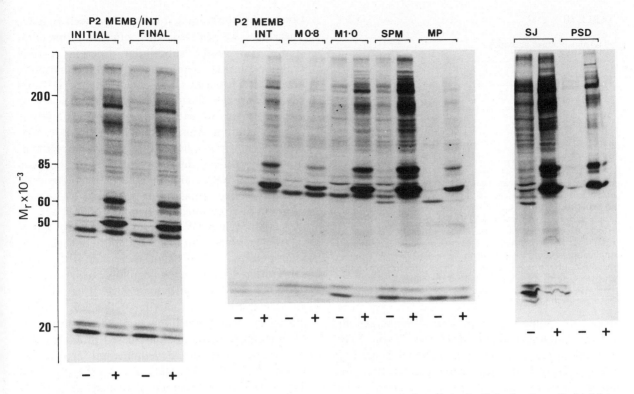

Fig. 3. Labeled subcellular fractions obtained from P2 membranes. Autoradiogram of purified subcellular fractions obtained from the INT-treated crude synaptic plasma membrane fraction (P2-M) that was phosphorylated and subsequently fractionated as described in Rostas et al. (1986). Left: INT-treated P2-M frozen at the beginning and end of the experiment to serve as a phosphatase control. Equal amounts of protein were run on the same gel and exposed for the same time. Centre: fractions obtained from the sucrose density gradient fractionation. The fractions floating on 0·8 M (M0.8), 1.0 M (M1.0) and 1.3 M (SPM) sucrose as well as the pellet (MP) are shown. Right: SJ and PSD fractions. + and − represent fractions obtained from membranes labeled in the presence and absence of calmodulin, respectively. SJ and PSD fractions were loaded at 15 μg and 5 μg respectively; all other fractions were loaded at 55 μg. Time of exposure for all fractions was the same.

by at least 1.7- and 6-fold, respectively. Selective phosphatase activity directed towards the 50K subunit cannot account for this discrepancy between the enrichment of the labeled kinase subunit and mPSDp (Table III; Rostas et al., 1986). Therefore, these results substantiate our previous findings that the majority of the mPSDp does not undergo autophosphorylation (Rostas et al., 1983) and extend them to show that the same is true in INT-treated P2 membranes which have not been exposed to detergent. The differential enrichment of the labeled and unlabeled forms of this protein could be due to:

(a) a different localization of the two forms (e.g. PSD versus membrane);

(b) a different mode of binding of the two forms such that the inactivation is a consequence of, or requirement for, one mode of binding; or

(c) a change in the detergent solubility of the protein as a direct consequence of phosphorylation.

What proportion of the 50K subunit in the PSD is inactive in vivo?

Our results clearly show that the great majority of the 50K subunit does not undergo autophosphorylation and therefore may be inactive as a kinase in isolated SJ and PSD fractions prepared by methods using INT. The INT treatment itself

TABLE III

50 K phosphatase activities

	Age		
	14 day	18 day	Adult
P2-S	17 (17)	20 (8)	9 (7)
S3	52 (40)	66 (40)	23 (18)
P2-M	10 (38)	21 (30)	35 (50)
P3	14 (27)	16 (45)	33 (33)

Phosphatase activity was measured at 37°C by adding 1 mM unlabeled ATP at the end of the standard 15-s labeling and allowing the incubation to proceed for 30 s before adding SDS stop solution. Quantitation was by densitometry of autoradiograms, which were within the linear range of the emulsion. Results are the average of two experiments each done in duplicate and are quoted as decrease in arbitrary O.D. units of the 50K subunit/mg fraction/30 s. The numbers in brackets give the percent decrease in O.D. of the band.

inactivates some of the enzyme (Weinberger and Rostas, unpublished), as does the Triton X-100 extraction, hence the proportion which is active in vivo is likely to be somewhat greater than that observed in the treated fractions. Indeed, while PSD fractions prepared by the method of Cohen et al. (1977) are obtained in lower yield, their calmodulin-stimulated kinase activity is higher than similar fractions obtained by the INT procedure. But can inactivation during isolation account for all of the observed results? We believe that they cannot. Even in adult P2-M and crude cytosolic (S3) fractions which have never been exposed to INT, detergent or incubation at 37°C, there is a great discrepancy between the relative kinase activities (see below) and the relative amounts of 50K subunit present in these fractions as determined by ^{125}I-calmodulin binding (Kelly and Vernon, 1985). This is consistent with there being a significant proportion of the 50K subunit that is inactive in vivo.

Change in distribution of calmodulin-stimulated protein kinase II during development in rat cerebral cortex

Unlike adult brain, from which it is possible to prepare highly purified and characterized subcellular fractions, the composition of subcellular frac-

tions from developing brain is less well defined. Therefore we carried out our developmental studies on crude subcellular fractions: crude synaptic plasma membranes (P2-M), presynaptic neuronal cytoplasm (P2-S), microsomes (P3) and whole brain cytoplasm (S3) (Fig. 2). In order to be able to do this we extended our previous analysis to show that it was possible to quantitate 50K subunit autophosphorylation from one-dimensional gels during development because, between day 10 and adult, and in all fractions, the 50K subunit of the kinase was the only significant calmodulin-stimulated phosphoprotein at its molecular weight (Weinberger and Rostas, 1986).

All fractions contained calmodulin-stimulated kinase activity and, as in the adult, the major calmodulin-stimulated phosphoproteins in all fractions were at 50K and 60K (Fig. 4). The autophosphorylation activity of the 50K subunit during postnatal development is shown in Fig. 5. Both membrane fractions increased to adult levels but showed different developmental profiles. In P2-M, 50K phosphorylation rose sharply from day 14 to day 18 and then plateaued, while in P3 it stayed constant till day 23 and then approximately doubled in the adult. The cytoplasmic fractions showed profiles markedly different from either of the membrane fractions: S3 and P2-S both rose to peak levels by day 18 and subsequently declined to adult levels.

The rates of dephosphorylation of the 50K subunit in each fraction varied during development (Table III) in a way very similar to that displayed by the autophosphorylation activity (Fig. 5). This indicates that the changes in the slopes of the curves in Fig. 5 represent changes in autophosphorylation activity. Correcting for the variation in phosphatase activity only accentuates the changes already observed. It is clear from Fig. 5 that, during development, there is a progressive increase in the proportion of the autophosphorylation activity that is present in the membrane compartment. This change in subcellular distribution is even more marked when the observed relative autophosphorylation activities are corrected for the differences in phosphatase activity between the fractions, and the fact that a large proportion of the PSD-associated kinase does not

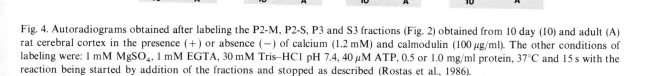

Fig. 4. Autoradiograms obtained after labeling the P2-M, P2-S, P3 and S3 fractions (Fig. 2) obtained from 10 day (10) and adult (A) rat cerebral cortex in the presence (+) or absence (−) of calcium (1.2 mM) and calmodulin (100 μg/ml). The other conditions of labeling were: 1 mM MgSO₄, 1 mM EGTA, 30 mM Tris–HCl pH 7.4, 40 μM ATP, 0.5 or 1.0 mg/ml protein, 37°C and 15 s with the reaction being started by addition of the fractions and stopped as described (Rostas et al., 1986).

autophosphorylate is taken into account. Thus, calmodulin-stimulated protein kinase II is primarily a soluble enzyme in immature rat brain, but changes to being a primarily membrane-bound one in the adult even though its observed activity, measured as autophosphorylation (Fig. 5) or labeling of exogenous (Kennedy et al., 1983) or endogenous (Weinberger and Rostas, 1986) substrates, is evenly distributed

between soluble and membrane fractions. These results suggest the possibility of a redistribution of enzyme during development by binding at specific membrane binding sites. The exact location of these membrane binding sites is unknown but, so far, the only membrane sites at which this enzyme has been positively identified are PSDs and synaptic vesicles. A similar apparent redistribution of kinase during development was found by Kelly

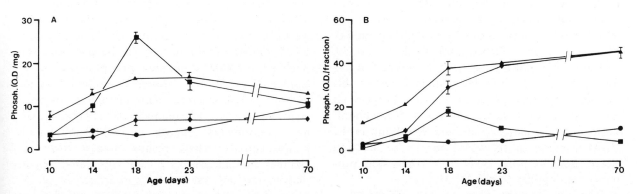

Fig. 5. Developmental changes in autophosphorylation activity of the 50K subunit in different subcellular fractions expressed as arbitrary O.D. units per mg protein in the fraction (A) and per fraction (B). ◆, P2-M; ■, P2-S; ●, P3; △, S3. Values are plotted as mean ±S.E.M. with a minimum of 4 animals at each age.

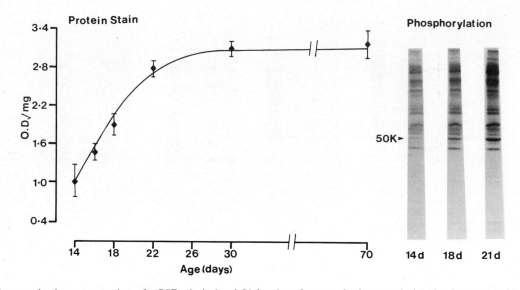

Fig. 6. Increase in the concentration of mPSDp in isolated SJ fractions from cerebral cortex during development (arbitrary O.D. units/mg protein) as determined by quantitative densitometry of protein-stained polyacrylamide gels and the increase in the autophosphorylation activity of the kinase in the same fractions as determined by autoradiography.

and Vernon (1985) by quantitation of ^{125}I-calmodulin binding to the 50K region of analogous subcellular fractions.

In order to determine whether the changes in kinase activity during development were due to changes in amounts of the kinase or changes in its regulation we needed to be able to measure the amount of kinase subunit independent of its autophosphorylation activity. This is possible in the SJ fraction where the 50K subunit is such a major protein that it can be quantitated from gels stained for protein. As can be seen from Fig. 6, the 50K subunit concentration rose steadily from day 14 to day 22 and reached adult levels by day 30. The phosphorylation of the 50K subunit in SJ fractions showed a parallel change. Thus, in this fraction, ^{32}P incorporation appears to give an indication of the relative amount of 50K subunit present. As the majority of the 50K subunit in the P2-M fraction is recovered in the SJ fraction (Kelly and Vernon, 1985), this conclusion probably also applies to the P2-M fraction.

The development of calmodulin-kinase II is quite different from that of the well-characterized cAMP-dependent protein kinases both in time course and in the relationship between enzyme concentration and substrate phosphorylation. Lohmann et al. (1978a) showed that both regulatory and catalytic subunits of cAMP-dependent protein kinases, soluble and membrane-bound, changed little during postnatal development. Similar results were found by Kelly (1982) in purified SPM and SJ fractions. Although no changes in regulatory subunits were found, Kelly (1982) found marked increases in cAMP-stimulated phosphorylation of endogenous proteins in SPM and SJ fractions, occurring in the first two weeks postnatally and reaching adult levels by day 15. A similar developmental profile has been reported for cAMP-stimulated phosphorylation of endogenous soluble proteins (Schmidt and Robison, 1972) whereas, using histone as an exogenous substrate, Lohmann et al. (1978a) found no developmental change in cAMP-stimulated kinase activity. These results suggest that the changes in endogenous cAMP-stimulated phosphorylation are due to the appearance of phosphoprotein substrates during development. This is in sharp contrast to the developmental changes seen with calmodulin-stimulated protein kinase II.

The autophosphorylation of the 50K subunit showed marked changes in all subcellular fractions except P3, which did not reach adult levels until after day 23. Also, there was a good correlation between the accumulation of the calmodulin-stimulated protein kinase II and the phosphorylation of other calmodulin-stimulated phosphoproteins, although the exact relationship between the amount of enzyme subunit autophosphorylation and substrate phosphorylation is not known.

The age at which the concentration of enzyme in P2-M reaches maturity is not known precisely. However, direct measurement of the concentration of the mPSDp in SJ fractions showed that adult levels had already been reached by day 30 (Fig. 6). Kelly and Vernon (1985) reported an increase in mPSDp concentration between day 25 and 90 which was over by day 50. Therefore, adult levels are probably reached at, or slightly before, day 30. This is roughly the same time at which the processes of synapse formation and maturation are complete, as judged by morphological and biochemical criteria (Calery and* Maxwell, 1968; Lohmann et al., 1978b; Barclay, 1979; Rostas et al., 1981; Blue and Parnavelas, 1983) although Wolff (1976, 1978) has suggested that synaptogenesis occurs even past day 30 in the cortex. In view of the fact that the most rapid phase of synaptogenesis occurs in the first 2 weeks postnatally but the increase in the levels of this calmodulin-stimulated kinase does not occur until after day 14, the enzyme in this fraction is more likely to be involved in the events involved with synaptic maturation rather than in synaptogenesis (Rostas et al., 1981) but an understanding of these roles must await further research.

It can be seen from Fig. 4 and Fig. 7 that the relative amount of radioactivity in the 50K and 60K subunits changed in all fractions during development although at any one age the ratios in all fractions were very similar. It is clear from the results of two-dimensional electrophoresis that this change was due to an alteration in the relative phosphorylation of the 60K subunit and not to a change in the minor contaminants (Weinberger and Rostas, 1986). In SJ fractions, where the kinase subunits have been shown to constitute the

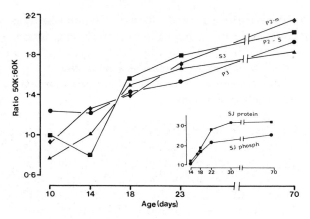

Fig. 7. Change in the ratio of the autophosphorylation activity in the 50K and 60K subunits of the kinase in different subcellular fractions during development. The inset shows the ratios for the SJ fraction as well as the ratios of the concentrations of the subunits as determined by densitometry of protein-stained polyacrylamide gels. Each point is the mean of at least 4 animals.

majority of the 50K and 60K protein bands (Kennedy et al., 1983; Kelly et al., 1984; Goldenring et al., 1984), the 50K:60K ratios in protein and radioactivity showed a very similar change (Fig. 7 inset), suggesting that the change in 50K:60K ratio probably reflects a change in the amounts of each subunit rather than an altered regulation of phosphorylation resulting in a differential molar incorporation of phosphate. This is supported by our recent finding that, in soluble calmodulin-stimulated protein kinase II purified from immature rat brain, the relative concentration of the 60K subunit was much higher than in adult with the 50K:60K ratio changing to the same degree when measured as autophosphorylation on silver staining (Rostas et al., 1986). This changing ratio could either be due to a continuously changing pattern of association of the two subunits, which is not consistent with biochemical mechanisms which operate in other tissues, or it could be due to the existence of at least two developmentally regulated isoenzyme forms in the cortex: an immature form which predominates at about day 10 and a mature form which predominates in the adult. The fact that in S3 from neonatal rats the ratio of 50K:60K remained constant at about 0.8 between day 2 and

10 (Weinberger and Rostas, unpublished) is consistant with the idea of two isoenzyme forms.

The relationship of changes in calmodulin-stimulated protein kinase II to the formation of postsynaptic densities

Our results have demonstrated that there is an increase in the amount of this calmodulin-stimulated protein kinase associated with PSDs during development, and particularly during maturation (Fig. 6). We have also shown that these changes are accompanied by changes in the morphology of the PSD (Rostas et al., 1984). Two major issues regarding the accumulation at the PSD remain: how the soluble kinase is modified to become the PSD-associated (largely inactive) kinase and how the kinase binds to the PSD.

How are the PSD associated subunits modified?

Assuming that inactive (non-autophosphory-latable) 50K subunit at PSDs is a modified form of the active 50K subunit, the question arises as to what sort of modification could bring about the differences in activity and solubility? The subunits

of the purified soluble kinase are indistinguishable from the mPSDp with respect to apparent molecular weight and isoelectric point. Thus, a proteolytic cleavage of the molecule cannot be involved because a minor clip is unlikely to be able to produce the large difference in solubility. Covalent and potentially reversible post-translational modifications such as methylation are a possibility, but since the purified (dephospho) form of the soluble enzyme and the inactive form of the mPSDp comigrate, this modification is unlikely to be phosphorylation itself. Another alternative is that the insolubility and inactivity are both brought about by an allosteric change in the enzyme subunits that occurs when they are bound to some other proteins. In view of the close association of the PSD with the cytoskeleton, and the capacity of cytoskeletal proteins to form insoluble complexes, this class of protein would be a prime candidate.

How does the kinase bind to the PSD?

The three general mechanisms that could account for the binding of soluble kinase to PSDs are illustrated in Fig. 8.

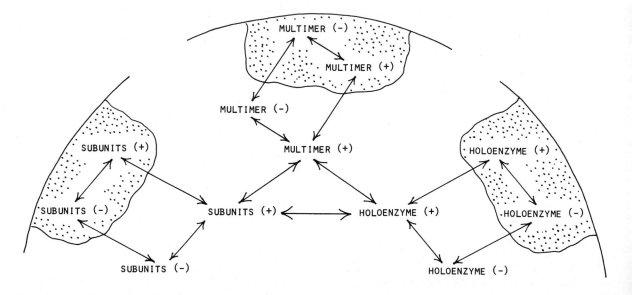

Fig. 8. Hypothetical scheme representing alternative ways in which the soluble calmodulin-stimulated protein kinase could associate with the PSD. + and − refer respectively to the active and inactive forms of the kinase as determined by autophosphorylation. See text for discussion.

In the cytoplasm, there must be an equilibrium between the individual kinase subunits and their stable multimeric form. Evidence for the existence of a smaller molecular weight multimer than the 550K holoenzyme is indirect:

(a) When the soluble enzyme from adult cortex, affinity purified on calmodulin–Sepharose, was applied to a Superose-6B column the peak of activity eluted with a molecular weight of approximately 550K but large amounts of activity were also recovered in lower molecular weight fractions. This enzyme activity of lower molecular weight bound less strongly to calmodulin–Sepharose and could be selectively removed by extensive washing but at all molecular weights, the 50K:60K ratio of autophosphorylation was constant (Rostas, Seccombe and Weinberger, in preparation).

(b) Sahyoun et al. (1985) also found that their calmodulin-stimulated kinase activity exhibited a broad range of molecular weights which changed with time suggesting a slow aggregation of multimers.

(c) The apparent subunit ratios in the kinase isolated from adult cortex, adult cerebellum and 10-day cortex vary greatly (Fig. 7; McGuinness et al., 1984). However, the apparent molecular weight of the purified holoenzyme is approximately 550K in each case. This could either be coincidence or an indication that 550K is merely the size of a stable aggregate which forms between the smaller multimers in vitro but that, in vivo, the multimers exist in a different form, perhaps bound in a large aggregate of similar size but with other proteins, e.g. cytoskeletal proteins.

The association of kinase subunits with the PSD could arise from either of these three forms of the soluble kinase. As our results have shown, the majority of the PSD-associated kinase is not able to undergo autophosphorylation in vitro and we have argued that this is likely also to be true in vivo. The generation of an inactive and an active pool in the PSD can happen in one of two ways: the inactivation may occur in the cytoplasmic compartment and the active and inactive forms could bind separately, or the active protein could

bind to the PSD and subsequently be inactivated. In either case this inactivation could be accomplished by binding to a protein, or modification by an enzyme, and the same two alternatives exist for the individual subunits, the stable multimer and the holoenzyme (Fig. 8).

The available experimental evidence does not allow us to definitely choose between these alternatives but the majority of the results favor the association being via some stable multimeric complex of 50K and 60K subunits rather than via an independent association of the separate subunits. The three major pieces of evidence are:

(a) There is a 60K protein band in adult SJ and PSD fractions which is composed mainly of the 60K subunit, which is about 3–5 times less abundant than the mPSDp band and which purifies in parallel with the mPSDp following detergent extraction of SPM (Cohen et al., 1977; Kelly and Cotman, 1978; Rostas et al., 1981, 1984; Gurd, 1982).

(b) The 50K:60K ratio of autophosphorylation was constant in all membrane subfractions even following detergent extraction (see above).

(c) The 50K:60K ratio was constant in all fractions at any age (Fig. 7).

The major piece of evidence in favor of the kinase subunits being incorporated independently is the observation that the only significant change in the relative concentration of the major proteins of SJ and PSD fractions during development is the large increase in the concentration of the mPSDp and that this is not accompanied by a corresponding change in the 60K region (Fu et al., 1981; Kelly and Cotman, 1981; Rostas and Jeffrey, 1981). At first sight it may seem that the change in 50K:60K ratio of both protein and phosphoprotein during development can account for this. However, despite the change in ratio, there is still an absolute increase in the 60K phosphorylation during this time (Fig. 6). For this to be reconciled with the notion of a multimer being incorporated into the PSD, one would have to propose that: (a) there is a major 60K contaminating protein in neonatal brain which disappears in the adult, or (b) there is a selective solubilization of the active

PSD-associated 60K subunit early in development. The particular susceptibility of immature synaptic junctions to disruption by detergents and mechanical factors has already been noted (Rostas and Jeffrey, 1981; Rostas et al., 1984) and it has also been shown that, under certain conditions, the 60K subunit of the cytosolic enzyme can be selectively removed from the holoenzyme (Fukunaga et al., 1982; Bennett et al., 1983).

Conclusions

There is a widespread assumption that only two forms of calmodulin-stimulated protein kinase II exist in cerebral cortex: a cytoplasmic and a membrane-bound form. The data in this paper clearly show that this simple notion is no longer tenable, since for each of these forms there are at least two further forms that can be recognized. The membrane compartment contains both active and inactive (by autophosphorylation) forms of the enzyme. Whether inactive enzyme also exists in the cytoplasm is not known. The soluble form can exist as multimers of varying size (at least in vitro) but whether the membrane-bound forms exist as multimers, the full holoenzyme or individual subunits is not clear. Finally, a different isoenzyme has been found to predominate in immature rat cerebral cortex and whether this form continues to be expressed in the adult is not known. It is likely that we will not fully understand the role of calmodulin-stimulated protein kinase II in neuronal function until we understand the properties of this enzyme in each of these forms and pools and the interrelationships that exist between them.

Acknowledgements

We are grateful to Marg Seccombe and Vicki Brent for research assistance, to Elinor Fitzsimmons for typing and Bruce Turnbull and Steve McInally for photographic assistance. This was supported by grants from the National Health and Medical Research Council of Australia. R.P. Weinberger is a Commonwealth Postgraduate Scholar.

References

Aoki, C., Carlin, R.K. and Siekevitz, P. (1985) Comparison of proteins involved with cyclic AMP metabolism between synaptic membrane and post-synaptic density preparations isolated from canine cerebral cortex and cerebellum. *J. Neurochem.*, 44:966–978.

Babitch, J.A. (1981) Synaptic plasma membrane tubulin may be an integral constituent. *J. Neurochem.*, 37:1394–1400.

Barclay, A.N. (1979) Localisation of the Thy-1 antigen in the cerebellar cortex of rat brain by immunofluorescence during postnatal development. *J. Neurochem.*, 32:1249–1259.

Beach, R., Kelly, P.T., Babitch, J. and Cotman, C.W. (1981) Identification of myosin in isolated synaptic junctions. *Brain Res.*, 225:75–95.

Bennett, M.K., Erondu, N.E. and Kennedy, M.B. (1983) Purification and characterization of a calmodulin-dependent kinase that is highly concentrated in brain. *J. Biol. Chem.*, 258:12735–12744.

Bloom, F.E. and Aghajanian, G.K. (1966) Cytochemistry of synapses: selective staining for electron microscopy. *Science*, 154:1575–1577.

Blue, M.E. and Parnavelas, J.G. (1983) The formation and maturation of synapses in the visual cortex of the rat. II. Quantitative analysis. *J. Neurocytol.*, 12:697–712.

Caceres, A., Payne, M.R., Binder, L.I. and Steward, O. (1983) Immunocytochemical localization of actin and microtubule-associated protein MAP2 in dendritic spines. *Proc. Natl. Acad. Sci. U.S.A.*, 80:1738–1742.

Caceres, A., Binder, L.I., Payne, M.R., Bender, P., Rebhun, L. and Steward, O. (1984) Differential subcellular localization of tubulin and the microtubule-associated protein map 2 in brain tissue as revealed by immunocytochemistry with monoclonal hybridoma antibodies. *J. Neurosci.*, 4:394–410.

Calery, D.W. and Maxwell, D.S. (1968) An electron microscopic study of neurons during post-natal development of the rat cerebral cortex. *J. Comp. Neurocytol.*, 113:17–44.

Carlin, R.K. and Siekevitz, P. (1983) Plasticity in the central nervous system: Do synapses divide? *Proc. Natl. Acad. Sci. U.S.A.*, 80:3517–3521.

Carlin, R.K., Grab, D.J., Cohen, R.S. and Siekevitz, P. (1980) Isolation and characterisation of post-synaptic densities from various brain regions: Enrichment of different types of post-synaptic densities. *J. Cell Biol.*, 86:831–843.

Carlin, R.K., Grab, D.J. and Siekevitz, P. (1981) Function of calmodulin in post-synaptic densities. III. Calmodulin binding proteins of the post-synaptic density. *J. Cell Biol.*, 89:449–455.

Cohen, R.S., Blomberg, F., Berzins, K. and Siekevitz, P. (1977) The structure of post-synaptic densities isolated from dog cerebral cortex. I. Overall morphology and protein composition. *J. Cell Biol.*, 74:181–203.

Cotman, C.W. and Kelly, P.T. (1980) Macromolecular architecture of CNS synapses. In C.W. Cotman, G. Poste and G.L. Nicolson (Eds.), *The Cell Surface and Neuronal Function*, Elsevier North-Holland Biomedical Press, Amsterdam, pp. 505–533.

Cotman, C.W. and Taylor, D. (1972) Isolation and structural studies on synaptic complexes from rat brain. *J. Cell Biol.*, 55:696–711.

Cotman, C.W. and Taylor, D. (1974) Localisation and characterisation of Concanavalin A receptors in the synaptic cleft. *J. Cell Biol.*, 62:236–242.

Cotman, C.W., Banker, G., Churchill, L. and Taylor, D. (1974) Isolation of post-synaptic densities from rat brain. *J. Cell Biol.*, 63:441–445.

Crick, F. (1982) Do dendritic spines twitch? *Trends Neurosci.*, 5:44–46.

Davis, G.A. and Bloom, F.E. (1973) Isolation of synaptic junctional complexes from brain. *Brain Res.*, 62:135–153.

Desmond, N.L. and Levy, W.B. (1983) Synaptic correlates of associative potentiation/depression: An ultrastructural study in the hippocampus. *Brain Res.*, 265:21–30.

Devon, R.M. and Jones, D.G. (1981) Synaptic parameters in developing rat cerebral cortex: Comparison of anaesthetised and unanaesthetised states. *Dev. Neurosci.*, 4:351–362.

Flanagan, S.D., Yost, B. and Crawford, G. (1982) Putative 51 000 M_r protein marker for post-synaptic densities is virtually absent in cerebellum. *J. Cell Biol.*, 94:743–748.

Foster, A.C., Mena, E.E., Fagg, G.E. and Cotman, C.W. (1981) Glutamate and aspartate binding sites are enriched in synaptic junctions isolated from rat brain. *J. Neurosci.*, 1:620–625.

Fu, S.C., Cruz, T.F. and Gurd, J.W. (1981) Development of synaptic glycoproteins: Effect of postnatal age on the synthesis and concentration of synaptic membrane and synaptic junctional fucosyl and sialyl glycoproteins. *J. Neurochem.*, 36:1338–1351.

Fukunaga, K., Yamamoto, K.M., Matsui, K., Higashi, K. and Miyamoto, E. (1982) Purification and characterisation of a calcium- and calmodulin-dependent protein kinase from rat brain. *J. Neurochem.*, 39:1607–1617.

Goldenring, J.R., Gonzalez, B. and DeLorenzo, R. (1982) Isolation of a brain calcium-calmodulin tubulin kinase containing calmodulin binding proteins. *Biochem. Biophys. Res. Commun.*, 108:421–428.

Goldenring, J.R., Gonzalez, B., Maguire, J.S. and DeLorenzo, R.J. (1983) Purification and characterisation of a calmodulin-dependent kinase from rat brain cytosol able to phosphorylate tubulin and microtubule-associated proteins. *J. Biol. Chem.*, 258:12632–12640.

Goldenring, J.R., Casanova, J.E. and DeLorenzo, R.J. (1984a) Tubulin-associated calmodulin-dependent kinase: Evidence for an endogenous complex of tubulin with a calcium calmodulin-dependent kinase. *J. Neurochem.*, 43:1669–1679.

Goldenring, J.R., Maguire, J.S. and DeLorenzo, R.J. (1984b) Identification of the major post-synaptic density protein as homologous with the major calmodulin-binding subunit of a calmodulin-dependent protein kinase. *J. Neurochem.*, 42:1077–1084.

Gordon-Weeks, P.R. and Harding, S. (1983) Major differences in concanavalin A binding glycoproteins of post-synaptic densities from rat forebrain and cerebellum. *Brain Res.*, 277:380–385.

Grab, D.J., Carlin, R.K. and Siekevitz, P. (1981) Function of calmodulin in post-synaptic densities. II. Presence of calmodulin activatable protein kinase activity. *J. Cell Biol.*, 89:440–448.

Groswald, D.E. and Kelly, P.T. (1983) Evidence that a cerebellum-enriched, synaptic junction glycoprotein is related to fodrin and resists extraction with Triton in a calcium-dependent manner. *J. Neurochem.*, 42:534–546.

Groswald, D.E., Montgomery, P.R. and Kelly, P.T. (1983) Synaptic junctions isolated from cerebellum and forebrain: Comparisons of morphological and molecular properties. *Brain Res.*, 278:63–80.

Guldner, F.H. and Ingham, C.A. (1979) Plasticity in synaptic appositions of optic nerve afferents under different lighting conditions. *Neurosci. Lett.*, 14:235–240.

Gulley, R.L. and Reese, T.S. (1981) Cytoskeletal organisation at the post-synaptic complex. *J. Cell Biol.*, 91:298–302.

Gurd, J.W. (1977) Identification of lectin receptors associated with rat brain post-synaptic densities. *Brain Res.*, 126:154–159.

Gurd, J.W. (1982) Molecular characterisation of synapses in the central nervous system. In I.R. Brown (Ed.) *Molecular Approaches to Neurobiology*, Academic Press, New York, pp. 99–130.

Hoff, S.F., Scheff, S.W., Kwan, A.Y. and Cotman, C.W. (1981) A new type of lesion-induced synaptogenesis. II. The effect of ageing on synaptic turnover in non-denervated zones. *Brain Res.*, 222:15–27.

Kelly, P.T. (1982) Protein phosphorylation in isolated synaptic junctional structures: Changes during development. *Brain Res.*, 247:85–96.

Kelly, P.T. and Cotman, C.W. (1977) Identification of glycoproteins and proteins at synapses in the central nervous system. *J. Biol. Chem.*, 252:786–793.

Kelly, P.T. and Cotman, C.W. (1978) Characterisation of tubulin and actin and identification of a distinct post-synaptic density polypeptide. *J. Cell Biol.*, 79:173–183.

Kelly, P.T. and Cotman, C.W. (1981) Developmental changes in morphology and molecular composition of isolated synaptic junctional structures. *Brain Res.*, 206:251–271.

Kelly, P.T. and Montgomery, P.R. (1982) Subcellular localisation of the 52 000 molecular weight major post-synaptic density protein. *Brain Res.*, 233:265–286.

Kelly, P.T. and Vernon, P. (1985) Changes in subcellular distribution of calmodulin kinase II during brain development. *Dev. Brain Res.*, 18:211–224.

Kelly, P.T., Cotman, C.W., Gentry, C. and Nicolson, G. (1976) Distribution and mobility of lectin receptors on synaptic membranes of identified neurons in the central nervous system. *J. Cell Biol.*, 71:487–496.

Kelly, P., McGuinness, T. and Greengard, P. (1984) Evidence that the major postsynaptic density protein is a component of a Ca^{++}/calmodulin-dependent protein kinase. *Proc. Natl. Acad. Sci. U.S.A.*, 81:945–949.

Kennedy, M.B. and Greengard, P. (1981) Two calcium/calmodulin-dependent protein kinases, which are highly concentrated in brain, phosphorylate protein I at distinct sites. *Proc. Natl. Acad. Sci. U.S.A.*, 78:1293–1297.

Kennedy, M.B., Bennett, M.K. and Erondu, N.E. (1983a) Biochemical and immunochemical evidence that the major postsynaptic density protein is a subunit of a calmodulin-dependent protein kinase. *Proc. Natl. Acad. Sci. U.S.A.*, 80:7457–7461.

Kennedy, M.B., McGuiness, T. and Greengard, P. (1983b) A calcium/calmodulin-dependent protein kinase from mammalian brain that phosphorylates synapsin I: Partial purification and characterisation. *J. Neurosci.*, 3:818–831.

Kuret, J. and Schulman, H. (1984) Purification and characterization of a Ca^{2+}/calmodulin-dependent protein kinase from rat brain. *Biochemistry*, 23:5495–5504.

Lohmann, S.M., Walter, U. and Greengard, P. (1978a) Protein kinases in developing rat brain. *J. Cyclic Nucleotide Res.*, 4:445–452.

Lohmann, S.M., Ueda, T. and Greengard, P. (1978b) Ontogeny of synaptic phosphoproteins in brain. *Proc. Natl. Acad. Sci. U.S.A.*, 75:4037–4041.

McGuiness, T.L., Lai, Y. and Greengard, P. (1985) Ca^{2+}/calmodulin-dependent protein kinase II: Isozymic forms from rat forebrain and cerebellum. *J. Biol. Chem.* 260:1696–1704.

Matus, A. and Walters, B.B. (1976) Type I and II synaptic junctions: differences in distribution of Concanavalin A binding sites and stability of the junctional adhesion. *Brain Res.*, 108:249–256.

Matus, A., Pehling, G., Ackermann, M. and Maeder, J. (1980) Brain post-synaptic densities: Their relationship to glial and neuronal filaments. *J. Cell Biol.*, 87:346–359.

Matus, A.I., Pehling, G. and Wilkinson, D. (1981) γ-aminobutyric acid receptors in brain post-synaptic densities. *J. Neurobiol.*, 12:67–73.

Matus, A., Ackermann, M., Pehling, G., Byers, H.R. and Fujiwara, K. (1982) High actin concentrations in brain dendritic spines and post-synaptic densities. *Proc. Natl. Acad. Sci. U.S.A.*, 79:7590–7594.

Nieto-Sampedro, M., Bussineau, C.M. and Cotman, C.W. (1982a) Isolation, morphology and protein and glycoprotein composition of synaptic junctional fractions from the brains of lower vertebrates: Antigen PSD-95 as a junctional marker. *J. Neurosci.*, 2:722–734.

Nieto-Sampedro, M., Hoff, S.F. and Cotman, C.W. (1982b) Perforated post-synaptic densities: Probable intermediates in synapse turnover. *Proc. Natl. Acad. Sci. U.S.A.*, 79:5718–5722.

Ouimet, C.C., McGuiness, T.L. and Greengard, P. (1984) Immunocytochemical localisation of calcium calmodulin-dependent protein kinase II in rat brain. *Proc. Natl. Acad. Sci. U.S.A.*, 81:5604–5608.

Ratner, N. and Mahler, H.R. (1983) Structural organisation of filamentous proteins in the post-synaptic density. *Biochemistry*, 22:2446–2453.

Rees, S., Güldner, F.H. and Aitkin, L. (1985) Activity-dependent plasticity of post-synaptic density structure in the ventral cochlar nucleus of the rat. *Brain Res.* 325:370–374.

Rostas, J.A.P. and Jeffrey, P.L. (1981) Maturation of synapses in chicken forebrain. *Neurosci. Lett.*, 25:299–304.

Rostas, J.A.P., Kelly, P.T., Pesin, R.H. and Cotman, C.W. (1979) Protein and glycoprotein composition of synaptic junctions prepared from discrete synaptic regions and different species. *Brain Res.*, 168:151–167.

Rostas, J.A.P., Shevenan, T.A., Sinclair, C.M. and Jeffrey, P.L. (1981) Markers for synaptic maturation in the central nervous system. In A.D. Kidman, J. Tomkins and R.A. Westerman (Eds.), *New Approaches to Nerve and Muscle Disorders*, Excerpta Medica, Amsterdam, pp. 23–26.

Rostas, J.A.P., Brent, V.A. and Dunkley, P.R. (1983) The major calmodulin-stimulated phosphoprotein of synaptic junctions and the major post-synaptic density protein are distinct. *Neurosci. Lett.*, 43:161–165.

Rostas, J.A.P., Brent, V.A. and Güldner, F.H. (1984) The maturation of post-synaptic densities in chicken forebrain. *Neurosci. Lett.*, 45:297–304.

Rostas, J.A.P., Brent, V.A., Heath, J.W., Neame, R.L.B., Powis, D.A., Weinberger, R.P. and Dunkley, P.R. (1985) The subcellular distribution of a membrane-bond calmodulin-stimulated protein kinase. *Neurochem. Res.*, 11:253–268.

Rostas, J.A.P., Seccombe, M. and Weinberger, R.P. (1986) Two developmentally regulated isoenzyme forms of calmodulin kinase II in rat forebrain. *Neurosci. Lett., Supp.* 23:S76.

Sahyoun, N., LeVine, H. III and Cuatrecasas, P. (1984a) Calcium/calmodulin-dependent protein kinases from the neuronal nuclear matrix and post-synaptic density are structurally related. *Proc. Natl. Acad. Sci. U.S.A.*, 81:4311–4315.

Sahyoun, N., LeVine, H. III, Bronson, D. and Cuatrecasas, P. (1984b) Ca^{2+}/calmodulin-dependent protein kinase in neuronal nuclei. *J. Biol. Chem.*, 259:9341–9344.

Sahyoun, N., LeVine H. III, Bronson, D., Siegel-Greenstein, F. and Cuatrecasas, P. (1985) Cytoskeletal calmodulin-dependent protein kinase. Characterization, solubilization and purification from rat brain. *J. Biol. Chem.*, 260:1230–1237.

Schmidt, M.J. and Robison, G.A. (1972) The effect of neonatal thyroidectomy on the development of the adenosine 3',5'-monophosphate sytem in rat brain. J. Neurochem., 19:937–947.

Sedman, G.L., Jeffrey, P.L., Austin, L. and Rostas, J.A.P. (1985) Turnover of proteins at the post-synaptic density. *Neurosci. Lett. Suppl.*, 19:S96.

Stewart, M.G., Rose, S.P.R., King, T.S., Gabbott, P.L.A. and Bourne, R. (1984) Hemispheric asymmetry of synapses in chick medial hyperstriatum ventrale following passive avoidance training: a sterological investigation. *Dev. Brain Res.*, 12:261–269.

Weinberger, R.P. and Rostas, J.A.P. (1986) Subcellular distribution of a calmodulin-dependent protein kinase activity in rat cerebral cortex during development. *Dev. Brain Res.* (In press).

Wolff, J.R. (1976) Quantitative analysis of topography and development of synapses in the visual cortex. *Exp. Brain Res. Suppl.*, 1:259–263.

Wolff, J.R. (1978) Ontogenetic aspects of cortical architecture: lamination. In M.A.B. Brazier and H.J. Petsche (Eds.), *Architectonics of the Cerebral Cortex*, Raven Press, New York, pp. 159–173.

Wood, J.G., Wallace, J.N., Whitaker, J.N. and Cheung, W.Y. (1980) Immunocytochemical localization of calmodulin and a heat-labile calmodulin-binding protein (CaM-BP$_{80}$) in basal ganglia of mouse brain. *J. Cell Biol.*, 84:66–76.

Yamauchi, T. and Fujisawa, H. (1981) A calmodulin-dependent protein kinase that is involved in the activation of tryptophan-5-monoxygenase is specifically distributed in brain tissues. *FEBS Letts.*, 129:117–119.

Yamauchi, T. and Fujisawa, H. (1983) Purification and characterisation of the brain calmodulin-dependent protein kinase (kinase II) which is involved in the activation of tryptophan-5-monoxygenase. *Eur. J. Biochem.*, 132:15–21.

W.H. Gispen and A. Routtenberg (Eds.)
Progress in Brain Research, Vol. 69
© 1986 Elsevier Science Publishers B.V. (Biomedical Division)

CHAPTER 28

Two-dimensional patterns of neural phosphoproteins from the rat labeled in vivo under anaesthesia, and in vitro in slices and synaptosomes

Richard Rodnight, Christopher Perrett and Soteris Soteriou

Department of Biochemistry, Institute of Psychiatry, De Crespigny Park, London SE5 8AF, U.K.

Introduction

The bulk of our knowledge of protein phosphorylating systems in nervous tissue has accumulated through subcellular studies, using $[\gamma\text{-}^{32}P]ATP$ as phosphate donor. This is entirely understandable, since information on the phosphorylating potential of neural tissue, and of factors that regulate protein phosphate turnover, such as cyclic nucleotides, calcium ions, calmodulin and lipids, can only be studied at this level and are an essential prerequisite to investigating the roles of protein phosphorylation in cell-containing tissue. In the intact respiring cell, protein phosphorylating systems are operating at a complex level of interaction and are subject to control mechanisms that cannot be reproduced or determined in broken cell preparations. Intact cell studies therefore constitute an essential complementary approach to subcellular studies.

Protein phosphorylation in intact cells may be studied both in vitro and in vivo. In vitro studies, using for example tissue slices, have the advantage of permitting precise control of the immediate chemical environment of the cell, but are limited by the essentially unphysiological state of the tissue. In the in vivo situation only very limited control over the cell environment is possible, but the tissue is subject to a degree of physiological regulation impossible to achieve in vitro. The actual extent of regulation clearly depends upon the state of the animal and at present systematic in vivo phosphorylation studies have been carried out almost entirely in anaesthetised animals (but see Mitrius et al. (1981) for an example of a labeling experiment in conscious animals).

When we commenced the studies reported in this chapter we set ourselves two technical objectives. The first was to develop methods for cell labeling that required, on the grounds of safety and economy, minimal amounts of ^{32}P radioactivity. For both in vitro and in vivo studies we found we could achieve this by drying the solution of carrier-free $[^{32}P]$orthophosphate and redissolving it in a suitable medium at a higher concentration than is available from commercial sources. The second objective was to employ methods of analysis that would ensure that no dephosphorylation of labeled proteins occurred during sample preparation. This precluded subcellular fractionation of the tissue and necessitated analysis by high resolution two-dimensional electrophoresis, in view of the complexity of phosphorylated substrates in whole tissue.

In vivo studies

In previous studies devoted to the labeling of cerebral phosphoproteins in vivo, one of two approaches has been used. In the first, labeling of the tissue was achieved by injecting $[^{32}P]$orthophosphate into the ventricles or subarachnoid space and allowing it to penetrate the tissue. In this approach high amounts of radioactiv-

374

ity are required, since the great majority of the isotope diffuses into the circulation or unwanted areas of the brain. For example, Berman et al. (1980) injected 1 mCi of ^{32}P per rat intraventricularly for subsequent analysis by one-dimensional electophoresis. For two-dimensional analysis even higher amounts would have been necessary.

In the other approach much lower amounts of radioactivity are infused directly into the brain tissue and the area adjacent to the cannula tip dissected out and analyzed. A procedure of this kind was first used by Mitrius et al. (1981). It has the advantage that a high degree of labeling can be achieved in a small area of tissue which can be defined by stereotaxic placement of the cannula. We have modified and developed the approach of Mitrius et al. in the following respects (for further details see Rodnight et al., 1985b).

(a) Since we were working with anaesthetised animals the prior implantation of stainless steel guides was unnecessary. The animal was held in a stereotaxic frame and the cannulae inserted in the desired position.

(b) By drying the ^{32}P solution as supplied (initially 10 mCi/ml) we were able to redissolve the radioactivity in isotonic medium, thus avoiding the injection of water directly into the tissue. In practice we found solution in isotonic sodium chloride gave the same results as solution in Krebs–Ringer bicarbonate buffer. Drying the radioactivity and redissolving it also permitted adjustment for decay and the injection of standard amounts of ^{32}P in the same volume over a period of weeks.

(c) A slow rate of infusion, mechanically controlled at a rate of about 0.1–0.13 µl/min (total volume 2–3 µl) was used in the present work.

(d) At the end of the experiment the animal was immediately frozen in liquid nitrogen and the brain tissue fixed while still frozen in trichloroacetic acid or lysis buffer containing sodium dodecylsulphate.

Materials and Methods

Acrylamide and Ampholines were obtained from LKB, Servalyt (pH 2–4) from Serva (Heidelberg,

F.R.G.), sodium dodecyl sulphate (SDS; 99%) and urea from British Drug Houses (Poole, U.K.). [^{32}P]orthophosphate (10 mCi/ml, carrier free in water) was obtained from Amersham International (U.K.). All other chemicals were the purest available. Wistar rats of either sex and weight 280–300 g were used.

The radioactivity was dried and redissolved essentially as described by Rodnight et al. (1985b). The infusion procedure followed the detailed description given in that publication, but with a few modifications to the equipment. Briefly, the 5-ml syringe drove two 25-µl microsyringes in parallel, thus enabling two areas of the brain to be injected simultaneously (Fig. 1). Also the microsyringes and about half the length of the polythene connecting tubes were filled with light liquid paraffin instead of dye solution. In the experiments reported in this work we infused 150–200 µCi of ^{32}P in 2 µl at a rate of 0.1 µl/min. The cannulae were left in position for a further 10 min after switching off the pump.

The fixation and sampling procedures used in the present study differed in certain respects from

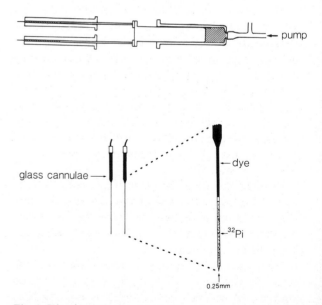

Fig. 1. Diagram of syringe assembly and arrangement of cannulae used for infusing radioactivity into two brain areas simultaneously in vivo. The syringes are filled with light liquid paraffin and the polythene connecting lines (not shown) with 0.2% Evans Blue dye in 0.9% NaCl.

those used by Rodnight et al. (1985b). Instead of decapitating the animal prior to freezing, the whole anaesthetised animal was dropped head-first into liquid nitrogen. The frozen heads were allowed to warm up to −10°C and then split sagittally with a sharp-pointed Stanley knife. The two halves of the brain were removed and frozen coronal sections, 0.6 mm thick, were cut across the area of the tissue marked by the dye using a hand-operated version of the McIlwain chopper. Discs of tissue 1.8 mm in diameter were cut out with a stainless-steel punch and either treated with 5% trichloroacetic acid as described before or by the following 2-stage procedure: The tissue disc was first homogenized in 40 µl of an isoelectric focussing sample solution containing 1% SDS, 12.5 mM lysine, 9 M urea and 2%(v/v) 2-mercaptoethanol and then diluted with 160 µl of a second solution of the same composition, but lacking SDS and containing instead 5% Nonidet NP-40. The final concentration of SDS was therefore 0.2% and of Nonidet 4%. The protein concentration of these extracts was about 1 µg/µl. The two procedures gave similar results in general,

but occasional difficulty was experienced in dissolving the protein pellet obtained with the acid precipitation method.

In our previous study (Rodnight et al., 1985b) a slab gel method based on the work of Burghes et al. (1982) was used for the isoelectric focussing stage of the two-dimensional electrophoresis procedure. This method gave good resolution and also possessed the advantage of permitting the quantitative entry of basic proteins into the focussing gel. In practice, however, we found this method unsuitable for routine use and for most of the present study we used a modified version of the O'Farrell (1975) procedure. The following ampholyte concentrations were used in the rod gels: pH 3.5–10 Ampholine, 1.87%; pH 5–7 Ampholine, 0.21%; pH 2–4 Servalyt, 0.21%. Autoradiography was carried out as before (Rodnight et al., 1985b).

Results

Typical autoradiographs prepared from two brain areas labeled in vivo are given in Fig. 2. It must be

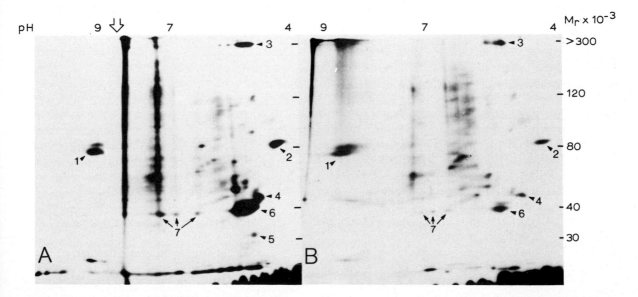

Fig. 2. Typical autoradiographs from two brain areas labeled in vivo. A: Caudate nucleus analyzed by the slab method for the isoelectric focussing stage. B: Parietal cortex using rod gels for the isoelectric focussing stage. In each case approximately 150 µCi of [^{32}P]orthophosphate was infused in 0.9% NaCl at a rate of 0.1–0.13 µl/min. The volumes infused ranged from 2–3 µl. Exposure times for autoradiography ranged from 8–24 h.

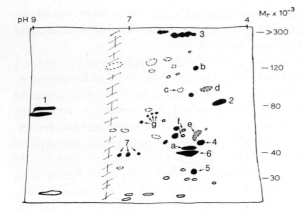

pH 9   7   4 $M_r \times 10^{-3}$

—>300

—120

—80

—40

—30

Fig. 3 Diagrammatic representation of the main phosphorylated peptides observed on autoradiographs from in vivo labeling experiments, based on the picture obtained with caudate nucleus. For provisional identification of the numbered polypeptides see Table I. Spots marked with a letter receive comment in the text.

emphasized that these patterns were obtained with relatively short periods of exposure (8–24 h); many more minor ^{32}P-polypeptides appeared on longer exposures, but at the expense of increased background labeling. The overall level of phosphorylating activity in the neocortex, neostriatum, hippocampus, amygdala and septum was higher

than observed in the cerebellum and mesencephalon, but with certain exceptions the general pattern of labeling was similar in all regions examined. There were, however, consistent variations, discussed below, in the relative intensity of the labeling of a number of polypeptides. Some variation was also observed in relative labeling when the same area was examined on different occasions, but these were much less than the regional differences.

To facilitate interpretation of the autoradiographs a diagrammatic representation of the general pattern is given in Fig. 3, based on that obtained with caudate nucleus using the O'Farrell method of focussing. The numbered spots are listed in Table I, where they are assigned provisional identities. These have been made on the basis of their isoelectric points, mobility in the second dimension and by comparison with phosphorylation patterns prepared from [^{32}P]ATP-labeled subcellular fractions of rat brain tissue and analyzed by the same procedure (unpublished data). The identities of numbers 1–3 (synapsin I, 82–87-kDa substrate of protein kinase C and MAP-2, respectively) are reasonably secure, since they occur at the outer margins of the gel. In fact, because of its basic nature, synapsin I does

TABLE I

Provisional identity of some [^{32}P]polypeptides on the autoradiographs

Number	Presumed identity	Cellular site
1	Synapsin I (1, 2)	Surface of synaptic vesicles (3)
2	82–87-kDa substrate (4) of protein kinase C (5)	Cytosolic (4, 6)
3	Microtubule-associated protein 2 (MAP-2) (7)	Mainly cytosolic; dendrites (6, 8, 9)
4	B-50 (45–47-kDa) substrate of protein kinase C (10, 11)	Presynaptic plasma membranes (12)
5	DARPP-32, 32–35-kDa substrate of cAMP-dependent protein kinase (13)	Postsynaptic cytosol; dopamine innervated regions (14)
6	40-kDa substrate of calcium/calmodulin-dependent protein kinase (15)	Occluded and non-occluded cytosol (6)
7	α-Subunit of pyruvate dehydrogenase (16, 17)	Mitochondria (16, 17)

1, DeCamilli et al. (1983a); 2, Sorensen and Babitch (1984); 3, DeCamilli et al. (1983b); 4, Wu et al. (1982); 5, Nishizuka et al. (1979); 6. Rodnight et al. (1985a); 7, Theurkauf and Vallee (1982); 8, Huber and Matus (1984); 9. Caceres et al. (1984); 10, Aloyo et al. (1983); 11, Cain and Routtenberg (1983); 12, Sorensen et al. (1981); 13, Walaas and Greengard (1984); 14, Ouimet et al. (1984); 15, R. Rodnight and C. Perrett, present paper and unpublished data; 16, Browning et al. (1981); 17, Morgan and Routtenberg (1980).

not always quantitatively enter the isoelectric gel using the standard O'Farrell method of focussing. It may be noted that synapsin I is the only major basic phosphoprotein present in grey matter; its in vivo state of phosphorylation has been studied by extraction and back-phosphorylation (Strombom et al., 1979).

We are also fairly confident about the identities of numbers 4, 5 and 7 (B-50 substrate of protein kinase C, the DARPP-32 substrate of cyclic AMP-dependent kinase and the α-subunit of pyruvate dehydrogenase, respectively). Thus they all possess the appropriate isoelectric points and mobilities and comigrate with these proteins derived from labeled subcellular fractions. In the case of spot 5, identity with DARPP-32 is reinforced by the observation that its labeling was prominent in the caudate nucleus and amygdala, but was absent or only very slightly labeled after injection of ^{32}P into the cerebral cortex and hippocampus; Ouimet et al. (1984) found that DARPP-32 was greatly enriched in areas of the brain innervated by dopaminergic terminals. The in vivo labeling of B-50 in immature rat brain was first shown by Oestreicher et al. (1982). Spot number 6 is probably a cytosolic 40-kDa substrate of calcium/calmodulin-kinase and is considered further later.

In preliminary experiments, in which radioactivity was injected into the cerebellum, we found relatively strong labeling of the highly acidic 82–87-kDa acceptor in relation to all others apart from the 40-kDa acceptor (number 6). The labeling of B-50 in the cerebellum was relatively faint. This result was also found in in vitro labeling of slices (see below).

The relatively minor spots marked with letters in Fig. 3 deserve some comment. The spot marked **a** may be a cytosolic substrate for cAMP-dependent protein kinase, since both occluded and non-occluded cytosol fractions labeled with [γ-^{32}P]ATP in the presence of cAMP exhibited a spot on two-dimensional electrophoretograms in this position. Spots **b** and **c** were prominent in autoradiographs made from synaptosomes labeled in vitro with [^{32}P]orthophosphate (see Fig. 5), except that in contrast to in vivo labeling, spot **c** in synaptosomal labeling was always as intense as spot **b**. The labeling of spots **d** and **e** was rather

variable, but they were seen more often in experiments on cerebral cortex and hippocampus; they were always characterized by a fuzzy outline. The two spots marked **f** occurred close to the position occupied by tubulin (as indicated by protein staining on the corresponding gels) but careful observation showed that both labeled spots always migrated to a slightly different position. The four spots collectively marked **g** have never been observed in any subcellular fraction labeled with [γ-^{32}P]ATP; the sharpness of the separation of these spots was a useful indicator of the quality of the separation.

In vitro studies

Methods

Micro-slices of rat brain were prepared as follows. The brain was divided sagittally and the cut surface of one half placed on a dry sheet of filter paper. The paper was then carefully moistened with incubation medium and mounted on the platform of a McIlwain chopper. Five or six transverse or longitudinal sections (0.36 mm) were cut across the appropriate area and the block of tissue transferred to a dish of medium. The sections were carefully teased out with brushes and the precise area required punched out with a 2.5 mm-diameter punch. The mini-slices weighed approximately 2 mg. They were transferred to tubes containing 100 µl of phosphate-free Krebs–Ringer bicarbonate buffer (Ca^{2+}, 1.2 mM) gassed with 95% O_2/5% CO_2 and incorporating 100 µCi of [^{32}P]orthophosphate. The tubes were incubated for 30 min at 37°C with occasional gentle shaking. Labeling was terminated by transferring the slices with a bent hypodermic needle to a glass mini-homogeniser and treating them with the two-stage sample buffer procedure described for in vivo labeled tissue.

A 'P$_2$' fraction enriched in synaptosomes was prepared ' by the procedure of Holmes and Rodnight (1981) except that the homogenizing medium was 0.32 M sucrose containing 1 mM EDTA. The pellet was washed with 25 ml of phosphate-free Krebs–Ringer bicarbonate buffer for each gram of original tissue represented. The washed pellet was then resuspended by gentle homogenization in 3.75 ml of Krebs–Ringer buffer per g of tissue and protein determined (Bradford, 1976). The protein concentration was adjusted to 5 mg/ml and 200 µl of the suspension added to a tube containing 400 µCi of dried ^{32}P solution. The incubation period was 45 min. The reaction was terminated by adding 0.25 ml of 5% trichloroacetic acid. The precipitated protein was spun out and dissolved in lysis buffer as before.

Results

Representative partial autoradiographs from slice tissue prepared from 6 brain regions are shown in Fig. 4. Exposure times were adjusted so as to give approximately equal intensity to the 40-kDa poly-

peptide (spot 6 in Fig. 3). The main features distinguishing the slice patterns from those obtained with in vivo labeling were a markedly higher *relative* labeling of polypeptides 6 and **a** (see Fig. 3) and relatively poor labeling of the B-50 polypeptide (spot 4 in Fig. 3) and of MAP-2 (not shown in Fig. 4). In the 3 regions of the forebrain analyzed (frontal cortex, caudate nucleus and hippocampus) the 82–87-kDa substrate of protein kinase C (spot 2 in Fig. 3) was also relatively poorly labeled in slices. However, in cerebellar slices, as in cerebellar tissue labeled in vivo, the 82–87-kDa substrate was strongly labeled with an intensity nearly equal to that of the 40-kDa polypeptide (see panel E, Fig. 4). A similar relatively high labeling of the 82–87-kDa polypeptide was observed in slices of superior

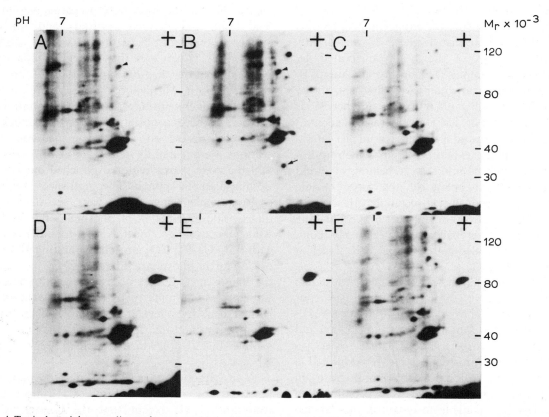

Fig. 4. Typical partial autoradiographs prepared from labeled slice tissue. A, Frontal cortex; B, caudate nucleus; C, hippocampus; D, superior colliculus; E, cerebellum; F, medulla oblongata. Slices from each area were incubated in 100 µl of phosphate-free Krebs–Ringer bicarbonate buffer containing 100 µCi of carrier-free [^{32}P]orthophosphate. Rod gels were used for the focussing stage. Exposure times for autoradiography were as follows: A, B and C: 12 h; D and E: 14 h; F: 48 h. Note that the basic and high molecular weight regions are not shown. In panel B the arrow indicates the putative DARPP-32 sport.

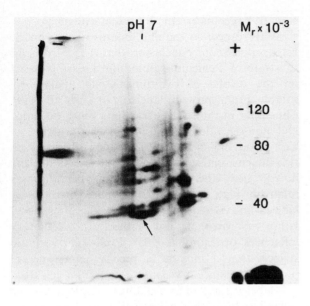

Fig. 5. A typical autoradiograph prepared from a labeled P_2 fraction (enriched in synaptosomes) from rat forebrain. The P_2 fraction was suspended in phosphate-free Krebs–Ringer bicarbonate buffer containing 2 µCi of [^{32}P]orthophosphate/µl at a protein concentration of 5 mg/ml. The incubation period was 45 min. The reaction was stopped with trichloroacetic acid and the labeled proteins prepared for electrophoresis as described in the text. Rod gels were used for the focussing stage.

colliculus and medulla oblongata (panels D and F in Fig. 4). Finally, spots **b** and **c** were usually of the same intensity in labeled slice tissue, whereas in tissue labeled in vivo spot **c** was always relatively faint.

When the P_2 was labeled under similar conditions the pattern obtained in Fig. 5 was obtained. The main feature of this pattern, compared with slice tissue, was the presence of a pronounced spot of M_r about 38 kDa and isoelectric point around neutrality (marked with an arrow in Fig. 5). The apparent absence of this polypeptide in labeled whole tissue suggests it may be highly concentrated in nerve terminals.

Discussion

Methodological considerations

The experimental procedures described in this chapter represent initial approaches to the study of protein phosphorylation in intact brain tissue and as such are clearly capable of refinement. In the in vivo labeling experiments parameters that require further exploration include the following:

The infusion rate and the volume of ^{32}P solution infused were arbitrarily chosen. We have not explored a range of different infusion rates, but it would be reasonable to assume that, using a standard quantity of radioactivity and within certain limits, the slower the infusion rate the higher the concentration of label in the tissue proteins contiguous to the cannula tip. The limits are set by (*a*) dilution of the infusate by the extracellular fluid and (*b*) the turnover rates of the tissue phosphoproteins. The possibility of causing local radiation damage to the labeled tissue through the accumulation of a high concentration of isotope in a very small volume of tissue, must also be considered. With regard to the volume of infusate we have tended recently to decrease this to 2 µl from the 4 µl volume originally used, thus reducing the danger of local tissue damage through edema. With this volume and an infusion rate of 0.1 µl/min efficient mixing with the extracellular fluid seems likely, a conclusion supported by the observation that infusing radioactivity dissolved in Krebs–Ringer buffer resulted in an identical protein phosphorylation pattern as obtained with our routine procedure of infusing 0.9% sodium chloride.

Fixation of the tissue. As is well known, immersion in liquid nitrogen is by no means an entirely satisfactory procedure for arresting metabolism and the possibility of some dephosphorylation occuring in deeper structures cannot be excluded. It is difficult to see how this problem can be overcome, considering the need to recover the brain intact for dissection. We have not investigated micro-wave fixation as used by Mitrius et al. (1981). Apart from the need to investigate systematically phosphorylation patterns in heated as compared with frozen tissue, we suspect that the safety problems of placing a highly radioactive animal in the micro-wave equipment would be greater than simply immersing it in liquid nitrogen; also in conscious animals the stress to the animal would be greater.

With respect to the in vitro labeling of micro-slices and synaptosomes, further work on the composition of the incubation medium, particularly in regard to the Ca^{2+} content, would be justified. In a one-dimensional study of synaptosomes, Dunkley and Robinson (Chapter 22) found that concentrations of Ca^{2+} above 0.1 mM progressively inhibited the incorporation of ^{32}P from orthophosphate into protein.

The importance of using two-dimensional electrophoresis for the analysis of labeled poly-peptides in whole tissue is generally accepted: the number of substrates for protein kinase activity in brain is far too large to allow more than very limited interpretations of one-dimensional separations. However, the present limitations of two-dimensional protein analysis must be recognized, particularly the relative inefficiency of the iso-electric focussing stage. Poor penetration of polypeptides into the focussing gel applies particularly to hydrophobic membrane proteins and to proteins associated with particulate structures such as the postsynaptic density. Therefore the pattern of polypeptides observed in extracts of whole tissue tends to be biassed in favor of soluble proteins. The development of better neutral solubilizing agents for iso-electric focussing may improve the situation, as will the appearance of a universal protein phosphatase inhibitor that permits the subcellular fractionation of labeled tissue.

Identities of labeled polypeptides

As already mentioned, further work is required to confirm finally the putative identities of the named polypeptides listed in Table I. Meanwhile, it is relevant to note that all of these are labeled relatively rapidly by $[\gamma-^{32}P]ATP$ in subcellular fractions. Other substrates that are rapidly labeled in subcellular fractions, but do not appear on autoradiographs from labeled intact tissue, include the 50-kDa and 60-kDa subunits of a calcium/cal-modulin-protein kinase (Kennedy et al., 1983) and the 52-kDa coated vesicle substrate (Chapter 21). The status of the labeling of proteins IIIa and IIIb of Greengard's group (Nestler and Greengard, 1983) and of the two tubulin subunits (Goldenring

et al., 1984) is uncertain on present evidence.

With respect to the one unknown polypeptide listed, spot 6, our conclusion that it is a cytosolic substrate of a calcium-calmodulin kinase is based on the results of two-dimensional analysis of soluble brain protein labeled with $[\gamma-^{32}P]ATP$. Thus only in the soluble fractions (both occluded and non-occluded) and only in the presence of Ca^{2+} and calmodulin was a spot observed on two-dimensional gels in this position. As already noted, the labeling of this polypeptide was relatively high in slices, as compared with tissue labeled in vivo, suggesting that its phosphory-lation in vitro is not subject to regulatory influences operating in vivo. Preliminary studies suggest that it may be a predominantly neural polypeptide, since it was not detected on gels from ^{32}P-labeled slices of liver, kidney or spleen. On the other hand, another major substrate observed on gels from labeled brain slices, namely spot **a** (which is probably a cytosolic substrate of cyclic AMP-dependent protein kinase, not listed in Table I), co-migrated with a major labeled poly-peptide on gels from labeled slices of liver and kidney, though not from spleen.

Regional variations in labeling pattern

These remarks apply mainly to regional variations in in vitro slice labeling since at present we have more information from these experiments than from in vivo labeling although, where available, basically similar patterns were observed in both experimental situations. Our limited observations on the regional distribution of the putative DARPP-32 polypeptide (spot 5) confirm the more extensive work of Ouimet et al. (1984). The relatively high labeling of the 82–87-kDa polypeptide (spot 2) in the phylogenetically more primitive brain areas is a new finding of particular interest. As already mentioned, the 82–87-kDa polypeptide almost certainly corresponds to the 87-kDa substrate of protein kinase C described by Wu et al. (1982), although it has yet to be established that its phosphorylation in intact tissue is catalyzed by the same enzyme. A protein with identical mobility characteristics was detected in slices of spleen tissue (C. Perrett and R. Rodnight, unpublished data) and apparently in adipocytes and fibroblasts (Chapter 16), where it may be related to growth factor action.

Acknowledgement

We are grateful to the Medical Research Council of the UK for support.

References

Aloyo, V.J., Zwiers, H. and Gispen, W.H. (1983) Phosphorylation of B-50 protein by calcium-activated phospholipid-dependent protein kinase. *J. Neurochem.*, 41:649–653.

Berman, R.F., Hullihan, J.P., Kinnier, W.J. and Wilson, J.E. (1980) Phosphorylation of synaptic membranes. *J. Neurochem.*, 34:431–437.

Bradford, M.M. 1976) A rapid and sensitive method for the quantitation of microgram quantities of protein utilizing the principle protein–dye binding. *Analyt. Biochem.*, 72:248–254.

Browning, M., Bennett, W. F., Kelly, P. and Lynch, G. (1981) Evidence that the 40 000 phosphoprotein influenced by high frequency stimulation is the alpha subunit of pyruvate dehydrogenase. *Brain Res.*, 218:255–266.

Burghes, A.H.M., Dunn, M.J. and Dubowitz, V. (1982) Enhancement of resolution in two-dimensional gel electrophoresis and simultaneous resolution of acidic and basic proteins. *Electrophoresis*, 3:354–363.

Caceres, A., Binder, L.I., Payne, M.R., Bender, P., Bebhun, L. and Steward, O. (1984) Differential subcellular localization of tubulin and the microtubule-associated protein MAP-2 in brain tissue as revealed by immunocytochemistry with monoclonal hybridoma antibodies. *J. Neurosci.*, 4:394–410.

Cain, S. and Routtenberg, A. (1983) Neonatal handling alters the phosphorylation of a 47K molecular weight protein in male rat hippocampus. *Brain Res.*, 267:192–195.

DeCamilli, P., Cameron, R. and Greengard, P. (1983a) Synapsin I (protein I) a nerve terminal-specific phosphoprotein. I. Its general distribution in synapses of the central and peripheral nervous system demonstrated by immunofluorescence in frozen and plastic sections. *J. Cell Biol.*, 96:1337–1354.

DeCamilli, P., Harris, S.M., Huttner, W.B. and Greengard, P. (1983b) Synapsin I (protein I) a nerve terminal-specific phosphoprotein. II. Its specific association with synaptic vesicles demonstrated by immunocytochemistry in agarose-embedded synaptosomes. *J. Cell Biol.*, 96:1355–1373.

Goldenring, J.R., Casanova, J.E. and DeLorenzo, R.J. (1984) Tubulin-associated calmodulin-dependent kinase: evidence for an endogenous complex of tubulin with calcium/calmodulin-dependent kinase. *J. Neurochem.*, 43:1669–1679.

Holmes, H. and Rodnight, R. (1981) Ontogeny of membrane-bound protein phosphorylating systems in the rat. *Dev. Neurosci.*, 4:79–88.

Huber, G. and Matus, A. (1984) Differences in the cellular distributions of two microtubule-associated proteins, MAP-1 and MAP-2 in rat brain. *J. Neurosci.*, 4:151–160.

Kennedy, M.B., Bennett, M.K. and Erondu, N.E. (1983) Biochemical and immunological evidence that the 'major postsynaptic density protein' is a subunit of a calmodulin-dependent protein kinase. *Proc. Natl. Acad. Sci. U.S.A.*, 80:7357–361.

Mitrius, J.C., Morgan, D.G. and Routtenberg, A. (1981) In vivo phosphorylation following [^{32}P]orthophosphate injection into the neostriatum or hippocampus: selective labelling of electrophoretically-separated brain protein. *Brain Res.*, 212:67–81.

Morgan, D.G. and Routtenberg, A. (1980) Evidence that a 41,000 dalton brain phosphoprotein is pyruvate dehydrogenase. *Biochem. Biophys. Res. Commun.*, 95:569–576.

Nestler, E.J. and Greengard, P. (1983) Protein phosphorylation in the brain. *Nature*, 305:583–588.

Nishizuka, Y., Takai, Y., Hashimoto, E., Kishimoto, A., Kuroda, Y., Sakai, K. and Yanamura, H. (1979) Regulatory and functional compartment of three multifunctional protein kinase systems. *Mol. Cell Biochem.*, 23:153–165.

O'Farrell, P.H. (1975) High resolution two-dimensional separation of proteins. *J. Biol. Chem.*, 250:4007–4021.

Ouimet, C.C., Miller, P.E., Hemmings, H.C., Waalas, S.I. and Greengard, P. (1984) DARPP-32, a dopamine and adenosine 3':5'-monophosphate-regulated phosphoprotein enriched in dopamine innervated brain regions. *J. Neurosci.*, 4:111–124.

Rodnight, R., Perrett, C. and Dosemeci, A. (1985a) Acceptors for cyclic AMP-dependent and calcium ion-dependent protein kinases in rat brain cytosol fractions: a comparison of occluded (synaptosomal) cytosol with non-occluded cytosol. *Neurochem. Res.* (in press).

Rodnight, R., Trotta, E.E. and Perrett, C. (1985b) A simple and economical method for studying protein phosphorylation in vivo in the rat brain. *J. Neurosci. Methods*, 13:87–95.

Sorensen, R.G. and Babitch, J.A. (1984) Identification and comparison of protein I in chick and rat forebrain. *J. Neurochem.*, 42:705–720.

Sorensen, R.G., Kleine, L.P. and Mahler, H.R. (1981) Presynaptic localization of phosphoprotein B-50. *Brain Res. Bull.*, 7:57–61.

Strombom, U., Forn, J., Dolphin, A.C. and Greengard, P. (1979) Regulation of the state of phosphorylation of specific neural proteins in mouse brain by in vivo administration of anaesthetic and convulsant agents. *Proc. Natl. Acad. Sci. U.S.A.*, 76:4687–4690.

Theurkauf, W.E. and Vallee, R.B. (1982) Molecular characterization of the cAMP-dependent protein kinase bound to microtubule-associated protein 2. *J. Biol. Chem.*, 257:3284–3290.

Walaas, S.I. and Greengard, P. (1984) DARPP-32, a dopamine- and adenosine 3':5'-monophosphate-regulated phosphoprotein enriched in dopamine innvervated brain regions. I. Regional and cellular distribution in the rat brain. *J. Neurosci.*, 4:84–98.

Wu, W.C-S., Walaas, S.I., Nairn, A.C. and Greengard, P. (1982) Calcium/phospholipid phosphorylation of a M_r '87K' substrate protein in brain synaptosomes. *Proc. Natl. Acad. Sci. U.S.A.*, 79:5249–5253.

W.H. Gispen and A. Routtenberg (Eds.)
Progress in Brain Research, Vol. 69
© 1986 Elsevier Science Publishers B.V. (Biomedical Division)

ADDENDUM

Comparison between the neural acidic proteins B-50 and F1

W.H. Gispen[1], P.N.E. De Graan[1], S.Y. Chan[2] and A. Routtenberg[2]

[1]*Rudolf Magnus Institute for Pharmacology and Institute of Molecular Biology, University of Utrecht, Padualaan 8, 3584 CH Utrecht, The Netherlands and* [2]*Cresap Neuroscience Laboratory, 2021 Sheridan Road, Evanston, IL 60201, U.S.A.*

The phosphorylation and dephosphorylation cycle is a common cellular mechanism by which the function of certain proteins can be regulated. The brain is especially enriched in protein kinase and phosphatase activity. Within the brain the regions rich in synaptic contacts comprise the major part of the endogenous phosphorylation activity (Weller, 1979). Weller and Rodnight (1970) demonstrated that cAMP stimulated the endogenous phosphorylation of brain phosphoproteins. Ueda et al. (1973) showed that of the many membrane phosphoproteins specifically a 80 kDa doublet protein band (protein IA and B) was stimulated by cAMP. A few years later DeLorenzo (1976) emphasized the importance of calcium in the regulation of some of the synaptic plasma membrane (SPM) proteins, previously shown not to be sensitive to cAMP. Presently, a number of protein kinases that are sensitive to different modulators and ion conditions are recognized (Nestler and Greengard, 1984). As more is becoming known about these kinases and their substrates it is increasingly clear that the regulation of protein function in the synaptic membrane by phosphorylation is far more complex than originally anticipated. For example, a given substrate protein may be phosphorylated at two different sites by two different kinases (Cohen, 1982).

The work of our laboratories has focussed on the characteristics and function of two major cAMP-independent, calcium-sensitive phosphoproteins in SPM. The Routtenberg group studies the protein referred to as F1 (see Chapter 18), whereas the Gispen group studies a protein termed B-50 (see Chapter 4).

B-50 and its endogenous protein kinase were isolated and purified from rat brain SPM (Zwiers et al., 1980). B-50 is an acidic phosphoprotein with a M_r of 48 kDa and a pI of 4.5. B-50 kinase has a M_r of 70 kDa and a pI of 5.5. The observed pI's were confirmed by the amino acid compositions of the two proteins (Zwiers et al., 1980). In subsequent experiments it was shown that the B-50 kinase is similar if not identical to protein kinase C (Aloyo et al., 1982, 1983). In line with this is the observation that dioctanoylglycerol and phorbol diesters but not 4α-phorbol stimulate B-50 phosphorylation (Eichberg et al., 1986; Chapter 4). B-50 is nervous tissue-specific (Kristjansson et al., 1982), predominantly localized in brain regions enriched in synaptic contacts (Oestreicher et al., 1981). Immunoelectron microscopical analysis using affinity-purified anti-B-50 anti-bodies and protein A–gold detection demonstrated that B-50 is predominantly present in presynaptic membranes (Gispen et al., 1985). In the developing brain of the fetal and neonatal rat B-50 is a major phosphoprotein component of neuronal growth cones, and is present in outgrowing neurites (De Graan et al., 1985; Oestreicher and Gispen, 1986).

Using chromatographic methods, protein F1 has been purified from rat synaptic membranes (Chapter 18; Chan et al., 1986). A phosphatidyl-serine-dependent phosphorylation of protein F1 by purified protein kinase C (Murakami and Routtenberg, 1985; Murakami et al., 1986) was also demonstrated. This property is consistent with previous studies using crude synaptic plasma membranes demonstrating phosphatidylserine and phorbol diester stimulation of protein F1 phosphorylation (Akers and Routtenberg, 1985). In growth cones, protein F1 is present as a major component and is probably identical to growth cone phosphoprotein pp46 (Nelson et al., 1985; Katz et al., 1985). Protein F1 and its kinase, protein kinase C, have been linked to and may play a crucial role in synaptic plasticity (Routtenberg, 1985a, 1985b; Akers et al., 1986).

In summary, evidence is accumulating that both B-50 and F1 may play a crucial role in transmembrane signal transduction, synaptic plasticity and growth. Furthermore, other groups have studied a protein that shares many characteristics of B-50 and F1. In brain SPM such proteins are $\gamma5$ (Rodnight, 1982), 47 kDa (Hershkowitz et al., 1982), p54(Ca)p (Mahler et al., 1982), and 48 kDa (Chapter 22). In growth cones and regenerating outgrowing neurites such proteins are referred to as GAP-43 (Skene and Willard, 1981), GAP-48 (Benowitz, 1983) and pp46 (Katz et al., 1985). In view of the increasing interest in neural acidic phosphoproteins with a M_r of 47–48 kDa in general, and the specific role that protein F1 and protein B-50 may play in regulating signal transduction, it was deemed of interest to carry out a cross-laboratory study to establish whether or not B-50 and F1 are identical proteins. The experiment involved SDS-PAGE immunoblotting of preparations enriched in F1 and B-50 using affinity-purified anti-B-50 immunoglobulins.

As source of the B-50 antigen, purified B-50 protein as described by Oestreicher et al. (1984) was used. The fraction containing F1 was a pooled DEAE column eluate, obtained from osmotically shocked rat brain synaptosomes (Chan et al., 1986). Aliquots of SPM-, B-50- and F1-containing

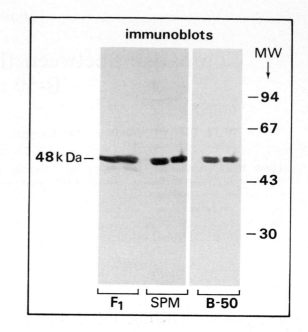

Fig. 1. Immunochemical comparison of B-50 and F1 (5 µl of a pooled DEAE column eluate: Chan et al., 1986), SPM (10 µg prepared according to Kristjansson et al., 1982) and B-50 (0.2 µg B-50 antigent purified according to Oestreicher et al., 1984) were subjected to 11% SDS-PAGE. Proteins were blotted onto nitrocellulose sheets and B-50-like immunoreactivity was detected with affinity-purified rabbit anti-B-50 immunoglobulins (serum 8420, dilution 1:2000) and peroxidase- conjugated swine anti-rabbit immunoglobulins (dilution 1:500) according to Schrama et al. (1984).

protein samples were subjected to 11% SDS-PAGE. The separated proteins were transferred onto nitrocellulose sheets and immunoreactivity was visualized according to Schrama et al. (1984) using affinity-purified anti-B-50 immunoglobulins (Oestreicher et al., 1983). With this procedure B-50 is the only protein cross-reacting in SPM (Oestreicher et al., 1983; De Graan et al., 1985; Fig. 1) In the F1-containing DEAE fraction only one single band, coinciding with the F1- band, cross-reacted with the anti-B-50 immunoglobulins (Fig. 1). This immunoreactive band migrated at the same height as purified B-50 and B-50 in SPM. Therefore, the present data add further evidence to the notion that F1 and B-50 are identical proteins.

References

Akers, R. and Routtenberg, A. (1985) Protein kinase C phosphorylates a 47 kD protein directly related to synaptic plasticity. *Brain Res.*, 334:147–151.

Akers, R.F., Lovinger, D.M., Colley, P.A., Linden, D.J. and Routtenberg, A. (1986) Translocation of protein kinase C activity may mediate hippocampal long-term potentiation. *Science*, 231:587–589.

Aloyo, V.J., Zwiers, H. and Gispen, W.H. (1982) B-50 protein kinase and kinase C in rat brain. *Progr. Brain Res.*, 56:303–315.

Aloyo, V.J., Zwiers, H. and Gispen, W.H. (1983) Phosphorylation of B-50 protein by calcium-activated, phospholipid-dependent protein kinase and B-50 protein kinase. *J. Neurochem.*, 41:649–653.

Benowitz, L.I. and Lewis, E.R. (1983) Increased transport of 44,000 to 49,000 dalton acidic proteins during regeneration of the goldfish optic nerve: a two-dimensional gel analysis. *J. Neurosci.*, 3:2153–2163.

Chan, S.Y., Murakami, K. and Routtenberg, A. (1986) Phosphoprotein F1: Purification and characterization of a brain kinase C substrate related to plasticity. *J. Neurosci.*, in press.

Cohen, P. (1982) The role of protein phosphorylation in neural and hormonal control of cellular activity. *Nature*, 296:613–619.

De Graan, P.N.E., Van Hooff, C.O.M., Tilly, B.C., Oestreicher, A.B., Schotman, P. and Gispen, W.H. (1985) Phosphoprotein B-50 in nerve growth cones from fetal rat brain. *Neurosci. Lett.*, 61:235–241.

DeLorenzo, R.J. (1976) Calcium-dependent phosphorylation of specific synaptosomal fraction proteins: possible role of phosphoproteins in mediating neurotransmitter release. *Biochem. Biophys. Res. Commun.*, 71:590–597.

Eichberg, J., De Graan, P.N.E., Schrama, L.H. and Gispen, W.H. (1986) Dioctanoylglycerol and phorbol diesters enhance phosphorylation of phosphoprotein B-50 in native synaptic plasma membranes. *Biochem. Biophys. Res. Commun.*, 136:1007–1012.

Gispen, W.H., Leunissen, J.L.M., Oestreicher, A.B., Verkleij, A.J. and Zwiers, H. (1985) Presynaptic localization of B-50 phosphoprotein: the ACTH-sensitive protein kinase substrate involved in rat brain polyphosphoinositide metabolism. *Brain Res.*, 328:381–385.

Hershkowitz, M., Heron, D., Samuel, D. and Shinitzky, M. (1982) The modulation of protein phosphorylation and receptor binding in synaptic membranes by changes in lipid fluidity: implications for aging. *Progr. Brain Res.*, 56:419–434.

Katz, F., Ellis, L. and Pfenninger, K.H. (1985) Nerve growth cones isolated from fetal rat brain. III. Calcium-dependent protein phosphorylation. *J. Neurosci.*, 5:1402–1411.

Kristjansson, G.I., Zwiers, H., Oestreicher, A.B. and Gispen, W.H. (1982) Evidence that the synaptic phosphoprotein B-50 is localized exclusively in nerve tissue. *J. Neurochem.*, 39:371–378.

Mahler, H.R., Kleine, L.P., Ratner, N. and Sörensen, R.G. (1982) Identification and topography of synaptic phosphoproteins. *Progr. Brain Res.*, 56:27–48.

Murakami, K. and Routtenberg, A. (1985) Direct activation of purified protein kinase C by unsaturated fatty acids (oleate and arachidonate) in the absence of phospholipids and Ca^{2+}. *FEBS Lett.*, 192:189–193.

Murakami, K., Chan, S.Y. and Routtenberg, A. (1986) Protein kinase C activation by *cis*-fatty acid in the absence of Ca^{2+} and phospholipids, *J. Biol. Chem.*, in press.

Nelson, R.B. and Routtenberg, A. (1985) Characterization of the 47 kD protein F1 (pI 4.5), a kinase C substrate directly related to neuronal plasticity. *Exp. Neurol.*, 89:213–224.

Nelson, R.B., Routtenberg, A., Hyman, C. and Pfenninger, K.H. (1985) A phosphoprotein (F1) directly related to neural plasticity in adult rat brain may be identical to a major growth cone membrane protein (pp46). *Soc. Neurosci. Abstr.*, 11:927.

Nestler, E.J. and Greengard, P. (1984) Protein Phosphorylation in the Nervous System. John Wiley & Sons, New York.

Oestreicher, A.B., Zwiers, H., Schotman, P. and Gispen, W.H. (1981) Immunohistochemical localization of a phosphoprotein (B-50) isolated from rat brain synaptosomal plasma membranes. *Brain Res. Bull.*, 6:145–153.

Oestreicher, A.B., Van Dongen, C.J., Zwiers, H. and Gispen, W.H. (1983) Affinity-purified anti-B-50 protein antibody: interference with the function of the phosphoprotein B-50 in synaptic plasma membranes. *J. Neurochem.*, 41:331–340.

Oestreicher, A.B., Van Duin, M., Zwiers, H. and Gispen, W.H. (1984) Cross-reaction of anti-rat B-50: characterization and isolation of a 'B-50 phosphoprotein' from bovine brain. *J. Neurochem.*, 43:935–943.

Oestreicher, A.B. and Gispen, W.H. (1986) Comparison of the immunocytochemical distribution of the phosphoprotein B-50 in the cerebellum and hippocampus of immature and adult rat. *Brain Res.*, 375:267–279.

Rodnight, R. (1982) Aspects of protein phosphorylation in the nervous system with particular reference to synaptic transmission. *Progr. Brain Res.*, 56:1–25.

Routtenberg, A. (1985a) Protein kinase C activation leading to protein F1 phosphorylation may regulate synaptic plasticity by presynaptic terminal growth. *Behav. Neural Biol.*, 44:186–200.

Routtenberg, A. (1985b) Phosphoprotein regulation of memory formation: Enhancement and control of synaptic plasticity by protein kinase C and protein F1. *Ann. N.Y. Acad. Sci.*, 444:203–211.

Schrama, L.H., Weeda, G., Edwards, P.M., Oestreicher, A.B. and Schotman, P. (1984) Multiple phosphorylation of pp30, a rat brain polyribosomal protein, sensitive to polyamines and corticotropin. *Biochem. J.*, 224:747–753.

Skene, J.H.P. and Willard, M. (1981) Axonally transported proteins associated with axon growth in rabbit central and peripheral nervous system. *J. Cell Biol.*, 89:96–103.

Ueda, T., Maeno, H. and Greengard, P. (1973) Regulation of endogenous phosphorylation of specific proteins in synaptic membrane fractions from rat brain by adenosine 3', 5'-monophosphate. *J. Biol. Chem.*, 248:8295–8305.

Weller, M. (1979) Protein Phosphorylation. The Nature,

Function and Metabolism of Proteins, which contain covalently bound Phosphorus. PION Ltd., London.

Weller, M. and Rodnight, R. (1970) Stimulation by cyclic AMP of intrinsic protein kinase activity in ox brain membrane preparations. *Nature (Lond.)*, 225:187–188.

Zwiers, H., Schotman, P. and Gispen, W.H. (1980) Purification and some characteristics of an ACTH-sensitive protein kinase and its substrate protein in rat brain membranes. *J. Neurochem.*, 34:1689–1699.

Subject Index